KERR AND ASH'S
ORAL PATHOLOGY
An Introduction to General and Oral Pathology for Hygienists

KERR AND ASH'S
ORAL PATHOLOGY

An Introduction to General and Oral Pathology
for Hygienists

Major M. Ash, Jr., B.S., D.D.S., M.S., Dr. h.c.
Marcus L. Ward Professor of Dentistry
The University of Michigan School of Dentistry
Ann Arbor, Michigan

Fifth Edition

Lea & Febiger   Philadelphia   1986

Lea & Febiger
600 Washington Square
Philadelphia, PA 19106-4198
U.S.A.
(215) 922-1330

Library of Congress Cataloging in Publication Data
Kerr, Donald A.
  Kerr and Ash's oral pathology.

  Rev. ed. of: Oral pathology / Donald A. Kerr, Major M.
Ash, Jr. 4th ed. 1978.
  Includes bibliographies and index.
  1. Teeth—Diseases. 2. Mouth—Diseases. 3. Pathology.
4. Dental hygiene. I. Ash, Major M., 1921–
II. Title. III. Title: Oral pathology. [DNLM: 1. Dental
Hygienists. 2. Mouth Diseases—pathology. 3. Tooth
Diseases—pathology. WU 140 K41o]
RK307.K47 1986   617'.522   86-2514
ISBN 0-8121-1025-0

First Edition, 1960
Second Edition, 1965
    Reprinted December, 1967
    Reprinted September, 1969
Third Edition, 1971
    Reprinted October, 1973
    Reprinted August, 1976
Fourth Edition, 1978
    Reprinted June, 1979
Fifth Edition, 1986

Copyright © 1986 by Lea & Febiger. Copyright under the International Copyright Union. All rights reserved. This book is protected by copyright. *No part of it may be reproduced in any manner or by any means without written permission from the publisher.*

PRINTED IN THE UNITED STATES OF AMERICA

Print number: 5 4 3 2 1

Donald A. Kerr,

who was not only a foremost pathologist and teacher,
but a friend to all of us who were fortunate to know him.

PREFACE

The practice of dentistry always reflects changes in patterns of disease as well as changes in the attitude of the public regarding its professional needs. Just as significant changes have occurred in the prevalence of dental caries and periodontal diseases, so that dental management now emphasizes their prevention rather than their correction, equally significant changes have occurred on the socioeconomic front. These include fourth-party payment for dental care, the clustering of dental practices, and megacorporate influences as well. The public's demands for corrective treatment will require more complex procedures, which can now be financed more easily than before. Dental professionals will become more involved in the diagnosis and treatment of such disorders as temporomandibular joint dysfunction, gerontologic problems, and secondary otolaryngologic symptoms. To meet these challenges, the dental hygienist must have a broad background in dentistry, medicine, and oral pathology.

The changing patterns of diseases are dynamic. One need only consider changes that have occurred within the past few years: the significance of hepatitis, the spread of acquired immune deficiency syndrome (AIDS), the explosive increase in temporomandibular joint complaints, and the reduction of caries in the general population. All individuals who work in the field of dentistry need some knowledge of the diseases that they are helping to treat, as well as information about systemic diseases that afflict their patients. Such knowledge will not only influence the welfare of the patient and help with dental treatment, but it will also help dental professionals avoid contracting transmissible disease from their patients.

This edition of *Oral Pathology* has been extensively revised and rewritten, not only to take into account the acquisition of new information about disease patterns, but also because our perception of oral diseases as simple infectious processes that conform to Koch's postulates is also undergoing revision. Unlike the situation in medical microbiology, the concept of "one microbe, one disease" has not been scientifically substantiated for dental caries or periodontal disease. Rather, infectious organisms might be viewed as being "associated" with these disorders instead of the sole cause of them.

As in past editions, Professor William Brudon of the Department of Anatomy has taken my sketches and turned them into excellent illustrations that bespeak his technical skill and will serve the reader well. The services of Ms. Marian Brokie and Ms. Sue Dexter are also gratefully acknowledged, as are the photographic services of Per Kjedel, Kerry Campbell, Lance Burghardt, Ellen Quinn, and Tom Oliver.

After the untimely death of Donald A. Kerr, coauthor of the preceding editions, I consulted with several teachers and students regarding the kind of text coverage that would be of most interest to them. I gratefully acknowledge the recommendations made by Doctors Richard Courtney, George Ash, and Carolyn Ash, and by dental hygiene teachers, Ms. Pauline Steele and Ms. Sally Holden. I also wish to acknowledge the use of several photographs contributed by Doctors J.L. Ash and H.D. Millard. The assistance of Ms. Sue Segar in verifying the references that appear at the end of each chapter is also greatly appreciated.

Ann Arbor, Michigan   M.M. Ash, Jr.

CONTENTS

Chapter 1
INTRODUCTION 1
  Scope of Oral Pathology
  Cellular Basis of Life and Disease
    Cell Structure and Function
    Tissues
    Intracellular Communication
    Cell Cycle
    Gene Expression
    Collagen Formulation
  Cellular Injury and Response
    Cellular Adaptation
    Cell Injury
    Clinical Correlates of Cellular Injury
  Summary

Chapter 2
AGENTS OF DISEASE 15
  Intrinsic Factors in Disease
    Genetic Factors
    Single Gene Disorders
    Chromosomal Disorders
    Polygenic Disorders
    Human Cancer
  Congenital Malformations
    Teratogenic Agents
    Radiation
    Chemicals and Drugs
    Microorganisms
    Prenatal Diagnosis
  Psychologic Factors
  Extrinsic Factors in Disease
    Physical Agents
    Infectious Agents
    Nutritional Factors
    Chemical Injury
    Environmental Agents
    Drugs and Hormones

Chapter 3
DEVELOPMENT DISTURBANCES 35
  Embryology of the Face
  Disturbances of the Upper Face
    Clefts
    Fissural Defects
  Disturbances of the Tongue
  Dentofacial Malrelations
  Embryology of the Teeth
  Surface Structures
  Disturbances of the Teeth

Chapter 4
RESPONSE TO INJURY 61
  Inflammation
    Cells in Inflammation
    Acute Inflammation
    Vascular Response
    Cellular Response
    Phagocytosis
  Hemostasis, Coagulation and Fibrinolysis
    Abnormal Clotting
    Bleeding Disorders
    Chronic Inflammation
  Healing: Repair and Regeneration
    Regeneration
    Healing by Primary Intention
    Healing by Secondary Intention
    Scar Tissue
    Bone Repair
  Summary

Chapter 5
IMMUNE RESPONSE AND IMMUNE
INJURY 76
  Immune System
    Antigens
    Immunity
    Characteristics of Immune Responses
    Genetic Control of Immune Response
    Blood Group Antigens

Antibodies
Complement System
Cells of the Immune System
  Macrophages
  Lymphocytes
  Humoral Immunity
  Cell-Mediated Immunity
  Interferon
Summary of Immune Responses
Immunopathology
  Immunodeficiency Diseases
  AIDS
  Hypersensitivity
  Organ Transplantation
  Autoimmune Diseases
  Rheumatoid Arthritis
Summary

Chapter 6
RESPONSES TO INCREASED FUNCTION, IRRITATION, AND INJURY . 92
Hyperplasia
Hypertrophy
Hyperkeratosis
Metaplasia
Reactive Oral Lesions

Chapter 7
AGING, RETROGRESSIVE CHANGES, AND DYSFUNCTION................... 103
Aging and Disease
  Theories of Etiology of Aging
  Organ Changes
Aging and Specific Diseases
  Alzheimer's Disease
  Osteoarthritis
  Immune Senescence
Retrogressive Changes
  Loss of Structure
  Atrophy
  Degenerations, Infiltrations, and Dysfunction
  Necrosis
  Mineral Metabolism
  Arteriosclerosis
  Pigment Metabolism

Chapter 8
NEOPLASIA 117
Definition
Epidemiology
Etiology
  Extrinsic Factors
    Viruses

Immunologic Defects
  Developmental Factors
General Characteristics
  Benign Characteristics
  Maligned Neoplasms
Classification
  Neoplasms of Epithelial Origin
  Neoplasms of Mesenchymal Origin
  Leukemias and Lymphomas
Cancer Therapy and Complications

Chapter 9
NUTRITIONAL DISTURBANCES 133
Necessary Nutrients
  Protein
  Carbohydrates
  Fats and Lipids
  Minerals
  Vitamins
Clinical Considerations

Chapter 10
DENTAL PLAQUE, MICROBIOTA CALCULUS, STAINS AND DISEASE 144
Clinical Aspects of Plaque
Ecologic Determinants of Plaque
Formation of Plaque
  Intraoral Pellicles
  Bacterial Colonization
  Subgingival Dental Plaque
  Colonization by Streptococcus Mutans
  Mechanisms of Colonization
  Adverse Influences
Pathogenicity and Virulence of Plaque and
    Microbiota
  Virulence Factors
  Potential Bacterial Mechanisms for Evading
      Host Defenses
  Potential Bacterial Mechanisms for Destruction
      of Periodontal Tissues
  Virulence Mechanisms of S. Mutans
  Microbial Resistance
  Host Responses to Plaque Components and
      Microorganisms
  Immune Responses to Plaque
  Saliva
  Crevicular Fluid
  Systemic and Local Responses to Plaque
  Summary of Host Responses
Plaque and Disease
  Nonspecific vs. Specific Plaque Hypotheses
Calculus
  Composition of Calculus

Saliva and Calculus
   Mechanisms of Calculus Formation
   Mineralization of Plaque
   Attachment of Calculus
   Significance of Calculus
  Stains
   Exogenous Stains
   Endogenous Stains
  Summary

Chapter 11
THE DENTIN-PULP COMPLEX AND DISEASE 166
  Dentin-Pulp Complex
   Innervation
   Pulp Circulation
   Dentin
  Pulp Disease
   Pulpitis
   Acute Pulpitis
   Chronic Pulpitis
  Sequelae of Pulp Disease
   Periapical Granuloma
   Periapical Cyst (Radicular Cyst)
   Cellulitis
   Periapical Abscess
   Parulis, Fistula, Gum Boil
   Osteomyelitis
  Summary

Chapter 12
DENTAL CARIES 178
  Epidemiology
  Prevalence of Caries
  Sites of Caries
  Target Populations
  Diet and Dental Caries
  Microbiology of Dental Caries
  Etiology of Caries
  Acid Production in Plaque
  Carious Lesions
  Control of Dental Caries
  Prediction of Caries

Chapter 13
PERIODONTAL DISEASES 196
  Periodontium
   Gingiva
   Periodontal Ligament
   Alveolar Bone
   Cementum
  Epidemiology
   Measurement of Periodontal Disease
  Etiology of Periodontal Diseases
   Initiating Factors
   Modifying Factors
  Pathogenesis of Periodontal Diseases
   Pathogens
   Bacterial Invasion
   Pocket Formation
   Host Defenses
   Immune Mechanisms in Periodontal Disease
  Histopathology of Gingivitis-Periodontitis
  Dento-Gingival Junction
   Junctional Epithelium
   Gingival/Periodontal Pockets
  Transition from Gingivitis to Periodontitis
   Normal Gingiva
   Gingivitis
   Periodontitis
  Classification of Periodontal Diseases
  Gingivitis
   Simple Gingivitis
   Complex Gingivitis
   Hyperplastic Gingivitis
   Necrotizing Ulcerative Gingivitis (NUG)
   Chronic Desquamative Gingivitis
   Traumatic Gingivitis
   Gingival Atrophy/Recession
  Trauma from Occlusion
  Periodontitis
   Chronic Destructive Periodontal Disease in the Adult
   Destructive Periodontal Disease in Young Individuals
   Juvenile Periodontitis
   Early Periodontitis
   Cyclic Neutropenia
   Chediak-Higashi Syndrome
   Papillon-Lefevre Syndrome
   Down's Syndrome
  Prevention of Periodontal Disease
  Summary

Chapter 14
STOMATITIS, INFECTIONS AND IMMUNOLOGIC DISTURBANCES 236
  Viral Infections
   Herpes Simplex Virus—Type 1
   Varicella-Zoster (VZ) Virus
   Coxsackie Viruses
   Mumps Virus
   AIDS Virus
  Recurrent Aphthous Stomatitis
  Systemic Diseases with Oral Manifestations
   Lichen Planus

Pemphigus
Benign Mucous Membrane Pemphigoid
 (BMMP)
Erythema Multiforme
Crohn's Disease
Bacterial Infections
 Gonorrhea
 Syphilis
Fungus Infections
 Candidiasis
 Histoplasmosis
 Coccidioidomycosis
Traumatic Stomatitis
 Mechanical Injury
 Thermal Injury
 Chemical Injury
Allergic Stomatitis

Chapter 15
ENDOCRINOPATHY AND METABOLIC DISEASES 254
Disturbances of Endocrine Function
 Pituitary Function
 Thyroid Function
 Parathyroid Function
 Hypoparathyroidism
 Hyperparathyroidism
 Adrenal Function
 Hypofunction of Adrenal Cortex
 Hyperfunction of Adrenal Cortex
Gonadal Dysfunction
 Hypogonadism
 Hypergonadism
Polyglandular Disorders

Multisystem Hyperfunction
Multisystem Hypofunction
Metabolic Diseases
 Diabetes Mellitus
 Metabolic Bone Disease
Summary

Chapter 16
HEMATOLOGIC AND HEMATOPOIETIC DISEASES 267
Formation of Blood Cells
Red Blood Cells
 Erythrocyte Disorders
White Blood Cells
 Leukemias
Bleeding
 Thrombocytic Disorders
 Vascular Factors
 Coagulation Disorders
Monocyte-Macrophage Disorders
Summary

Chapter 17
PATHOPHYSIOLOGY OF TEMPOROMANDIBULAR JOINTS AND MUSCLES OF MASTICATION 279
Masticatory System and Control
Epidemiology of TMJ/Muscle Dysfunction
Etiology
Signs and Symptoms
Trauma from Occlusion
Treatment
Summary

INDEX 295

1

INTRODUCTION

The oro-facial complex, including the mouth and its unique hard and soft tissues, consists of a number of diverse structures having closely integrated and coordinated activities for mastication, swallowing, and communication. These structures have an array of defense and repair mechanisms, as well as an adaptive capacity, to meet the wide range of biological, physical and emotional stresses to which the teeth and their supporting structures, joint muscles and neuromuscular system are subjected. Dental caries, periodontal diseases, congenital craniofacial anomalies, salivary gland diseases, malocclusion, sensory-motor dysfunctions and nutritional deficiencies only suggest the spectrum of oral diseases afflicting the oro-facial complex.

SCOPE OF ORAL PATHOLOGY

Even though the mouth is unique and intrinsically interesting, it should not be assumed that it is not a model of infections for other diseases found elsewhere in the body. Many of the features of dental caries and periodontal diseases are reflections of the interactions of pathogens and the immune system in a number of disorders of the body. Such slowly progressive or episodic disorders as heart disease, diabetes, arthritis and stroke may involve changes in the immune system; and periodontal diseases also exhibit many of the features of those chronic, debilitating diseases, as well as involving the immune system.

Although dental caries and periodontal diseases are virtually endemic problems, the scope of oral pathology extends to a wide variety of less frequent problems such as cleft palate, which may have more serious consequences for the individual patient. The genetic and environmental risks that threaten the normal development of the fetus are numerous. The scope of the problem of developmental disturbances is enormous: some cranio-facial malformations may be related to specific genetic or chromosomal disorders, others to malnutrition, drugs, or problems during pregnancy, but generally such malformations have a multifactorial basis. Genetic as well as environmental factors are important interactive processes in the development of the fetus, especially for cleft lip and palate. Gene-environmental interactions that predispose to the development of cleft lip, cleft palate, and other orofacial malformations are within the scope of oral pathology.

The scope of oral pathology also includes coverage of such common oral soft tissue diseases as recurrent canker sores (aphthous ulcers) where cause-and-effect relationships for infection by streptococcal organisms or immune mechanisms have yet to be proved; cold sores (fever blisters) where the infection is caused by herpes virus; and fungal diseases such as candidiasis (thrush) where Candida albicans infects the oral mucosa. Oral cancer and the adverse effects of surgery, chemotherapy, and radiation treatments are important aspects of oral pathology.

Intraoral symptoms may be related to a larger symptom complex such as Sjörgen's syndrome, i.e., dry mouth, dry eyes, and rheumatoid arthritis. Dry mouth (xerostomia) has a bearing on the exacerbation and treatment of dental caries. Rampant dental decay is a common problem in dry mouth caused by irradiation therapy. A number of common drugs cause dry mouth which can lead to increased caries activity. Dry mouth also increases with aging. Also intraoral symptoms may be related to endocrine disturbances such as diabetes, exocrine disturbances such as cystic fibrosis, blood dyscrasias such as hemophilia, and dietary deficiencies caused by treatment for systemic disease. Oral manifestations of systemic disease are important aspects of oral pathology.

It would be inappropriate in describing the scope of oral pathology not to include orofacial pain, including some of the chronic orofacial pain syndromes associated with the temporomandibular joints, craniomandibular muscles, neuralgias, and sensory-motor dysfunctions, especially those motor disorders related to the side effects of drugs, bruxism, and endocrine disorders.

The scope of oral pathology includes not only a range of diseases that may be found in the mouth as well as elsewhere in the body, but also those disturbances which involve soft and hard tissues unique to the mouth (Fig. 1–1). Oral pathology must be considered in terms of pathobiology and pathophysiology, not simply descriptions of the manifestations of oral disease. The full scope of oral pathology requires that clinical data be coupled with information about molecular,cellular, and genetic processes that govern growth, immune responses and

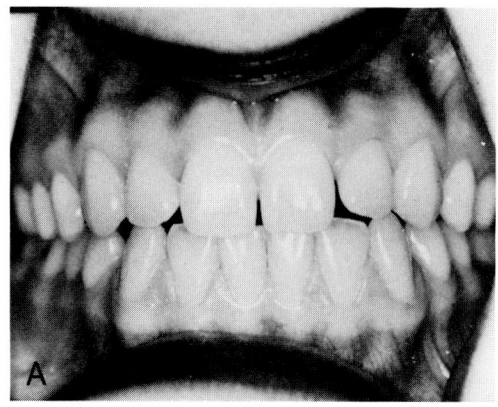

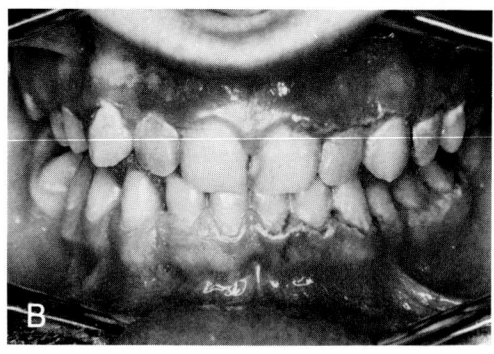

Fig. 1–1. *Pathophysiology of the oral tissues.* From the normal in *(A)* to the altered health in *(B)* lies the challenge of diagnosis, prevention and treatment. This challenge requires an understanding of those molecular, cellular, genetic, and psychophysiologic processes that govern cell function as well as human behavior.

cell function where such information enhances a better understanding of changing concepts of disease and goals for treatment.

It is no longer valid to consider disease in terms of a linear "one-way" cause-effect-treatment relationship. For example a host of factors other than bacteria, including genetic, nutritional, dietary, immunological, environmental and even social factors, shape the complex and uncertain pathways from the healthy tooth to a tooth with dental decay. And the operational definition of dental health as the absence of decay is in conflict with current knowledge of the carious process. At some point in time in the development of a carious lesion, the lesion can be reversed and thus intervention occurs without surgical treatment, i.e., without having to restore part of the tooth with amalgam, gold or composites, or to extract the tooth. Such prevention to avoid treatment is based on the implementation of current knowledge of causes, mechanisms, and progression of dental caries. Such knowledge falls within the scope of oral pathology.

CELLULAR BASIS OF LIFE AND DISEASE

The cell is the basic structural and functional unit of the body. In disease processes there are almost no new metabolic pathways occurring that have not been seen in normal cells. Exceptions are abnormal gene products resulting from mutations, usually lethal, and only occasionally heritable. The same molecular and cellular interactions that occur during development of the cell occur in disease. Small perturbations in the range of normal between health and disease are corrected by homeostatic servomechanisms. Cellular activity is dependent upon influences from internal control mechanisms and the environment. Thus disease is a reflection of a quantitative alteration of existing pathways involving metabolites, substrates, enzymes, or products that have been seen previously in normal cells.

Cell Structure and Function

Under the light microscope, the nucleus, cytoplasm and cell membrane boundaries are readily seen; however, organelles other than the nucleus and mitochondria may not be easily visualized and a composite illustration is used (Fig. 1–2). Cellular organelles (specialized parts of a cell having a definite function) include: nucleus, ribosomes, endoplasmic reticulum, and Golgi complex. Also cytoplasmic organelles include: mitochondria, lysosomes, microtubules, microfilaments, and centrioles.

The *nucleus* of the cell controls cellular activity. Inside the nucleus are the chromosomes which contain the *genes*. The genes, which are made up of deoxyribonucleic acid (DNA), control cellular replication and determine the type of protein made by the cell. Many of the cellular adaptations (changes in cell size, number, and type) are mediated by changes in gene expression. The nucleus contains one or more *nucleoli* which synthesize ribonucleic acid (RNA).

The *endoplastic reticulum* (ER) appears as a system of paired parallel membranes which separate the cytoplasm into two compartments or phases. Phase I is the ground cytoplasm or cytosol, Phase II is the area inside the ER. On the outside borders of the ER lie small granules or ribosomes which contain cytoplasmic RNA. Ribosomes which merge into strings are polyribosomes or polysomes. The ER with polysomes is called rough endoplastic reticulum (RER). This cytoplasmic organelle produces proteins and transports them through the cell. A smooth-surfaced ER (SER) is seen in cells that produce substances other than proteins such as hormones.

The *Golgi complex* appears as vesicles or larger vacuoles and flattened lamellae. The functions of the Golgi complex include the packaging and intracellular transportation of secretory proteins.

The *mitochondria* transform energy from foodstuffs into an energy-rich compound, adenosine triphosphate (ATP), which supplies the energy for the activities that take place in the cell.

The *lysosomes* exist in the form of a vacuole that contains a number of hydrolytic enzymes. This organelle is an intracellular digestive system capable of breaking down foreign material that enters the cell or digesting worn-out or damaged cell parts.

The *cell membrane* or *plasma membrane* consists of an organized trilaminar layering of lipids and proteins (Fig. 1–3). The inner and outer layers are usually protein and the middle one is a bimolecular layer of lipids. This membrane protects the cell from un-

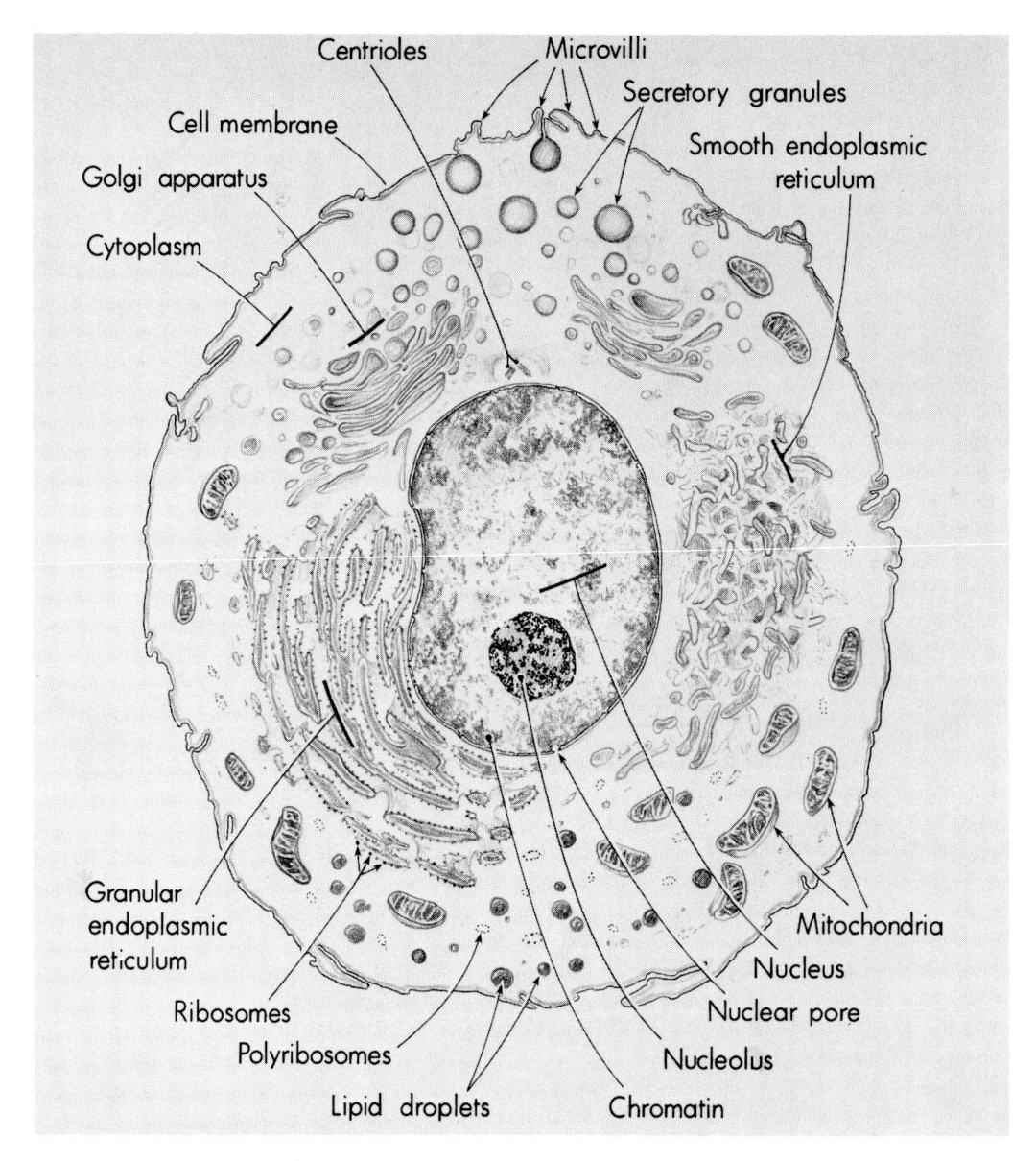

Fig. 1–2. Schematic representation of a composite cell showing in one cell most of the components (organelles) in the cytoplasm and the nucleus.

wanted substances and provides a mechanism of transport of materials coming in and out of the cell. The cell surface is surrounded by a fuzzy layer called the cell coat or *glycocalyx*. The cell coat contains sites for recognition of hormones, the ABO blood group and tissue antigens. This coat is also important for adhesion of bacterial cells to teeth. The movement of molecules and ions across the cell membrane occurs by a number of processes (Fig. 1–4): (1) passive diffusion or osmosis; (2) active transport (sodium and potassium via a calcium-magnesium-activated ATP (adenosine triphosphate) pump; (3) enzyme carriers; and (4) pinocytosis (Fig. 1–7) or phagocytosis. Interference with these transport mechanisms may lead to irreversible cellular changes.

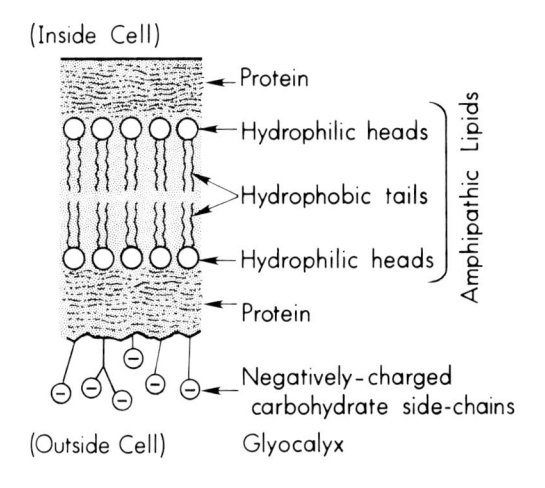

Fig. 1-3. *Cell membrane.* The trilaminar structure consists of a bilayer of phospholipids and cholesterol, as well as various proteins (lipoproteins and glycoproteins) which are an integral part of the membrane. Some of the proteins have a transport pore for the transport of lipid-insoluble materials in as much as the bilayer structure is essentially impermeable to all but the lipid-soluble substances.

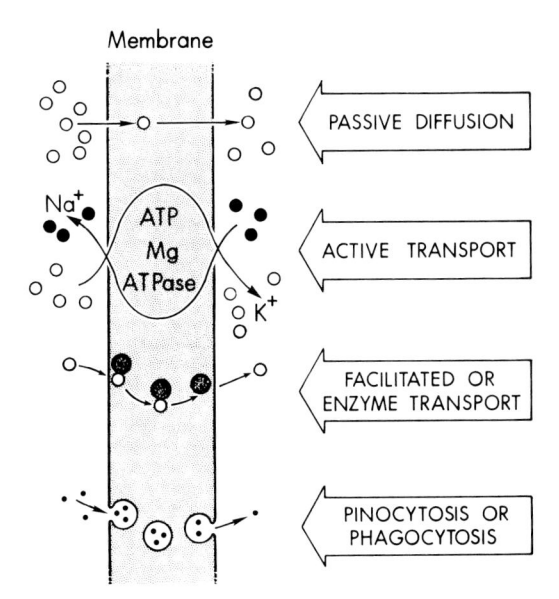

Fig. 1-4. *Mechanisms of cell membrane transport.* There are four basic mechanisms by which substances pass into a cell: passive diffusion (H_2O); active transport using an energy driven (ATP) pump; enzyme facilitated; and pinocytosis or phagocytosis.

Table 1-1. Classification of Tissues

Type	Location
Epithelium	Covering of body (skin)
	Lining of body cavities (mucous membranes of mouth, gingiva)
	Lining of blood vessels
	Lining of intestines
Connective Tissue	Bone, joints, cartilage, supporting tissues
	Hematopoietic tissues, blood cells, bone marrow, lymphoid tissue
Muscle	Striated muscles of locomotion and mastication attached to head, jaws, spine, long bones and flat bones
	Heart muscles
	Smooth muscle of intestinal tract, blood vessels, bronchi, bladder
Nervous Tissue	Central (brain and spinal cord) and peripheral nervous system

Absorption or entrance into the cell by bacteria viruses, drugs, hormones, antigens, antibodies, complement and other substances is possible because of specific attachment receptor sites on the membrane. Thus certain membrane receptors must first "recognize" the molecular structure before allowing passage in or out of the cell. For example each type of amino acid has a distinct chemical configuration which determines whether it is recognized and accepted by one transport system or another into the cell.

Tissues

The formation of different tissues is called cell differentiation. From the dividing and subdividing of the fertilized ovum a large number of different cell types are ultimately formed. Once a cell has reached a certain level of specialization consistent with the needs of a particular tissue, the cell type does not move back to a lesser degree of differentiation. Not all cells reach a particular state of specialization; a few serve as a stem cell source for continued replacement of cells throughout the life of the organism. Cancer may develop from stem cells or revert to an earlier stage of cell differentiation (p. 117).

All of the 100 or so different types of body cells are classified into 4 primary types: epithelium, connective tissue, muscle, and nervous tissue (Table 1–1). The adult body tissues originate from three layers in the initial form of the embryo: the ectoderm, mesoderm and the endoderm. The epithelium arises from all three embryonal layers, the connective tissue and muscle from the mesoderm, and the nervous tissue develops from the ectoderm. The term mesenchymal tissue refers to the precursor of connective tissue and is derived from the mesoderm. These types of tissue will be described in more detail in relation to location and function, viz., epithelium in relation to gingiva, muscle in relation to masticatory function, bone in relation to jaws, and nerves in relation to the neuromuscular system.

Intercellular Communication

Communication between cells occurs in one or more of four ways: through intercellular junctions, electrical impulses, hormones, and membrane receptors. The types of intercellular junctions include: desmosomes, hemidesmosomes, tight junctions, gap junctions, and several others found in specialized cells. These functions are shown schematically in Figure 1–5. The desmosome is the most common type of epithelial intercellular attachment (Fig. 1–6) found in gingival tissue and other stratified squamous epithelium. Hemidesmosomes are found at the base of epithelial cells, i.e., a hemidesmosome-basement lamina complex between the gingival epithelium and the subadjacent connective tissue (Fig. 1–7). Its relationship to the attachment apparatus of the tooth has not been clarified. Tight junctions provide for an area of low electrical resistance and also allow the transfer of small molecules between cells. The gap junctions are specialized for the transmission of electrical impulses between cells.

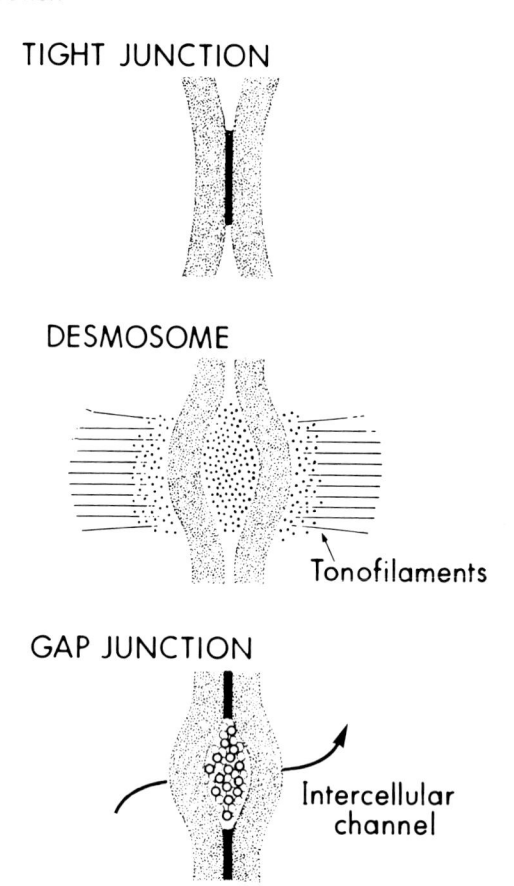

Fig. 1–5. *Intercellular junctions and communications.* Junctional areas which are more permeable than other areas of the cell are controlled by gating (cytoplasmic calcium). The upper two types of junctions make up the junctional complex. The epithelial desmosome acts as a bracing system.

Cell Cycle

The life cycle of most cells consists of nondivision (or interphase) and division (mitosis) phases. Just before and just after mitosis DNA synthesis ceases while RNA and protein synthesis occur. Between these pre- and post-mitotic phases, DNA replication occurs. Thus DNA is synthesized during a restricted period of interphase. During mitosis the nucleus divides and each daughter nucleus receives the same number and kind of chromosomes. Most tissues have three types of cell populations: those that continue to divide and move through the

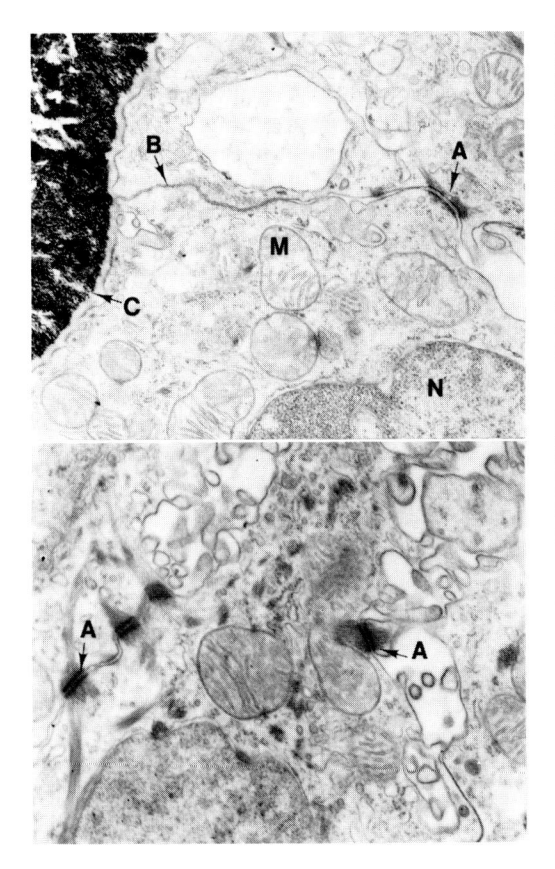

Fig. 1–6. *Upper, Ultrastructure of an odontogenic cell.* Desmosome (A), cell membranes of adjacent cells (B), outer surface of tooth (C), mitochondria (M), nucleus of cell (N). *Lower,* There are four desmosomes (A) present in the part of the cell represented. Two of the four desmosomes are indicated.

cycle; those that no longer divide; and those that become dormant, but may reenter the cell cycle (see Chapter 8).

Gene Expression

The main events for most cells involve dividing to make exact copies of themselves and the production of proteins, both dependent upon blueprints coded in genes, i.e., the germ material or DNA molecule. DNA is a large double-stranded helix which resembles a long rope ladder, twisted around and around into a corkscrew shape. The sides of the ladder are long chains of sugars and phosphates in re-

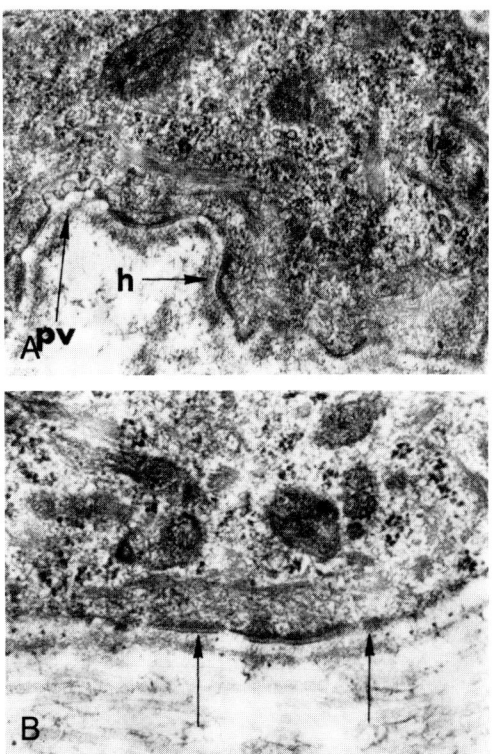

Fig. 1–7. *A,* Basal cell in basal layer of the gingiva. There are hemodesmosomes scattered along the basement lamina (h) and pinocytosis vesicles (pv) can be seen at the left of the figure ×34,000. *B,* Basement lamina with hemidesmosomes ×40,000.

peated sequences. The biochemical basis of heredity lies in the rungs of the ladder. Each rung is made up of two parts, i.e., each one-half of the rung of the ladder is made up of one of four types of molecules: adenine (A), cytosine (C), thymine (T), or guanine (G). These four bases and attachment segment of side chain are known as nucleotides. An A only couples with a T and a C only couples with a G. Thus a four-letter alphabet (A-T, T-A, C-G and G-C) can spell out messages. Prior to cell division the DNA ladder (double-helix) splits down the middle, i.e., the A nucleotides separate from the Ts and the Cs from the Gs, much like the separation of the two sides of a zipper. These nucleotides join with other nucleotides to create two ladders of DNA which

Steps in Protein Synthesis

```
      REPLICATION
           ①
        ↓
       DNA ←──┐
        │    ② TRANSCRIPTION
        ↓
      mRNA
        │          tRNA
        ↓           +
      rRNA ←── Amino Acid
                    +
                   ATP
        ↓
              ③ TRANSLATION
        ↓
     Protein
```

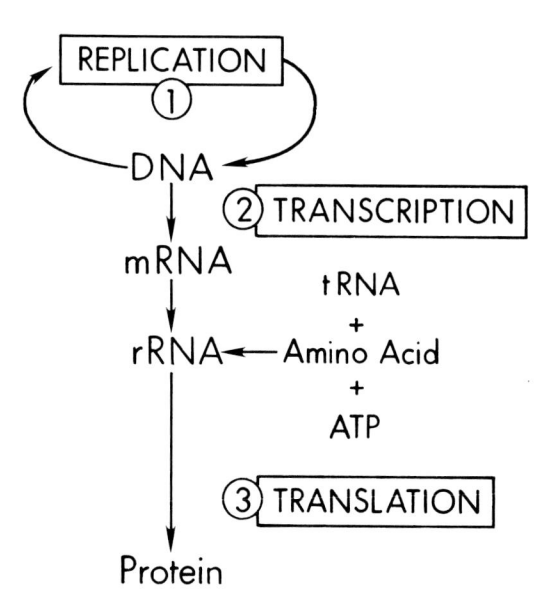

Fig. 1–8. Steps in the formation of protein. (1) Replication is necessary to provide for the conservation of one-half of the original DNA molecule and to provide a template for identical molecules; (2) The formation of mRNA involves complementary base pairing on a DNA template (transcription); (3) the production of a polypeptide (one of many to make up the protein) as directed by mRNA is called translation. tRNA transfers a specific amino acid to the ribosome so that it can be added at a specific place on a forming polypeptide chain.

are identical copies of the original. At this point the cell begins division.

The biochemical basis of heredity or genetic code lies in the sequence of bases found in the nucleic acid (deoxyribonucleic acid) or DNA molecule. One strand of a DNA molecule with its bases can serve as a template for creating a second strand that has a complementary set of bases. This exact *replication* is the copying mechanism for the genetic message (Fig. 1–8). In replication one of the strands of the double stranded DNA molecule serves as the template for the synthesis of new DNA. Thus each new molecule contains one-half of the original molecule.

In addition to the critical function of providing the blueprint coded in the genes for making exact copies of cells, these blueprints perform the function of making proteins. Each gene, or specific segment of a DNA strand, contains instructions for making one specific protein. These instructions are coded in an exact sequence of nucleotides. All living cells have the biochemical machinery to detect the sequence of bases in the DNA and to transcribe sections of DNA information into sequences of bases in the messenger RNA (ribonucleic acid). The messenger molecule (RNA) delivers the precise sequence of nucleotides containing the genetic instructions to the clusters of ribosomes where proteins are formed, i.e., the protein-making ribosomes decipher the precisely arranged string of nucleotides that contains the information required to describe the types of amino acids constituting the complex array of proteins needed to build the various tissues of the body. Some of these proteins are enzymes which catalyze biochemical reactions that result in the growth and function of the organism. Genetic material can be either nucleic acids alone (as seen in bacteria or viruses), or a nucleic acid in association with proteins (e.g., chromosomes).

Protein synthesis involves three forms of RNA (ribonucleic acid): ribosomal (rRNA), messenger (mRNA), and transfer (tRNA). RNA is usually single stranded but is similar in structure to DNA. Each form of RNA has a specific function in gene expression. The mRNA acts as a go-between for the permanent genetic information in the DNA and a forming polypeptide (ultimately the protein); the tRNA captures and transfers a specific amino acid to be added at a specific place in the developing polypeptide chain; and rRNA is part of the ribosomes which catalyze the incorporation of individual amino acids into the developing polypeptide chain. mRNA is produced with a structure which is complementary to one of the four bases: adenine (A), cytosine (C), guanine (G), and uracil (U). Individual amino acids in the polypeptide chain are coded by groups of three bases on a mRNA strand. These three bases (codons) are complements of the DNA template.

Protein synthesis begins when a ribosome becomes attached to an mRNA strand and moves along the strand with its codons to incorporate specific sequences of amino acids into a developing polypeptide (Fig. 1–10). Coding requires only 20 amino acids and since there are four possible bases (A,C,G,U) and thus 64 (4 × 4 × 4) possible codons, there are more than enough different signals for the genetic codes for the amino acids as well as two start and stop signals for protein synthesis.

The term plasmid refers to a short piece of DNA that normally codes for one of a few proteins and can often be transferred to another cell. It is usually separate from the DNA of the cell that carries the information for replication of the cell.

A recent advance in biological research has been the development of methods for cloning genes in bacteria. Defined segments of DNA from a variety of organisms can be spliced into appropriate plasmids and introduced into bacterial cells. On the basis of selected markers on the plasmid, colonies of bacteria can be isolated that carry a segment of foreign DNA. Single colonies carrying the gene of interest can be identified and used for preparing purified gene probes. Such probes can be used to study enamel proteins, virulence of bacteria involved in dental caries, the molecular basis of osteogenesis imperfecta, the human genome and molecular disorders (viz., phenylketonuria) or inborn errors of metabolism.

In summary the expression of the genetic message occurs when a single DNA strand is transcribed into the nucleic acid RNA and the RNA is translated into a chain of amino acids leading to the formation of a protein (Fig. 1–9). The process of mRNA formation involves *transcription* of the genetic information from the DNA molecule (Fig. 1–8). With this message the mRNA molecule travels to the site of protein synthesis in the cytoplasm. There the mRNA serves as a template for the production of identical polypeptide chains. This process is called *translation*. In order for translation to occur both rRNA and tRNA are required. The tRNA molecule recognizes and transfers to the ribosome a specific amino acid molecule to be added to the developing polypeptide chain at a specific site as directed by mRNA. Thus tRNA transfers amino acids to their proper site in the polypeptide chain. There is at least one tRNA for each of the 20 common amino acids.

Antibiotics such as penicillin G prevent the use of amino acids by staphylococcal microorganisms. Other antibiotics interfere with protein synthesis at the transcription or

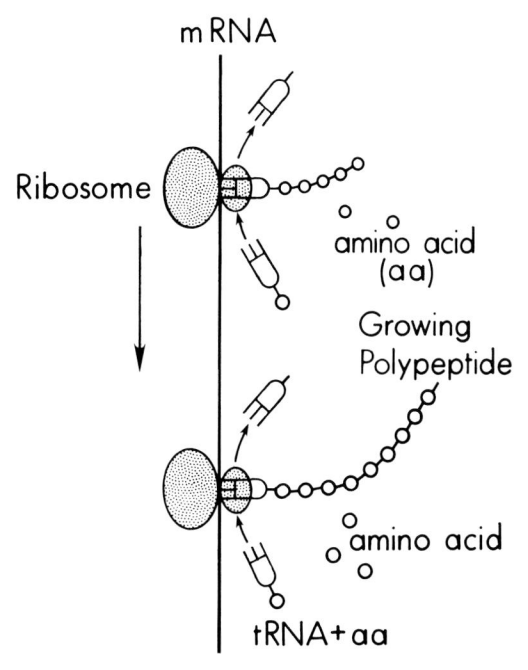

Fig. 1–9. *Protein synthesis*. The steps in the formation of protein involve (1) *activation* (aa combines with tRNA); (2) *initiation* (ribosomes, mRNA and the aa-tRNA come together); (3) *elongation* (amino acids are added to the growing polypeptide chain); and (4) *termination* (release of the polypeptide from its ribosomal-bound tRNA). The ribosome units move along the mRNA in one codon (three bases), starting with AUG (initiation codon) and ending with a nonsense codon.

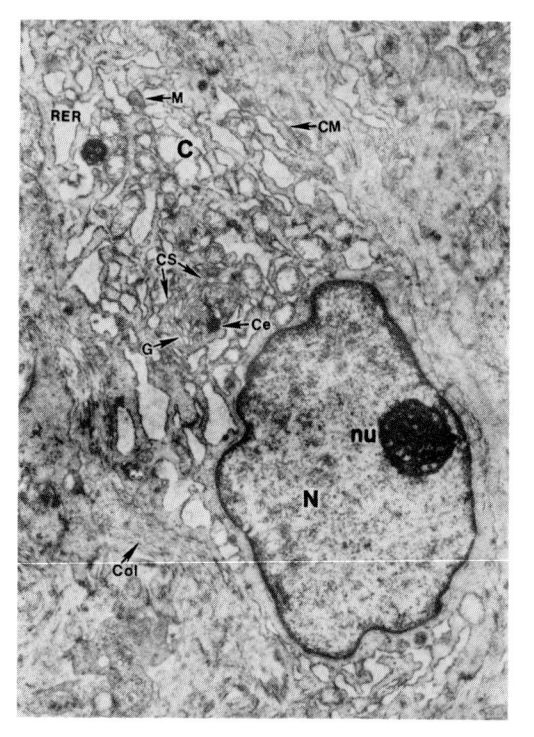

Fig. 1-10. *Ultrastructure of a differentiating cell.* The nucleus (N) contains a prominent eccentrically placed nucleolus (nu). The cytoplasm (C) contains dilated, rough endoplasmic reticulum (RER) and mitochondria (M). Since the section is through the center of the cell, the centrosphere area (CS) is present and demonstrates the Golgi apparatus (G) and a cross section through one of the centrioles (Ce). The cell is contained by the cytoplasmic membrane (CM). Strands and bundles of collagen fibers (Col) are found adjacent to the cytoplasmic membrane. Magnification approximately ×12,240.

translation level of protein synthesis. Another group of antibiotics acts on the osmotic barrier of bacterial membranes. Tetracycline interferes with protein synthesis at the translation level.

Collagen Formation

The formation of connective tissue such as the periodontal ligament (pdl) or periodontal membrane (pdm), which attaches the tooth to supporting bone, involves collagen biosynthesis (Fig. 1-10). A collagen fibril is made of three polypeptide chains of molecules coiled around each other in the form of a kinked helix (a kinked cork screw). Two different kinds of molecular chains are formed in the cell. Two chains of one kind (type $\alpha 1$) and one chain of another kind (type $\alpha 2$) combine with a carrier molecule as the intracellular precursor of collagen (procollagen). Collagen molecules are secreted from the cell where packing and orientation of the fibrils into bundles occurs. A collagen fiber is composed of smaller fibrils that make up a bundle. The cementing of individual collagen fibrils into a specific registration pattern (one-quarter stagger of the length of each collagen molecule) produces a formed collagen fibril. The synthesis of collagen is dependent upon vitamin C. The effects on the periodontal tissues of a deficiency of vitamin C in scurvy is described later (p. 140).

CELLULAR INJURY AND RESPONSE

The response of a cell to survive and maintain function under differing conditions requires a certain degree of adaptability. However, the challenge may exceed the cell's capabilities and changes in structure and function may occur.

Cellular Adaptation

Cells must be able to adapt to influences which tend to upset homeostasis. Cells adapt to increases in function and to changes in functional demands. Changes in cell type, size, and number may reflect an accommodation to a need and the presence of an appropriate stimulus. These changes do not occur independent of need or stimulus and cease when the need and appropriate stimulus are no longer present. Adaptive responses differ fundamentally from abnormal cell changes in cancer (p. 117).

The dividing line between reversible and irreversible changes and between what is cellular injury and what is an acceptable demand for changed function is not always apparent. Those influences or environmental cell stresses that lead to adaptation by causing changes in size, number, and type include atrophy, hypertrophy, hyperplasia, metaplasia, and dysplasia (p. 92).

Cell Injury

The response of a cell to injury reflects the degree to which the cellular and subcellular physiology is altered. There may be an increase or decrease in the size of its membrane pores, a change in the membrane structure, and a reduction or increase in the passage of molecular substances in and out of the cell. Disease affects primarily the cell membrane, mitochondria, and lysosomes.

The source of the injurious agent may be endogenous (defects in the genome), or more often involves exogenous factors such as nutritional deficiencies, chemical toxins, microbes, physical agents, immunological events, or lack of oxygen or nutrition at the cellular level.

Of particular importance in the response of a cell to injury is the control of cell organelles by nuclear DNA. The ability of the cell to respond by changing membrane transport, repairing damage by new protein synthesis, and other vital functions is determined largely by central control by DNA. Thus the nucleus in effect controls virtually all aspects of organelle response to injurious agents, including the interaction of the agent with the cell membrane, synthesis of structural and enzymatic proteins involved in the generation of energy in the mitochondria, regulation of the synthesis of the hydrolytic enzymes of the lysosomes, and control of the synthesis of enzymes necessary for cell division.

Injurious agents which are brought into the cell by pinocytosis or phagocytosis may be degraded by lysosomal enzymes. However, such degradation is not always possible, especially in an overwhelming infection. Some unwanted substances incorporated into the phagocytic lysosomal pathway may enter the cell by other transport processes and be degraded. Some substances, like tubercle bacilli, appear to be resistant to lysosomal degradation.

If the homeostatic control of adaptation to injury becomes impaired, several changes may be seen in the cell. If there is failure of the ion pump transport mechanism, water accumulates in the cytoplasm and appears microscopically as *cloudy* swelling. If water filled vacuoles accumulate in the endoplasmic reticulum, a more severe form of swelling called *hydropic degeneration* occurs. When protein synthesis fails due to ingestion of a substance such as carbon tetrachloride, fatty vacuoles and inclusions may occur. Many other materials may accumulate in cells with sublethal injury, i.e., lead, copper, glycogen, etc.

Adenosine triphosphate (ATP), which is obtained from the degradation of sugars (the glycolytic pathway), adequately supplies the energy for the resulting level of cellular activity. However, some cells and their specialized activities require increased ATP production via mitochondrial aerobic respiration (e.g., phagocytes) and are therefore particularly susceptible to injury from lack of oxygen (hypoxia), drugs, and nutritional deficiencies.

The chromosomal DNA is usually protected in the mitotic stage of cell division, but injury to chromosomes may occur during the prophase (translocation) and during the anaphase (disjunction). Damage to DNA results in cell death or mutation.

When the effects of cell injury are irreversible, death or *necrosis* of the cell, organ, or tissue occurs. As a result of cell death, changes in the cytoplasm and nucleus may be: liquification of the cell (liquification necrosis), which may be seen in the central part of an abscess; coagulation of cells into a firm mass (coagulation necrosis), which is found in coronary occlusion; and a cheese-like necrosis (caseous necrosis), which may be seen in tubercular lesions (tuberculosis). When a large area of tissue undergoes necrosis the term *gangrene* is applied.

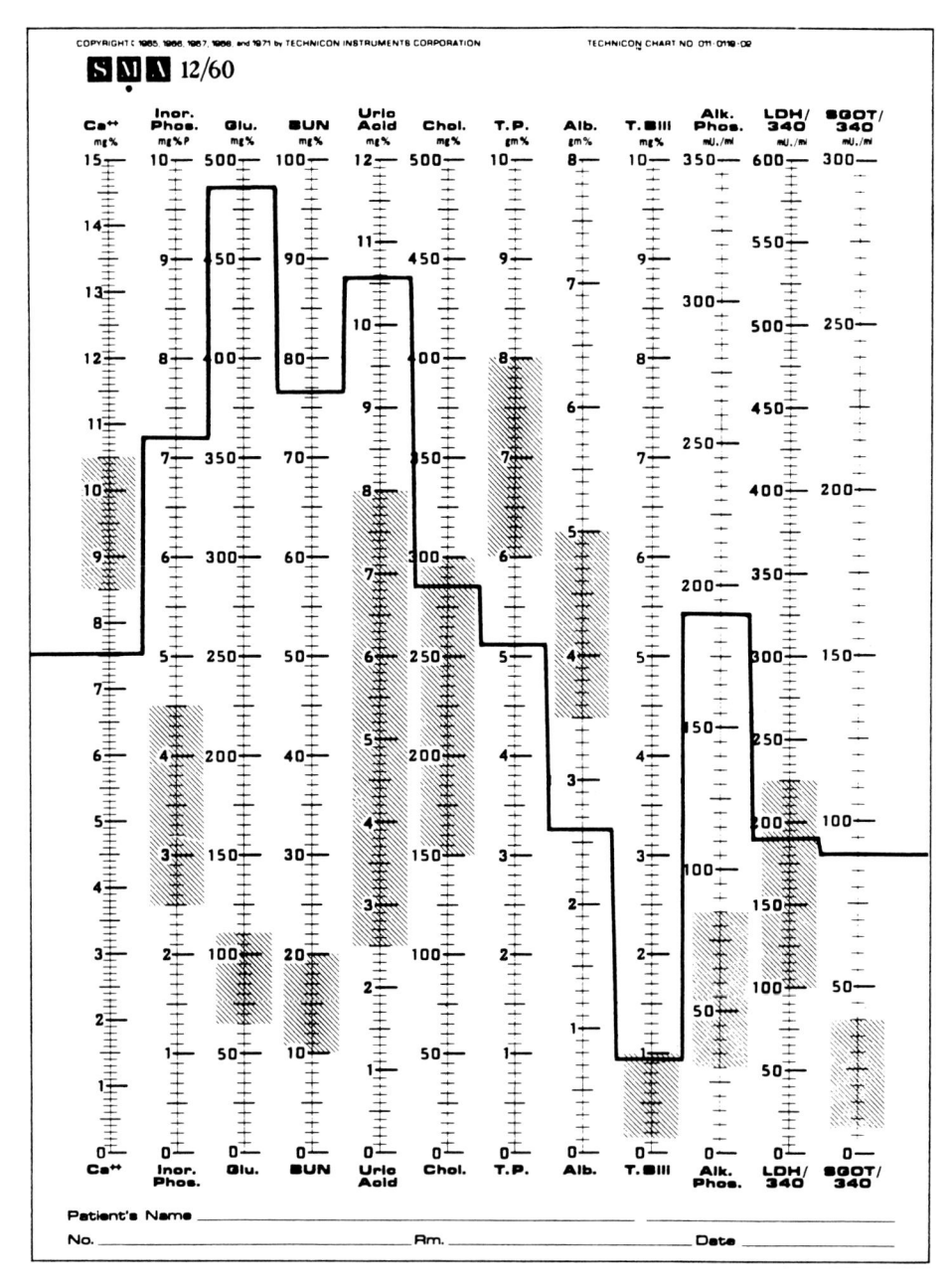

Fig. 1-11. Biochemical profile of serum findings made by an autoanalyzer. The solid line is that found for the patient; shaded areas indicate the range of normal. The profile is consistent with the clinical findings of diabetes mellitus, with associated kidney disease and secondary hyperparathyroidism.

Clinical Correlates of Cellular Injury

It should not be concluded that cellular injury is a purely local response. When a group of cells are injured, such as in the heart, liver, kidney, joints and skeletal muscle, trace materials are released from the cells which produce clinical manifestations. These manifestations include the direct effects of the cellular materials released from the injured cells and the response of the body, e.g., fever, perception of pain, increase in white blood cells (leukocytosis). Many substances cannot be detected, but others are of diagnostic value (Fig. 1–11), including enzymes in low concentrations, e.g., creatine phosphokinase (CPK) as an indicator of the size of heart muscle damage (myocardial infarcts). The CPK isoenzyme MB which is found in myocardial cells appears to be more reliable than other enzymes. CPK exceeds its normal values in 4–8 hours, reaches a peak in 24 hours, and returns to normal in 3–4 days. Other enzymes are lactic dehydrogenase (LDH) and glutamic-oxaloacetic transaminase (GOT).

There are a number of immunologic methods which provide evidence of past or present infection by the demonstration of substances (antibodies) in the blood serum or other body fluids (e.g., cerebrospinal fluid). Tests of serum (serologic tests) for antibody (cf. p.78) which reacts with a substance (antigen) under laboratory conditions only indicates that the patient has had a prior contact with the antigen or perhaps an antigen which is related closely. Such clinical laboratory tests have been found to correlate quite well with clinical findings provided the tests are conducted and interpreted correctly. The hepatitis B virus (HBV) surface antigen (HBsAg) is found on the outer coat of the virus and when found in the serum in measurable quantities is considered to be a diagnostic aid for HBV.

Other tests of cell injury and loss of function include changes in electrical activity detected by electroencephalography (brain waves) and electromyography (muscle function). The latter has been used in a number of ways to test dysfunction of jaw musculature.

SUMMARY

It is important to understand that it is the response of cell to injury that produces the manifestations of disease, not the injury itself although the signs of physical trauma may be obvious. In some diseases the injurious agent may not be identified although the manifestations may be readily seen, such as in cancer. The response to injury reflects a quantitative alteration (increase or decrease) in existing metabolic pathways. Alterations which exceed the adaptive capacity of the cell to correct for small perturbations via homeostatic servomechanisms may not be compatible with normal or continued existence of the cell. The sources of injury which require such adjustments by the cell include genetic errors which occur with gene disorders and chromosomal aberrations, as well as external agents of injury such as drugs, microorganisms (viruses, bacteria, fungi, etc.), trauma, heat, cold, nutrition, radiation, and immunologic reactions.

BIBLIOGRAPHY

Bender, G.A.: Virchow and cellular pathology. Therap. Notes, 68:149, 1961.

Farquhar, M.G. and Palade, G.E.: Junctional complexes in various epithelia. J. Cell Biol., 17:375, 1963.

Han, S.S.: *Cell Biology.* New York, McGraw-Hill Book Co., 1979.

Hartman, D.: The aging process. Proc. Natl. Acad. Sci. USA, 78:7124, 1981.

Hill, R.B. and LaVia, M.F.: *Principles of Pathobiology,* 3rd ed. New York, Oxford University Press, 1980.

Hirsch, J.G.: The phagocytic defense system. In: *Microbial Pathogenicity in Man and Animals.* pp. 59–74. Cambridge, University Press, 1972.

Kennedy, D.: *The Living Cell.* Scientific American Ed. San Francisco and London, W.H. Freeman and Co., 1965.

Listgarten, M.A.: The ultrastructure of human gingival epithelium. Amer. J. Anat., *114*:49, 1964.

Page, E. (ed.): Minisymposium on gap junctions. Am. J. Physical, Heart and Circulatory Physiology. *17*:H751, 1985.

Schroeder, H.E.: Ultrastructure of the junctional epithelium of the human gingiva. Helv. Odont. Acta, *13*:65, 1969.

Thilander, H.,and Bloom, G.D.: Cell contacts in oral epithelium. J. Periodont. Res., *3*:96, 1968.

Trump, B.F., Jesudason, M.L., and Jones, R.T.: Ultrastructural features of diseased cells. In B.E. Trump and R.T. Jones (eds.), *Diagnostic Electron Microscopy,* Vol 1, New York, John Wiley and Sons, Inc., 1978.

2

AGENTS OF DISEASE

Disease is caused by a wide variety of factors including changes that originate *within* the cell such as "genetic mistakes," and injury due to external agents such as microorganisms (bacteria, viruses, fungi, etc.), chemicals, drugs, radiation, trauma, heat, cold, nutrition, and immunologic reactions. The terms *genetic* or *inherited* are usually applied to disturbances involving genes or chromosomes. The term *congenital* simply means present at birth. It is not unusual to use the term congenital, or the terms congenital and developmental disturbances, to include all diseases that are inherited or acquired in utero. The agents of disease include both intrinsic (genetic, inherited) and extrinsic (e.g., trauma) causative factors.

INTRINSIC FACTORS IN DISEASE

A large percentage of birth defects are estimated to be the result of genetic disorders and the remaining 20% are the effects of infections, drugs, and physical injury to the fetus. More than 40% of all infant mortality is due to genetic factors. Seven per cent of all infants born alive in the United States have some mental or physical defect which become evident at birth or at a later time.

Manifestations of genetic inheritance may be due to single-gene disorders as well as polygenic disorders and chromosomal disorders. Almost 10% of all human malformations are due to single gene alterations. A gross chromosomal abnormality is present in 1% of all live births and 57% of stillbirths. Congenital disorders caused by environmental factors (teratogens) are not usually inheritable and affect only somatic cells or their progenitors. Genetic diseases may be categorized as *inborn errors of metabolism* (viz., specific protein deficiency, often enzymes) such as the error of metabolism seen in hemophilia, and *cytogenic disorders* (viz., chromosomal abnormalities) such as Down's syndrome (mongolism).

Genetic Factors

In the formation of new somatic cells, mitotic division, which is called *mitosis,* results in the production of two daughter cells, each of which has received a full complement of chromosomes. Each somatic (body) cell contains 23 pairs of chromosomes, one member of each pair being derived from the father and mother. Thus there are 22 autosome pairs and 2 sex chromosomes, i.e., the male possesses 22 autosome pairs and normally an X and Y chromosome, and the female 22 autosome pairs plus 2 X chromosomes. The human somatic cell contains 46 chromosomes and is the diploid number of the cell.

The genetic information survives the many processes of gamete (ovum and sperm) formation, fertilization, and cell divisions involved in the formation of a new organism from the single-celled zygote that forms from the union of the ovum and sperm.

Fertilization involves the fusion of the male and female germ cells to form a zygote and the development of a new person. Each germ cell has one-half the number (haploid) of chromosomes as the zygote or somatic (body) cells. Thus the production of ova and sperm cells requires the reduction of the chromosome number from 46 to 23. Then on fertilization the diploid number (46) chromosomes is reestablished in the new somatic cell.

The reduction in chromosomes from the diploid to the haploid number is called *meiosis*. During meiosis zygotes may be produced with an abnormal number of chromosomes, and result in congenital defects, for example, Down's syndrome (mongolism).

During fertilization the father contributes one of each pair of his chromosomes and the mother contributes one of each pair of her chromosomes and thus make up the pair of chromosomes in their offspring. Genes from each parent are located along the length of the chromosome; for each gene on a maternal chromosome there is a corresponding homologous gene in the same position on the paternal chromosome. For most of the time the two homologous genes are identical and common to the species. This arrangement is "normal" but sometimes an abnormal ("mutant") gene may be found along the line of genes on a chromosome. Mutation can occur at the level of individual genes or can involve whole chromosomes. In any case mutations usually occur when the DNA strand is dividing and may be the result of ionizing radiation or chemicals.

At a particular part of the DNA molecule, the genetic code may control an observable trait. This segment of the molecules is called a *gene locus*. Alternate codes at one gene location are referred to as *alleles*. Where the two alleles of a given pair at a gene location are the same (AA or aa), individuals are homozygotes. If the alleles at a gene locus are different (Aa), they are called heterozygotes. A dominant trait is expressed when the pairing is homozygous or heterozygous whereas a recessive trait is expressed only in homozygous pairing.

An abnormal gene produces no effect if it is dominated and suppressed by the corresponding normal gene on the other chromosome. Whenever a mutant (defective) gene is situated in the X or Y chromosome, whether or not an individual will be affected will depend upon that person's sex. The male has only one X chromosome and if he carries a mutant gene, he will exhibit the disease. If a female carries the mutant gene, whether she is affected depends upon whether the gene is dominant or recessive, and if she is homozygous or heterozygous (i.e., whether she has inherited a single or double dose of abnormal genetic material). All males who inherit the hemophilia gene on their X chromosome will have hemophilia. For the female to exhibit hemophilia, the defect would have to involve both X chromosomes, a rare event.

Single-Gene Disorders

Disorders of Mendelian or single-gene inheritance may be autosomal dominant, autosomal recessive, or X-linked recessive. In *autosomal dominant* disorders, including some disturbances of formation of the dental hard tissues such as dentinogenesis imperfecta (p. 57), an affected parent has a single mutant gene which is transmitted to the offspring regardless of sex. An affected individual has a 50/50 chance of transmitting the disorder to each offspring. In *autosomal recessive* disorders, including some cases of cystic fibrosis, sickle cell disease, and color blindness, the abnormal gene is expressed only when the gene is received from both parents, i.e., both members of the gene pair are mutant alleles. The recurrence risk in each pregnancy is 1 in 4 for an affected child. *Sex-linked* or X-linked inheritance, which is almost always the X or female chromosome, is predominantly recessive, as in classical hemophilia. The modes of inheritance of a few genetic diseases are shown in Table 2–1.

Chromosomal Disorders

Chromosomal disorders may occur during meiosis as already mentioned. In addition to accidental chromosomal abnormalities involving a change in number due to failure of separation of chromosomes (disjunction) during the formation of the ovum or sperm, aberrations in chromosomal structure may occur when there is a break in one or more of the chromosomes that is followed by deletion or rearrangement of the parts of the chromosomes. Breakage is caused by viral infections, chemicals, and ionizing (such as x rays) type of radiation. Down's syndrome, or trisomy 21, is the most common form of chromosomal disorder. Chromosomes are typed according to set standards for form and size. This karyotype of an individual (Fig. 2–1) is used in cytogenetics to study the structure and numerical characteristics of the cell's chromosomes. A decrease of one chromosome, i.e., monosomy (45 chromosomes), is usually lethal. An increase of one or more chromosomes is teratogenic and results in congenital malformations. In Down's syndrome there are 47 chromosomes, i.e., there are 3 autosomes of type 21 or an extra no. 21 chromosome. In mothers aged 35 to 40 the incidence is 1 in 200 compared to 1 in 2250 live births where the mother is under 30 years of age. Mongolism is characterized by mental retardation, upward slanting of palpebral fissures, flat nasal ridge, and macroglossia.

Polygenic Disorders

Polygenic inheritance refers to the inheritance of a general genetic package which predisposes individuals to certain illnesses and renders them more susceptible to environmental influences, viz., people with blood group type O are 40% more likely to develop a duodenal ulcer than those with other blood groups. In polygenic inheritance two or more genes or gene loci are influential in expressing the gene trait. Although polygenic traits cannot be predicted with the same degree of assurance as single-gene mutations, some patterns do exist. Congenital malformations tend to involve a single tissue or organ derived from the same embryologic developmental area and have an increased risk of occurring in future pregnancies. For example, there is an increased risk of having another child with cleft palate but not spinal defects. A number of conditions may be polygenic disorders, incuding congenital heart disease, allergies, and diabetes mellitus.

Human Cancer

Each human cell contains oncogenes, i.e., genes which have the potential to cause cancer. Ordinarily these genes carry out normal functions until activated by some mechanism which transforms the oncogene into a source of cancer. An oncogene may be activated by a "point mutation", i.e., a small segment of the gene is altered by radiation or a chemical carcinogen. It may also be activated by "amplification," that is,

Table 2–1. Modes of Inheritance of Some Genetic Disease

Dominant	Recessive	X-linked
Achondroplasia	Albinism	Color blindness
Congenital cataract	Cretinism	Hemophilia
Epiloia	Cystic fibrosis	Muscular dystrophy
Marfan's syndrome	Muscular dystrophy	(Duchenne)
Osteogenesis imperfecta	Phenylketonuria	
Polyposis coli	Sickle cell disease	

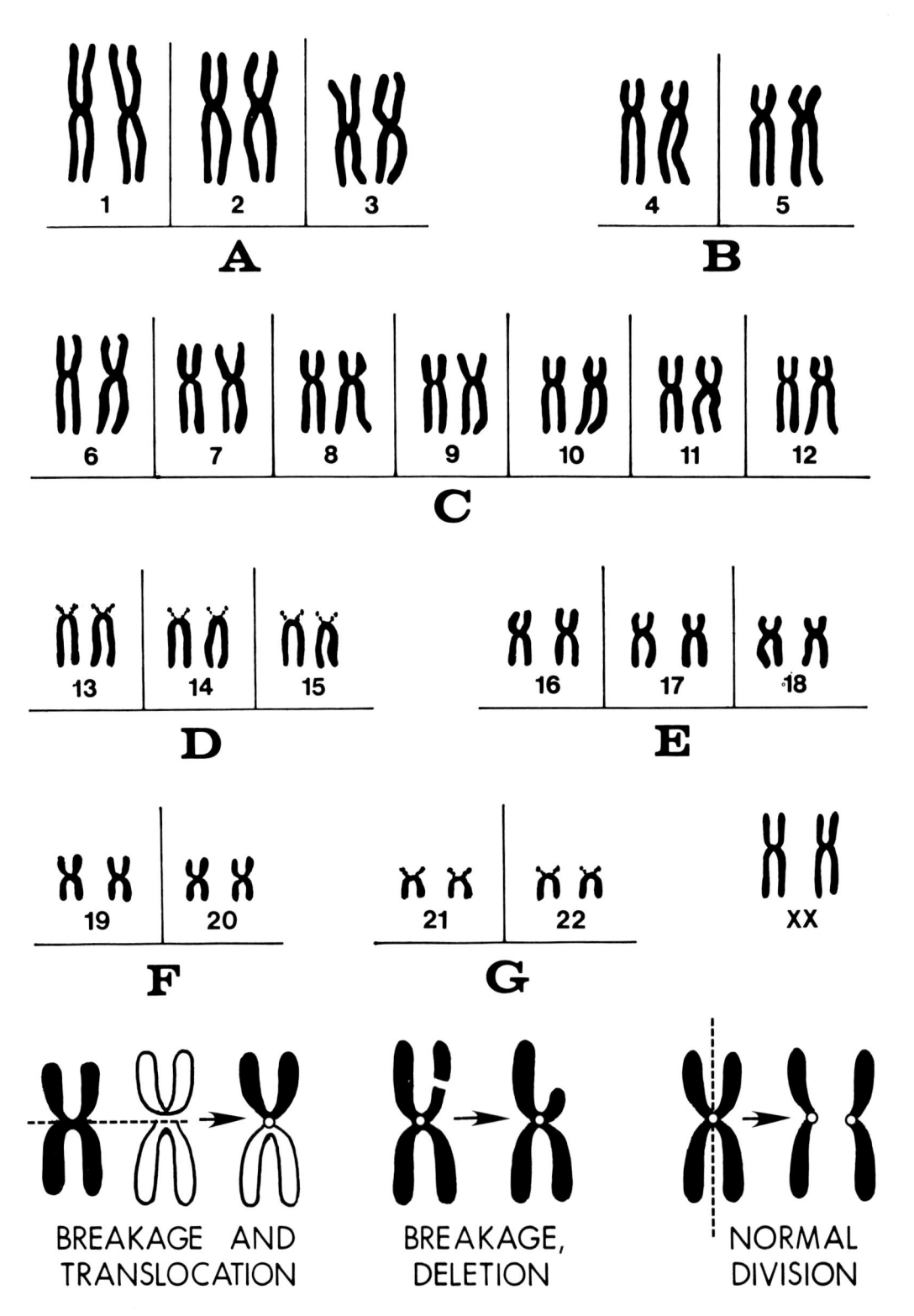

Fig. 2–1. Normal female karyotype. There are 22 pairs of autosomes and 1 pair of sex chromosomes (XX). In the female only one X chromosome is considered to be active in expressing genetic traits. Chromosome defects include changes in number and/or structure, e.g., breakage, translocation or rearrangement, and deletion of chromosome parts.

the oncogene is replicated many times resulting in several active copies of the gene being present in a single cell. An oncogene may be activated by incorporation into a retrovirus (a virus whose genetic material is made of RNA rather than DNA). Since few human tumors carry an oncogene in these ways, the role of the activating mechanisms is not clear. Another mechanism involves chromosome translocation, i.e., rearrangement of broken-off segments of chromosomes. This "trading" of chromosome segments could be a mechanism for activating oncogenes in the immune system (p. 76).

Examples of genetic factors in cancer related to simple gene inheritance and showing mendelian transmission are scarce. Single gene inheritance in cancer appears to occur only in one or two specific instances, e.g., retinoblastoma and polyposis coli. However, polygenic inheritance is probably important in the causation of cancer, i.e., genetic material favors the effect of environmental carcinogens on a specific organ. Although there may be a tendency to develop cancer at a specific site, there is not a tendency to develop cancer in general.

CONGENITAL MALFORMATIONS/ TERATOGENIC AGENTS

Congenital or developmental anatomic malformations may involve unfavorable environmental influence on the mechanism of polygenic inheritance. As with single gene mutations, degrees of "penetrance" (likelihood of manifestation) may occur in polygenic inheritance. The incidence of congenital malformations in siblings is 10 to 20 times higher than in the general population.

Teratogenic Agents

A number of agents produce malformations during the development of the fetus or embryo. These teratogens include viruses, irradiation, and drugs (Table 2–2):

Defective embryologic development occurs most frequently in most tissues and organs during certain weeks following conception. Significant adverse environmental influences during the first few weeks following fertilization may result in abortion. The susceptible periods for defective embryologic development involving the teeth and palate include the latter part of the sixth week as well as the seventh and eighth weeks following conception. Major morphologic abnormalities resulting from teratogenic agents occur in the third through the seventh week, e.g., teratogenic effects involving the central nervous system and heart occur during this period of time. Developmental disturbances of the teeth, tongue, palate and lips are discussed in Chapter 3.

Table 2–2. Some Teratogenic Agents That Can Cause Congenital Disturbances

Radiation	Pollutants
	Arsenic
Drugs or Chemicals	Mercury
Alcohol	Lead
Androgenic agents	Propylthiouracil
Anticonvulsants	Tetracycline
Methadiones	Thalidomide
Methotrexate	
Phenytoin	*Viruses*
Antitumor agents	Cyclomegalovirus
Aminopterin	Herpes simplex 2
Cyclophosphamide	Measles (rubella)
Oral contraceptives	Mumps
	Other Agents
	Toxoplasmosis

Radiation

Ionizing radiation includes particulate (alpha, beta, proton, and neutron particles) and electromagnetic (X and gamma rays) forms of energy. When ionizing electromagnetic radiation of high frequency, short wave length, and high photon energy interacts with matter (such as germ material), electrons are removed from atoms. DNA is the major target affected by ionizing radiation, although other parts of the cell are also damaged.

The amount of radiation absorbed by the tissues is measured in *rads*. The unit of exposure dose is the *roentgen*. A dose of 1 roentgen to living tissue results in the absorption of energy of 1 rad. The term *rem* has been used to indicate the equivalent biologic effect of irradiation by sources other than x rays. Thus 1 rem produces the same biologic effect as 1 rad.

The average gonadal dose from all sources of radiation (cosmic rays, gamma rays, medical-dental x rays, etc.) in 30 years is about 4 rems. If the whole body is irradiated with a dose of 300 to 500 rads, the dose is usually fatal. The effects of radiation are cumulative, i.e., each new dose must be added to previous doses of radiation.

Although DNA is the only component of the cell not freely replaceable and is probably being constantly repaired, injury by radiation leading to faulty replication at cell division can lead to inherited defects or even cell death. Ionizing radiation is not only teratogenic, but also mutagenic. Mutations that involve damage to the germ material or germ cells can be passed on to future generations of the organism; mutations in somatic cells of an organism may lead to organ dysfunction or in some cases to cancer. Evidence has been presented that shows an increased risk of cancer for children who are exposed to diagnostic x rays while in utero. Irradiating the pregnant abdomen has virtually been replaced by other diagnostic techniques.

Macromolecules may be damaged by direct action in which the molecules are ionized or by indirect action in which water or solute molecules are ionized and produce free radicals (H^+ and OH^-) that damage macromolecules in the nucleus (i.e., nucleic acids).

DNA in the process of replication is more vulnerable to ionizing radiation than resting DNA is. Therefore the effect of ionizing radiation is more damaging to tissues with rapidly dividing cells, viz., gastrointestinal tract, bone marrow, gonads, and lymphoid tissue.

Chemicals and Drugs

There are a number of potential teratogenic agents, but organic mercurials are some of the most important because of the severe defects, i.e., neurologic deficits and blindness. Sources of mercury that are particularly widespread are contaminated fish and water. The concern for mercury toxicity and hypersensitivity from amalgam restorations has not been substantiated.

Several teratogenic drugs have been suspected, but only a few documented. For example, one of the best known is thalidomide, which causes a wide range of malformations, including flipper-like appendages of arms and legs. Also the antibiotic tetracycline causes extensive staining of the teeth (p. 57). Fetal disturbances can be caused by other drugs such as antimetabolites used in the treatment of cancer, warfarin (an anticoagulant drug), several of the anticonvulsants, and ethanol (grain alcohol). Also, progestins which are found in several birth control tablets can cause virilization of the female fetus. A possible association between the use of diazepam in the first trimester of pregnancy and oral clefts has been suggested but not confirmed.

Microorganisms

Several microorganisms have been implicated as teratogenic agents, including herpes simplex 2 virus, cytomegalovirus, rubella, and toxoplasmosis. These infections can cause defects of the eyes and hearing, mental retardation, hydrocephaly and microcephaly. Screening for these infections utilizes infant serum to test for the presence of antibodies (p. 78).

Prenatal Diagnosis

Prenatal diagnosis of some of the genetic developmental disturbances can be accomplished by amniocentesis. A needle is inserted into the uterus through the abdominal wall and a sample of amniotic fluid is withdrawn for biochemical and chromosomal studies. Although not all hereditary defects can be detected in this way, amniocentesis is useful for detecting over 50 genetic disturbances. Because a defective fetus can be determined by the 16th or 17th week of pregnancy, it is possible to decide if termination of the pregnancy should occur. The test is especially useful when parents already have a child with chromosomal abnormalities, a parent is a carrier of a genetic disorder, or the mother is over 35 years of age and there is an increased risk that the baby will have Down's syndrome.

PSYCHOLOGIC FACTORS

Psychologic disturbances can be categorized as: (1) disorders of mind and behavior resulting from an observable pathologic condition of the brain; (2) functional psychoses in which there is no brain disease consistent with the symptoms (schizophrenia, manic-depressive disorder); and (3) disturbances in mind and behavior which reflect personality disorders and neurotic symptoms (anxiety states, phobias, panic disorder, obsessive-compulsive disorders, as well as somatoform disorders such as hysteria and conversion hysteria).

Schizophrenia and manic-depressive disorders are clinical disease entities, but they have no recognized neuropathy. *Schizophrenia* is a thought disorder characterized by confused associations, lack of logic, auditory hallucinations, detachment from reality, and delusions. The disease occurs most frequently between the ages of 15 and 45. There are four subtypes: *catatonia* (stupor, rigidity, mutism); *hebephrenia* (giggling, posturing, and gesturing for no apparent reason); *paranoia* (delusions of persecution and/or grandeur); and *simple schizophrenia* (social inadequacy, loss of ambition, initiative). The etiology of schizophrenia is not clear and several hypotheses have been suggested, including reaction to life stress, genetic factors, and functional excess of dopamine. There is no specific cure for schizophrenia.

Manic-depressive psychosis has an essential feature of periods of predominantly excessive disturbances of mood (elevated, expansive, or irritable). Three of the following symptoms must persist in mania: (1) increased activity; (2) flight of ideas, unusual verbosity; (3) inflated self-esteem; (4) decreased need for sleep; (5) easily distracted; and (6) excessive involvement in unproductive activities with untoward consequences, e.g., reckless driving, buying sprees, and foolish investments. Clinical manifestations include depression with lowered self-esteem and self-blame. The patient may complain of a physical symptom, typically chronic pain which fails to respond to treatment. Depression is diagnosed on the basis of: (1) change in appetite with gain or loss of weight; (2) insomnia or hypersomnia; (3) psychomotor agitation or retardation; (4) loss of interest in usual activities, decrease in sexual drive; (5) feeling of worthlessness, inappropriate guilt; (6) diminished ability to think; (7) loss of energy, fatigue; and (8) recurrent thoughts of death or suicide (Diagnostic and Statistical Manual of Mental Disorders DSM III, American Psychiatric Association). The etiology is not clear although there is good evidence for a genetic predisposition, but clearly nongenetic influences are involved. It has also been suggested that a deficiency of central nervous system neurotransmitters, particularly norepinephrine and serotonin, are involved in these affective (mood) disorders. Suicide precautions should be taken. Mania requires immediate treatment with hospitalization. Haloperidol may be used initially and then lithium carbonate started. Tricyclic antidepressants are usually considered for depression.

Panic disorder (anxiety neurosis) is characterized by attacks of extreme apprehension, accompanied by a sense of doom or fear of losing control. The symptoms include dyspnea (shortness of breath), palpitations, chest pain, sweating, faintness, trembling and choking sensations. The etiology is not clear although abnormal lactate levels may be linked to the cause of panic disorders. Treatment with the use of antianxiety (anxiolytic) drugs such as benzodiazepine or diazepam, and tricyclic antidepressants or monoamine oxidase inhibitors has greatly enhanced the control of panic attacks. A progression of stages for the disorder has been proposed: sub-panic symptom attacks, polysymptomatic attacks, hypochondriasis, single phobia, socia phobia, polyphobia, and depression. These attacks occur without provocation, whereas most cases of, for example, dental anxiety are exogenous, i.e., symptoms such as moist palms, fine hand tremors, and rapid heart beat occur in normal patients who experience stress or fear as in a dental office.

Phobias are irrational fears that can be triggered by virtually anything and are often associated with uncontrolled panic. Among the simple and complex phobias are: acrophobia (fear of heights), areophobia (fear of flying), agoraphobia (fear of open spaces), claustrophobia (closed spaces), cynophobia (dogs), gephyrophobia (bridges), and xenophobia (strangers). The etiology is obscure and does not usually yield to traditional psychotherapy. Antidepressant drugs and MAO inhibitors have been of value for treatment of phobias.

Hysteria is a somatization disorder in which physical symptoms, ranging from headache to paralyses, occur without known pathophysiologic cause. A variant, conversion hysteria, is characterized by the presence of a single symptom, usually of a single system (e.g., nervous system). Conversion includes blindness, amnesia, aphonia, and paralysis. Sexual and menstrual problems are usually present. Frequent surgery, hospitalizations, and diagnostic tests are found in the patient's past history.

Obsessive-compulsive neurosis as the name suggests is a disorder characterized by obsessions (recurrent ideas) and compulsions (repetitive, stereotyped acts) that follow the obsession. Thus, the patient has the obsession that some undesirable thing will happen unless some ritual is performed to prevent the happening. This kind of behavior becomes a psychiatric problem when it interferes with normal living. The etiology is not clear, and treatment has not been outstanding.

EXTRINSIC FACTORS IN DISEASE

Extrinsic disease is produced by etiologic factors brought to the cell from its environment rather than by transmission through chromosomes. Extrinsic factors may be considered as environmental factors if we think of environment in its broad sense—the environment of the individual cell as well as the environment of the organism as a whole. The extrinsic factors producing disease are more numerous than intrinsic factors and therefore are demonstrated more often in relation to disease.

The extrinsic factors in disease include physical agents of disease, infectious agents, nutritional factors, chemical injury, environmental agents, and drugs and hormones.

Physical Agents

Physical agents of injury include factors which disturb gas homeostasis, mechanical injury, and radiant energy.

OXYGEN, GAS HOMEOSTASIS. If the atmosphere is replaced by some other material, such as earth or water, the individual is prevented from obtaining oxygen and death results. When an individual is submerged in water, death is due to drowning, but if submerged in sand, death is due to suffocation. The individual may be deprived of oxygen if the air is replaced by another gas as sometimes occurs in deep wells or mines. If the air contains a high concentration of gas for which the hemoglobin has a marked affinity, it replaces the oxygen in the blood stream. An excellent example is carbon monoxide. Hemoglobin has several times the affinity for carbon monoxide than it has for oxygen, so when small quantities are present in the atmosphere, it is absorbed by the hemoglobin and prevents oxygen from being absorbed. The individual cells are thus deprived of oxygen and death is attributed to carbon monoxide poisoning. Death by asphyxiation occurs when individuals are trapped in smoke-filled rooms during a fire or stay in a closed garage while the car motor is running. Other substances for which hemoglobin demonstrates an affinity may combine with hemoglobin to form a stable chemical compound such as methemoglobin. Methemoglobin, produced in analine poisoning and many other chemical intoxications, does not have an affinity for oxygen and is incapable of transporting oxygen to and from the cells. Although the mechanism of oxygen deficiency associated with methemoglobin is different from low-oxygen tension in the atmosphere or carbon monoxide poisoning, the effect on the cell is the same, hypoxia. Some toxic agents damage and destroy the red blood cells which results in oxygen deficiency and death of the cells.

Oxygen toxicity occurs when excess oxygen is administered. Some years ago pure oxygen was given to premature babies and resulted in blindness.

Divers and to a lesser extent high flying circus crews need to take into account the effects of atmospheric pressure. To dive to low depths oxygen has to be mixed with helium. Trapping gas in closed places, including the teeth, may occur but can be avoided by slow controlled "decompression." The term "barodontalgia" is used to designate dental pain associated with changes in atmospheric pressure.

If decompression occurs too rapidly, nitrogen bubbles collect in joints and skeletal muscle ("bends"). Such nitrogen toxicity (Caisson disease) is avoided by slow decompression.

Cells of a limited area may die because of being deprived of oxygen and nutrients when the blood vessels to the area are obstructed. The local death of cells in a limited area of the body is designated *necrosis,* while the loss of the blood supply to the area leading to the death of the cells is called *ischemia.* The process of obstruction of an end-artery or the sole vein of an area and the resulting ischemic necrosis of the area is called *infarction.* The area of tissue that undergoes necrosis is called an infarct (Fig. 2–2). Obstruction of a vessel may occur as a result of thrombosis or embolism. *Thrombosis* is the intravascular clotting of blood. Most frequently it refers to the formation of a clot within a vessel owing to injury of the endothelial lining; such a clot is referred to as a thrombus. *Embolism* is the transportation of a substance or mass through vessels from one location to a second where it lodges. The mass is referred to as an *embolus.* The most common source of emboli are thrombi which become detached. Thrombosis is significant because of the possibility of occluding the vessels of vital tissues and organs of the body such as the heart. An individual is said to die of a "heart attack" or "coronary" if the coronary vessels of the heart are obstructed or occluded, and the heart muscle dies because of a lack of oxygen and other blood nutrients.

Clinical manifestations of a lack of oxygen (hypoxia) are shortness of breath (dyspnea), difficulty in breathing, and deep and rapid breathing. Absolute cellular *anoxia* probably does not occur at the cellular level because of some collateral circulation and local oxygen diffusion. Cyanosis may also be present and is due to an absolute increase in the amount of reduced hemoglobin in the blood. Cyanosis causes the skin and mucous membranes to be dusky blue color. The most common cause of generalized cyanosis is heart disease. Localized cyanosis, which is seen in gingivitis, is primarily due to local changes in circulation (venous congestion or passive hyperemia). *Passive hyperemia* refers to a decreased outflow or a stagnation of blood on the venous side of the circulation. An area so involved is not able to obtain its optimal requirements of oxygen and food. Venous congestion is a common feature of gingivitis. *Active hyperemia* refers to an increased flow of blood to the tissues and in part is responsible for increased heat and redness in inflammation.

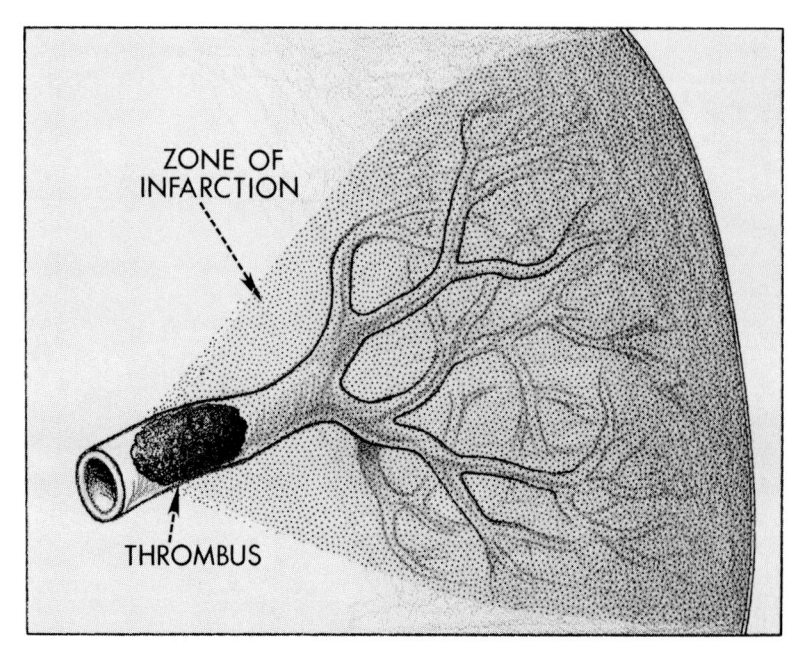

Fig. 2–2. Diagram demonstrating a thrombus and the resultant zone of infarction that might be produced by obstruction of a renal vessel.

TEMPERATURE CHANGES. Extremes of temperature, both heat and lack of heat (cold), produce tissue injury. The local application of rather mild heat to the skin causes a moderate increase in temperature resulting in redness and tenderness of the area to which the heat is applied. More intense heat results in the local accumulation of fluid within the tissues beneath the skin. The fluid causes a separation of the tissues and a thinning of the epithelium which results in a blister. If the heat is intense enough, it produces destruction of cells by coagulation of the cytoplasm or by actually burning and charring the tissues. An increase in the environmental temperature for long periods produces heat exhaustion because of the loss of chlorides through excessive perspiration. If the environmental temperature is high and water is unavailable, death from dehydration occurs in a short time.

The effects of cold are similar to those of heat. A mild reduction of temperature results in redness and swelling of the part (frostbite). Further reduction of temperature produces ice crystals which, on thawing, cause blisters in the tissues. If the temperature of a part of the body is reduced to a point where the blood vessels are injured so that the flow of blood into the part ceases, a clot forms within the blood vessels. The blood flow will not return to the part when the temperature returns to normal and the part dies (gangrene). General reduction of body temperature for prolonged periods results in gradual reduction of cell metabolism and death.

WATER BALANCE. Water as an extrinsic cause of disease is related to either too much or too little for the requirements of the body. Injury from too much water occurs only rarely, and then it is probably accidental in relation to intravenous or subcutaneous therapy. Insufficient water or excessive loss of water leads to dehydration. An individual may be dehydrated from excessive loss of water, from diarrhea, or from deprivation of water owing to insufficient intake. Infants or children who are sick may reject water or fluids and dehydration occurs. If dehydration progresses, death ensues.

Edema may be localized or generalized. Local edema is often due to inflammation and related to burns, infection, obstruction, allergy and hypoxia. Generalized edema is seen with protein deficiencies (starvation), cardiac failure, and hypothyroidism.

Deficiencies and excesses involving nutritional factors and metabolic imbalance are discussed in chapter 9, Nutritional Disturbances.

MECHANICAL INJURY. Mechanical force is a common cause of tissue injury. Its effects depend upon the site, intensity, and method of application. Tissue or parts may be crushed, torn, and/or abraded; bones may be fractured by mechanical or physical force. Injury produced by physical force is called *trauma*.

The injury produced by mechanical force depends on the area of the body to which the force is applied, the degree of the force, the method of application, and the duration of application. When a force is slight and tangentially applied, it may cause a shallow loss of skin or mucous membrane resulting in a wound called an *abrasion*. *Lacerations* are wounds with jagged margins produced by an irregularly shaped, hard object or by tearing of the tissues. When the physical trauma is produced by a sharp instrument, and the resulting wound has a smooth border, it is called an incisional wound or *incision*. Thin, sharp objects forced into the tissues produce *penetrating* wounds. A bullet may make a penetrating wound, or a perforating wound if it comes out the other side of the body forming two openings. *Contusions* or *bruises* are the result of forces applied by blunt objects which usually do not break the surface of the body but disrupt underlying tissues, viscera, or organs. A bruise is produced when soft tissue is impinged between two hard objects so that the blood vessels are injured and blood escapes into the tissues. This type of physical trauma results in a rather characteristic discoloration of the tissues, "black-and-blue" mark or "black eye." Similarly, a blow to the trunk of the body may rupture and bruise solid viscera like liver or spleen, or hollow viscera like the bladder or gut. Compressive forces produce the same results. Fractures of bones are produced by the sudden application of moderate or severe forces. Fractures vary in pattern, depending upon the area involved and the degree of force. When there is much displacement of the bone fragments and loss of continuity of soft tissue with exposure of bone, the injury is called a *compound fracture*. Microorganisms are frequently introduced into the tissue during mechanical injury producing infection which complicates the process of repair.

RADIANT ENERGY. The effects of irradiation on germ material and the developing fetus have already been discussed.

Irradiation by radiant energy may occur in several ways. The most common method is exposure to the rays of ultraviolet light or sunlight. These rays penetrate the skin, and when the exposure is intense and of sufficient duration tissue injury results. The initial changes are redness and slight swelling of the area, followed by blister formation if the exposure is intense and prolonged. The pigment of the skin provides some protection against irradiation by sunlight. By repeated minimal exposure, the skin pigment is increased (tanning), providing protection so that greater exposure to sunlight can be tolerated. Individuals with light skin and hair do not tolerate sunlight well because they do not tan to provide protection from and tolerance to sunlight. The repeated exposure of an individual with little natural pigment of the skin to sunlight conditions his skin to the development of skin cancer later in life. The majority of skin cancers on the surface of the body exposed to sunlight occurs in those individuals who have little natural tolerance to sunlight. (See Etiology of Neoplasia, Chapter 8.)

X-ray radiation is another form of radiant energy which produces cell damage. This type of radiation is much more damaging than ultraviolet rays. Even low doses of x rays used in diagnosis must be considered to be of significance, as all are additive. The routine taking of radiographs to evaluate for dental disease is no longer acceptable.

The initial changes due to significant x-ray irradiation include redness and slight swelling of the skin and loss of hair. These changes subside gradually if the irradiation has not been too intense. However, if the radiation is intense, cells are destroyed and an open sore frequently occurs called an x-ray burn. If the dose of x ray is intense but short causing tissue death, the acute tissue changes subside, but permanent injury to blood vessels and tissue is evident. The skin of the area is thin, slightly scarred, devoid of hair, and the superficial blood vessels are dilated and tortuous. The pale, scarred skin has delicate, red spider-web markings produced by the tortuous vessels (Fig. 2–3). If bone is irradiated, similar changes are present in its blood vessels and the metabolism and healing power of the bone is decreased. If such irradiated bone is subsequently subjected to injury or infection, necrosis occurs owing to the poor circulation. The necrotic bone is separated and expelled from the area (sequestration). Irradiation also results in reduced saliva production and subsequent rampant caries (Fig. 2–4). Prevention of root caries following radiation for cancer is discussed in Chapter 10, Dental Caries.

Small doses of x-ray irradiation over long periods condition the skin to the development of cancer. Various parts of the body are more severely affected by irradiation than others. The gonads are susceptible to x rays and exposure may produce sterility. Bone marrow is also sensitive to x-ray irradiation; and if there is total body exposure, the bone marrow may be destroyed. When the bone marrow is destroyed, the body is unable to cope with infection and death results. Irradiation from other sources of radiant energy, such as radium and radioactive materials, produces a similar type of injury.

Electrical energy causes damage to tissue. The severity of the damage depends upon the intensity of the current and the

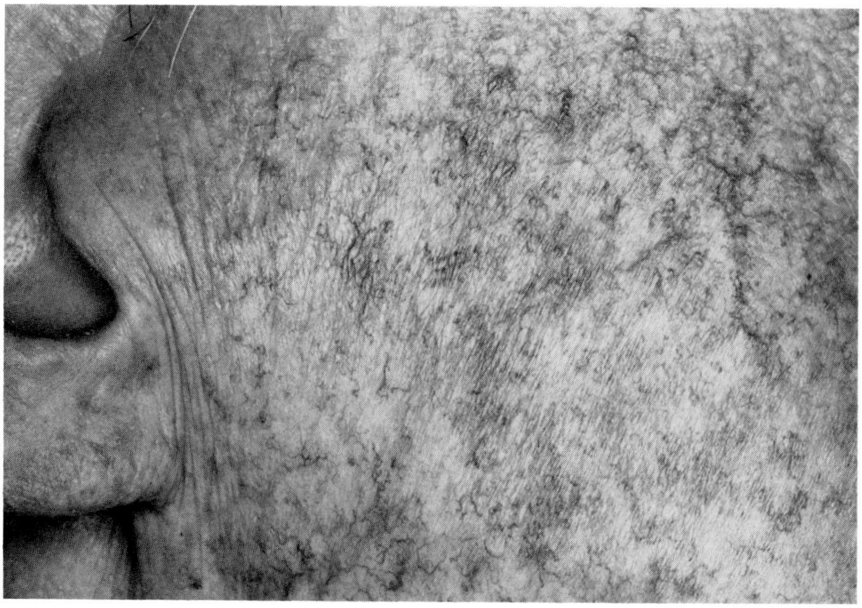

Fig. 2–3. *Chronic effects of irradiation.* In front of the ear the skin is atrophic and finely wrinkled. Below the ear it is smooth and depigmented. There is a "spider-web" effect produced by tortuous dilated vessels (telangiectasia).

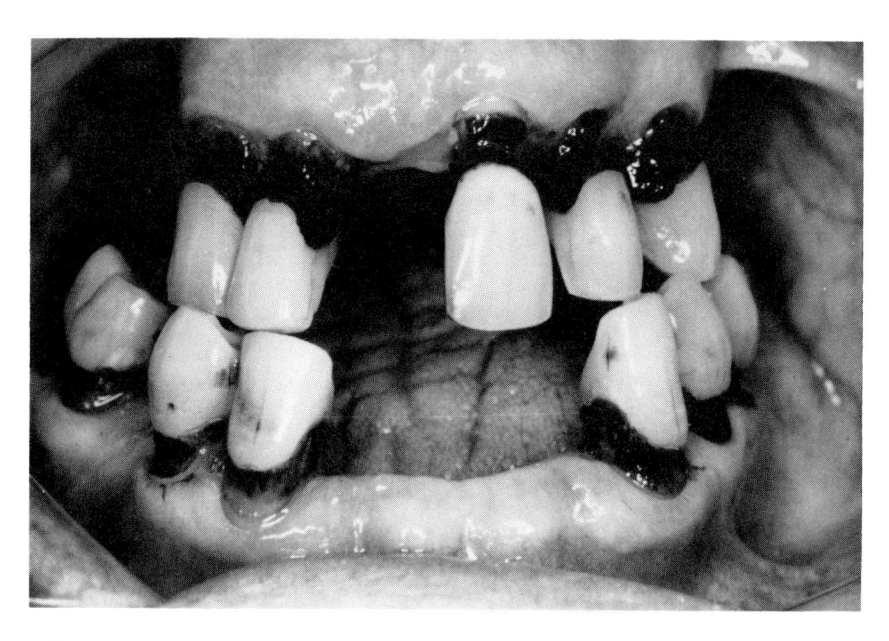

Fig. 2-4. Extensive cervical caries often result when there is intense irradiation of the oral region.

electrical resistance of the tissue. When a sufficiently high current passes through the body, death results because of paralysis of the respiratory center.

Infectious Agents

Much of human disease is caused by infection with microorganisms; however, balanced symbiosis between man and microorganisms is most often the case. *Infection* is a term which can mean the invasion of microbes and damage to tissues, or an imbalance in symbiosis, e.g., an increase in the population of resident microbial flora, and/or a reduction of defense mechanisms which normally limit the type and number of microorganisms present. The ability of an agent to infect is determined by the virulence (pathogenicity), number (dosage), and portal of entry of the microorganism. The major group of infectious agents includes bacteria, viruses, parasites (viz., rickettsiae, chlamydiae, protozoa, metazoa), and fungi.

An important aspect of infection is that a change in the population of the resident microbial flora has occurred and that the body mechanisms which normally limit the type and extent of the microbial flora present are deficient in some way. Ordinarily various bacterial species compete for an ecologic niche and successful symbiotes (i.e., bacteria that normally live in an area do not usually produce disease). Such symbiosis is important in preventing the colonization by other forms of bacteria, some potentially pathogenic. An appropriate amount of secretions from the skin and mucous membranes and from the salivary glands is important for control of the bacterial flora.

The interface between hard (teeth) and soft (gingiva) tissues is a strategic area for the control of bacterial colonization of the teeth and initiation of diseases of supporting structures of the teeth (p. 210). The defense against bacteria involved in diseases of the teeth (dental caries) and periodontal tissues (gingivitis and periodontitis) involves a number of naturally occurring mechanisms, as well as preventive measures taken by the patient and the professional (p. 208).

BACTERIA. Bacteria (0.5 to 8 μm) are traditionally divided into two groups on the basis of their staining reaction with Gram's stain, i.e., gram-positive or gram-negative.

They are also subdivided according to growth characteristics and shape, e.g., bacilli (rod-shaped) and cocci (spherical), and in various other ways. A bacterium is considered to be virulent and pathogenic when it has one of two properties, invasive capacity and toxicity. Bacteria release a number of enzymes which enable them to invade tissues, especially where there has been a breakdown in the normal protective mechanisms (e.g., break in the skin or mucous membranes).

Endotoxins and exotoxins are produced by bacteria and can produce extensive local as well as widespread systemic damage, e.g., in *botulism,* where deglutition and respiration are usually arrested and asphyxiation occurs, and in *Legionnaire's disease,* where the toxin from a gram-negative bacillus often causes death due to widespread damage to lungs, kidneys and the central nervous system (CNS). A number of bacteria are involved in periodontal diseases and dental caries and will be discussed in chapters related to these diseases.

Cocci are small, round organisms which grow in irregular grapelike clusters or in chains. There are two main types of pathogenic cocci: the staphylococci and the streptococci.

Staphylococci are natural inhabitants of the skin which are introduced into wounds or other areas of injury where they multiply and produce a strong exotoxin having an intense local necrotizing effect. Wherever the organisms gain a foothold and produce local necrosis, polymorphonuclear cells are attracted in large numbers to phagocytize the invaders. These cells in the area of liquefaction constitute pus, and the focal accumulation is an *abscess.* Because of this ability of the staphylococci to initiate pus production and abscess formation, they are termed pus-producing organisms. The invasion of a hair follicle or sebaceous gland duct by streptococci results in small abscesses called *furuncles* (pimples). They are common on the face, especially with the development of the beard associated with the beginning of sexual maturity. More extensive infections associated with hair follicles where pus extends into the deeper subepithelial areas with a large area of necrosis are *boils.* When the lesion involves many hair follicles and there are numerous areas of discrete necrosis and pus formation involving a large area, the lesion is a *carbuncle.*

The reaction of the tissues to the streptococci is basically the same in all areas and the disease process is named according to anatomic site, viz., tonsillitis, pharyngitis, endocarditis, nephritis. Streptococci frequently localize in the pharynx and tonsillar area to produce "strep sore throat." Streptococcus viridans produces subacute bacterial endocarditis when septicemia transports these organisms to previously injured heart valves. The avenue of invasion is often through the oral cavity following vigorous scaling or extraction of infected teeth. There is some question as to the part played by the streptococci in the production of rheumatic fever.

Bacilli are rod-shaped organisms of many varieties which produce widely different tissue reactions in many areas of the body. Bacilli are responsible for such disease processes as diphtheria, whooping cough, dysentery, tetanus, undulant fever, tularemia, and tuberculosis.

Diphtheria, whooping cough, and dysentery are acute infectious types of disease spread by droplets or by direct contact with infected individuals. They have specific symptom patterns and run short courses to terminate in spontaneous remission or death. Diphtheria and whooping cough are controlled well by immunization.

Tuberculosis is produced by a specific bacillus (tubercle bacillus) and is widespread in undeveloped countries where there are concentrations of people living in crowded conditions. This infection is spread by direct contact with persons having the disease. The disease also contaminates cattle, and milk obtained from infected animals produces the disease in man. Birds also are infected and avian tuberculosis may be transmitted to man.

The lung is the organ most often infected but the lymph nodes, intestine, kidney, brain, and bone, especially the spine, also are sites of infection. Pulmonary tuberculosis usually is acquired in childhood or early adult life owing to direct inhalation of infected sputum or dust. Tuberculosis of lymph nodes, stomach, and joints has been greatly reduced by the pasteurization of milk and the control of dairy herds.

Spirochetes are small spiral forms of microorganisms which are somewhat motile. They produce a variety of diseases, the best known of which is *syphilis*. Syphilis has been a widespread venereal disease of great importance in medicine and dentistry, but with the development of penicillin the disease has been more effectively controlled. Spirochetes also produce yaws, relapsing fever, rat bite fever, and acute necrotizing ulcerative gingivitis, which is discussed in Chapter 13, Periodontal Disease.

VIRUSES. Viruses vary in size from 10 to 400 nm (a nm is one millionth of a millimeter), are composed of a single- and double-stranded nucleic acid core (RNA or DNA, never both), and have a protein coat called a capsid. Viruses can only multiply within cells, but may survive outside cells in a resting form for prolonged periods of time. Viral diseases include smallpox, the common cold, herpes simplex 1 and 2, and a number of other diseases, incuding AIDS (cf. p. 236).

When the virus enters the tissues and damage occurs, cellular and humoral defenses are activated. Its needs for survival are very specific and as an intracellular inhabitant it competes for the metabolites needed by the host cells. Thus, viruses have an affinity for certain types of tissue, such as nerve or skin, and always localize in a specific tissue regardless of how they enter the body. This affinity for specific tissue is called *tropism,* and the virus is said to be neurotropic when it localizes in nerve tissue or dermatotropic when it localizes in skin. Rabies and poliomyelitis are examples of diseases caused by neurotropic viruses. The viruses producing chicken pox, smallpox, or warts are dermatotropic viruses. The common cold and associated upper respiratory infections are viral in origin.

Herpesvirus is incuded in the DNA virus groups. Herpesvirus infections include: *herpes simplex 1* (HSV$_1$), which is the cause of "cold sores"; *herpes simplex 2* (HSV$_2$), which is the cause of genitourinary tract infection and linked to cervical cancer; *herpes zoster,* which is responsible for "shingles"; and cytomegalic inclusion (CMV), which is the cause of the most common viral infection of the fetus and newborn.

Some of the more important viral diseases affect the central nervous system for which certain viruses (neurotropic) appear to have a marked affinity. One of the best known of the central nervous system viral diseases is poliomyelitis (infantile paralysis), an acute infection involving primarily the spinal cord and resulting in paralysis of muscles. The damage to the spinal cord is permanent, and since muscle function is never reestablished, muscle atrophy results. The "polio" vaccine is an effective preventive measure, and the incidence of the disease has been greatly reduced by its widespread use.

There is strong presumptive evidence that Burkitt's lymphoma, nasopharyngeal carcinoma, and T cell leukemia are caused by viruses, although the viral etiology of malignancy in humans has yet to be conclusively established. The Epstein-Barr virus (EBV), one of the herpesviruses, is the cause of infectious mononucleosis, is associated with Burkitt's lymphoma and nasopharyngeal carcinoma, and has been implicated in a faulty immune response in patients with rheumatoid arthritis (cf. p. 89). Oncornaviruses (oncogenic RNA viruses) are now called *retroviruses*. These viruses have been classed as *B* and *C* types. Type

A RNA viruses are not oncogenic (cancer producing). The virus implicated in *AIDS* (cf. p. 240) is a retrovirus.

Rabies is a viral disease transmitted by the bite of a rabid (infected) animal, usually a dog. The virus is introduced into a bite wound by saliva containing the virus. The virus is neurotropic and localizes in brain tissue producing a disease (hydrophobia) that is always fatal unless early treatment is initiated. The disease is characterized by muscular spasm, excitement, convulsions, coma, and death.

Some viruses affect the respiratory tract and produce a variety of reactions recognized as the common cold, influenza, and pneumonia. Influenza is the most common of the pulmonary viral diseases. It is periodically epidemic and results in severe disease and death. In the 1918 epidemic millions of deaths resulted from the almost universal infection which occurred. The manifestations of influenza vary from an asymptomatic infection to an infection with symptoms of fever, headache, chills, myalgia, and coughing. Only rarely are vomiting and diarrhea a clinical manifestation. There have been three well known pandemics of influenza since influenza type A virus was isolated in 1933: that of 1947, 1957 (Asian), and 1968 (Hong Kong). More recent flu strains include: Type A, USSR (1978–79); Type B, Singapore (1979–80); Type A, Bangkok (1980–81, 82, 83); Type B, Singapore (1982–83); Type B, USSR (1983–84); and Type A, Philippines (1984–85). Influenza appears to be *endemic* in large geographic areas yearly, *epidemic* in some regions, and *pandemic* every ten years when the disease occurs in all age groups in populations of most of the world. Such pandemics occur with the introduction of a new variant of one of the influenza viruses.

Pneumonia is the most frequent complication of influenza due to secondary bacterial infection. Other complications are encephalitis, congestive heart failure, Landry-Guillain-Barré syndrome ("French polio"), and Reye's syndrome.

The skin also is a common site for viral localization and common acute infectious diseases result. *Smallpox* (variola) is an acute infectious process spread by droplets from the respiratory tract or by direct contact with an infected individual. The symptoms are high fever, severe headache, and vesicles which become invaded by streptococci to produce pustules. The disease remits spontaneously in 2 to 3 weeks or is fatal owing to streptococcal septicemia and secondary pneumonia. Having contracted the disease provides a lasting immunity. Smallpox can be prevented by vaccination. At this time smallpox has been eliminated as a health problem throughout the world.

Acute viral hepatitis is a systemic infection involving predominately the liver. Two viruses have been implicated, viruses A and B. Hepatitis A is also called infectious hepatitis, short-incubation hepatitis and MS-1 hepatitis. Hepatitis B is called serum hepatitis, MS-2 hepatitis, and long-incubation hepatitis. Other viruses such as those termed non-A and non-B have been implicated also. At one time it was thought that hepatitis A had a shorter incubation period of 15 to 45 days, was highly contagious, and usually had a fecal-oral route of transmission; hepatitis B had an incubation period of 30 to 180 days, was less contagious, and was transmitted only by the parenteral route. However, these clinical and epidemiologic distinctions are no longer tenable. Specific serologic testing is necessary to distinguish between the various types of viral hepatitis.

The use of effective immunoglobulin therapy, immune serum globulin (ISG), prevents type A viral hepatitis when administered before or within 1 to 2 weeks of exposure. A prophylactic vaccine for hepatitis B virus has been developed. The nature of non-A and non-B hepatitis viruses, associated with most cases of post-transfusion hepatitis, has yet to be clarified.

Hepatitis B is now more often transmitted by contaminated needles used by drug addicts, by exposure to contaminated blood, and in the male homosexual population. Thus precautions against possible disease transmission are directed toward sterilization and prevention of transmission via contaminated blood or blood products, i.e., wear gloves, surgical masks, and eye glasses, and sterilize all instruments. Dental personnel dealing directly with patients should consider immunization. Available data at present show that AIDS is not transmitted by hepatitis B vaccination.

PARASITES. Parasites include rickettsiae, chlamydiae, protozoa, and metazoa. Reservoirs for these organisms include cats, dogs, rabbits, birds, fleas, ticks and mosquitoes.

Rickettsiae are larger than viruses but are like viruses in that they are resistant to heat and disinfectants. They contain RNA and DNA plus proteins, and only multiply within cells. These microorganisms cause such diseases as typhus and Rocky Mountain fever.

Chlamydiae are similar to Rickettsiae and cause *trachoma,* the leading cause of blindness in underdeveloped nations.

Protozoa are seen throughout the world. Protozoan agents of infection cause such diseases as amebic dysentery, malaria, and sleeping sickness.

Metazoa incude parasites which cause trichinosis, which is probably the most important *metazoan* disease in the United States. Other metazoan diseases are caused by infestations with tapeworms (pork, fish, dog), pinworms, and flukes.

FUNGI. Fungal infections include candidiasis (thrush), ringworm, and athlete's foot. Fungi do not often produce more than superficial disease in man, but serious infection may occur in debilitated patients. Such opportunistic infections are most likely to occur when there is suppression of normal flora by broad-spectrum antibiotics and compromised host defenses (p. 245).

NUTRITIONAL FACTORS. Nutrition is the summation of the dietary intake of food and its absorption, storage, and utilization by the tissues. Disturbances in nutrition result in a variety of disease processes, each having characteristic features and significance. Starvation results when the dietary intake does not meet the nutritional requirements of the individual. A deficient intake of food is compensated by utilization of the fat stored in the fat deposits of the body. After the fat is completely depleted, other tissues are utilized. The loss of fat and other materials causes a reduction in the weight and size of the individual. When the process is severe and all reserves are depleted, death results from starvation.

Anorexia nervosa is a term used to describe self-imposed weight loss which is beyond normal. In bulimia a patient eats excessively and then regurgitates the food in order to reduce his weight. These abnormal states can lead to nutritional deficiencies.

A National Institutes of Health consensus panel on the health implications of obesity has concluded that obesity is a potential killer. Everyone who is 20% or more overweight is considered to be obese. People who are obese are more likely to have high blood pressure, hypercholesterolemia, and diabetes. There are 34 million Americans who are at least 20% above their desirable weight. There is evidence that the signals to overeat may come from the fat cells themselves. (See Chapter 9 for Nutritional Disturbances.)

Chemical Injury

Injury by chemical substance may occur at the point of application (chemical burns) or the chemical may be carried to all parts of the body and produce injury (poisoning) to some or all of the body cells. Chemical burns are produced on skin and mucous membrane by the application of toxic materials such as phenol, silver nitrate, acids, strong bases (lye), and many other substances. The lesions produced may be areas of redness, blisters, or ulcers, depending upon the concentration of the chemical, its toxicity, and the length of time it was applied. Toxic substances enter the body by ingestion, injection, absorption, or inhalation and are transported to the cells by the blood. In this way many substances affect selected cells, organs, or the entire body and the effects are designated poisoning.

Toxic substances ingested or injected into the body produce effects locally or systemically as the result of their transportation by the blood to the cells. The most commonly injected poisons are from insect bites. The toxic material entering the tissue in the area of an insect bite is small in quantity but high in toxicity. The toxin from the insect produces a local reaction manifested as redness, swelling, and itching or pain. If larger quantities are introduced into the tissue, as in reptile bites, or if the toxin is potent, as in bites from black widow spiders, the effects are more widespread and death may result.

Toxic substances may be ingested and produce effects in the stomach resulting in nausea and vomiting, which eliminates the poison from the body. If the chemical substance does not produce vomiting, it may be absorbed into the blood and transported to cells. Some substances have a greater affinity for one tissue than for another and the effect produced is dependent upon the tissue affected; viz., some toxins are neurotoxins (coral snake venom and botulinal toxins), others are hemotoxins (rattlesnake venom). Poisons may be produced by microorganisms and have effects comparable to those produced by other chemicals. The bacterial toxins may produce gastric effects as in food poisoning (botulism) or the effects may be general as in diphtheria, tetanus, and other infections. The general effects of poisons are due to changes in the blood cells, the central nervous system, or vital organs.

Chemical substances injurious to the cells may be produced within the body or may enter from the outside. Many of the chemical substances produced by the body are toxic when present in too high a concentration or when in an area where they are not normally present. For example, if the fluid elaborated by the stomach escapes into the abdominal cavity, digestion of tissue occurs although no such effect to the lining of the stomach occurs. (See Chemical Injury, Chapter 14.)

Environmental Agents

A wide variety of environmental agents, from food additives to air pollution, are capable of causing disease. Many of these agents are taken into the body through such portals as the mouth and nose. They gain access to the tissues as a result of breaks in the continuity of the skin and mucous membranes.

Air pollution from automobile exhaust fumes can be a major health problem because the deleterious products contain nitrogen dioxide, whose primary components are nitric acid, nitrates, and ozone. Cigarette smoke contains carcinogens and is an allergen. A number of other agents such as asbestos, coal dust, and silica should be considered as air pollutants, and hazardous to the health.

Most fields of manufacturing, from paper to steel, have the problem of disposing of waste-containing solvents and other toxic materials. The discharging of industrial waste into the air, water, or land-fill has the potential for allowing toxic agents to be taken into the body via the water supply.

Fertilizers and insecticides contain arsenic or cyanide and can pollute streams, lakes and rivers with potentially profound deleterious effects. Also such toxic chemicals as PCB (polychlorinated biphenyl), Mirex and Kepone are potentially hazardous.

Workers in industrial plants are potentially subject to a number of hazardous chemicals, including acetone, carbon tetrachloride, and PVC (polyvinyl chloride). PVC has been implicated in cancer of the liver. It is a mutagenic chemical because it damages chromosomes.

Drugs and Hormones

Such common analgesics as salicylates can produce peptic ulcers and cause bleeding. Also phenacetin, which has been combined with caffeine and aspirin, is toxic to the kidney. A number of drugs interact with other drugs when used at the same time, producing adverse effects. For example, alcohol and barbiturates greatly increase central nervous system depression, and the prolonged use of laxatives when taking digitalis for the heart increases the toxicity of digitalis.

Antibiotics may produce an allergic response or act directly as a toxin even when used in therapeutic doses. For example, chloramphenicol (Chloromycetin) can cause a blood dyscrasia (agranulocytosis), actinomycin causes mutations, and metronidazole (Flagyl) causes leukemia in experimental animals. The latter amebocytic drug has also been used in the treatment of some forms of periodontal disease in humans.

Exogenous estrogens have been implicated in vaginal and cervical cancer, as well as in myocardial infarction. Also the oral hypoglycemic agent, Tolbutamide, which is used as an oral substitute for insulin therapy for diabetics, has been implicated in an increased incidence of myocardial infarction. ACTH or cortisone may produce a reduction of lymphocytes (lymphopenia).

SUMMARY

The causes of diseases can be divided into intrinsic factors and extrinsic factors. However, most diseases are not simply the result of a single causative agent, and even when a single factor is implicated, multiple host factors determine the response and the outcome of the disease. Thus, although etiologic factors are divided into intrinsic factors of disease (genetic) and extrinsic factors (physical, infectious, environmental, and chemical agents, as well as drugs and hormones), such a division has limitations.

Genetic disorders are responsible for 80% of birth defects whereas the remaining 20% are due to infection, drugs, and physical injury to the fetus. There are significant congenital defects in about 3% of all live births. More than 40% of all infant mortality results from genetic factors.

Malformations of the craniofacial area can be traced in a small proportion of cases to specific genetic or chromosomal disorders. Others may be due to potent environmental factors such as maternal disease, alcohol or other drugs, malnutrition, exposure to radiation, and difficulties in pregnancy and delivery. However, most craniofacial malformations have a multifactorial basis, i.e., an interactive process in which particular genes adversely influence the ability of the fetus to adapt to environmental factors. An illustration of these interactive processes is the evidence demonstrating an association between human genes of the major histocompatibility locus (HLA) and an increased susceptibility to clefting.

The prevention of congenital malformations at this time is approached by monitoring environmental agents and genetic counseling. Antiepileptic drugs and alcohol have been identified as potential risks to the fetus. The "fetal alcohol syndrome" is characterized by such disturbances as small head and widely spaced eyes and less than normal intelligence. Prevention of malformation due to rubella (measles) has been achieved by use of a vaccine.

The largest category of disease is provided by numerous extrinsic factors which are continuously active in the environment. Extrinsic factors are increasing in importance and number owing to our industrial advancement and the use of atomic energy. The continually changing pattern is due to the elimination or control of some disease factors and the development of new factors which cause disease. The pattern of disease changes with each generation. Heart disease, which 40 years ago was rated fourth or fifth as a cause of death, is now first. This shift in the position of heart disease as a cause of death is the result of the control of some diseases, such as smallpox, pneumonia, and typhoid fever, which in the past frequently caused death, and the conditions of tension under which we now live in our highly mechanistic society which predispose to heart disease.

BIBLIOGRAPHY

Andres, R.: Influence of obesity on longevity in the aged. Adv. Pathobiol., 7:238, 1980.

Dudgeon, J.A.: Infectious causes of human malformations. Br. Med. J., 32:77, 1976.

Erbe, R.W.: Principles of medical genetics. N. Engl. J. Med., 294:381, 1976.

Falconer, D.S.: The inheritance of liability to certain diseases estimated from the incidence among relatives. Ann. Hum. Genet., 29:51, 1965.

Fraser, D.W.: Legionnaire's disease: four summers' harvest. Am. J. Med., 68:1, 1980.

German, J.: Studying human chromosomes today. Amer. Sci., 58:182, 1970.

Gorlin, T.: Genetic disorders affecting mucous membranes. Oral Surg., 28:512, 1969.

Gorlin, R.J., Stallard, R.E., and Shapiro, B.L.: Genetics and periodontal disease. J. Periodont., 38:5, 1967.

Hanson, J.W., et al.: Fetal alcohol syndrome: Experience in 41 patients. J.A.M.A., 14:1458, 1976.

Harvey, E.B., et al.: Prenatal x-ray exposure and childhood cancer in twins. N. Engl. J. Med., 312:541, 1985.

Kohn, H.I. and Fry, J.M.: Radiation carcinogenesis. New Engl. J. Med., 310:504, 1984.

Kolata, G.: Why do people get fat. Science, 227:1327, 1985.

MacMahon, B.: Prenatal x-ray exposure and twins. N. Engl. J. Med., 312:576, 1985.

Marx, J.L.: Cytomegalovirus: A major cause of birth defects. Science, 190:1184, 1975.

Medical Research Council: The hazards to man of nuclear and allied radiations. London, Her Majesty's Stationary Office, 1960.

Naeye, R.L., and Blane, W.: Pathogenesis of congenital rubella. J.A.M.A., 194:1277, 1965.

National Institutes of Health: What are facts about genetic disease? Washington, D.C., U.S. Department of Health, Education and Welfare, Public Health Service, 1977.

Neel, J.V., and Schull, W.J.: Studies on the potential genetic effects of the atomic bombs. Acta Genet. (Basel), 6:183, 1956.

Ochoa, S.: The chemical basis of heredity—the genetic code. Bull. N.Y. Acad. Med., 40:387, 1964.

Poyton, H.G.: The effects of irradiation on teeth. Oral Surg., 26:639, 1968.

Rennie, D.: Give me air! But not much. N. Engl. J. Med., 297:1285, 1977.

Roizman, B. and Buchman, T.: The molecular epidemiology of Herpes simplex viruses. Hosp. Pract., 14:95, 1979.

Taussig, H.B.: The thalidomide syndrome. Sci. Amer., 207:29, 1962.

Tyler, P.E. (Ed.): Biologic effects of nonionizing radiation. Ann. N.Y. Acad. Sci., Feb. 28, 1975.

World Health Organization: Radiation hazards in perspective. Technical Report Series, No. 248, Geneva, 1962.

3

DEVELOPMENTAL DISTURBANCES

Because of the complex nature of the process of development of the body, unlimited possibilities for disturbances in development are present; these disturbances constitute important manifestations of disease.

A wide range of developmental disturbances occur, from those that are not clinically manifest to gross malformations, and from individual structures such as a tooth, to whole complexes such as the face. Terms used to describe developmental disturbances range from "anomaly" to specific descriptions such as dentinogenesis imperfecta. In a broad sense malocclusion is a developmental disturbance.

The face is a common location for developmental disturbances owing to its complex pattern of growth. Therefore a brief review of the embryology of the face and jaws will precede a discussion of the more common and important developmental disturbances of these areas.

EMBRYOLOGY OF THE FACE

The development of the facial region is a complex process of selective growth (proliferation) of parts which, as they grow, undergo changes in cellular detail (differentiation) to form the various structures of the face. The differentiation of the cells responsible for the formation of a part may depend upon some change in other cells of the immediate area. This process is called dependent differentiation, and it plays an important part in the development of the face. As the cells of the body proliferate they have the capacity to follow a particular pattern of growth to form a structure of specific architecture. This process is called morphodifferentiation and is evident in the formation of the face and oral structures (Fig. 3–1).

The head region of the embryo starts its development at about the fourth week of embryonic life by the development of a rounded prominence (the forebrain) on the cephalic (head) end of the embryo. This prominence folds forward and downward (ventral and inferior) to form a groove (the oral groove) representing the rudimentary oral cavity. The lower boundary of the groove is the first branchial bar. Lateral boundaries of the groove develop by proliferation of cells from the sides and top (lateral and superior) portions of the first branchial bar.

The first branchial bar forms the lower jaw (mandible) and the portions that develop

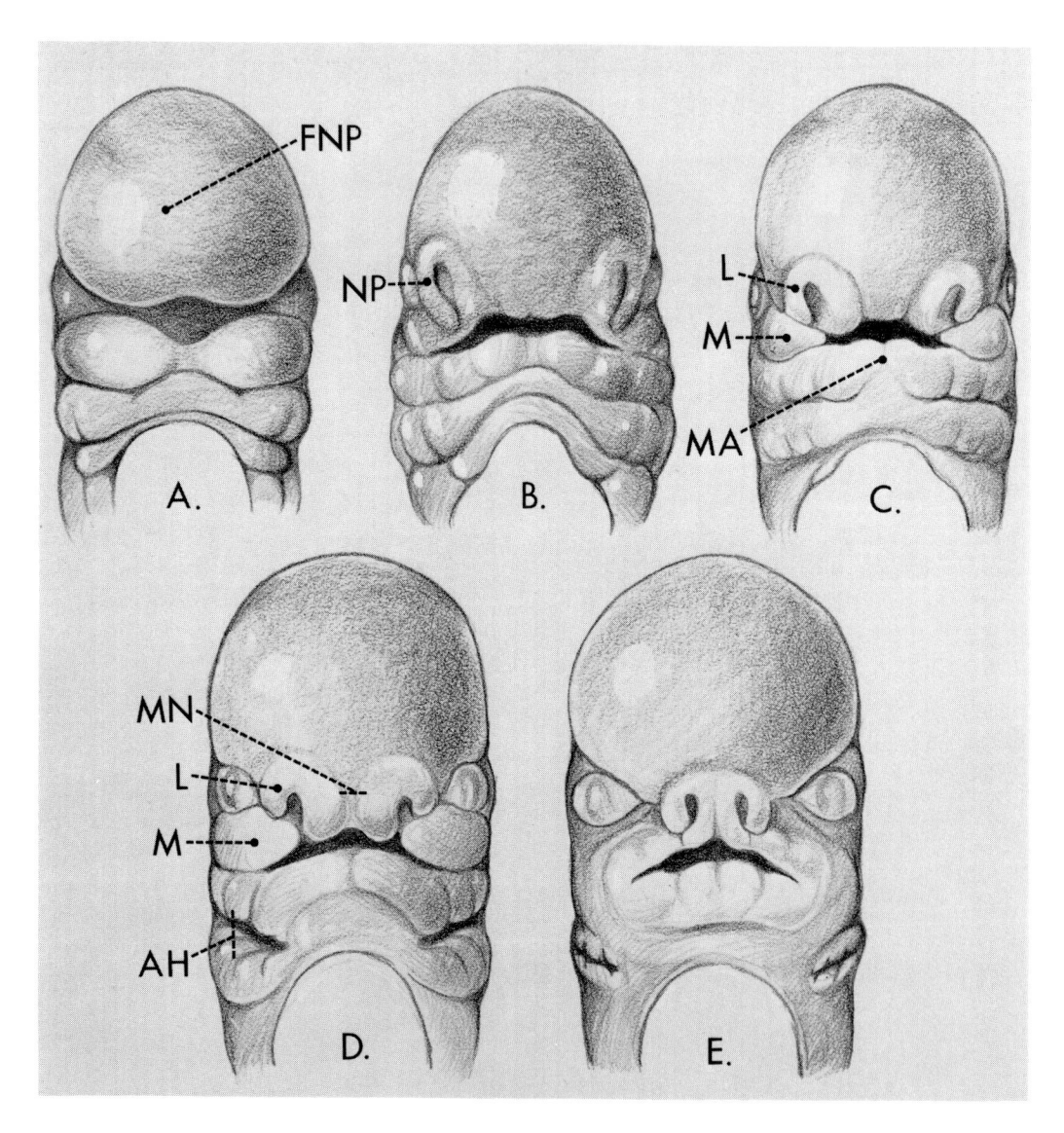

Fig. 3–1. *Development of the face.* A, Formation of stomadeum by anterior folding of the forebrain with development of frontal nasal process (FNP). Folds below rudimentary oral cavity are branchial bars. B, Development of globular processes from frontal nasal process and development of lateral nasal process (NP). C, Development of maxillary process (M) from superior portion of first branchial bar and nearly completed mandible (MA) from inferior portion of first branchial bar. D, More complete development of frontal nasal process to show medial and nasal process (MN) below which are the paired globular processes. Lateral nasal process (L), maxilla (M), and auricular hillock (AH). E, Nearly complete development of the face.

laterally grow forward to form part of the upper jaw (maxilla) and the roof of the mouth (palate). While these lateral processes are developing, there is an outgrowth in the center of the forebrain which grows downward between the two lateral processes of the developing maxilla. This outgrowth forms the middle part of the upper face and is called the median process. This process develops two lateral pits which separate the median process into two lateral processes and one medial process. They are the lateral nasal processes and the medial nasal process.

As the lateral nasal processes develop, they push the olfactory pits toward the midline and compress the medial nasal process to a thin strip. The lateral nasal processes form the sides of the nose, and the median process forms the center of the nose. The inferior portion of the median nasal process proliferates as a globular mass of tissue (the globular process) to form the upper midportion of the maxilla (the portion containing the central and lateral incisors). While the median nasal and lateral nasal processes are developing, the maxillary process grows forward to meet the globular process. When all the structures have developed and come in contact, they fuse to form the completed face. The face thus develops from several individual parts fusing together to form the final structure.

The two lateral halves of the maxillary process meet in the midline to form the posterior part of the palate. They fuse with the globular process to form the anterior palate. The opening of the oral cavity is produced by the incomplete fusion of the mandibular and maxillary processes of the face.

In a process as complex as the development of the face, there are many possibilities for some failure of formation to occur. Some of these occur quite frequently, whereas others are rare. The more common and most significant ones will be discussed in some detail.

DISTURBANCES OF THE UPPER FACE

Clefts

A cleft is one of the most frequently occurring disturbances resulting from the failure of fusion of the various processes from which the face develops. Any defect that results from failure of fusion of any of the facial processes is called a cleft. The most common clefts occur in the region of the upper lip and palate (Fig. 3–2). Clefts rarely occur in the lower jaw. Failure of the maxillary process to fuse with the globular process may result in a cleft on one or both sides of the midline. When the cleft is on one side of the midline, it is unilateral; when it occurs on both sides, it is bilateral. Such failure of fusion may involve only a portion of the lip or all of the lip. When all of the lip is involved, it may extend into the jaw and palate. Any combination and extent of cleft of the lip and palate may occur. In some instances only the two lateral portions of the maxillary process which form the palate may fail to unite and a cleft of the palate alone results.

Reports of the prevalence of clefts of the lip and palate indicate that some variation in their frequency occurs according to geographic regions and race. The frequency of occurrence is reported to be 1 out of 954 births in Holland (Sanders) and 1 out of every 700 live births in the United States. The etiology of cleft lip and cleft palate has not been definitely established, but it appears that heredity plays an important part. However, mechanical interference during development, and teratogenic agents such as radiation, drugs, hormones and infectious agents are implicated. Most teratogenic agents exert their adverse effects during the period of histodifferentiation and morphogenesis, i.e., between 4 and 8 weeks. Cleft palate is frequently associated with other types of developmental disturbances.

Infants born with oral clefts are usually able to live, but present many problems in

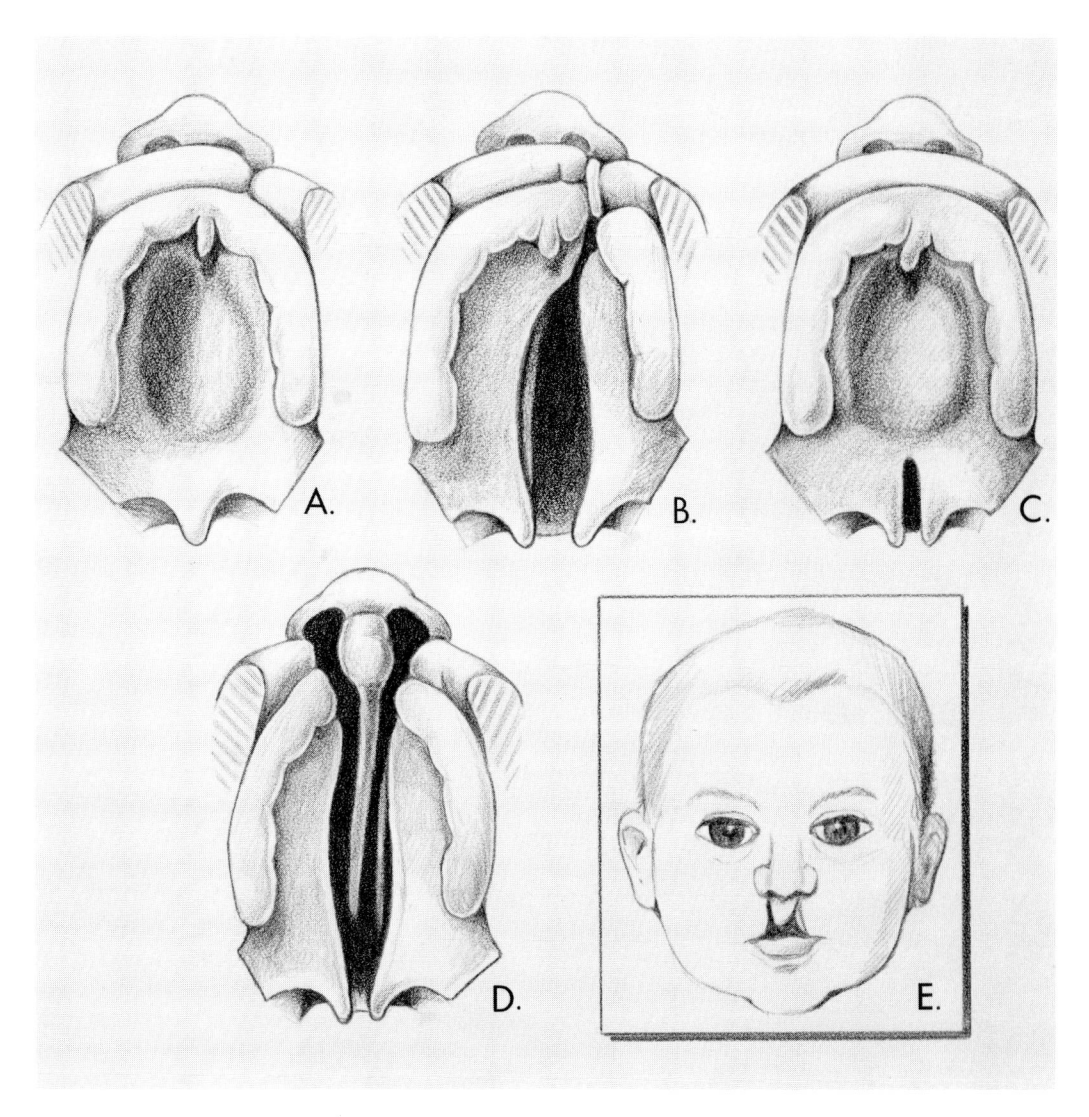

Fig. 3–2. *Cleft lip and cleft palate. A,* Cleft lip ony; *B,* cleft of lip, jaw, and palate; *C,* incomplete cleft of palate, bifid uvula; *D,* bilateral cleft of lip and jaw, extensive midline cleft of palate; *E,* front view of bilateral cleft.

care and treatment. Infants with clefts are unable to suckle well and present feeding problems. They have a tendency to aspirate food and therefore are susceptible to respiratory disease. Older children have problems of speech and esthetics as well as social and psychologic problems. To prevent the development of these problems during childhood and yet not interfere with growth centers, it is desirable to treat such individuals at an early age. Clefts of the lip usually are treated by surgical closure in the first few months of life, and cleft of the palate at about 18 months of age. In some instances, surgery is only partially successful and the clefts must be treated by prosthetic appliances and orthodontic procedures (Fig. 3–3). Today, in most large medical centers and in some states, special cleft palate clinics are staffed with teams of

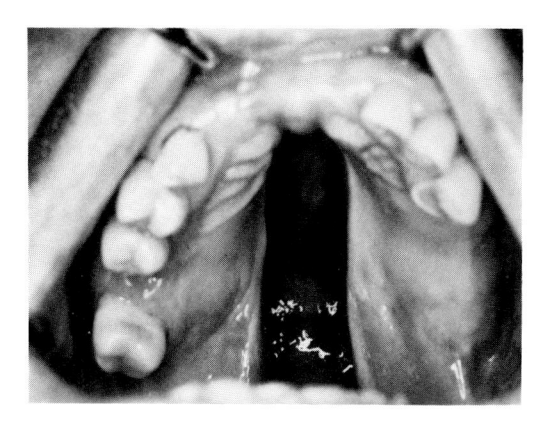

Fig. 3-3. Cleft palate.

surgeons, dentists, speech therapists, psychologists, and social workers to treat patients with clefts of the lip and palate.

Fissural Defects

In addition to the development of clefts from the failure of facial processes to fuse, less severe disturbances may occur in the lines of fusion. Facial processes are covered by epithelium which is obliterated at the time of fusion of the processes. In some instances, fusion may be complete, except for the persistence of epithelium in a small area of the line of fusion. Many variations of persistent epithelium occur. The epithelium may persist in a localized area through the full thickness of the line of fusion to produce an epithelial-lined tract from the outer to the inner surface of the fused processes. An epithelial-lined tube or tract open at both ends is called a fistula. The persistent epithelium may have continuity with only one surface to form a blind tract or tube with only one opening on one of the surfaces of the fused processes. This tract of residual epithelium with a blind end is called a *sinus*. When the persistent or residual epithelium forms a closed space in a line of fusion, the defect is called a *fissural cyst*.

CYSTS. Examples of fissural defects may be seen in various areas of the face and mouth. Cysts are by far the most common of the fissural defects and occur in the midline of the palate (midpalatine cyst) (Figs. 3-4, 3-5), in the line of fusion between the maxillary and globular processes (globulomaxillary cyst), or in the area of fusion between the two lateral portions of the palate and the medial nasal process (nasopalatine cyst) (Fig. 3-6). Fissural cysts may appear in front of the ear (preauricular cyst) owing to the persistence of epithelium between the superior and inferior halves of the first branchial bar. Sinuses occurring in this region are called preauricular sinuses and may be present bilaterally. Cysts also occur owing to the persistence of epithelium between the other branchial bars (branchial cysts) and are present beneath the angle of the jaw on the lateral surface of the neck. A cyst slowly increases in size due to an accumulation of tissue fluid within the cystic space, and thus produces a swelling and deformity necessitating treatment by surgical excision. If the removal is complete and all of the epithelial lining is removed, the condition is eliminated and there is no recurrence. However, if some of the lining is not removed, the cyst may re-form.

Other inclusions, usually some element of the skin, may occur in fusion lines. Sebaceous glands are frequently included in the line of fusion between the maxillary and mandibular processes. Such ectopic sebaceous glands (Fordyce's spots) are found just beneath the buccal mucosa along the line of occlusion of the teeth. They may present opposite the last molar, around the parotid papillae, sometimes near the angle of the mouth and occasionally on the gingiva. They usually occur bilaterally. These glands appear in the mucosa singularly or in groups as small (1 to 2 millimeters), slightly elevated chamois-colored spots (Fig. 3-7). When the inclusions are numerous and close together, they produce a yellowish, rough plaque. These glandular inclusions may be seen on the exposed vermilion border of the lip as extensions from the skin beneath the lip mucosa. About 80% of the adult population have these inclusions. Fordyce's spots are of no serious significance as far as the health of the patient

40　　　　　　　　　　　　DEVELOPMENTAL DISTRUBANCES

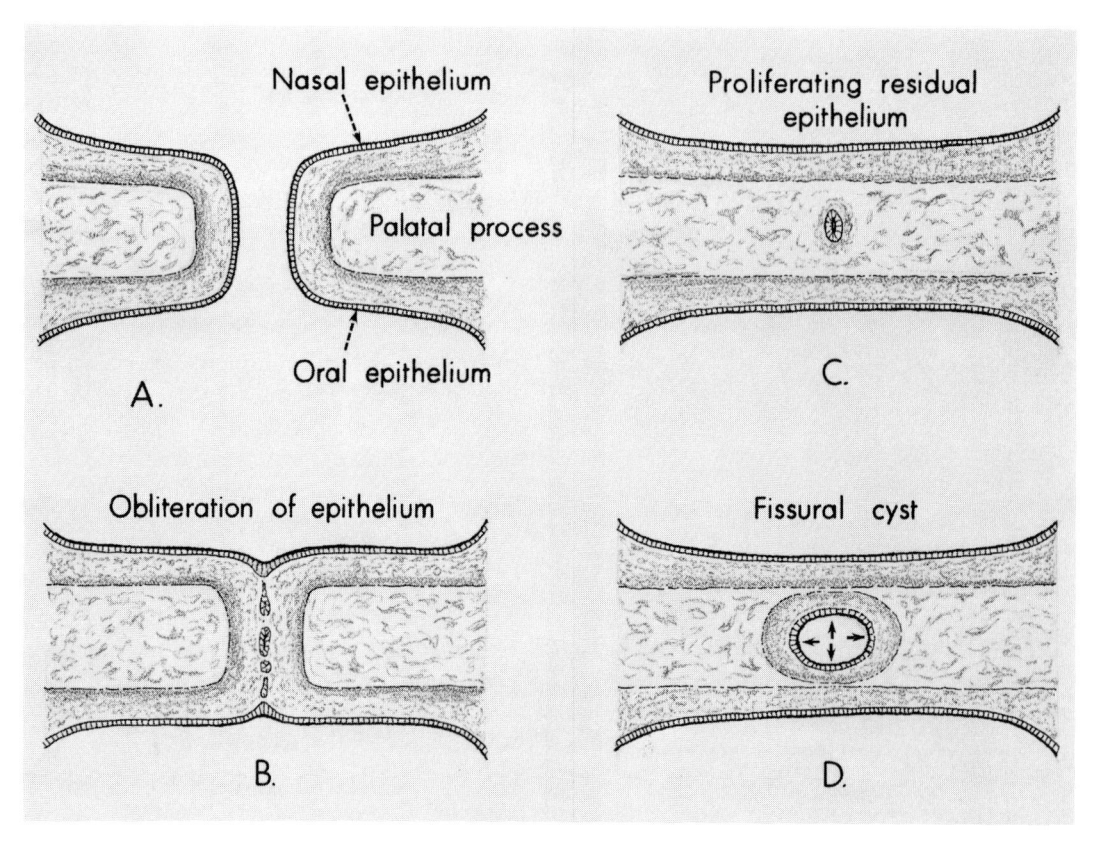

Fig. 3–4. Formation of fissural cyst in palate.

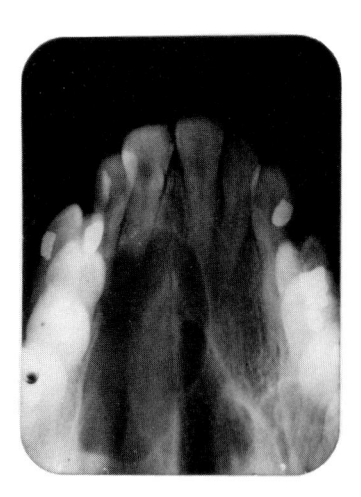

Fig. 3–5. *Fissural cyst of palate.* Cyst originates in midline but extends laterally as it meets floor of nose and maxillary sinus.

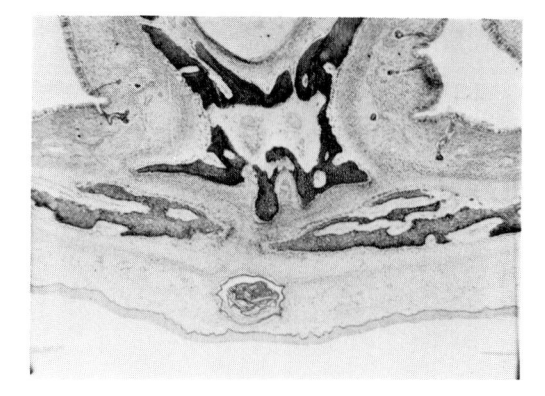

Fig. 3–6. Developing nasopalatine cyst beneath palatal mucosa at floor of nose. Nasal cavities can be seen at upper right and left of figure.

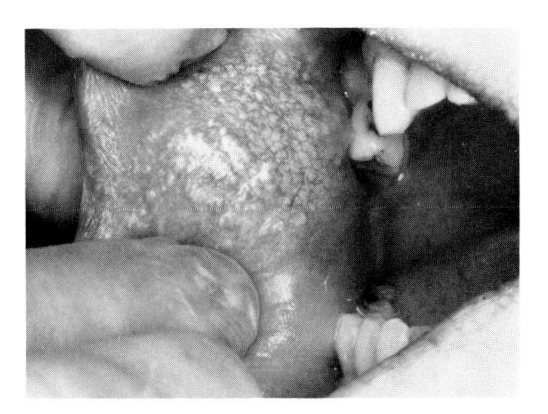

Fig. 3–7. Fordyce's spots in buccal mucosa.

is concerned, but may cause the patient to be alarmed when first noticed. They are not seen in children before puberty, inasmuch as sebaceous glands are a part of the secondary sex characteristics activated during puberty by hormonal stimulation from the gonads. Although no treatment is indicated, patients should be assured of the innocuous nature of Fordyce's spots.

DEVELOPMENTAL CYSTS. Developmental cysts may occur in association with the salivary glands, especially those located in the floor of the mouth (submaxillary and sublingual glands), and the submucosal glands (accessory salivary glands) of the lips, buccal mucosa, and palate. During the development of a major salivary gland, its ductal system may not develop completely so that some of the ducts within the gland do not establish communication with an excretory duct but end in the tissue as a blind tube. Because of the absence of an opening for excretion of the saliva, the secretions, chiefly mucin, accumulate in the duct. The accumulation of salivary secretions causes the duct to distend, which results in a space lined by ductal epithelium and filled with secretion. When this condition occurs in association with the major salivary glands, the distended epithelial-lined spaces filled with mucinous secretions are called *mucous retention cysts* (Fig. 7–12). Those arising from the same condition in the accessory glands are called *mucoceles* (Figs. 3–8, 7–10).

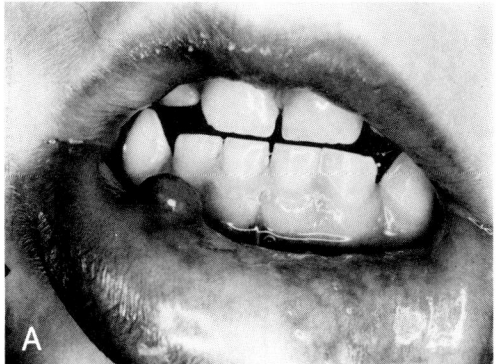

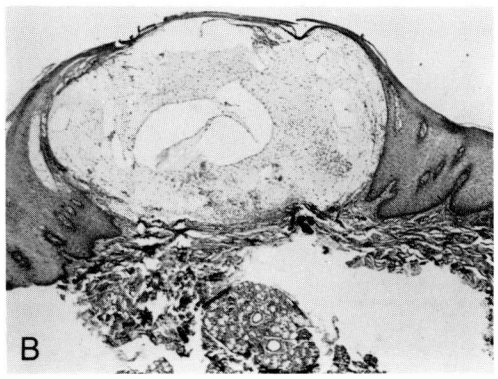

Fig. 3–8. *A,* Mucocele. *B,* Retention of mucin in epithelial tissue and underlying mucous gland.

Frequently the mucinous material escapes from the distended ducts into the surrounding tissues. In many instances, a mucous retention cyst or mucocele may be *acquired* owing to the plugging of a duct by a stone (sialolith) or by scar tissue following an injury. When the accumulation of mucin increases in ducts or tissues which are in close proximity to the surface of the mucosa, a visible swelling is produced. The accumulated mucin can be seen through the thin mucosa and imparts a blister-like appearance to the lesion. These lesions frequently rupture owing to pressure and injury, allowing fluid to escape into the tissue or the mouth. The ruptured area heals but the fluid accumulates again to produce a new swelling. These lesions may be eliminated by surgical removal.

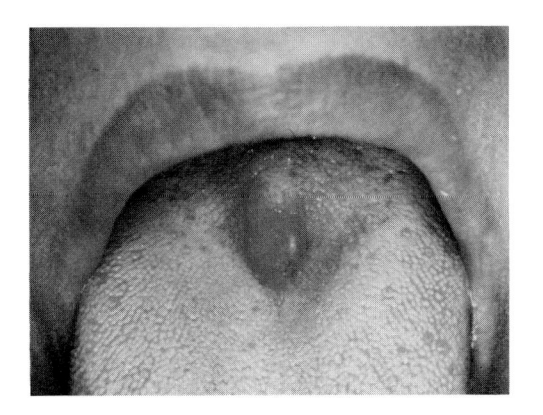

Fig. 3–9. *Median rhomboid glossitis.* Smooth rhomboidal elevation without papillae on the posterior one-third of dorsum of tongue.

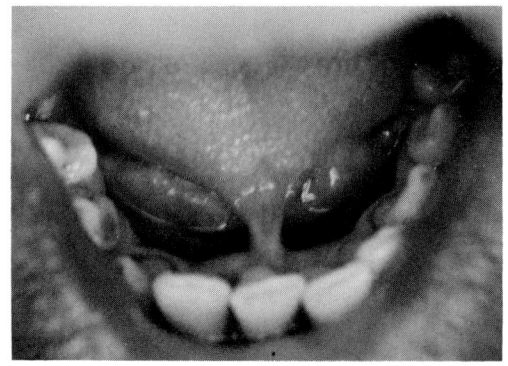

Fig. 3–10. *Ankylogossia.* Attachment of lingual frenum from tip of tongue to lingual aspect of gingiva.

DISTURBANCES OF THE TONGUE

The tongue develops from the posterior and lateral internal surfaces of the first, second, and third branchial bars as three nodular swellings. The middle nodule, arising from the posterior area, develops into the base of the tongue, whereas the two lateral nodules develop into the body of the tongue. In the early stages of development of the tongue, the growth of the medial portion is much more advanced than the lateral portions. However, as development progresses the lateral portions usually outgrow the medial portion so that the medial portion is not evident in the mature tongue. In less than 1% of the population, a part of the outline of the medial portion persists as a smooth, elevated, mamelonated, rounded or flat, rhomboid zone in the midline of the posterior part of the tongue just anterior to the circumvallate papillae. This abnormality is called *median rhomboid glossitis* (Fig. 3–9). Rarely the two lateral portions of the tongue do not completely fuse resulting in a notched or forked tongue. This is manifest as an irregular V-shaped notch in the tip of the tongue called *bifid tongue.*

The anterior one-third of the tongue is usually free or partially attached to the floor of the mouth by a thin strip of tissue extending from the midline of the ventral surface of the tongue to the floor of the mouth (lingual frenum). In some instances the frenum is short and attached too near the tip of the tongue so that the tongue is bound tightly to the floor of the mouth, preventing normal mobility (Fig. 3–10). This abnormality, *tongue tie* or *ankyloglossia,* sometimes causes difficulty in suckling, eating, or speaking. In such cases it is necessary to clip the frenum to permit the tongue to move freely.

Normally the tongue is smooth in its contour and is covered by fine projections, papillae, which give it a slightly shaggy appearance. Food and cell debris entrapped in these fine hair-like papillae produce a somewhat velvet-like appearance to the

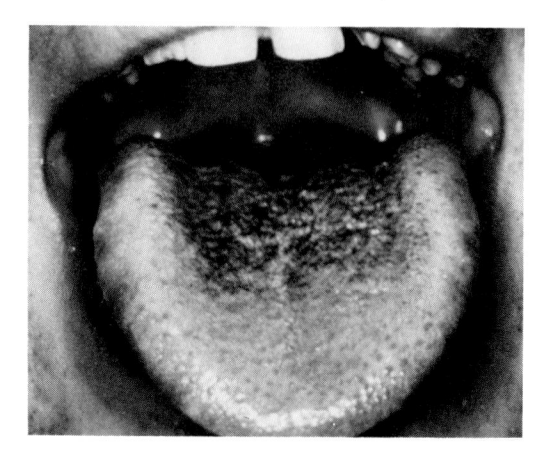

Fig. 3–11. *Black hairy tongue.* Accentuated filiform papillae on posterior one-third of the dorsum of tongue simulate coarse hairs.

tongue, designated the "coat of the tongue." The coating of the tongue varies in color and amount depending upon the abundance of saliva and the texture and the color of foods eaten. The coat is usually grayish-yellow but may be brown from coffee, tea, or smoking; red from colored candy; green from chlorophyl lozenges or certain toothpastes; or other colors depending upon the substance taken into the mouth. A "coated tongue" is generally of little dental or medical significance except as it relates to oral hygiene. In fact, the absence of coating may be of significance in anemias and vitamin deficiencies.

So-called *hairy tongue* is perhaps only an exaggerated form of coated tongue, but the retained filiform papillae are longer and are localized to a limited area of the tongue (Fig. 3–11). The retained filiform papillae are like hair in both texture and color, usually being dark-brown or black in color and a few millimeters to a centimeter in length. When the papillae are long, the patient may feel their presence, but usually they are discovered by observation. The retention of the papillae is enhanced by the use of hydrogen peroxide as a mouthwash, use of antibiotics, and presence of yeast in large numbers in the oral flora; in some instances there is no identifiable cause.

Furrowed tongue is an abnormality of the tongue present in about 25% of the population in which the dorsum of the tongue develops heavy folds (Fig. 3–12). The folds may follow a regular geometric pattern or they may be irregular, without pattern. The entire dorsum of the tongue is involved, and the deep furrows between the folds may extend onto the lateral borders. The depth of the furrows may not be readily discernible until the tongue is extended or mildly stretched. Geographic tongue is superimposed upon furrowed tongue in many instances. Irritation in the furrows has been suggested as a possible cause of geographic tongue. Some writers believe that furrowed tongue is congenital, whereas others think that it is acquired. In favor of its

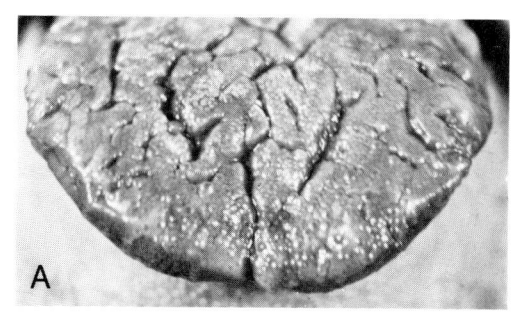

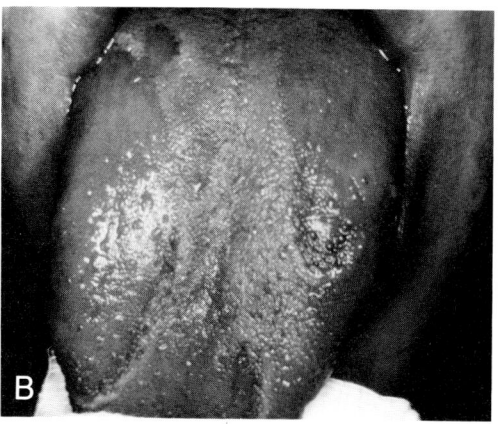

Fig. 3–12. *A, Furrowed tongue. B,* Geographic tongue superimposed on furrowed tongue.

being acquired is the fact that it rarely occurs in children.

Another anomaly of the tongue present in about 5% of the population is *geographic tongue* also designated wandering rash or glossitis migrans (Fig. 3–13). This condition is frequently associated with furrowed tongue, but may be seen on a smooth tongue. When associated with furrowed tongue, the change usually starts as a loss of filiform papillae about a fissure. The loss of papillae extends from the fissure in a widening arc and the zone of separation from the normal surface of the tongue appears as a white line. When the papillae are completely lost, the epithelium is thin and the underlying tissue is near enough to the surface of the tongue to be seen readily and to give the narrow area involved a reddish appearance. The epithelium then regenerates and new papillae start to form; this process produces a smooth, slightly pur-

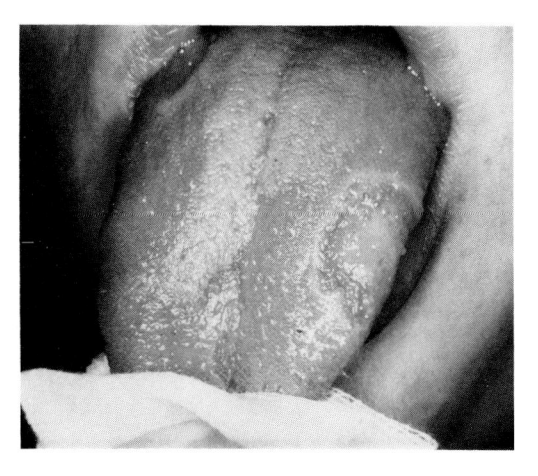

Fig. 3-13. *Geographic tongue.* There is an active lesion on the lateral border indicated by the white circular and arcuate boundaries. The lesion is superimposed on a larger area of previous desquamative activity.

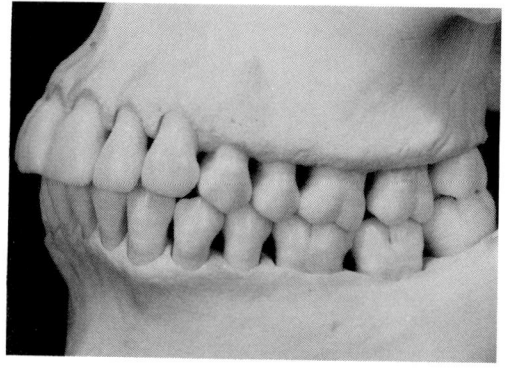

Fig. 3-14. Normal occlusion (Angle Class I). Mesial buccal cusp of maxillary first molar occludes in the buccal groove of the mandibular first molar.

plish zone. The process of depapillation, thinning of the epithelium and its regeneration, extends progressively outward from a fissure for a variable distance and then ceases, only to start again in the same or another area. Because some lesions are healing while new ones are starting, there usually are several areas of variable size and shape which present a continually changing picture to the tongue so it appears different each time it is observed. The pattern of involvement is suggestive of a map and for this reason it has been designated geographic tongue. Geographic tongue occurs in children as well as adults and may be present for a lifetime. It rarely produces symptoms and the patient usually becomes aware of it only through observation. In a few cases a smarting or burning sensation may be present, especially when eating highly seasoned or hot foods. The cause of this condition is believed to be associated with the action of bacteria in the coat of the tongue or in the fissures of furrowed tongue where food debris or organisms are trapped and produce irritation. This condition is of little or no significance to the individual and treatment is not indicated. When treatment is attempted, it usually is unsuccessful.

DENTOFACIAL MALRELATIONS

The most common disturbance in the development of the jaws is the cleft of the jaw and palate, discussed under clefts of the face. Other disturbances in the jaws are associated with alterations of growth due to injuries to the jaws at birth as the result of forceps deliveries or to infections of the ear and about the jaws. Injury or infection in the region of the condyle may prevent growth, which results in a lack of development of the mandible (micrognathia). In this case the individual has a receding chin or appears to have no chin. There may be unequal growth of the two sides of the jaws resulting in an asymmetry of the face. Overgrowth of the mandible or lack of development of the maxilla results in a protrusion of the mandible, giving a pugnacious appearance to the individual. The jaws may fail to develop sufficiently to provide adequate space for accommodation of the teeth, resulting in an irregularly formed arch and crowding of the teeth.

Malocclusion is a term used to describe dentofacial malrelations involving the teeth and facial bones. The most common features are: "buck" teeth, protruding (prog-

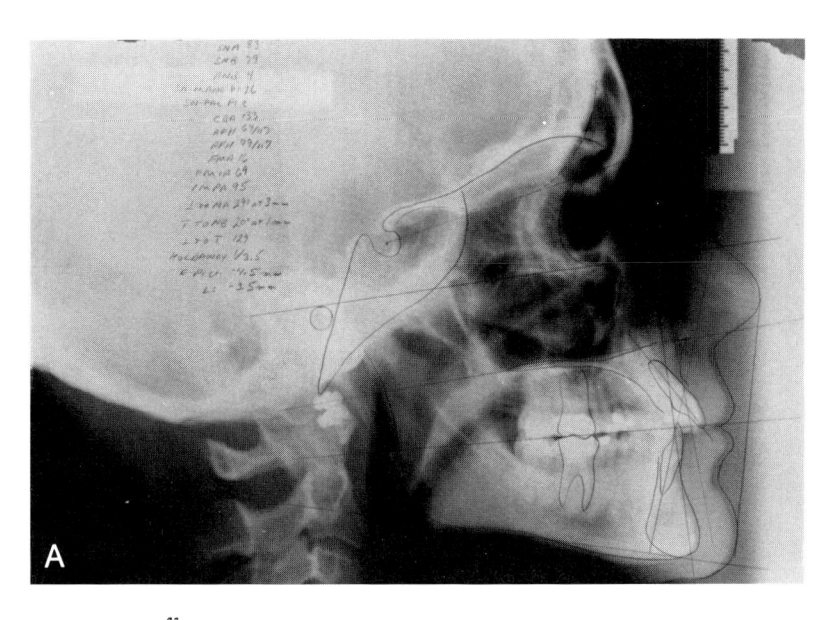

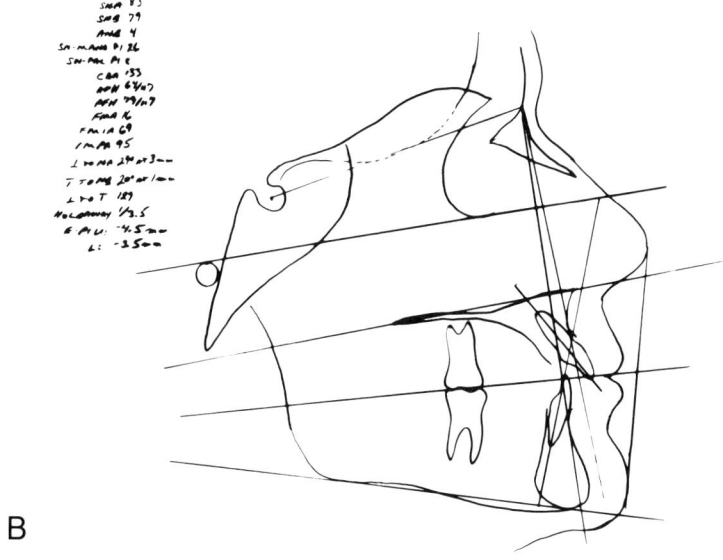

Fig. 3–15. Orthodontic evaluation of dentofacial malrelations includes an analysis of characteristic angles on cephalograms *(A)* and tracings *(B)*.

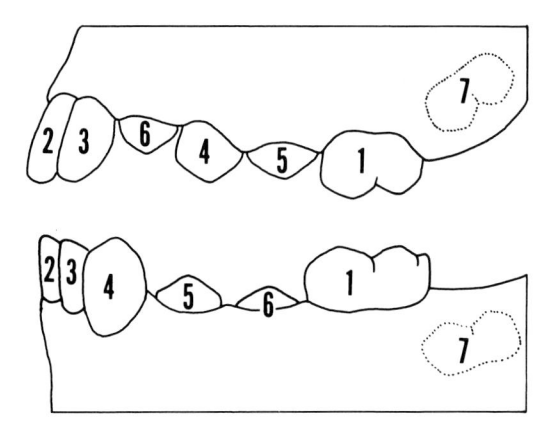

Fig. 3–16. Favorable sequence of tooth eruption for normal occlusion.

nathic) jaw, retruding (retrognathic) jaw, i.e., underdeveloped lower jaw, and crowding of teeth. Malocclusion has been classified by Angle as Class I (normal) relationship of the first molars (Fig. 3–14); Class II (retrognathic) and Class III (prognathism) malocclusion. Orthodontic evaluation makes use of radiographs (cephalograms) that allows facial angles and growth patterns to be evaluated (Fig. 3–15). The most favorable sequence of eruption of the permanent teeth is shown in Figure 3–16 and is considered to favor normal occlusion, i.e., favor proper alignment of teeth and jaw relations.

Dentofacial malrelations can occur on the basis of genetic disturbances and environmental factors. As already indicated in chapter 2, environmental factors operate in utero and after birth. Physical forces such as that produced by intrauterine molding by a limb pressed against the face of the fetus may cause facial malformation. Postnatal influences include abnormal breathing habits, trauma, and oral habits such as thumb sucking.

EMBRYOLOGY OF THE TEETH

About the sixth week of embryonic life the development of the teeth starts as a proliferation of the cells on the crest of the rudimentary jaw (Fig. 3–17). This selectively localized growth of cells on the crest of the ridge produces a strand of epithelium called the dental lamina. At about the tenth week, certain areas of the dental lamina proliferate more rapidly than others and bud-like swellings are produced. Each of these bud-like masses of epithelium represents the beginning of the formation of an individual tooth and is termed the tooth bud.

Cells in different areas of the tooth bud proliferate at different rates, making some of the cells of the dental lamina appear as if they are growing into or invaginating the surrounding tissues. In effect, the differential growth rate results in the formation of a cap-like appearance of the developing tooth bud (cap stage) (Figs. 3–18, 3–19). Further growth and selective proliferation of the peripheral cells change the appearance of the tooth bud to a bell-like structure (bell stage) (Fig. 3–20). This process of selective growth of cells to provide a characteristic shape to a structure is morphodifferentiation. The process of proliferation and morphodifferentiation of the epithelium also influences the proliferation of mesenchymal tissue in contact with the inner aspect of the epithelium of the bell-like tooth bud. This area of mesenchymal tissue within the bell-like arrangement of the epithelium is the dental papilla (Fig. 3–20). The epithelium arranged in the bell-like fashion is designated the enamel organ. The enamel organ and the dental papilla constitute the tooth germ. The enamel organ is now divided into distinct layers with the cells of each layer having a characteristic pattern. (1) The epithelium forming the outer surface of the bell-like tooth bud is the *outer enamel epithelium*. (2) The epithelium forming the inner aspect of the bell-like structure is the *inner enamel epithelium* (Fig. 3–20).

As the tooth germ increases in size, cells of the inner enamel epithelium change in shape and become columnar. Cells of the outer enamel epithelium retain their original shape, while cells between the inner and outer enamel epithelium increase in number and develop a stellate character. This change in shape and accompanying pro-

DEVELOPMENTAL DISTURBANCES 47

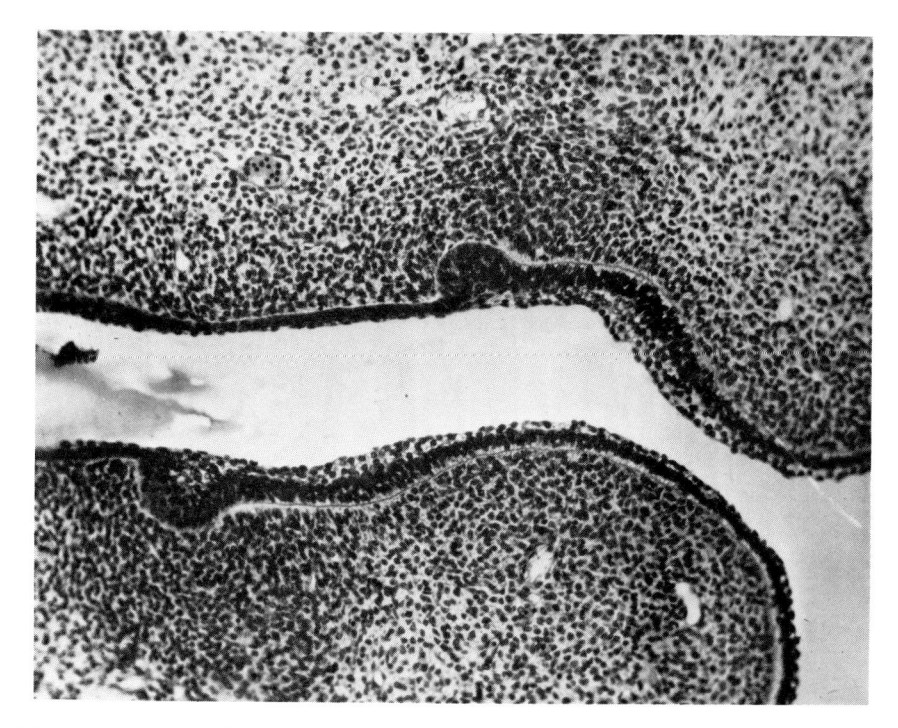

Fig. 3–17. *Dental lamina.* Initial development of tooth buds in embryo of six weeks.

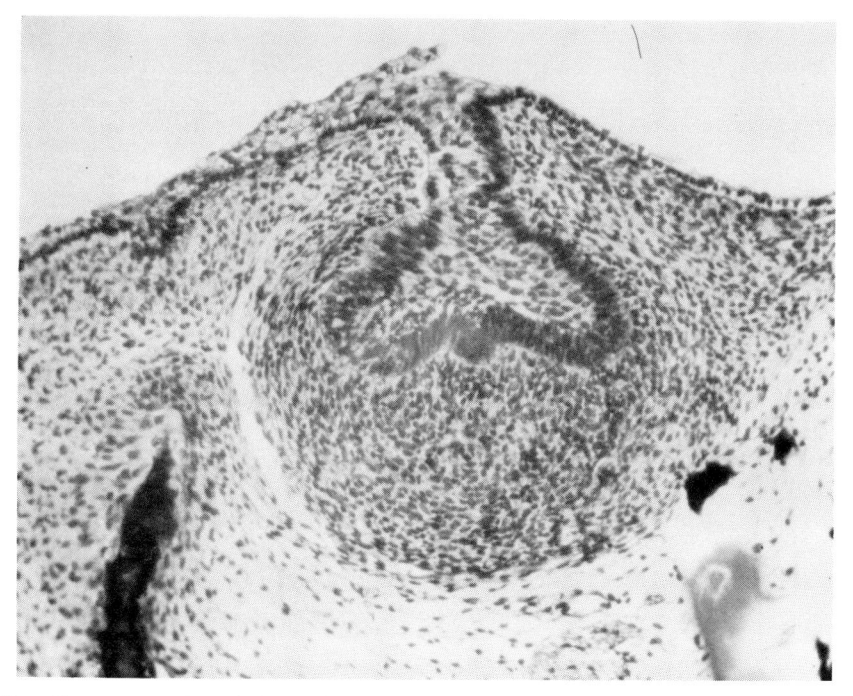

Fig. 3–18. *Cap stage of tooth bud.* Note concentration of mesenchymal cells around tooth bud indicating initial formation of dental sac and dental papillae. Black areas at right and left are developing bony crypt.

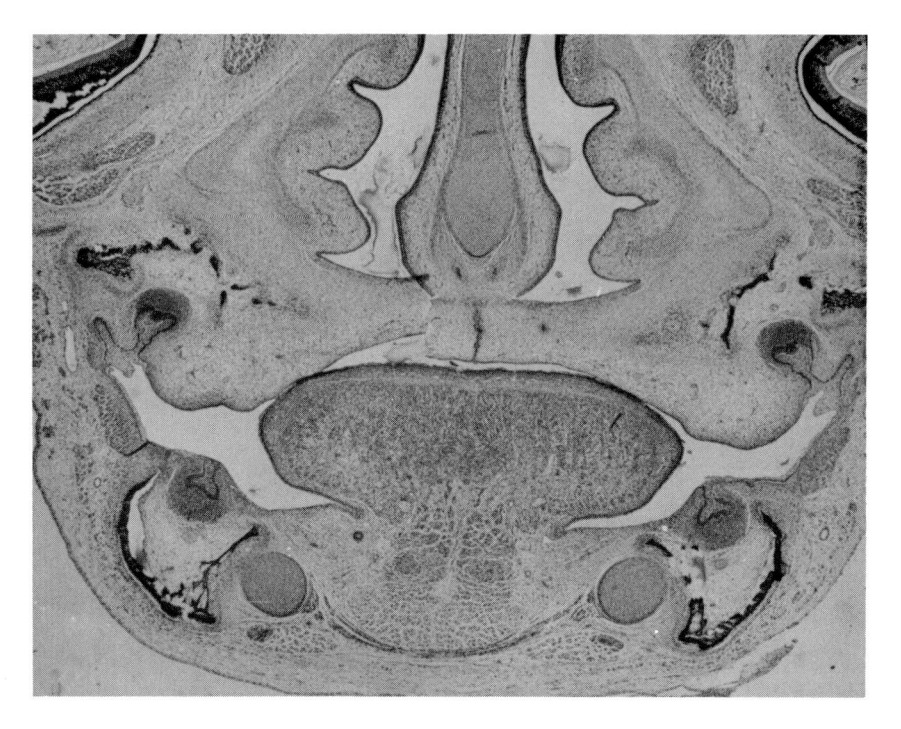

Fig. 3-19. Frontal section through face of embryo of seven weeks. Note relation of tooth germ to oral cavity; early development of mucobuccal fold lateral to the dental lamina; outline of developing mandible.

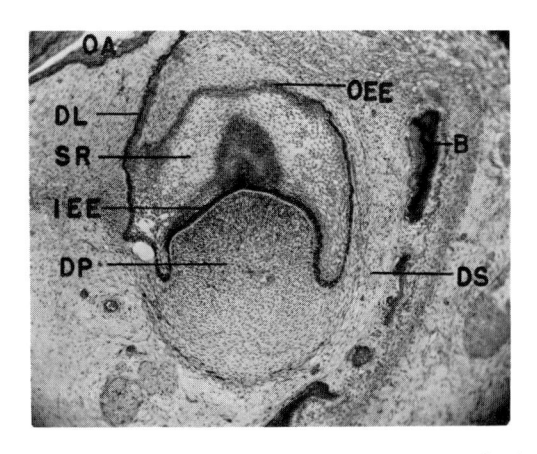

Fig. 3-20. *Bell stage of developing tooth.* Oral cavity (OA), dental lamina (DL), outer enamel epithelium (OEE), stellate reticulum (SR), inner enamel epithelium (IEE), dental papillae (DP), dental sac (DS), bone (B) of developing jaw.

liferation is histodifferentiation. As the inner enamel epithelium develops, its cells differentiate into two layers: (1) The inner-most layer composed of a single row of tall columnar cells (the ameloblasts), and (2) An outer layer of polyhedral cells four to six cells in thickness (the stratum intermedium). The outer-most layer of the enamel organ retains the character of squamous epithelium. Between the outer and inner enamel epithelium the cells become stellate with numerous long intercellular processes producing a mesh-like pattern (the stellate reticulum). As proliferation progresses, morphodifferentiation continues and the configuration of a particular tooth becomes evident. One enamel organ develops the configuration of an incisor, another a cuspid, and another a molar. At the same time, histodifferentiation continues in both the ameloblastic layer of the enamel organ and the dental papilla. The ameloblasts become tall and are arranged parallel to each other

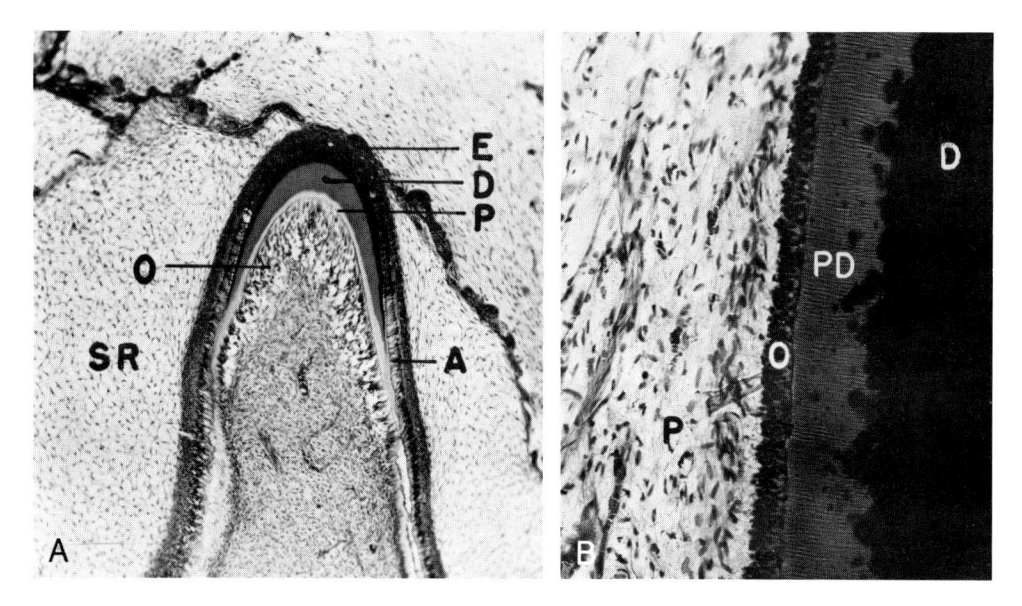

Fig. 3–21. *Dentin formation. A,* Initial enamel and dentin formation over tip of cusp; dentin (D), predentin (P), odontoblasts (O), enamel matrix (E), ameloblasts (A), stellate reticulum (SR). *B,* Later stage of dentin formation; odontoblasts (O), predentin with dark spherical areas of calcification (PD), calcified dentin (D), dental pulp (P).

and perpendicular to the border of the dental papilla. The basement membrane of the ameloblasts in contact with the dental papilla thickens and is designated the dento-enamel membrane, which is the landmark for the future dento-enamel junction.

The formation of the dento-enamel membrane influences the peripheral cells of the dental papilla to differentiate into columnar cells oriented perpendicularly to the enamel membrane. These cells are the odontoblasts, responsible for the formation of dentin (Fig. 3–21). After the odontoblasts differentiate and start to form dentin, the ameloblasts become functional and produce enamel. Each ameloblast forms an individual enamel rod as it moves away from the dento-enamel junction toward the outer enamel epithelium. The movement of the ameloblasts toward the outer enamel epithelium compresses the stellate reticulum, causing it to undergo atrophy (Fig. 3–22). When the full thickness of the enamel is completed, the ameloblasts of the inner enamel epithelium unite with the outer enamel epithelium. The completed enamel of the

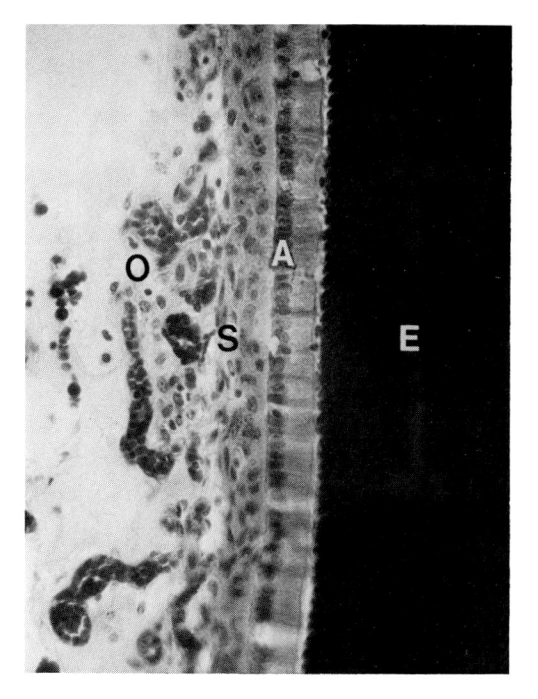

Fig. 3–22. *Formation of enamel.* Enamel (E), ameloblasts (A), stratum intermedium (S), outer enamel epithelium (O) about capillaries.

crown of the tooth is now covered by a single layer of squamous epithelium (the reduced enamel epithelium). The reduced enamel epithelium remains on the surface of the tooth as it erupts into the oral cavity.

The *reduced enamel epithelium* has been defined in several ways. The standard definition refers to the reduced enamel epithelium as an atrophied or degenerated tissue on the basis of its having completed its function with the formation of the enamel. However, another definition refers to the reduced enamel epithelium as enamel epithelium containing ameloblasts from early maturation to those that have been transformed to squamous epithelial cells. The latter definition suggests that the cells of the reduced enamel epithelium actively participate in the process of enamel maturation and the formation of junctional epithelium. The term *junctional epithelium* (cf. p. 210) is used in place of such terms as epithelial attachment and epithelial cuff when used to describe the specific epithelium responsible for the union of the gingiva to the tooth structure. Junctional epithelium may originate from reduced enamel epithelium or de novo formation from oral epithelium.

The term *epithelial attachment* is used to describe in a general way the structural system responsible for the attachment of epithelial cells to the surface of a tooth. It is the biologic mechanism uniting epithelial cells to the tooth surface.

While the enamel is being formed, the odontoblasts form dentin as they move inward from the dento-enamel junction. As dentin is formed it surrounds the dental papilla now designated the dental pulp. The process of dentin formation becomes slower when dentin reaches its normal size, but continues as long as the pulp is vital.

During the time the enamel organ is undergoing proliferation, morphodifferentiation, and histodifferentiation, the connective tissue surrounding it proliferates and differentiates into the dental sac, responsible for the formation of the supporting mechanism of the teeth, i.e., the cementum, the periodontal membrane, and the alveolar bone.

Also during the period the teeth are developing, they are surrounded by the bone of the developing jaws. The cavity within the bone in which the tooth is being formed is the dental crypt. The first teeth formed from the dental lamina are the deciduous or primary teeth. After the primary teeth are partially formed the dental lamina sends off secondary buds, which develop in the same manner but more slowly than primary teeth to form the permanent or succedaneous teeth (Fig. 3–23).

All permanent teeth are called succedaneous except the molars. The dental lamina proliferates posteriorly to form the tooth buds of the permanent molars (Fig. 3–23). All of the enamel organs do not develop at the same rate of speed; thus some teeth are completed before others are formed. The result is different times of eruption for various groups of teeth. Groups of teeth develop at specific rates so that the times of eruption follow a definite chronologic order. Their appearance in the mouth can be anticipated at specific ages (Table 3–1).

Because of the complex nature of odontogenesis wherein cells undergo morphodifferentiation and histodifferentiation and where the changes in one group of cells are dependent upon another group of cells, there are many possibilities for disturbances in the development of the teeth. These disturbances may be in the formation or eruption of one or of all the teeth.

Surface Structures

Several terms describing structures of developmental origin covering the enamel have become obsolete but still are found in the literature. *Nasmyth's membrane* is a term that probably describes many organic structures so diverse as to be impossible to specify in a meaningful way. *Primary enamel cuticle* was thought to be a secretion of the ameloblasts after the amelogenesis was completed, but this structure has not been identified as such. The *secondary en-*

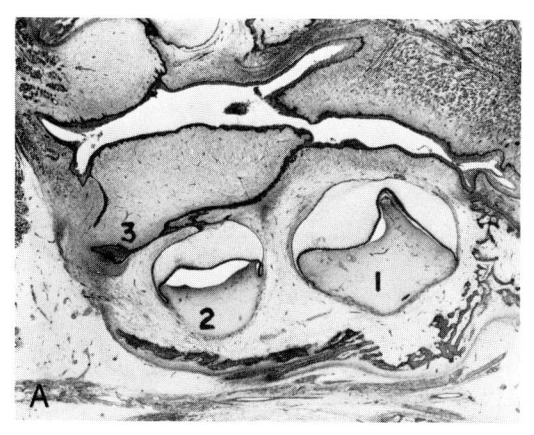

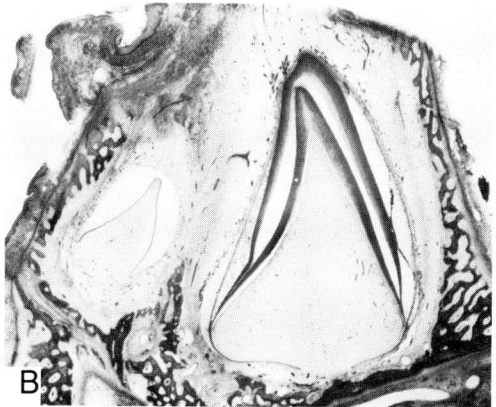

Fig. 3–23. *Enamel organ.* A, (1) Beginning dentin formation at tip of cusp of first deciduous molar; (2) advanced bell stage of second deciduous molar; (3) posterior proliferation of dental lamina with initiation of tooth bud for first permanent molar. B, Partial development of enamel and dentin of crown of deciduous incisor, and development of enamel organ of succedaneous incisor.

Table 3–1. Chronology of Permanent Teeth

Teeth	Eruption (Years)
	(Upper/Lower)
Central Incisor	7–8/6–7
Lateral Incisor	8–9/7–8
Canine	11–12/9–10
First Premolar	10–11/10–12
Second Premolar	10–12/11–12
First Molar	6–7/6–7
Second Molar	12–18/11–13
Third Molar	17–21/17–21

amel cuticle was described as the keratinized product of the outer enamel epithelium. However, it is not made of keratin nor is its origin determined. Because of the uncertainty of the nature of a nonmineralized cuticular structure seen at the dento-epithelial junction to which the term dental cuticle might apply, this term is still of conditional use.

The structures of developmental origin occurring on the surface of the enamel include the reduced enamel epithelium, patchy coronal cementum, and a subsurface enamel matrix. The enamel cuticle also may be considered to be of developmental origin if it is accepted as a secretory product of the junctional epithelium. These structures will be encountered again in later discussions of dental plaque and periodontal diseases.

DISTURBANCES OF THE TEETH

Developmental disturbances of the teeth may be manifest by variations in number, position, size, shape, eruption, or structure. Such disturbances may occur in association with some more generalized disorder or may occur independently. Some of the more common developmental anomalies will be discussed.

Disturbances in the *number* of teeth may occur when all or some of the teeth fail to develop (agenesis or anodontia) or because too many teeth develop (hyperodontia or supernumerary teeth). Agenesis may occur with any disturbance of ectodermal tissue which prevents its proliferation and differentiation into highly specialized cells (ectodermal dysplasia). In such instances, all or some of the teeth may fail to develop. This disturbance is associated with anhidrotic ectodermal dysplasia manifestated by a failure to develop the specialized skin appendages such as sweat glands, hair follicles, and nails. In other instances, a single tooth or type of tooth may fail to develop. This type of anodontia usually is hereditary and both parent and offspring may have the same teeth absent. The third molars, maxillary lateral incisors, and the first bicuspids are the most frequently congenitally absent teeth, in the order named.

In some hereditary diseases an individual may develop more than the normal number of teeth. The extra, or supernumerary, teeth are most often the maxillary incisors or molars. Supernumerary teeth are usually abnormal in size and shape and may or may not erupt. If eruption occurs it is usually associated with abnormal position. They may fail to erupt and prevent the eruption of adjacent normal teeth. From time to time patients report they know of someone with a third dentition; however, no authenticated case of a third dentition has been reported. Occasionally babies born with teeth have also been reported. Usually they are not true teeth but are tooth-like structures formed from the mucosa over the area from which the dental lamina is initiated. Such "teeth" may be shed quickly or may have to be removed. They represent overzealous proliferation of oral epithelium in the region of the dental lamina.

Disturbances in eruption may be manifest as precocious or delayed eruption. The primary teeth may erupt earlier than normal, usually followed by early shedding of primary teeth and early eruption of the permanent dentition. Early eruption of teeth may be due to hyperfunction of the pituitary or thyroid glands.

Delayed eruption of teeth may involve all or part of the dentition. The entire primary dentition may be delayed as well as a corresponding delay in the eruption of the permanent dentition and is usually associated with delay in the general growth of the individual. Individual teeth may be delayed in eruption because they develop in an abnormal position and impinge against adjacent teeth. This is especially true of third molars and occasionally the maxillary cuspids. Such teeth are designated *impacted teeth*.

Delay in shedding the primary teeth and

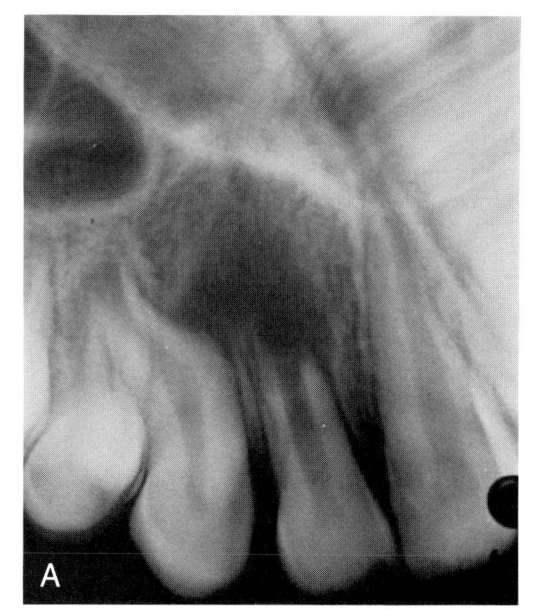

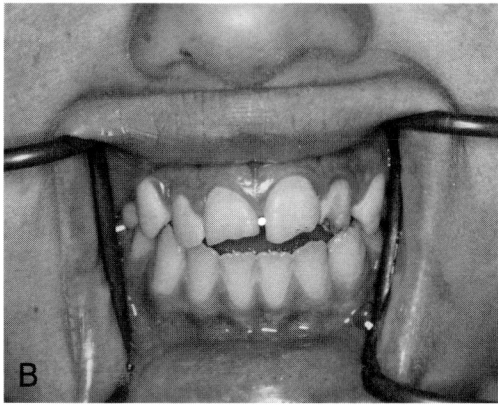

Fig. 3–24. Dilaceration of cuspid (A) resulting from periapical lesion associated with pulpitis secondary to traumatic fracture of lateral incisor (B).

eruption of the permanent teeth accompanied by the presence of supernumerary teeth and failure of the bones of the face, the skull, and the clavicle to develop properly is a hereditary mesodermal dysplasia, *cleidocranial dysostosis*. The presence of some primary teeth, a few permanent teeth, and absence of other teeth in an individual who has reached his late teens is very suggestive of this condition. Radiographs will demonstrate the presence of supernu-

DEVELOPMENTAL DISTURBANCES 53

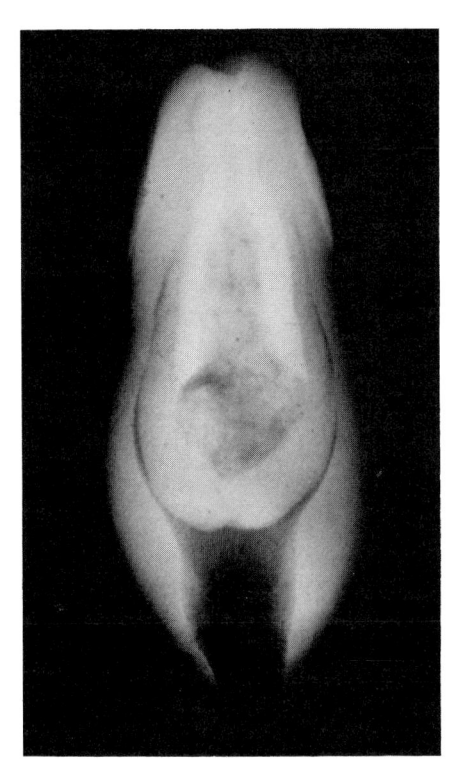

Fig. 3–25. *"Dens in dente."* Incisor with enamel lining a central cavity extending to apex of root. A configuration of a tooth appears to be within the pulp chamber.

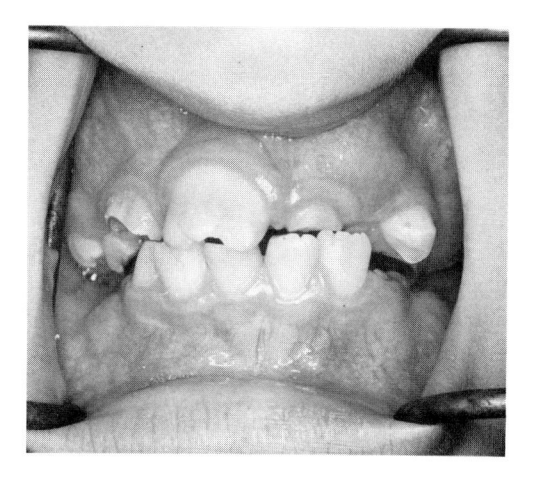

Fig. 3–26. *Giantism.* Marked variation in size of teeth. The permanent central incisor is three times the width of the deciduous central incisor.

merary teeth and the failure of the bones to develop.

Dilaceration is a condition in which the long axes of the crown and root are not in the same plane. The long axis of the root forms an angle with the long axis of the crown. This deviation of the root is usually due to crowding of the teeth during development, or it may be due to a blow which displaces the crown when root formation is beginning. The root continues to form in the original axis, while the crown remains in the displaced position (Fig. 3–24).

"Dens in dente" is an anomalous development from invagination of the enamel into the area of a natural pit or groove. It most often occurs in the maxillary lateral incisors as an invagination of the enamel into the lingual pit. The enamel invagination may extend a short distance or to the apex of the root. Radiographically, the radiopaque enamel of the crown is continuous with enamel surrounding a central space. With enamel on both the outside and inside of the tooth, it has the appearance of a tooth within a tooth (Fig. 3–25). These teeth are frequently lost early owing to organisms or debris passing through the central space to the apical area where an inflammatory process is initiated similar to that which develops at the apex of a tooth with pulp disease.

Disturbances in the *position* of teeth may be caused by insufficient space on the arch for the size of the teeth resulting in crowding, especially of anterior teeth. In some instances, there may be transposition of teeth, i.e., the positions of the lateral incisor and cuspid may be reversed. Anomalous position of teeth may affect the esthetics of the teeth and the physiognomy of the individual to the extent that it is desirable to correct the position by orthodontic procedures.

Teeth may be too large (giantism) or too small (dwarfism). Giantism (Fig. 3–26) may involve all of the teeth, pairs of teeth, or the crown or root of a single tooth. Dwarfism involves the teeth similarly but is more common than giantism. Most often third molars and maxillary lateral incisors are dwarfed.

54   DEVELOPMENTAL DISTRUBANCES

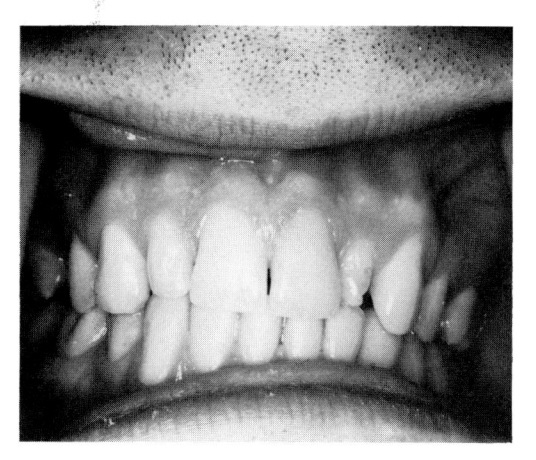

Fig. 3–27. *"Peg Lateral."* Both maxillary lateral incisors are narrow; the left incisor is conical and shows hypoplasia of enamel.

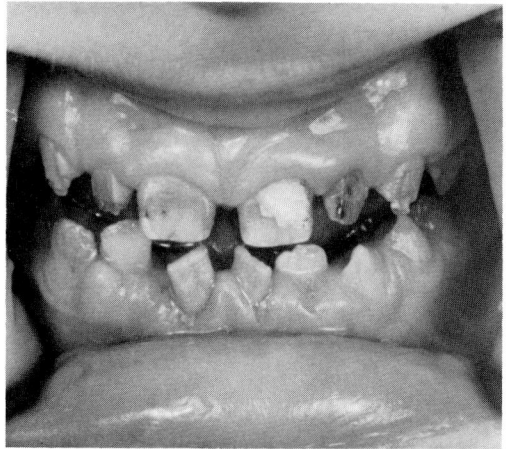

Fig. 3–28. Amelogenesis imperfecta with almost complete absence of enamel on many teeth.

Dwarfed teeth frequently are abnormal in shape, especially the lateral incisor which may be represented as only a small peg-shaped tooth called a *"peg lateral"* (Fig. 3–27).

Disturbances in the *formation* of teeth occur at any stage of odontogenesis and involve any of the developing cellular components. Some defects in tooth development are genetic in origin and therefore usually involve all teeth and both dentitions. Such defects may be associated with dysplastic processes in other tissues developing from the same germ layer.

Amelogenesis imperfecta is a hereditary disturbance of enamel formation which may be associated with other evidence of ectodermal dysplasia. This disturbance, which involves all teeth in both dentitions, is the result of a defect in the formation of the enamel matrix or in the calcification and maturation of enamel. The severity of the defect in the formation of enamel varies in different patients, different teeth, and even different areas of the same tooth (Fig. 3–28). Thus, the clinical appearance is rarely duplicated, although the basic defect of the enamel is the same in all cases. The characteristic findings are due to a failure of the formation of enamel matrix of one or more teeth or a portion of a tooth. The complete absence of enamel matrix results in teeth having the shape, size, and yellow color of the dentin core. Some variation in color is produced by staining from substances taken into the mouth. In teeth where areas of the enamel matrix is formed but not calcified, the surface of the defective enamel has a normal contour, but the enamel has a yellowish color and a soft, chalky consistency. In other areas the enamel is calcified and mature, so the enamel is normal in color and consistency. In spite of the poor formation of a portion of the enamel, such teeth have a low caries susceptibility and are not subject to marked attrition. However, these teeth are esthetic problems and, because of this, may cause psychologic problems necessitating the replacement or crowning of most of the teeth.

Enamel hypoplasia is a disturbance in the formation of the enamel matrix from a variety of causes, resulting in defective enamel of one or several teeth (Fig. 3–29). The hypoplastic defects vary in size, shape, and severity depending upon the etiology of the hypoplasia and the degree of tooth development reached at the time the defect was initiated. Hypoplasia is usually manifest as a series of irregular to round pits of varying size in the enamel. The pits are frequently

DEVELOPMENTAL DISTURBANCES 55

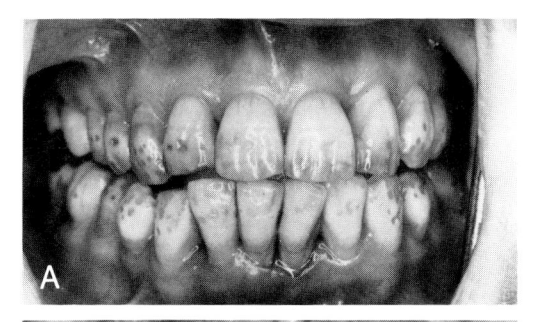

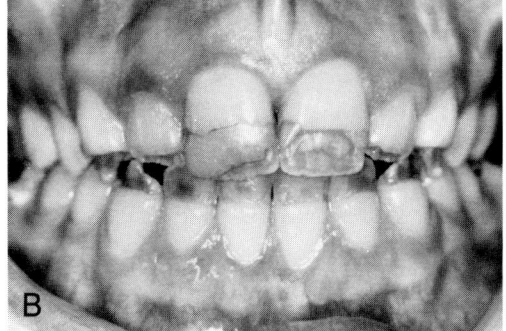

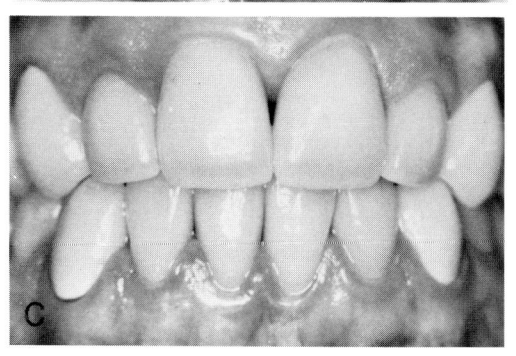

Fig. 3–29. *Hypoplasia of enamel. A,* Nearly all teeth show hypomaturation of enamel and numerous small hypoplastic pits. *B,* Hypoplasia of incisal one-third of anterior teeth. *C,* Teeth restored to improve esthetics.

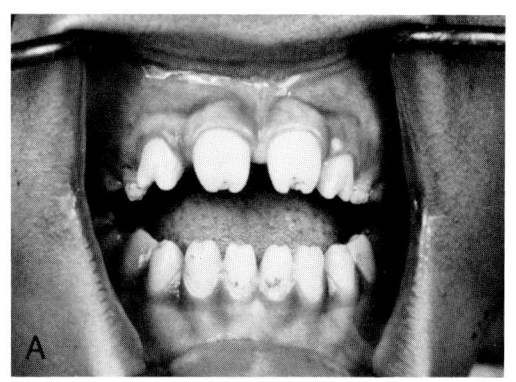

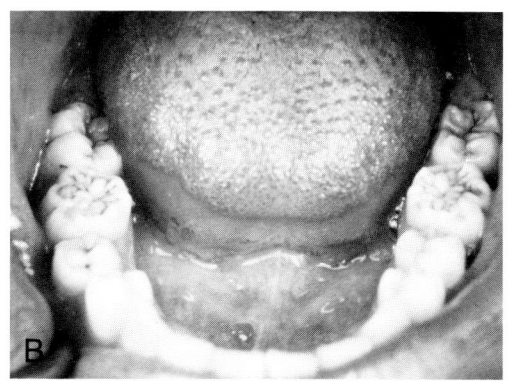

Fig. 3–30. *A, Hutchinson's incisors.* Maxillary central incisors are typical and are usually the only teeth involved. However, the lower incisors are also affected in this instance. *B, Mulberry molars.* Both lower first molars show the small nodules of enamel resembling the surface of a berry.

arranged in a row parallel to the incisal or coronal surfaces of the labial or lingual surfaces of the teeth. They follow the pattern of the imbrication lines. When the defect occurs in several teeth, it follows the chronologic pattern of tooth development. For example, hypoplastic defects may be present on the incisal one-third of the central incisors and the incisal tips of the cuspids, whereas the lateral incisors are not involved. This variation in involvement is due to the difference in time at which the various teeth develop, viz., the formation of the enamel of the central incisors and cuspids occurs before that of the lateral incisor teeth. The defects are usually stained brown to black. No particular immunity or susceptibility to caries is associated with enamel hypoplasia.

Hypoplasia may be caused by high fever, acute infectious diseases characterized by a rash (measles, chicken pox), dietary deficiencies, irradiation, local or generalized infection, or the ingestion of toxic substances. The nature of the defect is not always characteristic of a particular etiology. However, hypoplasia of the enamel can be correlated with a specific cause if the pa-

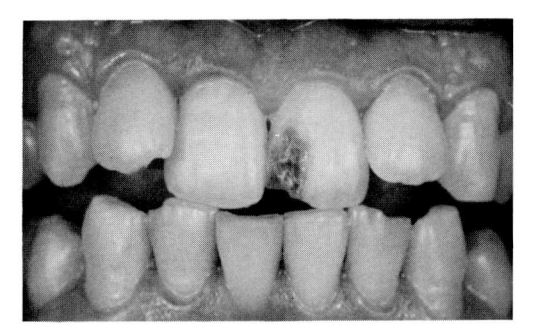

Fig. 3–31. *Turner's tooth.* Focal hypoplasia of a portion of labial enamel of central incisor.

tient's history indicates that an etiologic factor was present during the time the defective parts of the teeth were being formed. In some cases, the type of defect is characteristic of a particular disease, such as syphilis or periapical infection of a deciduous tooth.

In congenital syphilis, hypoplasia may involve the maxillary central incisors and the first permanent molars. The incisors have a notch in the incisal edge and a mesio-distal narrowing of the incisal portion of the crown. This produces a shape like the notched blade of a screw driver (Fig. 3–30A). Such incisors are called *Hutchinson incisors* and are very suggestive but not positive evidence of congenital syphilis. Involved molars have a slight constriction of the occlusal surface which is composed of small nodular masses of enamel simulating the surface of a raspberry or mulberry and therefore are designated mulberry molars (also Pfluger molars) (Fig. 3–30B). Often the small nodular masses of enamel are poorly attached to the dentin and they fracture, exposing the dentin of most of the occlusal surface. The appearance of the molars, like that of the incisors, is very suggestive but not positive evidence of congenital syphilis.

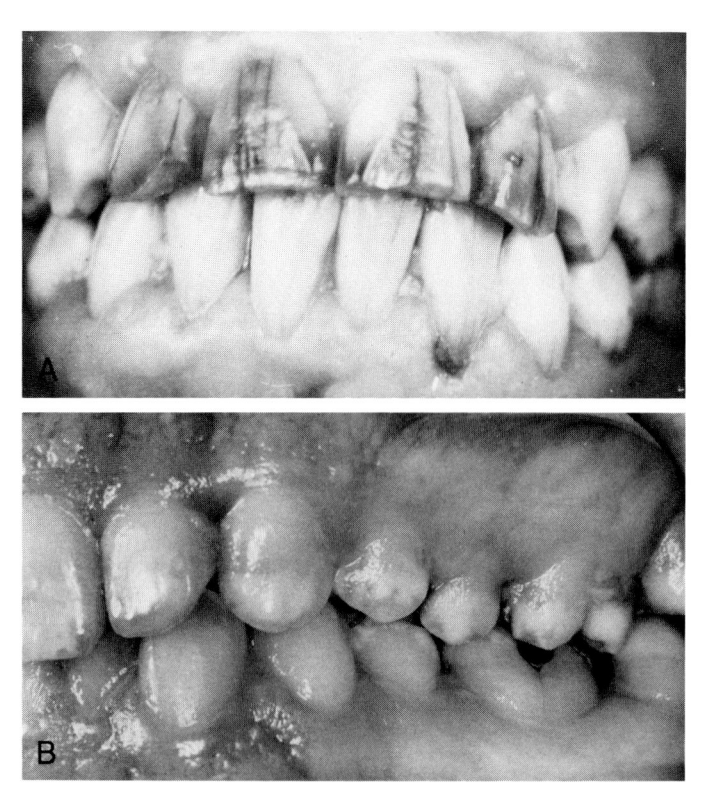

Fig. 3–32. *Mottled enamel.* A, Some opacity and incisal wear with cracking and dark-brown staining of enamel. B, Patchy white mottling due to intense hypomaturation of enamel.

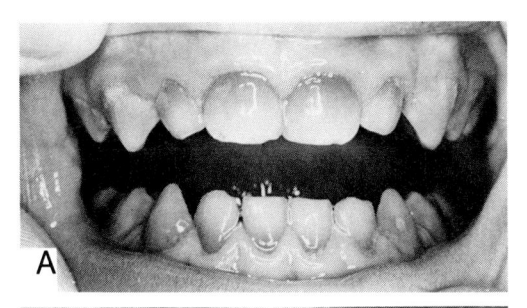

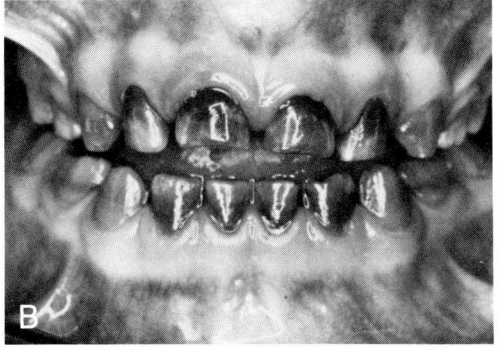

Fig. 3–33. *Tetracycline pigmentation.* A, Mild effect with yellow to brownish pigmentation showing at the cervical one-third of the teeth. B, Intense effect with the entire tooth discolored. Note distribution is the same as A with greatest intensity at the cervical margins.

When the pulp of a deciduous tooth is diseased, the presence of a periapical lesion may involve a part of the enamel organ of the succedaneous tooth and produce a defect in a limited area of the developing enamel of a permanent tooth. In this case, there is a defect involving a portion of a single surface of a single tooth (Fig. 3–31). Teeth so involved are characteristic and are named *Turner's teeth* after the investigator who first reported their occurrence and etiology.

Fluorosis or *mottled enamel* is a particular type of hypoplasia produced by the ingestion of water containing more than two parts per million of fluoride during the time when the enamel was forming. The fluorine incorporated into the forming enamel prevents its complete maturation and produces an opacity and porosity to the enamel (Fig. 3–32). The enamel is irregularly whitish-gray to brown with some exaggeration of the lines of imbircation. Mottled teeth are immune to caries, but are susceptible to enamel fracture and attrition. The loss of enamel with exposure of dentin sometimes causes the teeth to become hypersensitive. Enamel fluorosis or mottling may be severe and unattractive but usually presents no esthetic problems in localities where it is common or endemic. However, mottled enamel does present a problem in individuals who move to a locality where it is uncommon. To overcome hypersensitivity and to improve the esthetic appearance, mottled teeth may have to be extracted and replaced or covered by crowns.

Pigmentation of a developing dentition may occur as the result of ingestion of the antibiotic tetracycline during critical periods of tooth development. Such pigmentation may involve both the primary and permanent dentitions. This disturbance is a frequent complication in cystic fibrosis. Mild pigmentation shows as a yellow discoloration at the cervical margins of the teeth (Fig. 3–33A). In severe pigmentation the entire dentition may be stained brown to bluish-violet (Fig. 3–33B). Depending on the stage of dental development, staining may involve only a portion of the dentition.

Disturbances in dentin formation may accompany those produced in enamel, but are usually not clinically evident because they are hidden by the enamel covering the crowns. *Dentinogenesis imperfecta,* or hereditary opalescent dentin, like osteogenesis imperfecta, is considered to be a mesenchymal defect. Both may occur independent of the other but an association occurs frequently. Dentinogenesis imperfecta has been classified into three types (Shields et al., 1973). Type I is dentinogenesis imperfecta (D.I.) without osteogenesis imperfecta (O.I.). Type II (hereditary opalescent dentin) is D.I. without O.I. Type III involves an isolated inbred kindred in Maryland. Dentinogenesis imperfecta type II is inherited as an autosomal dominant trait that affects both the primary and permanent dentitions. Dentinogenesis imperfecta is

58 DEVELOPMENTAL DISTRUBANCES

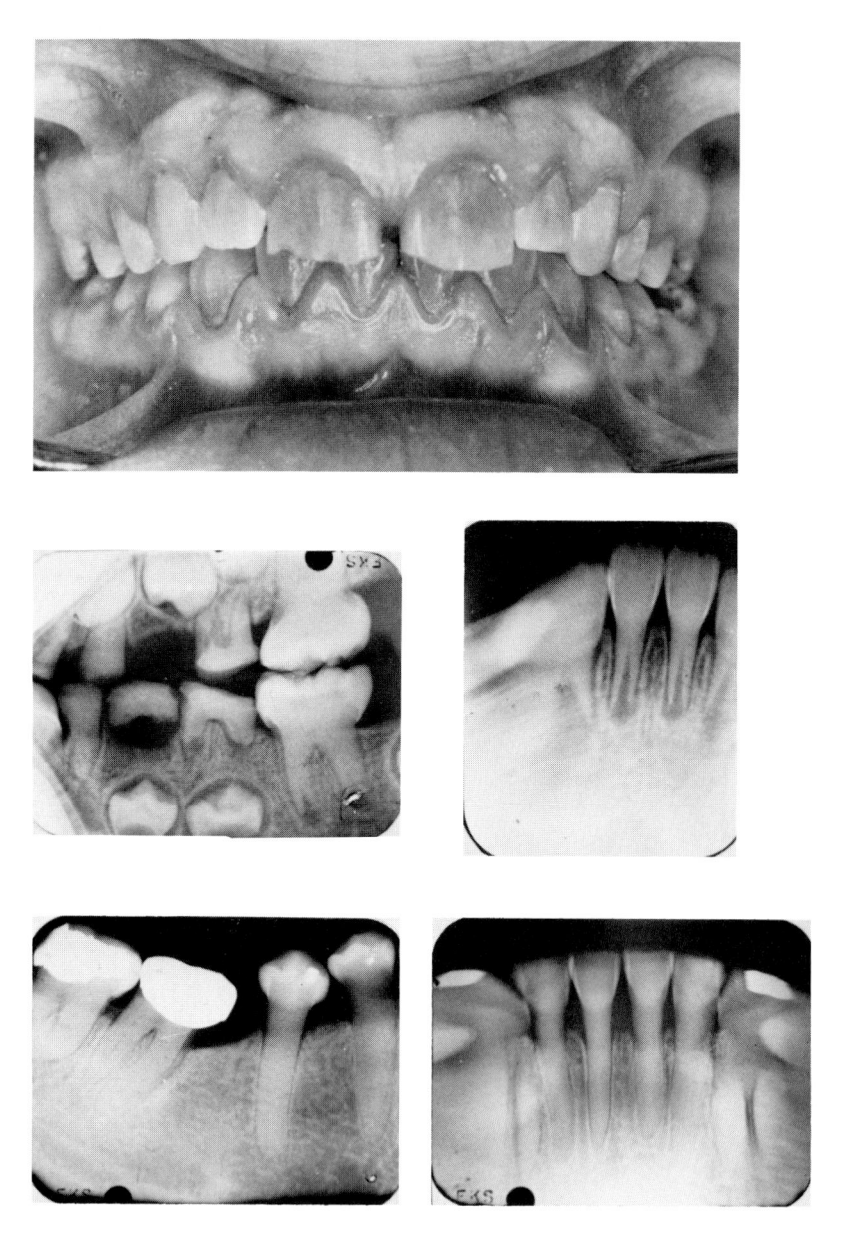

Fig. 3–34. *Dentinogenesis imperfecta*. A, Opalescent color and incisal abrasion. B, Radiographs of erupted deciduous and developing permanent teeth showing obliteration of pulp chamber and extensive occlusal wear. C, Radiographs of permanent teeth of same patient ten years later showing characteristic configuration of root and obliteration of pulp chamber.

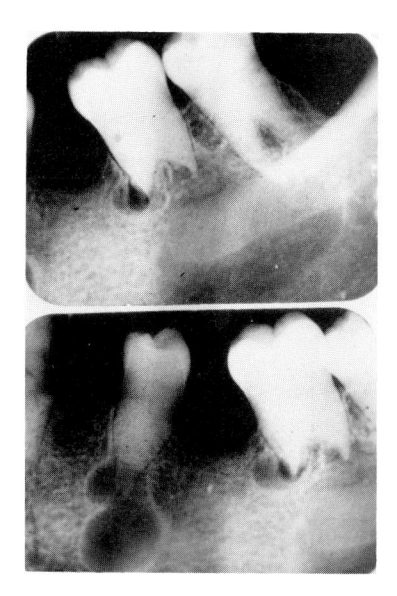

Fig. 3–35. *Dentin dysplasia*—typical findings. Both dentitions are involved and show limited root formation with periapical radiolucency. The molar roots are square and show no tendency for bifurcation. The pulp chambers are absent.

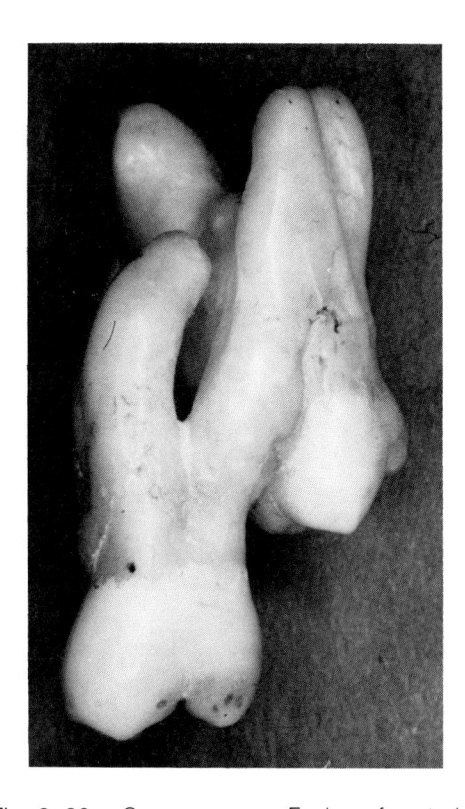

Fig. 3–36. *Concrescence.* Fusion of roots by excess deposition of cementum.

characterized clinically by opalescent teeth with short roots, obliteration of pulp chambers, shortening of canals, and gross attrition at an early age (Fig. 3–34).

In *dentin dysplasia,* another defect of the dentin, the crowns of the teeth appear normal in shape and color. The teeth are usually malposed owing to distorted, blunt, or absent roots. The pulp chambers are frequently absent, and there are rarefied areas in the bone at the apex of the peculiarly shaped roots. Radiographically, the rarefied areas resemble periapical cysts (Fig. 3–35).

Disturbances in cementum may occur, but are very rare and are not clinically discernible. When present, they are associated with premature shedding of the teeth.

Concrescence is the union of two teeth by cementum (Fig. 3–36). It most frequently occurs in the maxillary molar region between the second and third molars with the third molar in an abnormal position so that the roots of the teeth are in close contact. Excess deposition of cementum about mal-

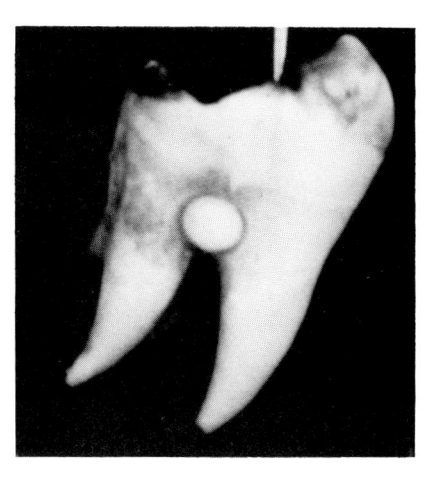

Fig. 3–37. *Enamel pearl.*

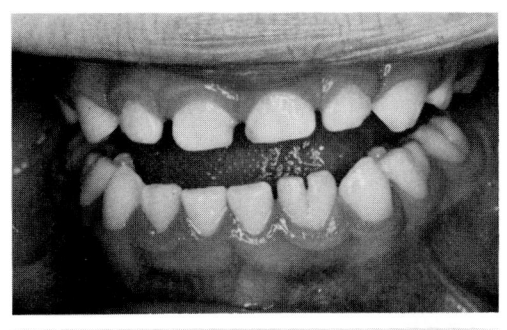

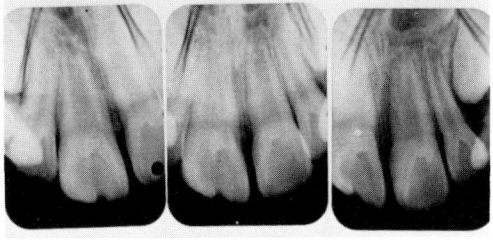

Fig. 3–38. *Geminism. Upper,* Almost complete division of crown. Radiographs show there is a common root. *Lower,* Radiographs of maxillary central incisors showing slight division of crown with common root.

posed teeth fuses the roots together. They present a considerable problem in extraction because the condition is not usually evident on clinical examination.

Enamel pearls are small masses of tooth material covered by enamel and are attached to the surface of the root. These malformations most often occur in the bifurcation of multi-rooted teeth as small (1 to 4 millimeters) globular masses of enamel partially covered by cementum (Fig. 3–37). They are formed by persistent amelogenic activity of a localized area of Hertwig's sheath. The enamel pearl may present a problem in the treatment of a periodontal pocket that has extended beyond the attachment of the enamel pearl.

During development, a single enamel organ may divide partially to form a tooth appearing to have two crowns (geminism). This defect may occur only as an incisal notch. Radiographs of geminism show that a single root and pulpal canal are present (Fig. 3–38). The normal number of teeth are present counting the divided crown as one. *Fusion* is a malformation produced by the union of two developing adjacent teeth. Fusion occurs most often when a normal tooth becomes fused with a supernumerary tooth. Radiographs of fusion show a double root with two pulp canals.

BIBLIOGRAPHY

Ash, M.M., Jr.: *Wheeler's Dental Anatomy, Physiology and Occlusion.* 6th ed., Philadelphia, W.B. Saunders Co., 1984.

Colby, R.A., Kerr, D.A., and Robinson, H.B.G.: *Color Atlas of Oral Pathology,* 3rd ed. Philadelphia, J.B. Lippincott Co., 1971.

Lassi, A., and Partin, P.: The inheritance pattern of missing, peg-shaped and strongly mesio-distally reduced upper lateral incisors. Acta Odont. Scand., 27:563, 1969.

Logan, J., Berk, H., Silverman, A., and Pindborg, J.J.: Dentinal dysplasia. Oral Surg., 15:317, 1962.

Sander, J.: Inheritance of harelip and cleft palate. Genetica, 15:433, 1934.

Shafer, G.G., Hine, M.K., and Levy, B.M.: *Textbook of Oral Pathology,* 3rd ed., Philadelphia, W.B. Saunders Co., 1974.

Shields, E.D., Bixler, D., and El-ka frawy, A.M.: A proposed classification for heritable human dentine defects with a description of a new entity. Arch. Oral Biol., 18:543, 1973.

Stewart, D.J.: The effects of tetracyclines upon the dentition. Br. J. Derm., 76:374, 1964.

Ten Cate, A.R.: *Oral Histology, Development, Structure, and Function.* St. Louis, C.V. Mosby Co., 1980.

Witkop, C.J., Jr.: Hereditary defects of dentin. Dent. Clin. North Am., 19:3, 1975.

4

RESPONSE TO INJURY

The ability of the body to sustain injury, resist infectious agents, and repair damaged tissues is the hallmark of pathology. These functions are dependent upon inflammation and immune responses. The essential aspects of inflammation are injury and cellular damage with associated normal inflammatory, hemostatic, and immune responses, followed by resolution or reparative response.

Although the inflammatory response can be initiated by a variety of agents, the basic events that follow are remarkably similar for all types of injury. Most definitions simply specify that inflammation is a local reaction of living, vascularized tissues to injury by a nonspecific injurious agent. Most simply defined, inflammation is a local multicellular response to injury.

However, the response to injury is more complex than the simplistic definition suggests. It is often complex and interrelated among a number of pathways involving vascular, and cellular, as well as coagulation and enzyme systems that complement the response. The response of white blood cells and tissues to injurious agents leads to the production of chemical substances which mediate and control both inflammatory and immune responses. The purpose of these mediators involving multicellular responses is the destruction or neutralization and removal of injurious agents and the facilitation of repair of the injured tissues.

INFLAMMATION

The presence of inflammation in a tissue or organ is designated by adding the suffix -itis to the anatomic site, i.e., gingiva - gingivitis; appendix - appendicitis, nerve - neuritis, and dermis (skin) - dermatitis.

Local manifestations of inflammation include redness (rubor), heat (calor), swelling (tumor), pain (dolor), and loss of function (functio laesa). These manifestations occur primarily in relation to hemodynamic changes at the site of injury.

Systemic manifestations such as fever may occur secondary to the local reaction to injury, especially in response to some infectious agents, although other endogenous pyrogens (fever producing substances) may also cause fever. There is also an increase in white blood cells (WBC), especially with bacteria in the blood (septicemia). Bacteria gain access to the blood on a transient basis (transient bacteremia) even when brushing the teeth but do not cause fever unless bacterial endocarditis occurs.

Cells in Inflammation

Leukocytosis is an increase in white cells in the circulating blood following injury. The increase is made possible by the release of leukocytes from tissue pools such as the spleen and bone marrow. These tissues are stimulated by leukocyte releasing and mobilizing factors, as well as additional blastogenic factors released from the site of inflammation. Thus a number of factors released at the site of injury are capable of stimulating the division and maturation of primordial stem cells.

There are two types of leukocytes, *granular* and *nongranular leukocytes*. The granulocytes contain cytoplasmic granules and the nucleus has a distinctive multilobar (3–5 lobe) shape (Fig. 4–1). If the granules do not stain with an acid or basic dye in the laboratory, they are called *neutrophils* or polymorphonuclear leukocytes (PMNs). In acute inflammation, PMNs are the first leukocytes to reach the site of injury, attracted

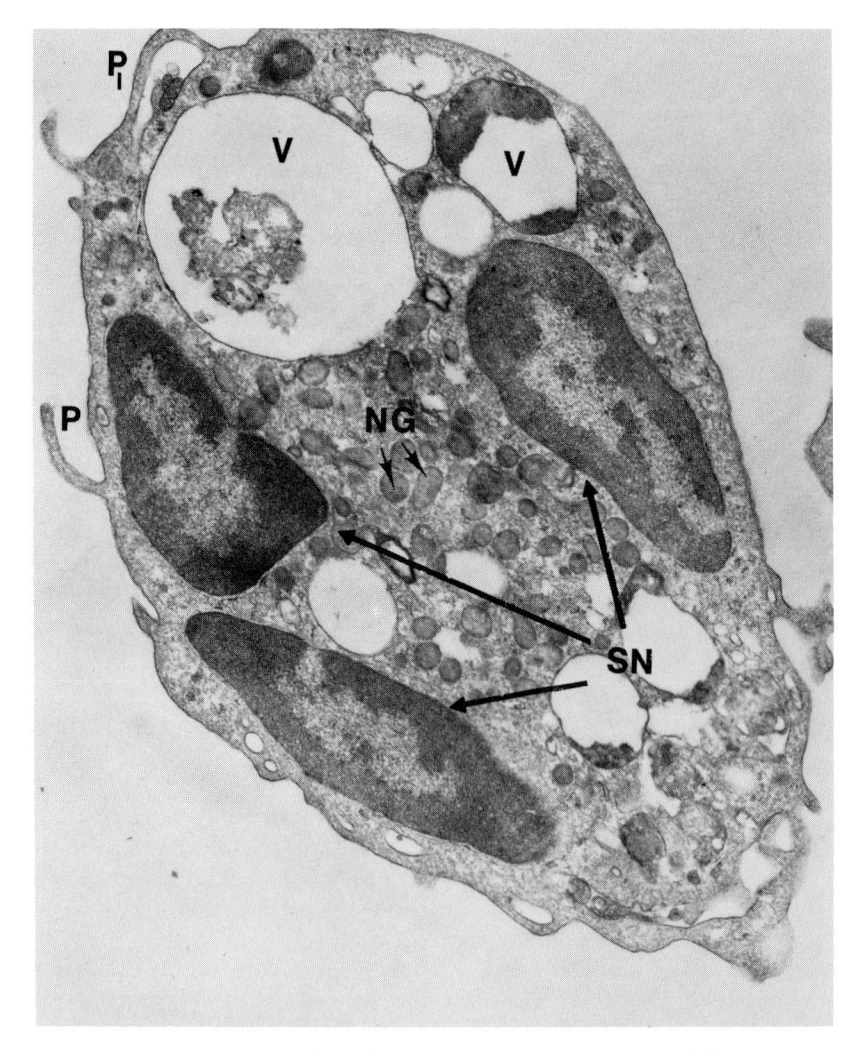

Fig. 4–1. *Ultrastructural characteristics of a polymorphonuclear neutrophilic leukocyte*. The segmented nuclei (SN) are present, but the linking nucleoplasm is not present in this section. Numerous neutrophilic granules (NG) are present throughout the cytoplasm. Large vacuoles (V) are seen which may represent the residual elements of phagocytized material. The peripheral cytoplasm is specialized into projections (P) which fold over and re-unite with the cytoplasm to capture material (P_1). Magnification approximately ×10,000. (Courtesy of Dr. David Krutchoff.)

by substances from the blood plasma, bacteria, and tissues. A significant reduction in the number or in the functional ability of the neutrophilic granulocyte, such as occurs in agranulocytosis and/or certain kinds of leukemia, may lead to potentially lethal disturbances.

PMN, which are also called microphages, release enzymes that can damage bacteria, cause tissue destruction, release plasmin (fibrinolysin) in blood clotting, generate prostaglandins (which are vasodilators and increase vascular permeability), and release kinin (which is a permeability factor).

PMNs constitute 60 to 70% of the total count of white blood cells (WBC). If the granules stain red with acid dye eosin, they are called *eosinophils* and constitute 1 to 3% of the WBC. Eosinophils may control immediate hypersensitivity reactions (p. 87) and are increased in some parasitic infections. If the granules stain blue with basic dye, the granulocytes are called *basophils* and constitute 0.3 to 0.5% of the total WBC. They may leave the blood stream and participate in an inflammatory reaction such as delayed type hypersensitivity reactions including contact dermatitis. They have similar characteristics as the tissue mast cell.

Mast cells are found in extravascular tissues. They contain chemical mediators of inflammatory and immune responses, including histamine, serotonin, lysosomal enzymes, and prostaglandins.

The nongranular leukocytes include *monocytes* and *lymphocytes*. The monocyte constitutes about 3 to 8% of the total number of white blood cells in the circulating blood. On leaving the blood the monocyte acts as a macrophage in the area of inflammation. The monocytic macrophages phagocytize fibrin, dead PMNs, cellular debris, and foreign protein. *Lymphocytes* constitute about 20 to 30% of the number of white blood cells. There are two types of lymphocytes, B cells and T cells, as well as differentiated B cells called plasma cells. The lymphocyte plays a major role in immunologic defense reactions (p. 76). Monocytes

Table 4–1. Differential White Blood Cell Count (WBC)

	Normal	Acute Infection
Total WBC/mm^3	5–10,000	15–20,000
PMNs %	65	85
Stabs	—	12
Lymphocytes %	25	12
Monocytes %	2	1

and lymphocytes are considered to reflect chronic inflammation, although considerable overlap is always present. Generally the presence of many PMNs indicates an acute response, whereas increased numbers of monocytes and lymphocytes indicates a chronic response. Tissue cells will be discussed in relation to tissue and immune responses.

During an acute bacterial infection a differential white cell count (Table 4–1) will show an increase in white blood cells but a disproportinate increase in the neutrophils, including immature forms called "stabs."

Acute Inflammation

Inflammation is designated as acute or chronic, depending upon whether it lasts a few days or months or longer, and upon the type of white blood cell present. Inflammation can be considered in relation to the vascular as well as the cellular response to injury. Vascular responses may be immediate as occurs with direct damage to the tissues, delayed for 6 to 8 hours as is the case with radiation injury such as sunburn, or longer with x rays, bacterial toxins and various chemicals.

Vascular Response

The initial response of the tissue to injury is vascular, i.e., there is an initial constriction of vessels that lasts for 20 to 30 seconds and then the vessels gradually increase in size until they are larger than before injury (Fig. 4–2). The transitory constriction of the arterioles is an autonomic, neurogenic response of unknown cause.

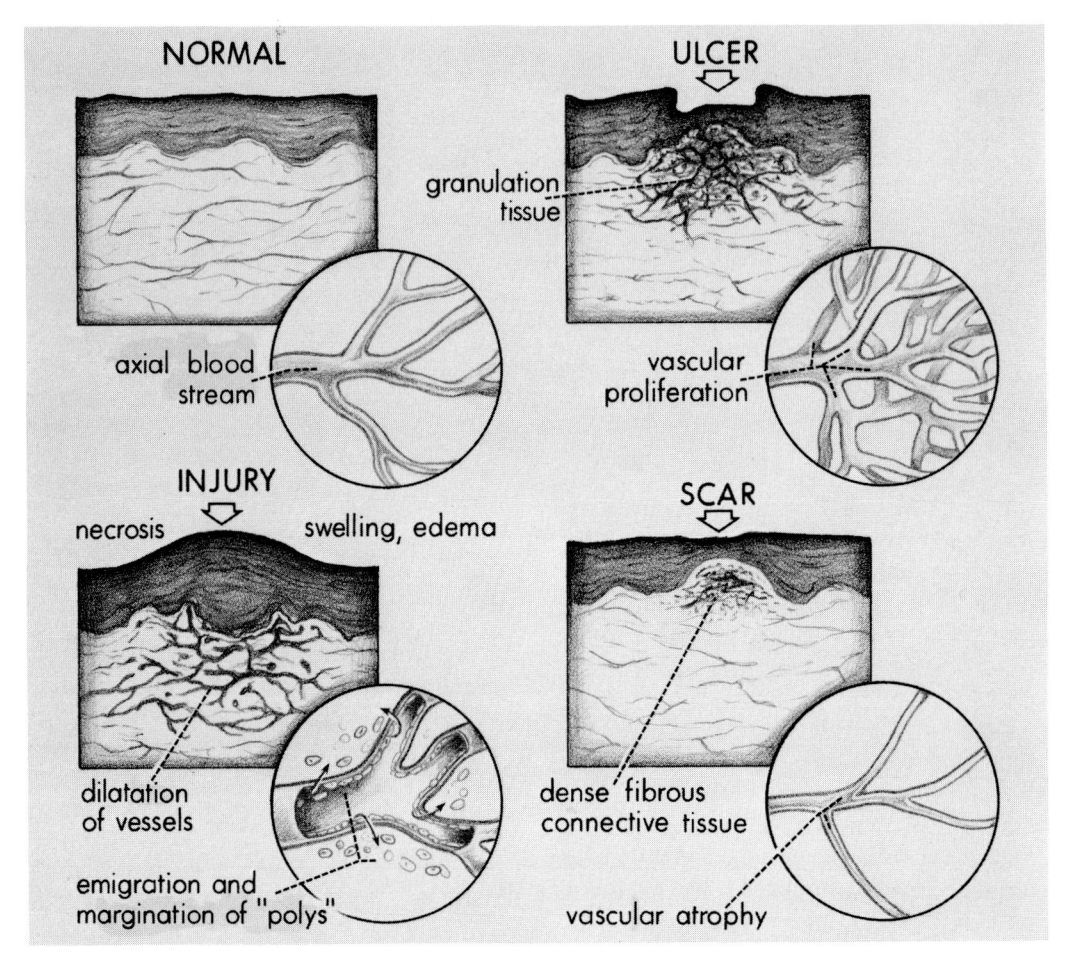

Fig. 4–2. Response to injury. Schematic representation of vascular, cellular and reparative processes.

The vasodilatation accompanying increased permeability of postcapillary venules results in passage of fluids (transudation) into the surrounding tissues where the fluid tends to accumulate (edema). By definition transudates are low-protein extravascular fluids with a specific gravity of less than 1.012. The shift of water, ions and small amounts of serum proteins, and cells is called *exudation*, and the combination of fluid, proteins, and cells is called an *exudate*. By definition exudates are high-protein fluids having a specific gravity of more than 1.020 and contain cells.

The vascular response to injury involves vascular dilatation and a decrease in the velocity of blood flow through the microvascular system. At the same time there is an increase in vascular permeability, and increased lymph flow. These reactions provide plasma proteins for the isolation of infectious organisms, as well as antibacterial substances and mediators of the inflammatory process.

Changes in vascular permeability result from a number of factors, including direct injury to the vessels as a result of the irritant, increased hydrostatic pressure in the microvascular system, and an increase in the size of the junctions between the endothelial cells lining the inner aspects of the walls of postcapillary venules. Ordinarily these small vessels are permeable only to small molecules, salt, and water necessary for local tissue function. But with an injury the junctions between the endothelial cells open, allowing plasma proteins and large molecules to escape into the tissues. Interendothelial gaps in venules result primarily because the endothelia of venules behave like smooth muscle, that is, they contract via microtubules and fibrils, which involves the contractile protein actomyosin. Probably cAMP (cyclic adenosine triphosphate), with the enzyme which forms it, adenyl cyclase, regulates the contraction process.

Biochemically active substances which may mediate the early increase in vascular permeability are primarily the vasoactive amines, *histamine* and *serotonin*. Histamine is found in mast cells and serotonin in blood platelets. *Prostaglandins* (PGE) are also mediators of the vascular permeability and are often present during the later stages of inflammation. Other chemical mediators of the vascular response are *thromboxanes* (platelet aggregating and vasoconstrictor factor) and *leukotreines* (factors involved in leukocyte adhesion to vessel walls, neutrophil chemotaxis, and vascular permeability).

The principal mediators in the blood plasma that affect vascular permeability are kinins and plasma-protein fractions of complement (p. 80). Following injury or exposure to an irritant, these mediators activate precursors of other mediators such as histamine in the granules of tissue mast cells. Thus, inactive precursors of the initial phase of acute inflammation are activated when the appropriate stimulus (injury) is present. However, the concept that the mast cell functions essentially by releasing granules containing histamine and other mediators is highly simplistic. Tissue mast cells are also effectors of certain hypersensitivity reactions which may follow a bee sting or penicillin injection in an allergic individual (p. 87).

In summary, the mediators of the vascular events in the micro-circulation during acute inflammation include an amine such as histamine, a peptide such as the kinins or complement fragments, or an acidic lipid such as a prostaglandin. The activation of the complement system (p. 80), whether by immune complexes or non-specific reactions, results in the release of mediators which are important to the inflammatory reaction. These mediators result in increased vascular permeability as well as activation of the PMNs and macrophages.

Cellular Response

After vasodilatation occurs and more blood flows into an area (active hyperemia), the rate of flow decreases and white blood cells migrate to the periphery of the vessels (margination) where they appear to adhere to the walls of the vessels (endothelium). The white blood cells (PMNs) move through the vessel wall (emigration), which is made possible by increased permeability of the vessel wall, and migrate to the site of injury (Fig. 4–2). The migration of leukocytes reaches a peak in 4 to 6 hours and then gradually declines. The migration of monocytes starts in about 4 hours and reaches a peak in 20 to 24 hours. White blood cells are directed toward the area of injury or injurious agents by a process called *chemotaxis*. The chemotactic factors are derived from cells, plasma, and tissues. The most active chemotactic substances for neutrophilic granulocytes include complement, kinins, prostaglandins, lysosomal products from neutrophils, lymphokines, and bacterial products. Most of these substances are also chemotactic for monocytes.

At the site of injury the cellular infiltrate (initially PMNs and later monocytes and lymphocytes) is mobilized to neutralize, destroy, and surround the injurious agent; however, viruses tend to bypass the PMN phase. A significant aspect of the cellular response is phagocytosis by both neutrophils and monocytes.

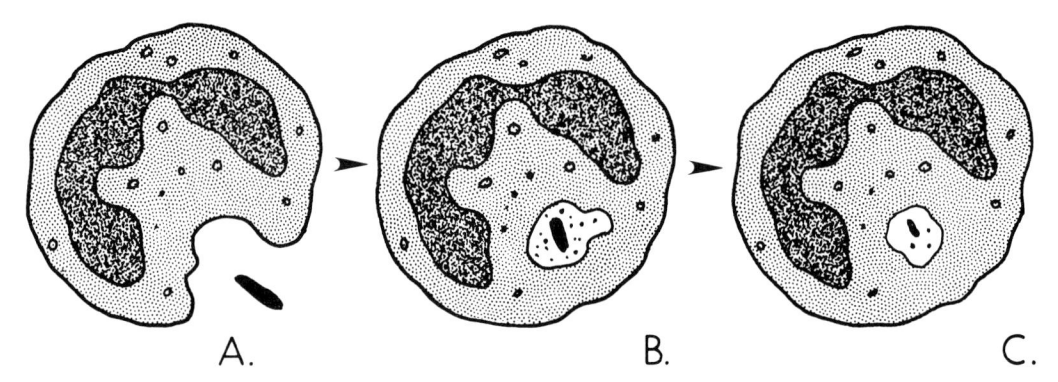

Fig. 4–3. Phagocytosis by polymorpholeukocyte. A, small bacterium is engulfed after coming into contact with the PMN. B, the cell membrane of the PMN invaginates and encloses the bacterium. C, then lysosomes fuse within the invagination, releasing cytocidal agents.

Phagocytosis

Phagocytosis is the ability of certain cells to engulf and degrade bacteria and larger particles in an area of injury (Fig. 4–3). There are two major cells which are capable of phagocytosis: macrophages and polymorphonuclear leukocytes; the latter are sometimes referred to as microphages. Macrophages are derived from monocytes which are formed from a precursor cell in the bone marrow. Monocytes spend about 20 to 30 hours in the blood stream. The monocyte enters a variety of tissue compartments to become macrophages. Thus, macrophages are found as free cells in connective tissue and in dispersed collections referred to as the mononuclearphagocyte system (also reticuloendothelial system or lymphoreticular system) which includes central lymphoid tissues (thymus and bone marrow) and peripheral lymphoid tissues such as the spleen, tonsils, liver, lymph nodes, and gastrointestinal tract lymphoid tissue (e.g., Peyer's patches). In contrast to polymorphonuclear leukocytes, which uually die soon after phagocytosis and destruction of bacteria, macrophages may survive for months or even years with phagocytosed material in them. Macrophages engulf much larger particles than the PMN, are capable of mitotic division in the area of inflammation, and can resynthesize the enzymes and structures lost during phagocytosis and digestion.

Bacteria or particles are digested by lysosomal enzymes, of which there are more than 40. Phagocytes require at least three basic types of lysosomal enzymes: A lipase to break down the lipid cell membrane; an acid protease to break down protein; and nucleases to break down the nucleic acids DNA and RNA. Bacteria are killed intracellularly by a number of mechanisms, including high acidity in phagosomes, free halide radicals (iodide or chloride), hydrogen peroxide and lysosomes.

During the engulfing of bacteria some of the lysosomes from the phagocyte may be secreted extracellularly into the tissues of the host instead of simply engulfing microorganisms. Thus tissue damage in acute inflammation is caused primarily by lysosomal enzymes released from neutrophils, not by the direct action of the microorganisms.

Polymorphonuclear leukocytes and macrophages ingest bacteria and foreign particles without having previous contact with foreign substances. However, phagocytosis is enhanced when the foreign particle or microorganism is coated with chemical substances (antibodies) which have been produced by the body in response to contact with the alien particles (immune response). Therefore phagocytosis is en-

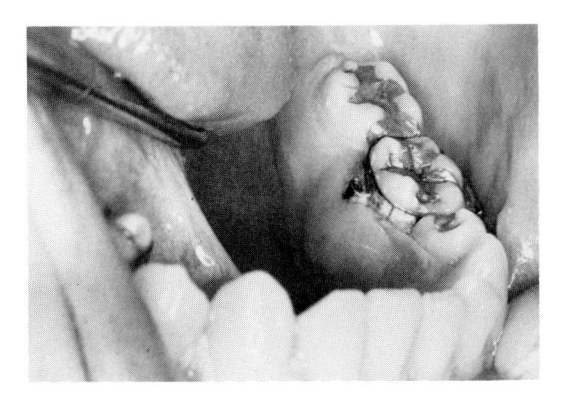

Fig. 4-4. Periodontal abscess resulting from position of orthodontic band on the mandibular first molar.

hanced if the targeted antigen (bacteria, particle, debris, etc.) is covered by host derived protein substances (antibody) which act as "glue" or an attachment mechanism between the particle and the phagocyte (see Fig. 5-4).

At the site of injury, enzymes are liberated into the tissues that digest the fibrin precipitated from the tissue fluid as well as dead cells and bacteria in the area. At the same time macrophages are ingesting cellular debris and foreign material. The liquefaction of the fibrin, dead cells, and bacteria, and the elimination of the cell debris by the macrophages, cause the area of injury to soften and become fluid in character. This liquefied material, which contains large numbers of dead neutrophils and cell debris, is *pus*. The process of forming pus is called *suppuration*. An *abscess* is the accumulation of pus in a localized area (Fig. 4-4). If an abscess develops near the surface of the skin, mucosa or gingiva, the accumulated pus may escape or drain to the exterior and thereby provide for rapid elimination of the dead material. If the pus is deep in the tissues and cannot escape, the fluid portion diffuses into the blood vessels and lymphatics to be carried from the site of injury to other parts of the body for complete destruction. An extensive accumulation of pus in the facial spaces associated with pulp disease and an alveolar abscess may require surgical incision and drainage.

Basic types of inflammatory response are indicated by the nature of the exudate produced and are designated accordingly. A *serous exudate* is due to an outpouring of a large amount of fluid in the early stage of the response. It is high in protein but low in fibrinogen. This process typically occurs in body cavities lined by serosa. It is the type of response produced by the pleura, the pericardium, and the peritoneum. In other responses there is abundant fluid but the fluid is high in fibrinogen so that fibrin is precipitated onto a tissue surface. Such an exudate is designated a *fibrinous exudate* and is seen in the same locations as serous exudates. If an exudate contains many red cells, it is a *sanguineous* or *hemorrhagic exudate*. This is produced when the permeability of the vessels is intense. *Mucinous* or *catarrhal exudates* are produced by tissues having the ability to produce mucin. Large quantities are produced by the cells to protect a body surface against irritants. It is seen in the respiratory and digestive tracts where the mucosa normally produces mucin and the physiologic capacity is exaggerated in response to mucosal injury. Upper respiratory infection with bronchitis is an excellent example of a catarrhal inflammation.

Purulent inflammation in some cases results in an intense liquefaction process and diffuse spread of the inflammation through the tissue which has been called cellulitis. When mucosal surfaces are injured by highly toxic agents, intracellular coagulation necrosis results and abundant fibrin is precipitated in the necrotic tissue and on the surface to form a membrane-like covering to the area of injury. This process may be initiated by the toxin of the diphtheria bacilli. The process is diphtheritis and the covering membrane is a pseudo- or diphtheritic membrane. Such a pseudomembrane typifies diphtheria and acute necrotizing ulcerative gingivitis (Fig. 4-5).

Any of the inflammatory responses may

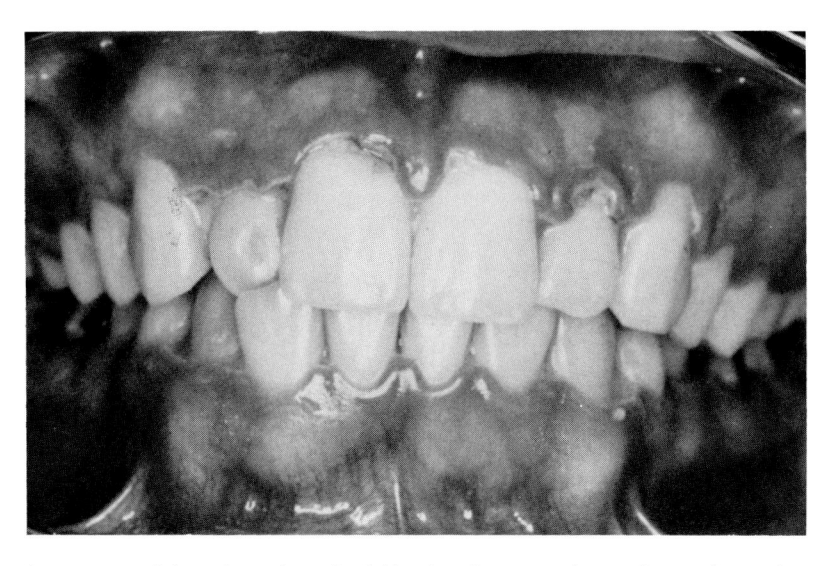

Fig. 4–5. Acute necrotizing ulcerative gingivitis showing pseudomembrane formation.

be present at various stages of activity. If only the alterative and exudative processes are present, the stage of inflammation is acute, the course is rapid, and the classical signs that are evident are often associated with sudden, intense constitutional symptoms. The process may subside or may progress to a subacute or chronic inflammation.

Subacute inflammation demonstrates active acute inflammation with some evidence of fibrous proliferation heralding the beginning of repair. It is an intermediate stage between acute and chronic.

HEMOSTASIS, COAGULATION, AND FIBRINOLYSIS

An important aspect of the vascular response in inflammation is the activation of several homeostatic mechanisms which facilitate repair of the tissues. The formation of fibrin resulting from the process of blood coagulation serves to retard the spread of infectious agents by blocking the lymphatics leading away from an area of inflammation, and to provide a scaffolding for macrophages and a framework for the repair process, i.e., fibrin acts as a scaffolding on which fibroblasts lay down collagen.

Hemostasis can be divided into stages: transient neurogenic vasoconstriction of the injured vessel, formation of a platelet plug, blood coagulation, clot retraction, and clot dissolution.

The process of hemostasis begins with the constriction of the size of the vessel and reduction of blood flow. The next phase results in the adherence of platelets to the vessel wall and formation of a mass of platelets (platelet or hemostatic plug) in the vessel. The platelet plug is cemented together with the fibrin clot which then contracts to pull the walls of the injured vessel together.

Platelets are cytoplasmic fragments from bone marrow cells (megakaryocytes) that find their way into the circulating blood. The primary function of platelets is adhesion, i.e., the sticking of platelets to a nonplatelet surface. When the endothelial lining of a vessel is injured blood platelets become sticky and adhere to the site of vessel injury; the platelets release their granules in response to such factors as plasmin, collagen, thrombin, and antigen-antibody complexes; and a platelet activating factor is released by basophils and mast cells. In a normal vessel a substance is present which prevents platelet aggregation by increasing

Table 4–2. Coagulation Factors

Factor I	Fibrinogen
Factor II	Prothrombin
Factor III	Tissue thromboplastin
Factor IV	Calcium
Factor V	Labile factor
Factor VI	No longer designated
Factor VII	Stable factor
Factor VIII	Antihemophilic globulin
Factor IX	Plasma thromboplastin component, Christmas factor
Factor X	Stuart-Prower factor
Factor XI	Plasma thromboplastin antecedent
Factor XII	Hageman factor
Factor XIII	Fibrin stabilizing factor

the concentration of cyclic adenosine monophosphate (cAMP).

The role of platelets in inflammation includes contributions to clotting, i.e., release of lysosomes, clot promoting factors and serotonin, temporary sealing of vessels which provides a basis for endothelial repair, and production of prostaglandins.

After the formation of the platelet plug the third stage of hemostasis involving blood coagulation occurs. In the process of coagulation strands of fibrin are formed which create a meshwork for cementing components of the blood together. The process of blood coagulation is a stepwise procedure involving twelve factors (Table 4–2) which involve activation of intrinsic or extrinsic pathways or both (Fig. 4–6). The intrinsic pathway occurs in the blood vessels and the extrinsic pathway occurs in the tissues. The intrinsic pathway is activated when the blood makes contact with the wall of the injured vessel, and the extrinsic pathway is activated when the blood is exposed to the tissue fluids.

Coagulation is activated by Hageman factor XII and has been described as the cascade sequence. Activated factor XII (XIIa) in turn activates factor XI which functions as a proteolytic enzyme and converts factor IX into an active enzyme (IXa). Then factor IXa combines with factor VIII, and the presence of divalent calcium ions, platelet factor 3 (platelet phospholipid) and factor V, factor X is activated. Factor X can be activated also by interacting with factor VII,

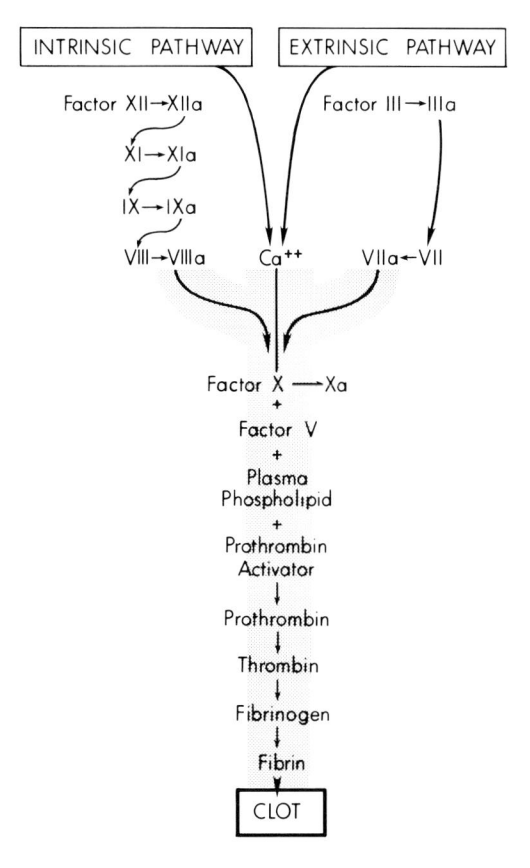

Fig. 4–6. Blood coagulation. Schematic representation of intrinsic and extrinsic pathways in blood coagulation. The final steps for both pathways converts fibrinogen to fibrin and the matrix of the blood clot.

calcium, and thromboplastin. Tissue thromboplastin comes from injured cells of several types. The activated factor X, whether derived from the intrinsic or extrinsic pathway or both, forms a complex with factor V, calcium ions and platelet factor 3 which converts prothrombin to thrombin. The thrombin converts fibrinogen into fibrin. The second enzyme involved in the transformation of soluble fibrinogen to insoluble fibrin is factor XIII.

Factor XII is also critical for activating kinins for vasodilatation, complement in the complement cascade (p. 80), and for activation of plasmin (fibrinolysin). Plasmin is the active form of plasminogen, the proenzyme for the fibrolytic process. Plasmin (fibrinolysin) degrades fibrin and results in dissolution of the clot. Plasmin also degrades factor V and VIII as well as hormones such as ACTH. Thus the fibrinolytic system is necessary for the eventual removal of fibrin and elimination of fibrin which has been a temporary basis for repair and fibrosis.

Abnormal Clotting

Clotting disorders include those related to hypercoagulation and bleeding disorders. Hypercoagulation disorders include disturbances in number and function of platelet and acceleration of clotting. Hemostasis is dependent upon an adequate number of functioning platelets, functional endothelium and a complete coagulation system.

Platelet activity is increased in atherosclerosis, diabetes mellitus, smoking, and elevated levels of blood cholesterol. Factors that increase the activity of the coagulation system include, disturbed blood flood and alterations in coagulation components. For example, blood coagulation factors are increased in women using oral contraceptives, and myocardial infarction and stroke are more frequent in women using oral contraceptives. Also malignant diseases increase clotting activity and contribute to increased incidence of thrombosis (p. 23). The basis of the platelet thrombus is the platelet adhesion-agglutination reaction. Low doses of aspirin seem to decrease the risk of thrombus formation, i.e., low doses of aspirin inhibit thromboxane synthesis. Thromboxane is a potent platelet aggregating agent.

Bleeding Disorders

Defects in platelets and coagulation factors can also result in bleeding disorders or impairment of blood coagulation. Platelet function may be impaired if there is a severe reduction of the number of platelets in the circulation (i.e., 20,000 compared to 200,000/mm^3 of blood). A number of drugs interfere with platelet production or function, including alcohol, antihistamines, anticancer drugs, aspirin, diuretics, lidocaine, nonsteroidal anti-inflammatory drugs, penicillins, propranolol, quinidine, sulfonamides, tricyclic antidepressants and vitamin E. Thrombocytopenia (reduced platelet numbers) may occur because of decreased production in the bone marrow or excessive pooling of platelets in the spleen (i.e., more than 40%). In splenomegaly (enlarged spleen) up to 70 to 80% of the platelets may be pooled in the spleen.

Abnormalities of blood coagulation may occur from impaired coagulation factors synthesized in the liver, and factor VIII which is synthesized in endothelial cells. Factors VII, IX, X and prothrombin require the presence of vitamin K for normal function. A deficiency of vitamin K may occur with continued use of broad spectrum antibiotics that significantly reduces the intestinal flora, which is important for synthesis of vitamin K. Vitamin K deficiency may also result if there is impaired absorption of vitamin K due to gallbladder or liver disease.

Disseminated intravascular clotting (DIC) is a complication of a number of disorders in which blood coagulation, clot dissolution and bleeding all take place at the same time. About 50% of patients with DIC have obstetric problems. DIC may occur with burns, malignant disease, shock and other diseases.

Hereditary defects in coagulation factors include most commonly: disturbances in factor VIII (classic hemophilia), factor IX (Christmas disease) and factor XI (hemophilia C). Factor VIII defects account for three-fourths of all cases of hemophilia, and Christmas disease for about 15 to 20% of hemophilia.

Chronic Inflammation

Chronic inflammation is a persistent inflammatory response which occurs when the body defenses are inadequate or because of the nature of the irritant; however, the dividing line between acute and chronic inflammation is not always clear. In many

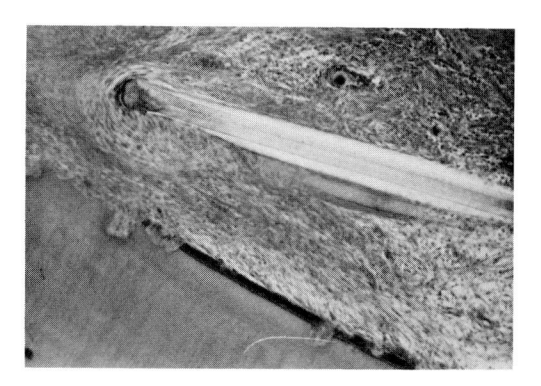

Fig. 4–7. Giant cell response to toothbrush bristle in gingiva adjacent to tooth.

cases an immune response is involved, the purpose of which is to identify and bind the irritant, treat it as a foreign substance (antigen), and activate macrophages. When the causative agent is nonantigenic (does not cause an immune response) such as an insoluble substance, macrophages (multinucleated giant cells) are present in large numbers. Generally lymphocytes, monocytes and plasma cells are the predominant cells in chronic inflammation. Chronic inflammation is seen in a number of diseases such as periodontal diseases, rheumatoid arthritis, and tuberculosis.

Recurrent attacks of acute inflammation may extend over years with bouts of pain and fever. Such organs as the gallbladder, kidney, and large intestine are prone to this kind of chronicity. However, except for evidence of healing between the episodes of inflammation, the tissues show primarily what would be expected to be presented following subsidence of acute inflammation.

The picture of other types of chronic inflammation may reflect less connection with acute inflammation, i.e., no significant infiltration of polymorphonuclear leukocytes into the area of injury and the absence of cardinal manifestations of inflammation. Rather, the response of the tissues is the proliferation of fibroblasts and vascular structures, not the formation of exudates.

In a form of chronic inflammation, which is called *granulomatous inflammation,* the

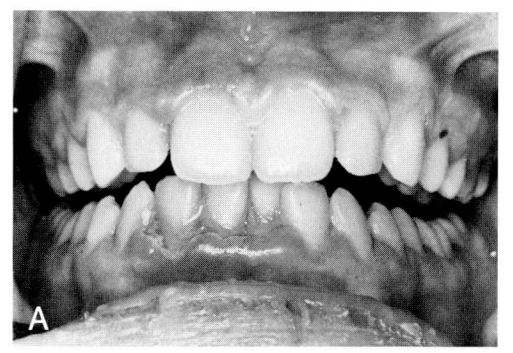

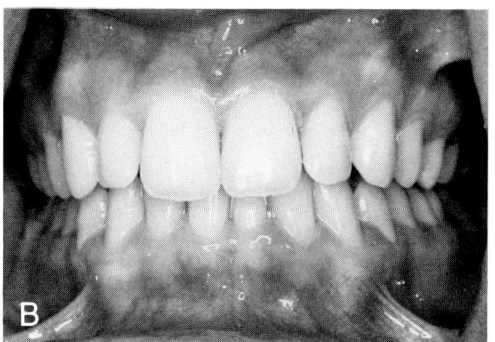

Fig. 4–8. Resolution of acute inflammation and repair. A, acute necrotizing ulcerative gingivitis. B, resolution of inflammation and repair of periodontal tissue following removal of plaque and calculus from the teeth.

typical lesion is composed of monocytes and their derivatives, i.e., macrophages (epithelioid cells), often in the form of multinucleate cells, and lymphocytes. There is a proliferation of connective tissue which eventually encapsulates the lesion and isolates it. These lesions are called *granulomas.* The classic granuloma-associated disease is tuberculosis. Chronic inflammation is associated with foreign bodies such as splinters, sutures, and toothbrush bristles (Fig. 4–7), as well as with diseases caused by microorganisms, including syphilis, leprosy, fungal infections, and parasitic infestations.

HEALING: REPAIR AND REGENERATION

The resolution of inflammation and the degree to which the tissues can be restored to normal architecture is very much dependent upon the extent to which the parenchymal cells can be replaced and arranged as they were originally. Repair may involve regeneration of mesenchymal and epithelial elements to the extent that the normal architecture is approximately restored (Fig. 4–8). If regeneration is not possible because of inherent characteristics of the cells or because of tissue factors, healing will occur by fibrinous replacement of normal structures by scar tissues. When injured tissues are replaced by functional tissue of the type destroyed, it is regeneration.

Regeneration

The complete regeneration of highly specialized tissues such as the heart, kidney, brain, and lung is not possible although partial regeneration of some specialized tissues like skeletal muscle is possible. Each type of cell possesses different abilities to undergo regeneration. The principal requirement for complete regeneration of the epithelial cells of the lung, kidney, and glands is an intact basement membrane. Regeneration of the liver depends upon a number of factors, including the blood supply and the size of the area of injury. Connective tissue, blood vessels, surface epithelium, and blood forming tissues have a marked ability to regenerate. Nerves, bone (not bones), and cartilage (not cartilaginous structures like the nose or joint discs) have a moderate ability, but nerve cells of the central nervous system have no ability to regenerate nor do adult cardiac muscle cells. When regeneration is not possible, scar tissue usually develops.

Fibroblasts have the ability following injury to divide to form new cells and regenerate their tissue architecture, synthesize collagen, become a tissue histiocyte capable of phagocytosis, or become a lipid-storing cell.

Healing by Primary Intention

Healing by first intention refers to healing of wounds in which there is minimal tissue

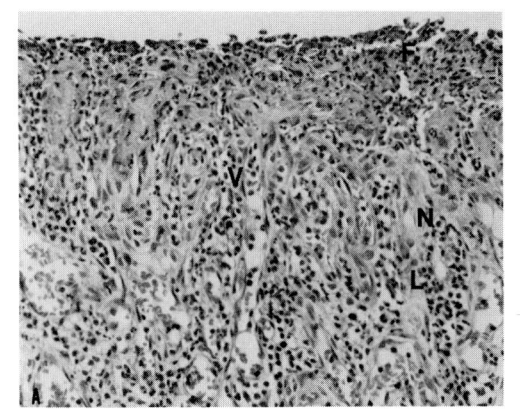

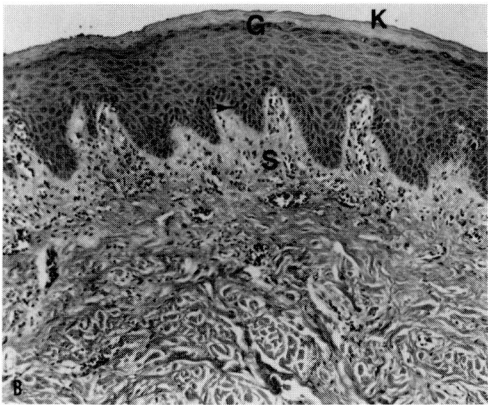

Fig. 4–9. *A, Granulation tissue of an ulcer;* fibrin membrane with entrapped cell debris (F); newly formed vascular channels growing into fibrin (V); new fibroblasts (N); leukocytes (L), chiefly polymorphonuclear cells. *B, Mature scar* surfaced by hyperplastic hyperkeratotic epithelium; keratin layer (K), granular layer (G), division figure (→), maturing scar (S) in subepithelial layer.

loss, i.e., a surgical incision with clean, apposable edges that can be closed with sutures. Such wounds quickly fill with fibrin and platelet clot which is infiltrated in a matter of 1 to 2 days with PMNs and then in the next day or two with mononuclear cells. By the fifth day newly formed collagen is present. Thus the wound is closed by fibroblast migration in the fibrin clot formation of new connective tissue and blood vessels, and by covering of the surface with new epithelium which forms from the epithelium at the periphery (sutured edges).

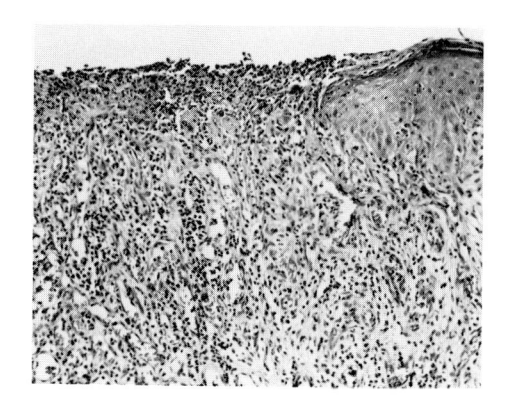

Fig. 4–10. *Granulation tissue* at the border of a healing ulcer. *Regenerating epithelium* at upper right.

Healing by Secondary Intention

When there has been significant loss of tissue so that the skin or mucous membranes or organ tissues cannot be approximated by sutures, the wound heals by secondary intention, i.e., granulation tissue (Fig. 4–9A) fills the defect and then the surface is re-epithelized, beginning at the edge of the wound and migrating to the center (Fig. 4–10). The repair begins with elimination of dead cells by monocytic phagocytes and proliferation of fibroblasts on the fibrin scaffold. Also there is a proliferation of capillary endothelial buds with the developing fibroblasts. The presence of monocytes and lymphocytes aids the immune response.

Scar Tissue

When organization of the wound is complete and the defect has been replaced with granulation tissue, there is an increase in extracellular collagen, the inflammatory cells disappear, and the small blood vessels eventually disappear as well (Fig. 4–9B). The collagen matures and shortens, leading to contraction of the wound. Finally, scar tissue consists of much collagen, few blood vessels, and when involving the skin, may have only a thin covering of dermis which does not have the same coloration as adjacent skin. An excess of granulation tissue is sometimes referred to as "proud flesh." Continued production of scar tissue results in a *keloid*. Where an exudate involves two contacting surfaces of body cavities, organization of the two surfaces may lead to union of the surfaces and is called *adhesion*. Adhesions occur chiefly in pericardial and pleural cavities and adhesions here may cause pain and other complications.

Bone Repair

The term *bone* is used to identify a specialized form of mesenchymal tissue, i.e., an osseous form of connective tissue. It is also a term for bones, i.e., specific bones such as the lower jaw bone (mandible) or a long bone of the leg such as the femur. Three forms of functional bone cells are recognized: *osteoblasts* which provide the asteoid matrix which becomes mineralized; *osteocytes* which transform into osteoblasts when necessary for formation of bone, and which are sequestered in bony lacunae until needed; and *osteoclasts* which are active in the process of bone resorption, i.e., dissolution of mineralized and lysis of bone matrix.

Fractures of bones are healed by two processes: flat bones or solid bones are healed by intramembranous ossification and long bones by endochondral ossification (Fig. 4–11). Healing of a long bone occurs in stages: (1) formation of a *procallus,* i.e., a form of granulation tissue produced by fibroblasts and capillary buds and involved in the organization of the hemorrhage associated with the fracture; (2) the development of the *fibrocartilaginous callus,* i.e., entry of osteoblasts into the area to form fibrocartilage; and (3) conversion of the fibrocartilaginous callus into osseous bone or *osseous callus*.

SUMMARY

Inflammation is a multicellular response to injury that involves vascular and cellular phenomenon directed toward the isolation and elimination of the injurious agent and

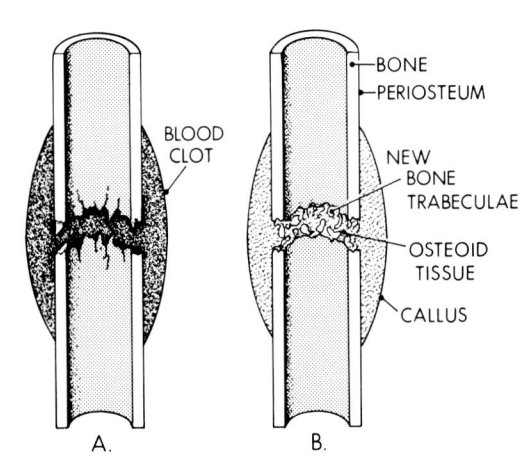

Fig. 4–11. Repair of a long bone which has been fractured. The fracture (A) heals by endochondral ossification (B) arising from cartilage. Initially the healing involves the organization of the hemorrhage (A) and the formation of a procallus from invading fibroblasts and budding capillaries. Osteoblasts are derived from the periosteum and new cartilage and osteoid are formed, converting the procallus to a fibrocartilaginous callus which is converted to osseous callus.

the repair of injured tissues. The initial phase of acute inflammation consists of a hemodynamic phase wherein capillary permeability is increased and there is an increase in white blood cells (e.g., polymorphonuclear leukocytes) in the area. A number of chemical mediators are responsible for changes in vessel permeability as well as attracting phagocytic leukocytes (PMNs) to the injurious agents such as bacteria. Much of the tissue damage done during acute inflammation is a consequence of the release of lysosomal enzymes from the polymorphonuclear leukocyte (neutrophil, PMN). Lymphocytes also release chemical mediators (lymphokines) which are important in the immune response (cf. p. 83) as well as in inflammation.

Acute inflammation may be resolved with a self-limiting injurious agent or one that is controlled satisfactorily by the defense mechanisms. When the injury is perpetuated, the inflammatory process may last for weeks, months, or years. Such chronic inflammation is seen when the body defenses are inadequate. Usually an immune response is involved and lymphocytes and plasma cells predominate. In some instances where the injurious agent is not an allergic substance or antigen (cf. p. 77), macrophages may be present in large numbers. In chronic inflammation there is proliferation of vascular structures and fibroblasts rather than exudates (e.g. purulent, hemorrhagic, serous) which occur in acute inflammation. A special kind of chronic inflammation is granulomatous inflammation which is seen in infections with microorganisms such as the tubercle bacillus. Macrophages (giant cells) are seen frequently in the granulomatous inflammatory response.

The vascular response to injury includes hemostasis whereby bleeding is arrested by vasoconstriction, formation of a platelet plug, development of a fibrin clot, and clot retraction. This sequence of steps is integrated with the dissolution of the clot, reestablishment of blood flood, and repair of the tissues. Bleeding disorders associated with impaired platelet function, impaired synthesis of coagulation factors, hereditary defects, vascular disorders, and drugs may impair hemostasis and complicate responses to injury, especially when the injury is direct physical trauma.

Healing of injury to the body is dependent upon the replacement and organization of parenchymal cells. If these cells are fully replaced both structurally and functionally by the same or similar cells, regeneration of tissues, organs, and parts occurs. Tissues vary in their ability to regenerate according to the type of cells involved. Epithelial cells of the skin and gastrointestinal tract regenerate continually, whereas some cells like those in the liver only regenerate when the necessary stimulus is present, and some others cannot regenerate such as nerve cells. When a tissue is injured and connective tissue replaces the injured tissue because regeneration is not possible, the result is scar tissue. The response to injury may result in progressive and exaggerated reactive tissue changes which are discussed in Chapter 6.

BIBLIOGRAPHY

Ake, N., and Landt, H.: Hyperplasia of the oral tissues in denture cases. Acta Odont. Scand., 27:481, 1969.

Adams, D.O.: The granulomatous inflammatory response. Am. J. Pathol. 84:164, 1976.

Adams, D.O.: Macrophage activation and secretion. Fed. Proc., 41:2193, 1982.

Black, M.M., and Wagner, B.M.: *Dynamic Pathology*. St. Louis, C.V. Mosby Co., 1964.

Bostick, W.L.: The vascular-cellular dynamics of inflammation. Oral Surg., 2:425, 1949.

Bryant, W.M.: Wound healing. Clin. Symp. 3:1, 1977.

Dunphy, J.E., and Udupa, K.N.: Chemical and histochemical sequences in the normal healing of wounds. N. Engl. J. Med., 253:847, 1955.

Editorial: Reticuloendothelial function. J.A.M.A., 199:419, 1967.

Mason, R.G. and Saba, H.I.: Normal and abnormal hemostasis—an integrated view. A review. Am. J. Pathol., 92:775, 1978.

Menkin, V.: *Dynamics of Inflammation*. New York, The MacMillan Co., 1940.

Pierce, C.W.: Macrophages: modulators of immunity. Am. J. Pathol., 98:10, 1980.

Resistance to Infection. Therap. Notes, 73:8, 1966.

Robbins, S.L. and Cotran, R.S.: *Pathologic Basis of Disease*. Philadelphia, W.B. Saunders Co., 1979.

Rogers, P.D.: *Influenza Alert*. Philadelphia, F.A. Davis Co., 1976.

Ryan, G.E. and Majno, G.: Acute inflammation. A review. Am. J. Pathol., 86:247, 1977.

van Furth, R.: An approach to the characterization of mononuclear phagocytes involved in pathological processes. In: *Future Trends in Inflammation*. Vol. 2. J.P. Giroud (Ed.). Birkhäuser Verlag. Basel, Switzerland, 1976.

Warren, K.S.: A fundamental classification of granulomatous inflammation. In: Seventh International Conference on Sarcoidosis and Other Granulomatous Disorders. Louis E. Siltzbach, ed. Ann. N.Y. Acad. Sc., 278:7, 1976.

Wissler, R.W., Fitch, F.W., and Lavia, M.F.: The reticuloendothelial system in antibody formation. Ann. N.Y. Acad. Sci., 88:134, 1960.

Wound healing. Therap. Notes, 71:68, 1964.

5

IMMUNE RESPONSE AND IMMUNE INJURY

All living cells have imbedded in their surfaces molecules (recognition markers) that are uniquely specific, i.e., they are markers of biologic individuality. The recognition of the odor and taste of food is possible because molecules in the food fit the shape of specific receptors in our nose and taste organs. The same is true of a wide range of body processes which are controlled by the hormones which lock onto target cells through recognition molecules.

Such genetically determined recognition molecules are also basic to the body's immune system, i.e., the mechanisms by which the body defends against the introduction of molecularly identified structures that appear to post a threat to the internal environment of the host. If it were not for the body's ability to recognize its own cells through marker recognition molecules on cell membrane surfaces, the body might destroy itself. Immunologic recognition largely decides the fate of transplanted organs and tissues and is a significant part of the immune response to invading bacteria and viruses.

When bacteria and viruses gain entrance in a host, they are recognized as unwanted intruders by a group of molecules called antibodies (Ab). Thousands of different types of antibodies are produced by the immune system, each type of antibody formed to recognize a specific intruder. These antibodies (Ab) circulate through the body and bind to the foreign substances, whereupon immunocompetent cells (cells of the immune system capable of responding) engulf and digest the intruders or destroy them by secreted substances.

Of course the foregoing description of the immune system's response to agents of disease is an oversimplification of a complex network of interacting processes, and further clarification is necessary. An important aspect of the immune response involves *autoimmune diseases* where there is a problem in recognizing one's own body cells, and *immunodeficient* states where the immune response is compromised or inadequate to cope with an agent of disease.

IMMUNE SYSTEM

The *immune system* is a network of complex cellular and fluid (humoral) components that respond to the introduction of substances (including microorganisms) which are recognized as foreign to the host's internal environment. It has an important role in inflammation and repair and is the primary mediator in a number of diseases. Both the inflammatory response and immune reactions are defense mechanisms. Not only does the immune system protect against invasion by infectious agents, it may also protect against the proliferation of mutant cells. But paradoxically, all immunologic responses may not be beneficial, e.g., hypersensitivity (or allergy) reactions such as hay fever, bronchial asthma, contact dermatitis, and graft or transplanted organ rejection.

Cellular components of the immune system arise from stem cells in the bone marrow and differentiate into lymphocytes and monocytes. These cells respond to foreign substances such as infectious agents by provoking a humoral response or by interacting directly with the foreign substances to destroy or neutralize them. The *humoral* components of the immune system are substances produced by certain lymphocytes that participate in the defense reaction in a number of ways, e.g., neutralization of bacterial toxins (antitoxin), forming a "coating" (opsonization) on the surface of bacteria thereby facilitating their elimination (viz., phagocytosis), and activation of certain plasma proteins (complement) which damage cell membranes and cause lysis of bacterial cells.

Antigens

An immune response involves an interaction between the foreign agent (antigen or immunogen) introduced into the body and the production of antibodies (immunoglobulins). An *antigen* (Ag) is a foreign substance, usually a protein "recognized" as foreign, that induces an immune response. Common antigens include serum proteins, lipoproteins, food proteins, and polysaccharides on surfaces of bacteria. Some agents become antigenic if combined with a carrier protein. These types of antigens are called *haptens* and include such agents as house dust, plant pollens, and animal danders.

Immunity

Immune responses can be active or passive. The development of immunity against a specific agent may be achieved by actively having the disease *(active immunity)*. *Passive immunity* refers to a temporary immunity conferred on the basis of injections of an antiserum which contains antibodies for a specific disease. *Natural immunity* is species specific, i.e., humans do not have certain animal diseases and are thus immune to these diseases.

Characteristics of Immune Responses

From the foregoing it is obvious that the immune system must have three characteristics: (1) *self-recognition,* i.e., capability of distinguishing between "self" and "nonself," otherwise, the system would form antibodies against the body's own tissues (proteins); (2) *Immunologic memory,* i.e., the capability of the immune system to respond to an antigen even though a period of time has elapsed since the antibody was first formed in response to an antigen; and (3) *specificity,* i.e., recognition mechanisms by which an antibody reacts with a specific antigen. The antigenic determinants involve a small area of an antigen molecule which is the mirror image of a specific binding site on an antibody molecule. These complementary sites provide for binding of antigen to antibody and this antigen-antibody coupling mechanism results in the formation of an immune complex whereby the antigen is processed.

Genetic Control of Immune Response

The surfaces of most cells of the body contain surface antigens which are genetically determined by a single region of genes called the major histocompatibility complex (MHC). These surface antigens are markers by which the cells of an individual "recognize" and accept other cells from the same individual but at the same time reject cells from another person. The human major histocompatibility complex

CHROMOSOME 6

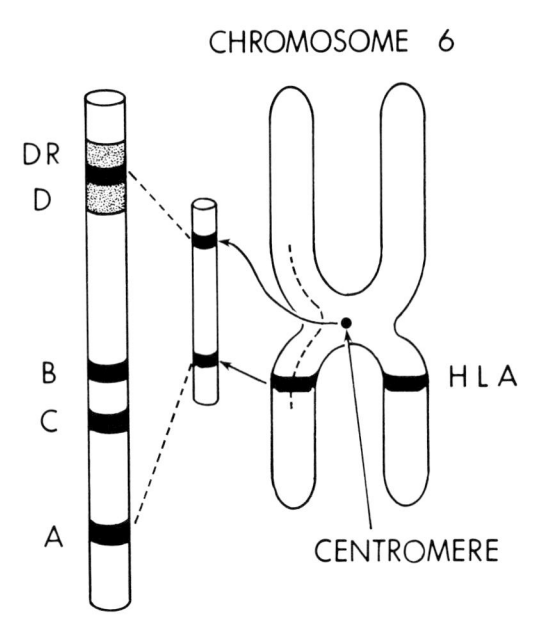

Fig. 5–1. The human leukocyte antigen (HLA) located on chromosome 6. The genes of the HLA system include four loci (HLA-A, B, C, and D) which control histocompatibility determinants. Each gene loci has multiple alleles. Associations and linkages have been established between a number of human diseases and the HLA system.

(HLA or human leukocyte antigen is the logo for the human MHC) comprises gene loci on chromosome 6 and designated as HLA-A, B, C and HLA-D/DR (Fig. 5–1). HLA-A, B, C are Class I molecules found on almost all cells. HLA-DR, and others such as MB, MT are class II molecules which are found on B cells and some monocytes but not T cells which are resting (not immunologically active).

HLA antigens are coded for each locus and are numbered. For example, the specific HLA antigen for ankylosing sypondylitis is HLA-B27 and is observed in 90% of the persons having the disease. The mechanism by which HLA inheritance determines disease has not been clarified, but the HLA complex provides the antigenic basis for disease susceptibility, regulatory effects on immune responses, and tissue transplant rejection. Genes of the MHC predispose to the development of autoimmune diseases (cf. p. 88), i.e., multiple genes influence immune responses in ways which depend on different combinations of genes from MCH loci. There is increasing evidence that multiple inherited factors are involved in the development of these diseases. The tendency for combinations of genes to be inherited together more than would be predicted by chance is known as *linkage disequilibrium*.

The typing of HLA in tissue grafting and organ transplantation is important in order to reduce the risk of organ or tissue rejection. An understanding of histocompatibility genes and their products may provide a mechanism for controlling immune responses that cause transplant rejection, as well as allergic (atopic) and autoimmune diseases.

Blood Group Antigens

Blood group antigens indicate the connection between specific blood types or blood group systems and the presence of antigens on the surface of red blood cells. The major groups making up the ABO system are A, AB, B, and O. It is important to identify specific blood types to avoid transfusion reactions. Another blood group system is Rh, which is important in hemolytic disease of the newborn. When a mother who has a Rh negative blood group is sensitized by red blood cells from a first baby with Rh antigens at the time of the birth because of the release of red blood cells into the mother via a placental bleed, antibodies are formed which cross the placenta at a subsequent pregnancy. The latter reaction causes hemolysis of the blood cells of the newborn and is called hemolytic disease of the newborn (erythroblastosis fetalis).

Antibodies

Antibodies, which are serum proteins called immunoglobulins (Ig), are produced by the body in response to the introduction of foreign substances (antigens). The immunoglobulin molecule consists of two parts or cleavage fragments that bind (attach to) antigen, called Fab (fragment an-

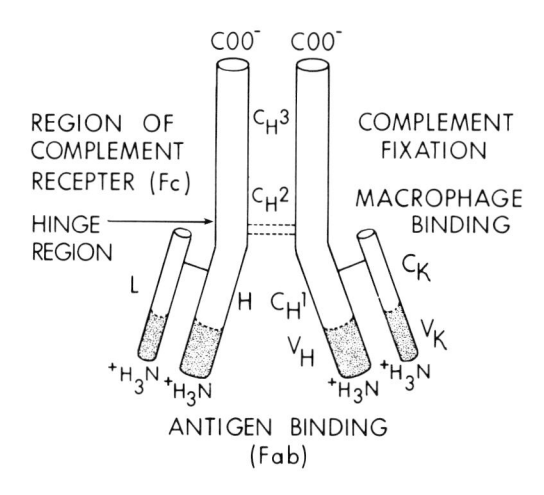

Fig. 5-2. Prototypic structure for an IgGl (κ) human antibody molecule. Each immunoglobulin contains at least one basic unit (monomer) composed of four polypeptide chains: two heavy chains (H) and two light chains (L), joined by disulfide bonds (dotted lines). The hinge region separates the Fab region from the Fc region. The variable (V) region (shaded area) and constant (C) region relate to the considerable heterogeneity and enormous diversity with respect to antigen binding and different biologic activities. Antigen binding activity is associated with Fab regions (V_H and V_L) whereas the Fc region is involved in the initiation of a number of secondary phenomenon, such as complement fixation (classic), release of histamine by mast cells, and passive binding of antibodies by macrophages which are then "armed" to function in a cytotoxic fashion.

tigen *binding*), and a third fragment, fragment complement (Fc), is the complement receptor region (Fig. 5-2). The ability of the immune system to generate enormous variants of the immunoglobulin structure that binds antigen—the variable region—sets it apart from all other biologic systems. Antibody producing lymphocytes use a language that consists of four symbols: V_H, V_L, C_H, and C_L, which are protein structures that are encoded genetically in the form of DNA. In DNA, V_L consists of two letters: V genes and J genes. And correspondingly for the two L chains (κ and λ) there are $V_κ$, $V_λ$, $J_κ$ and $J_λ$ genes. A similar alphabet encodes the V region of the H chains. A third group of letters consisting of D_H genes partici-

pates in forming the H chain variable region. A massive rearrangement of the immunologic alphabet occurs during differentiation of B lymphocytes, e.g., the cells destined to form antibodies. Rearranging a few hundred V, J and D genes provides for antibody specificities. The distinguishing feature of B cells is the rearrangement of immunoglobulin genes inasmuch as all other cells have the usual germ-line configuration. The molecular biology of immunoglobulin genes has clinical importance, viz., the identification of neoplastic lymphocytes that lack the conventional markers of either B or T cells-null cells (cf. p. 83). New methods of DNA hybridization can be used to distinguish B cells from T cells and B cells from cells that the pathologist cannot identify (e.g., a metastatic melanoma). DNA hybridization has led to a precise definition of lymphomas (see p. 129).

Five classes of immunoglobulins are found: IgA, IgG, IgM, IgD, IgE. IgA is the primary component of the defense mechanism of the mucous membranes. It is found in secretions from the mucous membranes in all parts of the respiratory and digestive tracts and provides local immunity by neutralizing infectious agents. IgA prevents bacterial adherence to mucous membranes and, more specifically, of S. mutans to dental plaque. IgG is the major component in most antibody responses. It functions as an antitoxin, opsonin, and neutralizes viruses in the blood stream. IgM is effective in complement activation (fixation) and thus aids in bacteriolysis. It is also important for agglutination (clumping) of bacteria. IgD is thought to play a role in immune tolerance, i.e., state in which substances normally considered to be antigenic fail to stimulate an immune response. IgE is the primary mediator of immediate hypersensitivity (p. 87), and is of importance in the defense against intestinal parasites.

Complement System

The complement system consists of serum proteins found in the circulating

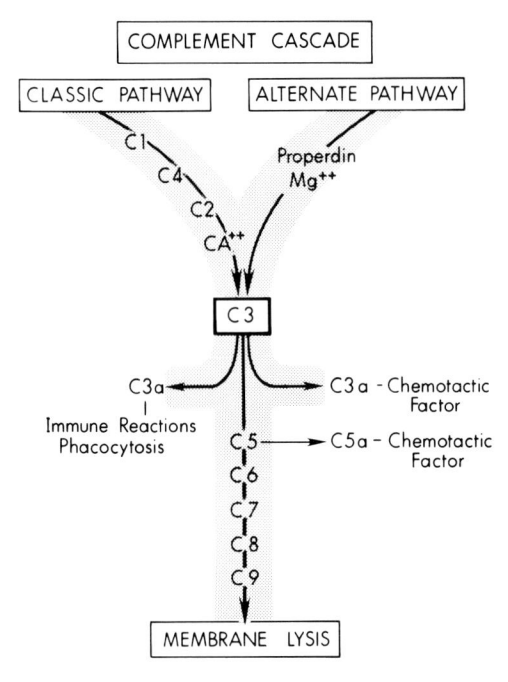

Fig. 5-3. The complement system consists of serum proteins that can lyse bacterial cells as a consequence of an antibody response. In addition to the antibody dependent system another system (alternate or properdin system), which is not dependent upon antibody, subserves a humoral cytolytic function which may be required to combat bacterial or viral infections before an antibody response is expressed. The end-point of this sequential array is the destruction of a target cell and while en route substances are produced that are involved in inflammations. C1 is the recognition unit (recognizes antibody and fixes to the F_c portion of the immunoglobulin).

blood in an inactive form that complement or cooperate with antibodies to destroy certain bacteria, mediate vascular responses (increase permeability) and recruit phagocytic cells (PMNs and macrophages). The major components, C1, C4, C2, C3, C5, C6, C7, C8, and C9, can be divided into a recognition unit, C1, in the classic pathway (Fig. 5-3), an activation unit, C4, C2, C3, and the membrane unit, C5 through C9.

When antibody combines with antigen or a microorganism the resultant antibody/antigen (Ab/Ag) complex triggers the cascade of reactions involving C1 through C9. The activation of complement, sometimes referred to as complement fixation because once started it continues until activity in a particular serum sample is no longer demonstrable, may occur via the "classical" or alternate pathway. The latter is triggered by the presence of a substance not of antibody nature. The cascade is in effect a cascade of enzyme reactions culminating in the activation of an esterase which can attack and dissolve the phospholipid wall of the membrane of cells and bacteria (cell lysis). Comparable cascades occur in blood clotting (coagulation), kinin formation, and fibrinolysis (p. 69), and like the complement system, have a complex system of inhibitors to control the potentially destructive nature of unregulated enzyme activities.

Cells of the Immune System

The cells of the immune system include not only those cells discussed in the inflammatory reaction, but also mononuclear phagocytes-*macrophages* and two other cells which have specific receptors for antigen and are responsible for specific immune responses. These two cells are: *B-lymphocytes,* which are involved in humoral immunity, and *T-lymphocytes,* which are effectors of cell-mediated immunity.

Macrophages

Mononuclear phagocytes, including monocytes and macrophages, are closely related to lymphocytes in the immune response. Macrophages are not only involved in phagocytosis, but "present" antigen to the lymphocyte, an essential step in the activation of the lymphocyte. In effect the phagocytosis and killing of microorganisms by macrophages occurs in response to sensitized lymphocytes (T-cells). Macrophages are involved in tissue repair, antigen recognition, and proliferation of lymphocytes.

There are two phases to phagocytosis: an attachment phase where the antigen (bacteria, viruses, etc.) is bound to the surface of the macrophage, and a phase where the antigen is taken into the macrophage and lysed. Phagocytosis is facilitated if the antigen has been coated (opsonized) with antibody and complement so that antigen can be bound by the Fc and C3 receptors on its surface (Fig. 5–4).

The surface of the phagocyte contains two special binding sites or receptors for opsonins; the Fc receptor which binds the IgG and IgM antibodies (p. 79) and the C3 receptor which attaches to the C3 component of complement (Fig. 5–4). Thus

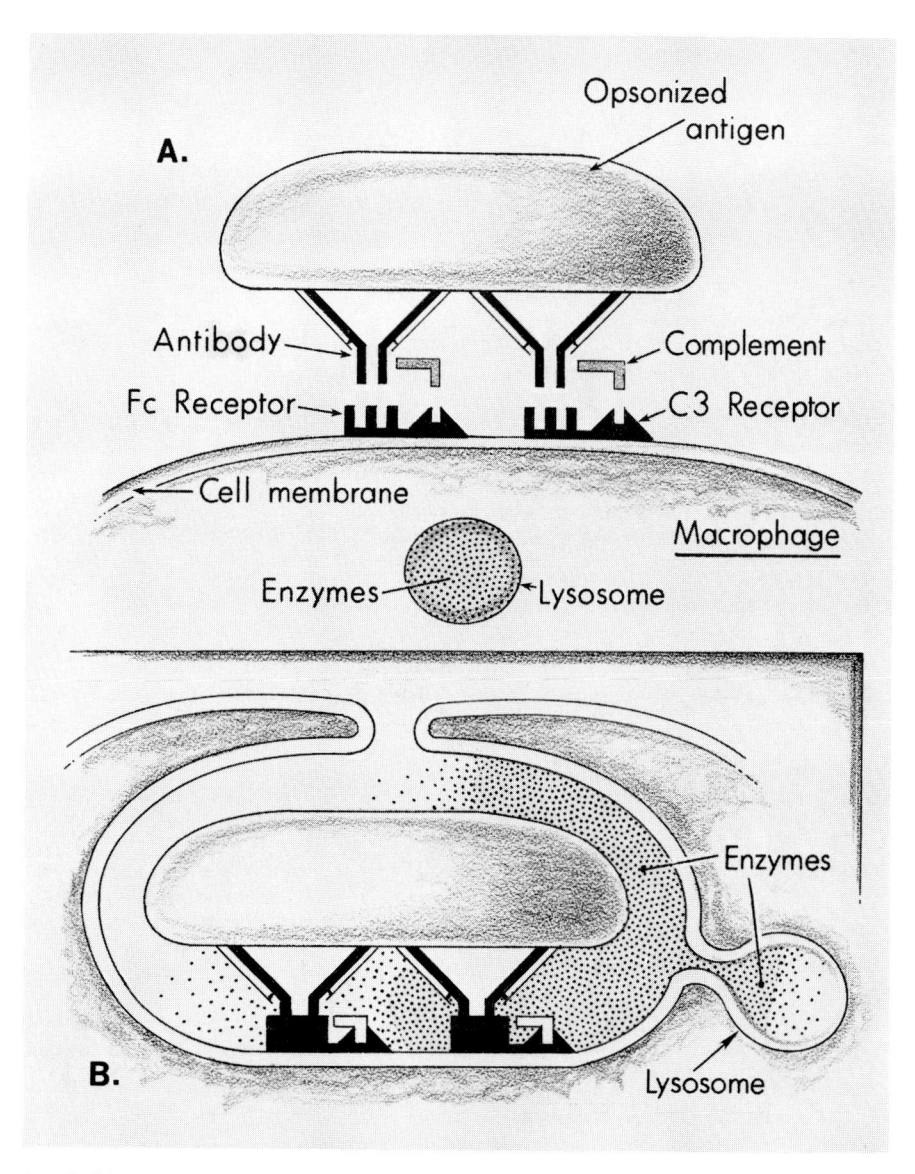

Fig. 5–4. *A*, Phagocytosis occurs with attachment through its cell membrane receptors (F$_c$ and C$_3$) to an antigen (microorganism, protein). This binding is facilitated by coating with antibody and complement (opsonization). *B*, after attachment to the membrane of the macrophage, the antigen is interiorized by invagination of the macrophage membrane and formation of a vacuole which merges with a lysosome. Lysosomal enzymes digest the antigen and fragments eliminated from the cell. A few adhere to the cell membrane of the phagocyte. Thus the macrophage is an antigen-processing and antigen-presenting cell.

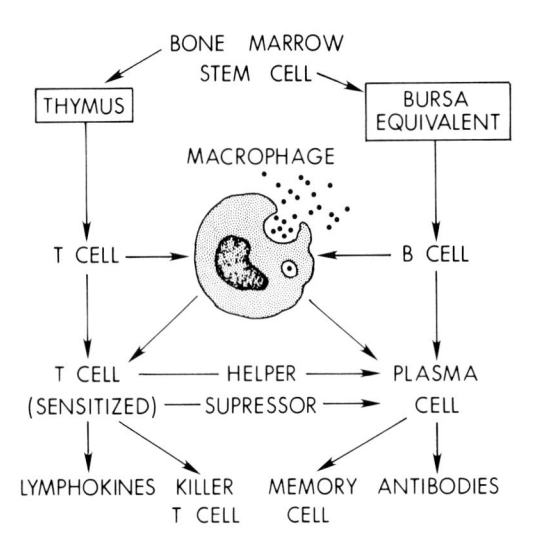

Fig. 5–5. Basis of cellular and humoral immunity (see text).

when opsonized material is bound to specific Fc receptors on the surface of the phagocyte a number of responses are triggered, including phagocytosis.

Bacteria or particulate matter are engulfed into the cytoplasm of the phagocyte by invagination of the cell membrane (Fig. 5–4) and formation of a cell-membrane lined vacuole (phagosome). Adjacent lysosomes, which are cytoplasmic vesicles filled with digestive enzymes, fuse with the phagosome, discharging the enzymes into it and forming a phagolysosome.

Lymphocytes

Lymphocytes arise from stem cells in bone marrow and then migrate either to the thymus or to a presumed equivalent of the bursa of Fabricius in birds, which is now thought to be bone marrow in humans (Fig. 5–5). In the thymus, *T-lymphocytes* (T-cells) acquire receptors by which antigens are recognized. After processing by the thymus, T-cells appear in peripheral lymphoid tissues (e.g., lymph nodes, spleen). Some T-cells circulate in the blood and lymphatic systems to maintain immunologic surveillance or "keep watch" for the need for increased defense activity. *B-lymphocytes* (B-cells) differentiate under the influence of the presumed human homologous bursa organ (bone marrow?) and then migrate to peripheral lymphoid tissue where they differentiate into plasma cells and become involved in antibody synthesis. T-cells are the basis for cell-mediated immunity and B-cells are the basis for humoral immunity.

It has been reported that the skin, like the thymus, might be a site where certain types of T-cells undergo maturation. Thus the skin is an integral and active element of the immune system.

On the surface of the T-cell are antigen-specific receptors which are not immunoglobulin (Ig) receptors, but the nature of the antigen-binding receptor remains to be clarified. Antigen binding by B-cells involves receptor sites which are antigen-specific immunoglobulin receptors on the surface membrane of the cell. When an antigen contacts and becomes bound to a receptor site of either B-cells or T-cells, a general cellular activation called blast transformation is triggered and proliferation of new cells occurs. The result of proliferation is the formation of antibody producing plasma cells from the B cells and sensitized lymphocytes derived from T-cells. The process of forming new cells in response to contact with an antigen also includes the proliferation of clones of memory and effector T-cells as well as clones of memory and effector B-cells.

There are two populations of T lymphocytes which are involved in cellular immune responses: *Regulator* T cells and *effector* T cells (Fig. 5–4). The regulator T cells either enhance or suppress the action of B cells, i.e., they develop into helper T-cells which enhance the proliferation of stimulated B-cells, or into suppressor T-cells that suppress proliferation of stimulated B-cells.

Effector T-cells include lymphocytes that release lymphokines (cf. p. 83) when they encounter antigen toward which they are sensitized, and cytotoxic T-cells (CTL) which kill target cells when, after immunization, the CTL responds to antigenic determinants (specific antigen and HLA or MHC antigen) on the target cell.

There are killer (K) cells which constitute a cytotoxic lymphocyte population that do not require immunization but depend for their effect upon the recognition and interaction with an appropriate antibody that has coated the target cell. These cells have receptors on their surface specific for the Fc portion of IgG molecules (Fc receptors) and permit T-cells to bind to target cells coated with IgG antibodies. K-cells kill nonspecifically, importantly tumor cells.

Another effector of immunologic cytolysis is the natural killer (N_K) or "null cell." The K and N_K cells have the same properties and, except for the circumstances which determine the function expressed, may be manifestations of the same cell. The natural killer cell mediates a cytotoxic reaction and appears without the need for sensitization, i.e., "naturally". It has been suggested that N_K cells, along with macrophages, provide the first line of defense against malignant cells. Null cells have been termed "non-T, non-B cells."

Humoral Immunity

When an antigen is first introduced into the host, a primary response occurs during which recognition of the antigen by the antibody occurs and a clone of plasma cells that will produce the antibody develops. The level (titer) of antibody in the blood reaches a peak about the time recovery from many infectious agents occurs. On a second exposure to the antigen the antibody titer reaches a higher level sooner. In addition to the antibody producing plasma cell, another cell called a "memory" cell is produced. This cell records the information necessary to produce specific antibodies at a subsequent exposure to the same antigen. A "booster shot" causes an almost immediate rise in antibody titer which is sufficient to prevent the disease.

Humoral or antibody-mediated immunity provides defensive reactions involving antibodies so that: (1) bacteria or other antigens may be more easily ingested and digested by macrophages; (2) bacterial toxins can be neutralized; (3) agglutination (clumping) of bacteria can help clear the blood stream; (4) complement activation can take place with subsequent lysis of bacterial cells; and (5) viruses are prevented from entering cells.

Cell-Mediated Immunity

Some microorganisms like the tubercle bacillus and certain viruses have developed the capacity for living and multiplying within cells of the host. The defense against organisms such as these is dependent upon cell-mediated immunity in which the effector cell is the sensitized lymphocyte, i.e., the T-lymphocyte. However, killing of these organisms is done within macrophages which have been activated by the specifically sensitized T-cells. Thus this kind of immune response does not depend upon conventional antibodies (Ig) or complement, but upon a subtle interplay between T-cells and macrophages. The interaction between macrophage and T-cells is essential.

Two processes are involved in the interaction of the macrophage with the T-lymphocyte: presentation of antigen and secretion of biologically active molecules. After the antigen has been ingested and partially degraded some of the antigen is fixed in or near the surface of a macrophage (which is now in a strongly immunogenic state) and is associated with the antigens of the major histocompatibility complex. At this stage the macrophages present antigen on their surface to antigen-sensitive lymphocytes. This interaction results in the formation of T cells which elaborate lymphokines, those which recruit and activate cells of the mononuclear-phagocyte system, or those which become cytotoxic and produce lysis of target cells.

Lymphokines are soluble factors released by activated lymphocytes that nonspecifically modulate immunologic and inflammatory responses by regulating target cells. These factors include a macrophage migration inhibition factor (MIF), a macrophage activating factor (MAF), interferon (inhibits viral replication), bastogenic factor (stimulates nonsensitized lymphocytes), chemotactic factor (localizes macrophages), mitogenic factor (for T-helper function), and a lymphocyte inhibitory factor (LIF)-T cell suppressor function. Similar factors produced by other cell types, together with lymphokines, are called *cytokines*, e.g., *interleukin-1* (formerly called leukocyte activating factor), *interleukin-2* (formerly called T cell growth factor), and *interferons*. Interleukin-1 (Il-1) is a macrophage factor that promotes short-term proliferation of T cells. Interleukin-2 (Il-2) is probably a lymphocyte-derived factor that promotes long term proliferation of T cells in culture. Interferons inhibit virus replication and have antiproliferative activities, as well as immunoregulatory activities.

An example of cell-mediated immunity to virus infection is serum hepatitis. In serum hepatitis or hepatitis caused by B hepatitis virus (BHV), the invading virus does not damage the liver cells in which it proliferates. However, the cell-mediated response kills liver cells along with the virus which inhibits the liver cell. In effect the immune response produces virtually all of the manifestations of the disease. In addition the blood vessels of the kidney may be damaged by antibody-mediated circulation complexes of viral antigen and IgG.

Several diseases are associated with viruses that appear to be able to avoid the immune defenses of the body. Herpes viruses (p. 236) are this type and seem to exist, for example, by inducing the host cell to form Fc receptors which bind and inactivate antiherpes IgG. A number of other such mechanisms could account for the ability of viruses to survive, as well as immunodeficiency disturbances involving host defense mechanisms.

Some viruses persist for long periods of time in a subclinical state but may not cause disease. "Slow viruses" cause disease many years after infection. Slow progressive diseases (SPD) may be the consequence of abnormal RNA processing—possibly secondary to some viral infection. It has been suggested that multiple sclerosis (MS) may be linked to a previous measles infection and the development of a slowly progressive autoimmune-like response.

Interferon

An important antiviral defense mechanism apparently not harmful to the host is interferons. Interferons are proteins produced by viruses and other stimuli. The interferon is released from infected cells and inhibits the protein synthesis of the virus but not that of the host cell. Thus proteins elaborated by infected host cells protect noninfected cells from some viruses. Interferon also acts as a second signal together with antigen in the regulation of a number of immune responses.

SUMMARY OF IMMUNE RESPONSES

Bacteria and viruses are recognized as "foreign" because of the presence in the host's internal environment of circulating molecules (antibodies) which are capable of binding to the intruders and to defensive cells (monocytes) of the mononuclearphagocyte system or the reticuloendothelial system (RES). The coating (opsonization) of the bacteria with antibody facilitates the ingestion (phagocytosis) of the intruders by mononuclear phagocytes (macrophages). Monocytes (white blood cells) become activated into aggressive macrophages when the coated bacteria come into contact with monocytes.

With destruction of the bacteria the recognition markers (antigenic determinants) appear on the surface of the macrophages. With this "processing" the macrophages "present" the antigen to another type of white blood cell (lymphocyte) which is part of the immune system's line of defense.

Some of the lymphocytes (T-cells) have

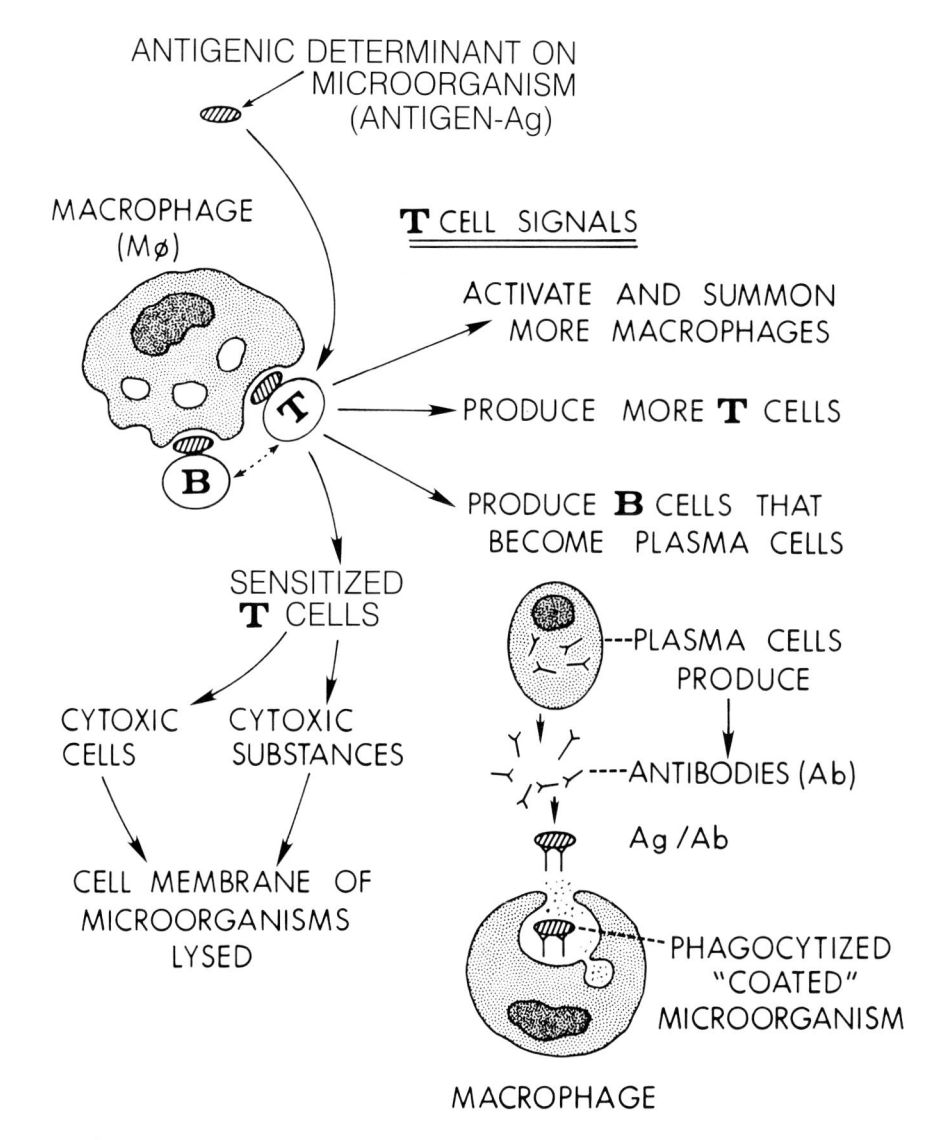

Fig. 5-6. Composite view of immune responses to an antigen (Ag). Attachment to monocytes results in macrophage (Mφ) transformation, antigen processing and interaction with T-cells. The linkage of antigen, macrophage and T-cells stimulates the T-cells to signal for more macrophages, more T-cells, and for B-cells to proliferate and become plasma cells. The latter produce and release antibodies (Y-shaped molecules) which attach to the intruder (antigen, bacteria) which facilitates the phagocytosis.

antigen specific receptors on their surfaces for attaching to the intruding bacteria and macrophages. As a result of this linkage and presentation of antigen to the T-cell, three responses occur: (1) more macrophages are activated and attracted to the site of the interaction between the macrophage, T-cell and antigen; (2) more T-cells are produced; (3) another type of lymphocyte (B-cell) is stimulated to proliferate and become plasma cells (Fig. 5-6).

Plasma cells produce and release specific antibodies (Y-shaped molecules). The yoke end of the antibody (Ab) attaches to the antigen (Ag) or bacterium and the shaft end to the macrophage. Thus antibodies lock onto intruder molecules (antigen) on the surface of the bacteria and link the yoke of the Y to them. The shaft of the Y attaches to the macrophage. This facilitates ingestion by macrophages. In addition some T-cells attack the intruder directly or by releasing cytotoxic substances which cause cell lysis.

IMMUNOPATHOLOGY

The immune response is a normal protective mechanism; however, deficiencies in the immune mechanisms associated with white blood cells and complement, as well as with hypersensitive or allergic states, may allow or cause injury to the injury. Thus an immune response may be: (1) deficient (immunodeficient disease); (2) inappropriate (hypersensitivity or allergy), or (3) misdirected (autoimmune diseases).

Immunodeficiency Diseases

Immunodeficiency diseases can affect virtually every component of the immune system, from gross deficiencies of immune cells to subcellular alterations in cellular mechanisms. Defects may involve phagocytosis, cell-mediated responses, and antibody synthesis. Immunodeficiency states are often primary congenital diseases. They may also be associated with a number of systemic diseases, including diminished leukocyte mobilization sometimes seen in steroid therapy, diabetic acidosis, and alcohol ingestion.

AIDS

The acquired immunodeficiency syndrome (AIDS), as defined clinically by the Centers for Disease Control (CDC) surveillance, is characterized by opportunistic infections and malignant diseases in patients without a known cause for immunodeficiency. There is strong evidence that the etiologic agent is a lymphocytotrophic retrovirus or a closely related group of such retroviruses, designated by the National Cancer Institute as HTLV-III (human T-cell lymphocytotrophic virus III; HTLV-III/LAV).

AIDS is seen almost exclusively in certain "at-risk" groups. Most of the patients in developed countries are homosexually active men. Also at risk are intravenous-drug abusers and patients who are recipients of blood, especially hemophiliacs receiving factor VIII concentrates. The epidemiologic pattern resembles the spread of hepatitis B and suggests a transmissible agent in the blood and other body fluids. There is a frequent occurrence of Kaposi's sarcoma in AIDS, and a number of opportunistic infections have been observed. Characteristically AIDS is associated with a depletion of T-cells. Therapeutic approaches have been largely empirical.

The epidemiologic aspects of AIDS indicate that patients have been detected in the majority of the United States and in Canada and Europe. Most cases reported are residents of large cities (New York and San Francisco), 90% are 20 to 49 year olds (94% males), and by late 1983, over 3,000 cases were reported in the United States compared to 267 in Europe. By mid 1985 over 9,000 adults and 113 children were diagnosed as having AIDS. Of the patients diagnosed before 1983, 75% are known dead. The most common marker diseases noted have been Pneumocystis Carinii pneumonia, Kaposi's sarcoma, or both. Cytomegalovirus and herpesviruses cause marker diseases.

The incubation period for AIDS ranges from 3 to 18 months or longer. As of this writing there is currently no specific laboratory test for AIDS, but the diagnosis is made on the basis of history and microbiologic and immunologic methods relating to a deficiency in cell-mediated immunity.

The health risks for health-care personnel who treat patients with AIDS has not been clarified at this time. Guidelines for treatment of suspected or diagnosed AIDS patients have been developed by the Council of the American Dental Association on Dental Therapeutics following recommendations of CDC and include: (1) wear masks, gloves and eye glasses; (2) sterilize all instruments with methods known to kill all life forms; (3) scrub surfaces in the operatory with detergent solution; and (4) sterilize all contaminated materials before discarding.

The possibility of the development of a vaccine for AIDS is dependent upon the solution of problems common to all retroviral diseases. An enzyme-linked immunocompetent assay (ELISA) has been developed to detect antibodies to HTLV-III. A confirmed positive test indicates that a person has been exposed to the virus, not whether the person currently harbors the virus.

Hypersensitivity

Hypersensitivity or allergy refers to immune responses which are identical to those that destroy microorganisms, but under certain circumstances produce tissue damage. There are several varieties of hypersensitivity, but most commonly four main categories are described.

Type I (immediate hypersensitivity) reactions include atopic allergies such as asthma, hayfever, and urticaria (hives) but less commonly anaphylaxis. This response is mediated by IgE which causes the release of histamine and slow reacting substances (SRS-A) from mast cells. The response in the tissues is leaking of the vessels leading to inflammation, contraction of smooth muscles and narrowing of the bronchi and other abnormalities of the airways that lead to asthma. In some instances anaphylaxis or anaphylactic shock may occur with a collapse of the general circulation and pulmonary edema. Common causes of anaphylaxis are stinging insects, seafoods, radiographic contrast media, drugs such as penicillin, and vaccines.

Type II (cytotoxic reactions) involve the activation of the complement cascade and eventual lysis of host cells, including red blood cells (hemolytic anemias), white blood cells (agranulocytosis), endothelium (purpura), and platelets (thrombocytopenic purpura). Initially the reaction involves the combining of antibody (IgM or IgG) with cell surface antigens which results in direct damage to the cell as the consequence of activation of C8 and C9. Cytotoxic injury includes transfusion reactions in which IgM antibodies are formed against ABO antigens (cf. p. 78), hemolytic disease of newborn in which there is a cytotoxic reaction to the Rh blood group on fetal red blood cells, and certain drug sensitivities involving injury to platelets. The surfaces of cells may be rendered antigenic when a drug or chemical binds to the host tissues and makes an otherwise innocuous protein antigenic (i.e., forms a hapten). As already indicated, if a drug such as phenacetin is used continuously for some time, it may form an antigenic complex with the surface of red blood cells and cause the formation of antibodies which are cytotoxic for the drug-cell complex and results in hemolytic anemia. Similar cytotoxic reactions may lead to agranulocytosis from the use of quinidine or amidopyrine.

Type III (toxic immune complex) hypersensitivity reactions involve complexes formed in the circulation, body fluids or spaces or on vascular basement membranes. These circulating antigen/antibody complexes become held up in the basement membrane of vessel walls or joints where the addition of complement, if not already present, to the immune complex (antigen and IgG or IgM) initiates or aggravates a local inflammatory response. When the complement system is activated PMNs are attracted chemotactically to the immune complexes which are phagocytized. In the process lysosomal enzymes are released causing injury to vessel basement membranes with resulting inflammation, thrombosis, hemorrhage, and necrosis. Examples of this type of hypersensitivity include rheumatoid arthritis, systemic lupus erythematosus, serum sickness and the Arthus reaction.

Type IV (cell mediated or delayed) hypersensitivity reactions involve T lymphocytes that have been sensitized to locally deposited antigens in contrast to the previously discussed types of hypersensitivity which involve circulating antibody. In addition Type IV hypersensitivity reactions are not evident until 24 to 48 hours after the sensitized host is challenged with antigens. Because of this delay Type IV reactions are referred to as delayed hypersensitivity. This type of hypersensitivity is also called specific cell-mediated immunity. The reaction is mediated by the release of lymphokines and/or direct cytotoxicity. Delayed hypersensitivity reactions are usually associated with such infections as tuberculosis, and viral, fungal and parasitic diseases. Other such reactions include graft rejection and tumor rejection.

Organ Transplantation

A limiting factor in replacing damaged organs and tissues by transplantation is immunologic rejection. To avoid the cytotoxic effects of the immune system of the recipient on the donor tissue or organ, the immune system is suppressed using corticosteroids, cytotoxic drugs, and lymphocyte-depleting techniques. However, the suppression of the defenses leave the host open to infection, and methods of more specific immunosuppression methods, including total lymphocyte irradiation and the use of cyclosporine. Irradiation of selected lymphoid tissue areas favors suppressor functions at the expense of effector ones whereas cyclosporine selectively inhibits the helper T cells secreting lymphokines. Thus the immune apparatus may be sufficiently intact to fight most inflations when such immunosuppression is needed. Immune suppression is used for the management of unwanted immune reactions involved in transplantation tolerance and autoimmune disease, e.g., juvenile-onset diabetes, multiple sclerosis and systemic lupus erythematosus.

Autoimmune Diseases

As already indicated (cf. p. 77) a requirement of the immune system is to recognize body cells as "self" and to prevent the recognition of these components as antigens. When self-antigens, or antibodies that react to self are produced, the loss of self-tolerance may lead to autoimmune diseases. The probable mechanisms to explain autoimmune disease are many and at this time there is no generally accepted concept. However, one of the most commonly advanced mechanisms is that there is a general deficiency of suppressor T cells. Several considerations support this concept, including evidence that deficient suppressor T cell population may be a factor in systemic lupus erythematosus (SLE). It is also evident that persistent viral infection may be associated with autoimmune mechanisms. There is a strong association of some HLA subtypes with autoimmune diseases.

The spectrum of autoimmune diseases ranges from organ-specific (e.g., thyroiditis) to generalized systemic diseases (e.g., rheumatoid arthritis). There is a tendency for more than one autoimmune disorder to occur in the same individual and the disorders to fall within the same spectrum. Thus autoimmune thyroid disease occurs together with pernicious anemia at the organ-specific end of the spectrum, and systemic lupus erythematosus occurs together with rheumatoid arthritis at the non-organ-specific end of the spectrum more frequently than would be expected in a random population.

Some of the autoimmune diseases with oral manifestations include recurrent aphthous stomatitis (RAS)—a minor type called canker sores and a major type called periadenitis mucosae necrotica, Behçet's syndrome, Sjögren's syndrome, systemic lupus erythematosus, and pernicious anemia. These disturbances are discussed in the chapter on Stomatitis (cf. p. 236). Most autoimmune diseases may have oral manifestations, and in some instances the oral manifestations may be the reason that the patient first seeks an evaluation. Significant oro-facial manifestations of auto-immune disorders include TMJ/muscle dysfunction associated with rheumatoid arthritis, loss of masticatory muscle function in myasthenia gravis, and lesions of the oral mucosa in systemic lupus erythematosus.

Rheumatoid Arthritis

Rheumatoid arthritis (RA) is a chronic systemic disease of unknown etiology. There appears to be a susceptibility for RA which is influenced by a genetically determined response, i.e., the histocompatibility antigen HLA-DR is found in 70 percent of the patients with RA. The type of immune response involved in RA suggests it is an autoimmune disease. The majority of patients with RA have antibodies in the serum and joint fluid which is specific for the F_C fragment of IgG (rheumatoid factors). The disease appears commonly in the fourth decade, more commonly in women than men.

RA may involve the skin, voluntary muscle, heart, blood vessels, and connective tissue of other organs, as well as the peripheral joints (Fig. 5–7).

It has been hypothesized that a deficiency in some aspect of the immune response in RA permits B cells infected with Epstein-Barr virus (ubiquitous member of the herpes virus family) to proliferate. Epstein-Barr virus (EBR) is usually countered by cytotoxic T cells which destroy B cells carrying EBV, and by T helper cells which produce interferon which inhibits the virus from infecting new B cells. The hypothesis suggests that RA patients have a weakened T helper cell/interferon mechanism.

Joints that are freely movable contain synovial membranes which secrete synovial fluid which has the consistency of egg white and serves as a lubricant. In RA there are inflammatory changes involving the synovial membrane that ultimately lead to reactive hyperplasia and replacement of the synovial membrane of the joint with a painful mass of granulation tissue and collagen called a pannus. In time the articular cartilage is destroyed and the joint capsule

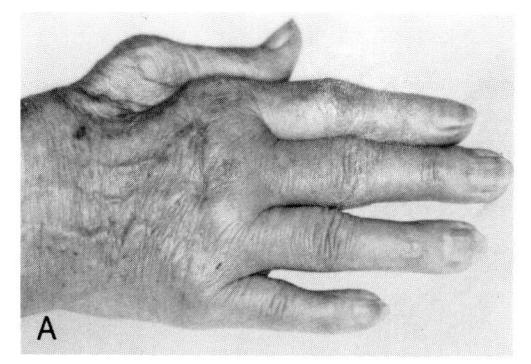

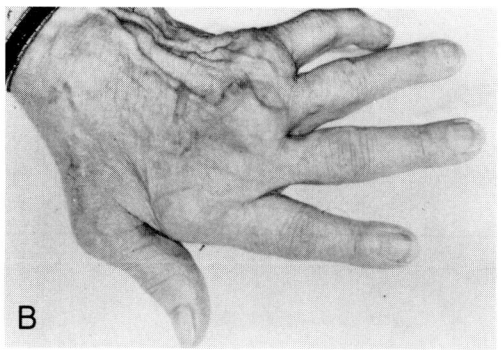

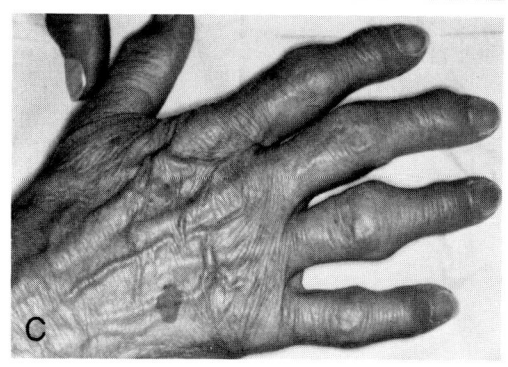

Fig. 5–7. Rheumatoid arthritis. A, synovial proliferation of metacarpophalangeal joints and somewhat the proximal interphalangeal joints. B, advanced deformities with subluxation and ulnar deviation of the metacarpophalangeal joints. There are swan deformities of the fingers and hyperextension of the proximal interphalangeal joints. C, primary involvement in the interphalangeal joints.

and ligaments are involved in the destructive process. As the articular cartilage is destroyed the underlying bone is exposed and ankylosis may occur. One manifestation of RA are subcutaneous nodules located over the extensor surface of the elbows or less commonly over the extensor surfaces of the fingers.

When RA is associated with dry eyes (xerophthalmia conjunctivitis) and dry mouth (xerostomia), the symptom complex is referred to as *Sjögren's syndrome.* The decrease in tears and saliva is referred to as sicca syndrome.

SUMMARY

The immune system provides protection against foreign substances, infectious agents, and proliferation of mutant cells. An immune response involves an interaction between antigens (e.g., bacteria) and antibodies (immunoglobulins) as well as reactive lymphocytes (T or B cells). The antibodies produced against the antigens facilitate phagocytosis, prevent entry or viruses into cells, and neutralize bacterial toxins.

Macrophages process and "present" antigens to lymphocytes, which in the case of B cell/antigen interaction results in a clone of plasma cells that produce antibody for that specific antibody or produce memory cells which carry the information needed for antibody production at a later time when the host is exposed to the same antigen again; or which in the case of T cell/antigen interaction results in the blastogenic transformation of the lymphocyte into subpopulations of regulatory and effector T cells, as well as memory cells.

Regulatory T cells either help (enhance) or suppress B lymphocytes. One kind of effector T cell is capable of killing cells (via lymphokines), and another type (killer T cell) is cytotoxic without being sensitized by antigen. The T cells are responsible for cell-mediated immunity and B cells for humoral immunity.

Certain genes, which are referred to as the major histocompatibility complex (MHC), are concerned with the expression of cell surface antigens (HLA) and are closely linked to genes that predispose to or protect against infectious and immuno-pathologic disease. Differences in HLA antigens are the antigenic basis for tissue transplant rejection, and for regulatory effects on immune responsiveness and disease susceptibility. A number of diseases have been related to HLA antigens, and associations are particularly strong for some of the rheumatic diseases and for certain diseases that are characterized by chronic inflammation and aberrant immunologic responses, including insulin-dependent diabetes mellitus (p. 263), Sjögren's syndrome, and multiple sclerosis.

HLA associated disease does not mean the disease itself is inherited, but rather a susceptibility to the environmental factors which cause it. The gene determining disease susceptibility does not have to be the HLA gene but a gene close to the HLA gene that are transmitted together on the same piece of DNA (via linkage disequilibrium, p. 78). For example, close to the DR gene locus is the gene that codes for the second and fourth components of complement (p. 80) and possibly responsible for autoimmune disease.

Immune responses, such as hypersensitivity and allergic reactions, involve antigens (environmental agents, food or drugs) usually considered harmless. The basic types of responses are: (1) Type I responses such as seen in hay fever and asthma, (2) Type II responses found in blood transfusion reactions, (3) Type III responses that cause local tissue injury, e.g., serum sickness, and (4) Type IV responses in which sensitized T lymphocytes react with an antigen to cause inflammation and tissue injury, e.g., from insect bites and contact dermatitis (e.g., poison ivy).

In autoimmune diseases the host becomes sensitized to its own tissues or to cross-reacting antigens. These disorders can involve T cells, B cells or the complement system, and any of the tissues of the body. Rheumatoid arthritis, systemic lupus erythematosus, and possibly recurrent aphthous stomatitis are examples of an autoimmune disease.

BIBLIOGRAPHY

Adams, J.M.: The organization and expression of immunoglobulin genes. Immunol. Today, 1:10, 1980.

Bona, C.A. and Kohler, H.: Immune Networks, Conference held November 29–December 1, 1982. Ann. N.Y. Acad. Sci. 418, Dec. 29, 1983.

Cerottini, J.C.: Lymphoid cells as effectors of immunologic cytolysis. In F.J. Dixon and D.W. Fisher (eds.), *Biology of Immunologic Disease,* Sunderland, MA, Sinauer Assoc. Inc., 1983.

Cumbo, V., et al.: HLA -A, B, C, DR, MT and MB antigens in recurrent aphthous stomatitis. Oral Surg. 59:364, 1985.

Dausset, J.: The major histocompatibility complex in man. Science, 213:1469, 1981.

Edelson, R.L. and Fink, J.M.: The immunologic function of skin. Sci. Am., 252:46, 1985.

Herberman, R.B., and Ortaldo, J.R.: Natural killer cells: their role in defense against disease. Science, 214:24, 1981.

Kaliner, M.: The Mast cell—a fascinating riddle. N. Engl. J. Med., 301:498, 1979.

Landesman, S.H., et al.: The AIDS epidemic. N. Engl. J. Med. 213:421, 1985.

Pierce, C.W.: Macrophages: modulators of immunity. Am. J. Pathol., 98:10, 1980.

Robertson, M.: The life of a B lymphocyte. Nature, 283:332, 1980.

Roitt, I.M. and Lehner, T.: *Immunology of Oral Diseases.* Oxford, Blackwell Scientific Publications, 1980.

Rosenthal, A.S.: Regulation of the immune response: role of the Macrophage. N. Engl. J. Med., 303:1153, 1980.

Selikoff, I.J. et al (eds.): Acquired Immune Deficiency syndrome. Conference, New York Academy Science, November 14–17, 1983. New York, Ann N.Y. Acad. Sci., December 29, 1984.

Strober, S.: Managing the immune system with total lymphoid irradiation. In F.J. Dixon and D.W. Fisher, *Biology of Immunologic Disease.* Sunderland, MA, Snauer Assoc, Inc. 1983.

Tan, E.M.: Autoantibodies to nuclear antigens: Their immunobiology and medicine. Adv. Immunol. 33:157, 1982.

Unanue, E.R.: The regulation of lymphocyte functions by the macrophage. Immunol. Rev. 40:227, 1978.

Unanue, E.R.: Macrophages as regulators of lymphocyte function. In F.J. Dixon and D.W. Fisher (eds.), *The Biology of Immunologic Disease.* Sunderland, Mass., Sinauer Assoc., Inc., 1983.

World Health Organization Workshop: Conclusions and Recommendations on Acquired Immunodeficiency Disease. Leads from the MMWR. Vol. 34, Nos. 18, 19, 20, 1985, Center for Disease Control, Atlanta, J.A.M.A., 253:3385, 1985.

6

RESPONSES TO INCREASED FUNCTION, IRRITATION, AND INJURY

The tissues of the body may respond to increased function, irritation, or injury by reactive changes which range from protective measures and functional adaptation to exaggerated proliferative lesions that serve no usual purpose. Such reactive responses include hyperplasia, hypertrophy, keratosis, and metaplasia. The reactive oral lesions include pyogenic granuloma, traumatic fibroma, peripheral fibroma, giant cell granuloma, tori, amputation neuroma, and traumatic hemangioma (varix).

Hyperplasia

Hyperplasia is the response of a tissue or organ to increased function and is a physiologic process characterized by an increase in the number of cells making up the tissue or organ. This response may occur in organs, especially in glands, when there is a demand for greater functional activity. It also occurs in the epithelium covering the surface of the body, such as the skin, mucous membrane of the oral cavity, nasal mucosa, and the mucosa of the respiratory and gastrointestinal tracts. Supporting tissue may also increase its functional activity in an attempt to meet functional demands by increasing the number of supporting cells in an area of increased activity. Supporting tissue hyperplasia often accompanies hyperplasia of surface epithelium.

Hyperplasia of the tissues of the body surface is usually a response to the demand of these tissues for increased protection against surface irritation. It is demonstrated in the skin in areas of pressure and functional irritation, such as occurs on the hands or fingers when an object such as a golf club, shovel, or periodontal instrument is held tightly. Under the areas of pressure and friction, the epithelium thickens, and the resulting lesion is designated a *callus*.

Hyperplasia of the gingival tissue may occur from wearing ill-fitting dentures (Fig. 6–1). As the dentures move, the tissue is rubbed and compressed which results in an increase in thickness of the epithelium to protect against injury (Fig. 6–2). The increase in size of the gingiva related to the ill-fitting denture is due to an increase in quantity of both epithelium and connective tissue. An increase in size of the gingiva may be due to other sources of irritation (p. 219).

Hypercementosis occurs on teeth which

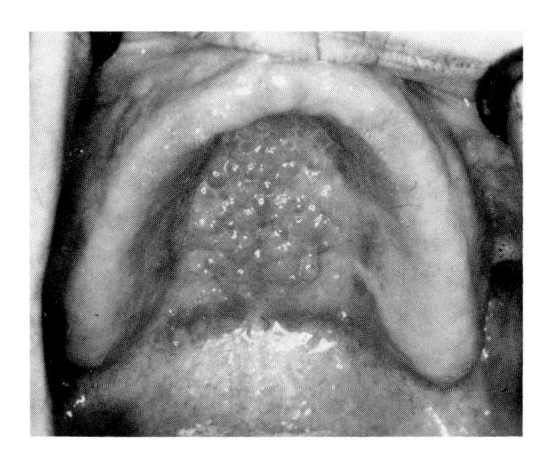

Fig. 6-1. *Hyperplasia.* Palatal hyperplasia associated with ill-fitting dentures.

are in heavy use or around the roots in areas of chronic inflammation. The response to heavy use or inflammation stimulates an excessive deposition of cementum about the apical one-third or one-half of the root (Fig. 6-3). This increase in cementum produces a bulbous appearance to the root. The enlargement of the root end makes extraction difficult.

Hypertrophy

Hypertrophy is the increase in size of a part owing to an increase in the size of the cells which constitute the part. Because both hyperplasia and hypertrophy imply an increase in size of a tissue or organ, their use is frequently confused.

Hypertrophy like hyperplasia is a response to meet an increased functional demand. It may commonly be exhibited in muscle and usually reflects a physiologic response of the muscular tissues to an increased functional demand. Hypertrophy per se occurs only in those tissues or cells with limited ability to reproduce themselves and therefore can only be demonstrated orally in such structures as the tongue and muscles of mastication. Gingival enlargement or hyperplasia should not be described as gingival hypertrophy.

Hyperkeratosis

Hyperkeratosis is a change occurring in squamous epithelium in response to irritation. It is an attempt by the body to protect the tissue beneath an area of irritation by changing the character of the surface. To fully understand this protective mechanism, it is advisable to discuss briefly the physiology of squamous epithelium. The hard palate and the gingiva are the only areas of the oral mucosa which normally exhibit any degree of protective keratinization.

The layer of epithelial cells immediately in contact with connective tissue is called the basal layer or stratum germinativum (Fig. 6-4). The cells of this layer have the ability to undergo cell division; this they do continuously at a slow rate unless stimulated by irritation or injury to increase the rate of new cells being formed. As new cells are formed and move toward the surface, changes in morphology occur; they become larger, polyhedral, and develop small projections (spinous process) which unite them with adjacent cells. At this stage of maturation, the cells form a layer called the prickle cell layer or stratum spinosum, which may be several cells in thickness (Fig. 6-4). At this point maturation may be directed toward the formation of protective keratinization in response to surface stimuli, as in the hard palate and gingiva, or toward nonkeratinization and desquamation, as in

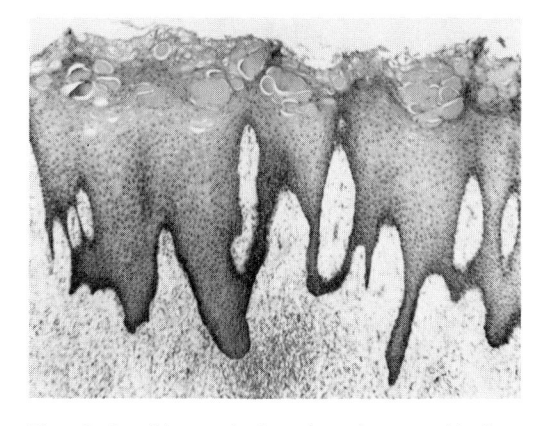

Fig. 6-2. Hyperplasia of surface epithelium with branching and fusing of rete ridges. The epithelium at the surface shows exaggerated formation and retention of intraepithelial hyalin.

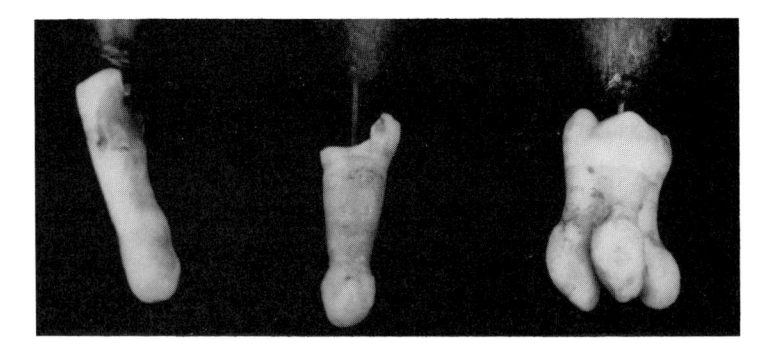

94   RESPONSES TO INCREASED FUNCTION, IRRITATION, AND INJURY

Fig. 6-3. *Hypercementosis.* Apical deposition of cementum in response to increased functional demand.

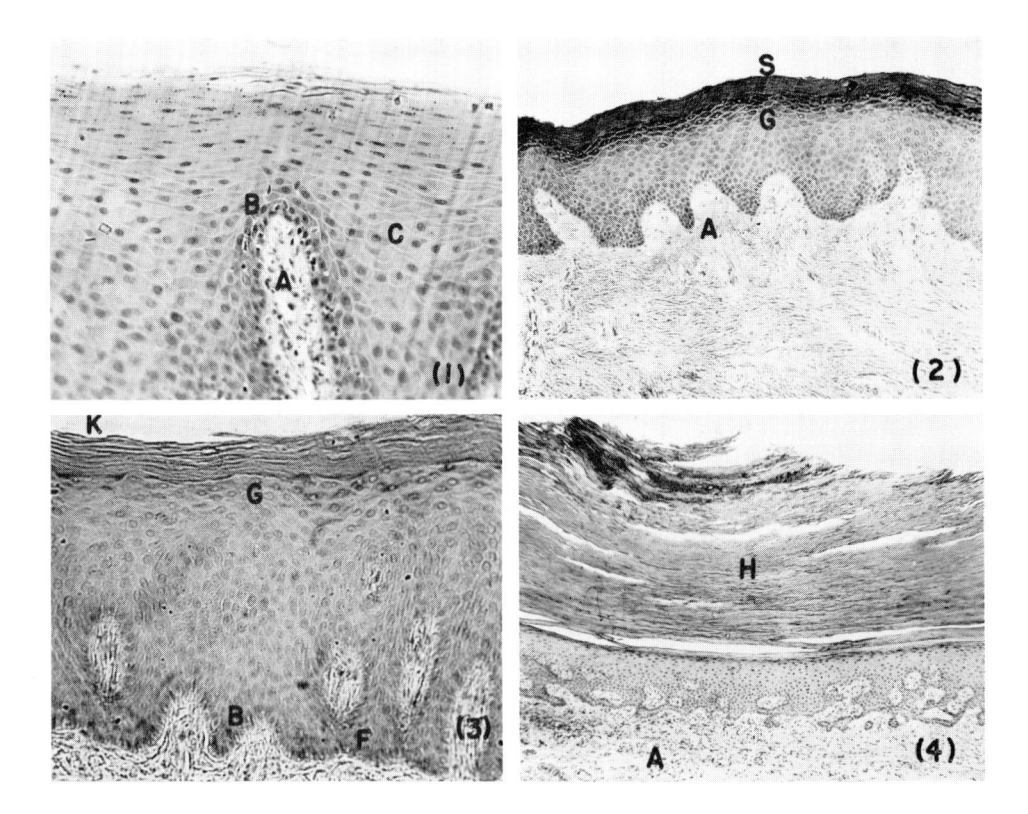

Fig. 6-4. *Epithelial response to irritation.* (1) Nonkeratinized mucosa; connective tissue papillae (A), basal cells (B), stratum spinosum (C) with wide intercellular spaces. (2) Skin; stratum cornium (S), stratum granulosum (G), lamina propria (A). (3) Gingival mucosa showing protective keratinization and hyperplasia; thickened keratin layer (K), increased granular layer (G), increased basal cell proliferation (B), fusion of rete pegs (F). (4) Focal hyperkeratosis of buccal mucosa; heavy production of keratin (H), atrophic epithelium (A).

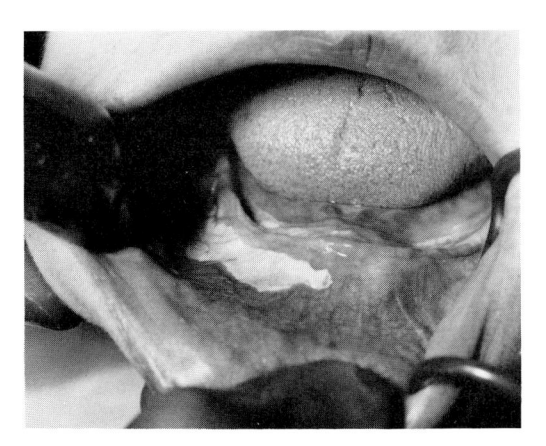

Fig. 6–5. *Hyperkeratosis*. Large white patch of hyperkeratosis of the gingival and alveolar mucosa due to denture irritation.

the normal buccal mucosa. (The process of keratinization may be initiated in the buccal mucosa in response to surface irritation.) If maturation is directed toward keratinization, the intracellular hyalin increases in quantity. All the squamous cells, at this point of maturation, contain increased amounts of hyalin. In the skin, with the loss of the spiny process of the prickle cell layer, a somewhat translucent layer is present called the stratum lucidum. This layer may be several cells in thickness in the skin but is absent in the oral mucosa. The cells containing intracellular hyalin undergo further degeneration or maturation as evidenced by fragmentation of the nucleus (karyorrhexis), dissemination of chromatin particles throughout the cell, loss of distinctness of the cell boundary or membrane, and the increased compactness of the cytoplasm (Fig. 6–4). The outer cells lose their cell boundaries, the nuclear fragments disappear, and the cells become flat flakes of keratin on the surface of the skin. This outer layer is the stratum corneum. The small flakes of keratin gradually separate from the surface and fall away (desquamation). This continuing formation, degeneration, and loss of epithelial cells is a slow but constant process which provides a constantly changing covering for the body.

Irritation to the body surface acts as a stimulation for an increased production of new epithelial cells; this activity results in a thicker layer of keratin on the surface of the body. In some areas of the body's surface, the keratin layer is normally very thin or absent, but owing to an increase in the rate of proliferation and degeneration of the squamous epithelium, an accumulation of keratin may occur. This increase in the thickness of keratin on a naturally keratinized surface, or the appearance of keratin on a surface which does not normally become keratinized, is called hyperkeratosis (Fig. 6–5). The increased production of epithelial cells and the resultant thickening of the keratin layer provide a harder and more protective surface against injury. Hyperkeratosis may or may not accompany hyperplasia. In a *callus* both hyperplasia and hyperkeratosis are present. Hyperkeratosis of the oral mucosa may or may not be associated with hyperplasia. A localized increase in keratin on the oral mucosa gives a white or grayish appearance to the mucosa and is called focal hyperkeratosis.

Focal hyperkeratosis occurs when the tissue is irritated by rough, sharp, or irregular teeth, by poorly fitting dental appliances, or by habitual chewing of the lips and cheeks. It is also produced by chemical and thermal irritation associated with heavy smoking of tobacco or the use of highly seasoned foods. The protective process of keratinization is a physiologic one, but under some situations it does not follow the normal pattern of epithelial maturation but becomes altered so it is no longer beneficial. Such a nonbeneficial alteration then becomes a part of an abnormal process called leukoplakia.

Metaplasia

Metaplasia is a tissue reaction to injury in which the epithelium or connective tissue is transformed into epithelium or connective tissue of another type of lower order (Fig. 6–6). An example of metaplasia is the transformation of respiratory epithelium to strat-

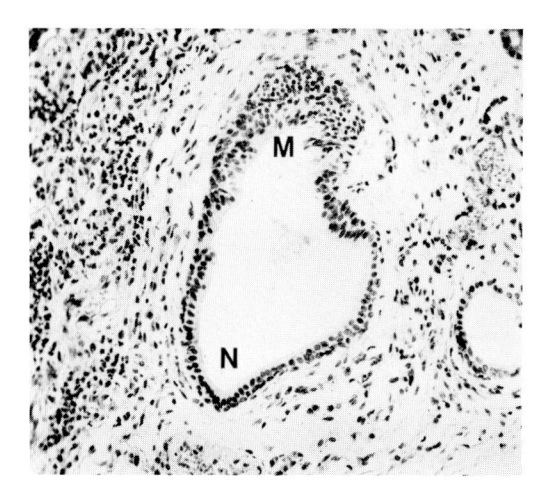

Fig. 6–6. *Metaplasia* of accessory salivary gland duct. Normal ductal epithelium (N), metaplasia of columnar epithelium to squamous type (M).

Table 6–1. Reactive Oral Lesions

Pyogenic granuloma
Traumatic fibroma
Peripheral fibroma
Peripheral ossifying fibroma
Peripheral giant cell granuloma
Central giant cell granuloma
Tori—palatinus, mandibularis, exostosis
Amputation neuroma
Traumatic hemangioma (varix)

ified squamous epithelium. The respiratory epithelium is composed of more highly differentiated cells which are less resistant to injury than the less differentiated squamous epithelium. For example, chronic irritation of the columnar epithelium of the respiratory passages of the lungs and the excretory ducts of the salivary glands may result in the replacement of the columnar epithelium by squamous epithelium. Squamous epithelium is less highly specialized than columnar epithelium (ductal and respiratory epithelium). Squamous epithelium has a greater protective ability than columnar epithelium; therefore, the conversion of columnar epithelium to a less specialized squamous type of epithelium may be a protective reaction of the tissues.

REACTIVE ORAL LESIONS

Reactive lesions are progressive proliferations in response to injury. Every act of injury incites a process of repair in which various types of cells play a part. The proliferative activity of the various tissue elements normally occurs in a definite physiologic proportion to injury, producing just the right amount of tissue to eliminate the defect. In some processes of repair there is an overzealous proliferation of one tissue element resulting in an exuberant process of repair. Progressive proliferation beyond the normal limits of repair results in the development of tumor-like configurations, which are progressive and permanent in nature. Because the lesion is characterized by proliferation which progresses beyond the normal demand and results in tumescences, it exhibits some of the tendencies of neoplasia. However, these lesions are not autonomous nor are they capable of unlimited growth and cannot be considered as neoplasms (cancer or tumor).

Reactive lesions are common in the oral cavity because of the frequency with which the oral tissues are injured. They have characteristic features in specific locations. The *reactive* lesions seen in the oral cavity are listed in Table 6–1.

Pyogenic granuloma is a distinct clinical entity which occurs as a sudden exuberant growth of highly vascular granulation tissue (Fig. 6–7). The vascularity imparts a red or bluish color and a soft consistency to the lesion. The proliferation occurs in the area of surface injury and results in a nodular, usually pedunculated lesion ranging in size from a few millimeters to a centimeter or more. The lesion may occur suddenly and grow rapidly to a certain size, and then remain static for an indefinite period.

A *pregnancy tumor* is a pyogenic granuloma arising from the gingival tissue of a patient who is pregnant (Fig. 6–8). Because the lesion receives hormonal stimulation during pregnancy, it may grow more rapidly during this period and may regress when

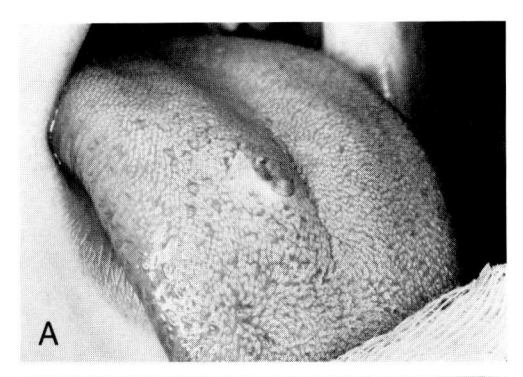

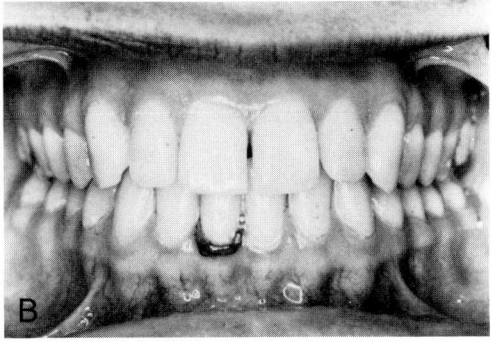

Fig. 6–7. *Pyogenic granuloma.* A, This is an early lesion with the granulation tissue herniating through a distinct circular defect in the mucosa. The border of the lesion is elevated and rolled. The ulcerated surface is free of fibrinous membrane which is present on the surface of most ulcers. B, Smooth, red, sharply defined ring of granulation tissue at the free gingival margin.

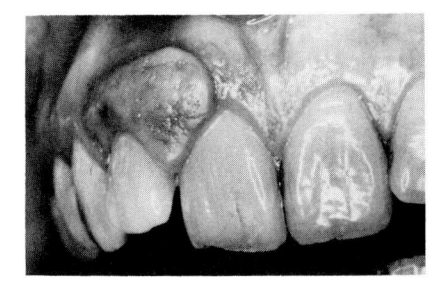

Fig. 6–8. *Pregnancy tumor* (pyogenic granuloma). This soft red pedunculated mass arising from the interdental and subgingival area is flattened and ulcerated by the pressure of the lip. This lesion demonstrated a rapid increase in size during the third month of pregnancy.

the hormonal stimulation is reduced with the termination of the pregnancy.

Traumatic fibroma is a slightly elevated nodule of dense scar which is pale, smooth, and firm and varies in size from about 3 to 10 millimeters (Fig. 6–9). The lesion occurs in the buccal mucosa, the lateral border of the tongue, the lip, and the palate, in the order named. The lesion is due to a scar in the repair of a small perforating or crushing wound produced by biting or by impingement of tissue against teeth. In rare cases it results from the spontaneous healing of a pyogenic granuloma. Because the lesion is asymptomatic and of limited size, it is not recognized or treated, and therefore the history indicates it was present for a long time.

Peripheral fibroma results from the excessive proliferation of fibrous connective tissue of mature character in response to gingival injury or irritation. Subgingival calculus or a foreign body in the gingival sulcus is the most frequent source of irritation. The origin of the lesion from the gingival sulcus results in a nodular lesion below the gingival margin or interdental papillae (Fig. 6–10). The lesion is firm and covered by normal gingival mucosa so there is little alteration in color. The lesions are asymptomatic and may be present for a long time.

Peripheral ossifying fibroma (Fig. 6–11) arises from the gingiva in the same area as the peripheral fibroma. It appears as a firm, pale nodule with a broad base arising from the marginal or papillary gingiva. It projects more abruptly from the gingiva and is firmer in consistency than the peripheral fibroma because the center of the lesion is composed of bone. The bone originates as the result of chronic irritation to periosteum or periodontal membrane, inciting bone formation. The lesions grow slowly without symptoms and rarely exceed a centimeter in size.

Peripheral giant cell granuloma is a lesion of gingiva produced by injury to periodontal membrane or bone, probably with associated hemorrhage and bone resorption (Fig.

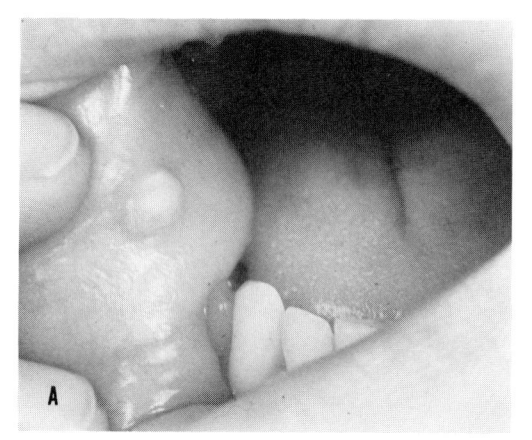

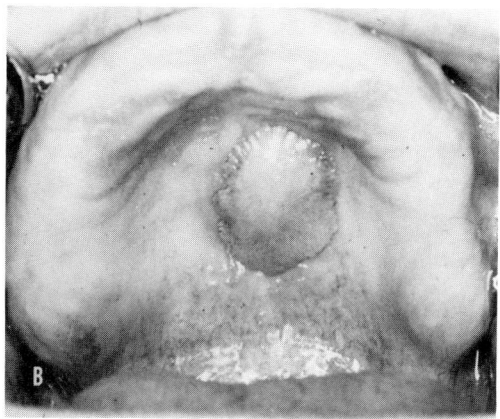

Fig. 6-9. *Traumatic fibroma.* A, The elevated smooth nodule, which is broadest at its base, lighter in color, and firmer than the surrounding mucosa, is typical of this trauma-induced lesion. B, The leaf-like mass attached to the palate by a slender stalk is flattened by the pressure from a denture. The lesion is firm and pale except at the crenated border, which shows a mild inflammatory response. These lesions are often associated with a relief chamber in the denture.

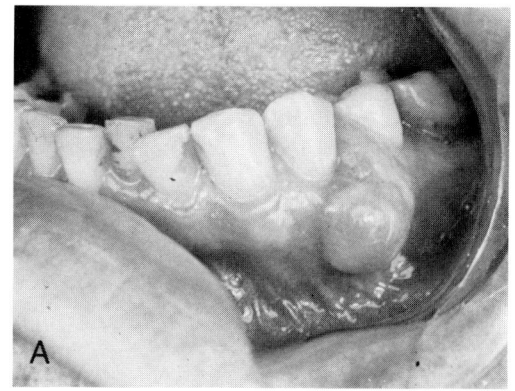

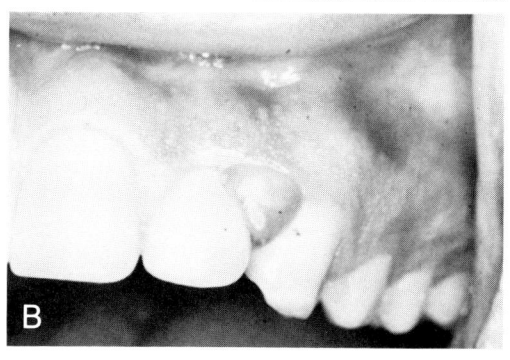

Fig. 6-10. *Peripheral fibroma.* A, Focal gingival hyperplasia resulting from irritation in gingival sulcus. B, The triangular lesion in the interdental area is the result of proliferation of epithelium and connective tissue due to irritation in the gingival sulcus. The lesion is intensified in color and slightly softer than the normal gingiva.

6-12). In the process of osseous repair there is destruction of bone by specialized cells which develop from connective tissue for the specific purpose of resorbing bone. These cells are large multinucleated cells resembling osteoclasts which characterize this lesion and give it the name of giant cell granuloma.

The giant cell lesion arises as a smooth tumescence of gingiva or interdental tissue, but as it increases in size, it may become somewhat lobulated. Since the lesion is highly vascular, it is soft in consistency and intensified in color, varying from bright- to bluish-red depending on the state of the vascular supply. There is a tendency for the lesion to bleed on manipulation, frequently the only symptom presented. The lesion appears fixed to underlying bone.

The histologic features are proliferating fibroblasts and endothelium and occasional inflammatory cells.

Osteoclastic-like giant cells are present in varying numbers. They are usually in focal zones scattered throughout the vascular stroma. The lesion contains varying quantities of phagocytized blood pigment at the site of origin as well as a zone of productive osteitis. The presence of the os-

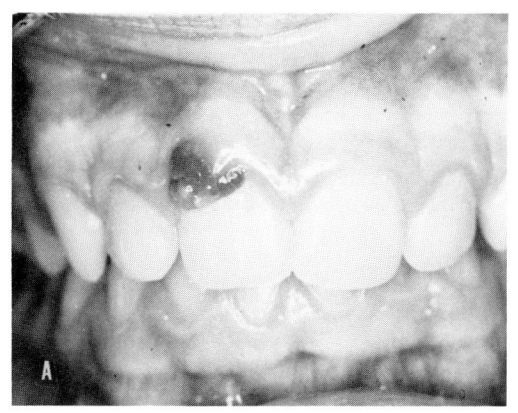

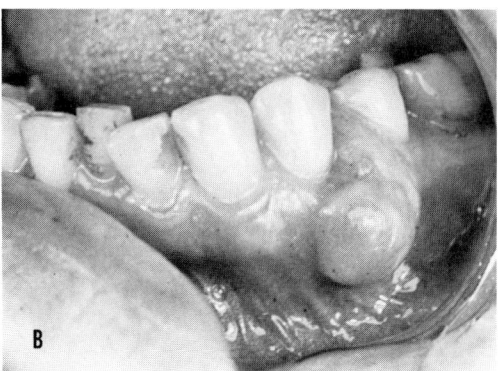

RESPONSES TO INCREASED FUNCTION, IRRITATION, AND INJURY 99

Fig. 6–11. *Peripheral ossifying fibroma. A,* This lesion arising from the marginal gingiva is due to injury of the alveolar crest. *B,* This hard nodular mass having the same color as the surrounding gingiva is attached by a small stalk to the attached gingiva. The lesion is composed of fibrous tissue with central ossification arising as the result of injury to the periosteum.

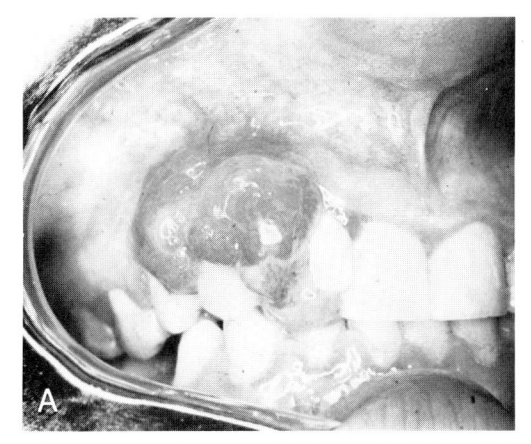

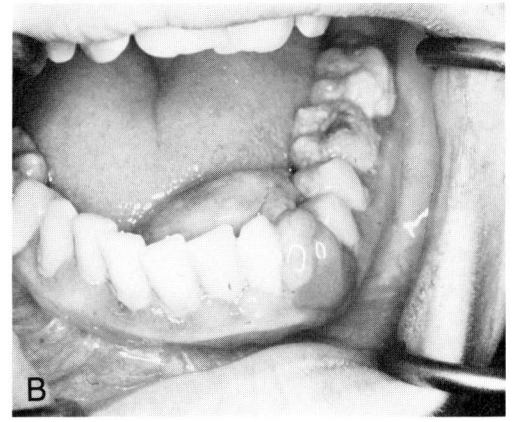

Fig. 6–12. *Peripheral giant cell granuloma. A,* This nodular soft red lesion is contoured by the pressure of lip and cheek to fill the canine fossa and the embrasure between the teeth. *B,* This lesion arising from the embrasure and extending slightly to the buccal and extensively to the lingual has been present for nine months. The lesion is soft and has been molded by the pressure of the lips and tongue. The lesion is intensely red and the sublingual portion shows surface ulceration.

teoclastic-like cell associated with the evidence of hemorrhage and bone repair is an indication of the etiology of the lesion. The exuberant production of the giant cells is evidence of the overzealous repair which places the lesion in this group of reactive lesions.

Central giant cell granuloma is a lesion associated with the overzealous repair in bone (Fig. 6–13). The lesion arises from the center of the bone rather than from its surface. The peripheral lesion arises from the periosteum; the medullary (central) lesion arises from the endosteum. Like the peripheral lesion it is characterized by proliferation of connective tissue and endothelium to produce a granulomatous tissue with varying numbers of giant cells. The phagocytized hemosiderin and the productive osteitis are also a characteristic feature of the lesion. All of the changes present indicate the reactive nature of the lesion. Microscopically, the peripheral and central lesions are identical. The central lesion probably arises as the result of trauma with

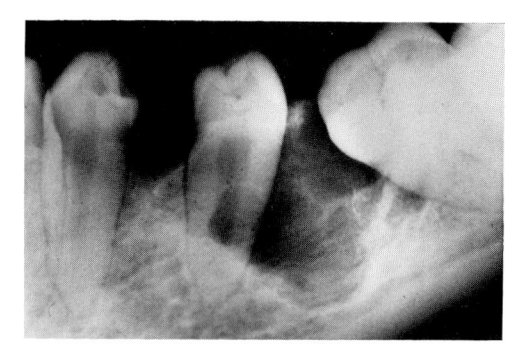

Fig. 6-13. *Central giant cell granuloma.* The lobulated area of radiolucency has a sharp arcuate border and is partitioned by delicate trabeculae giving it a multilocular or "soap bubble" appearance.

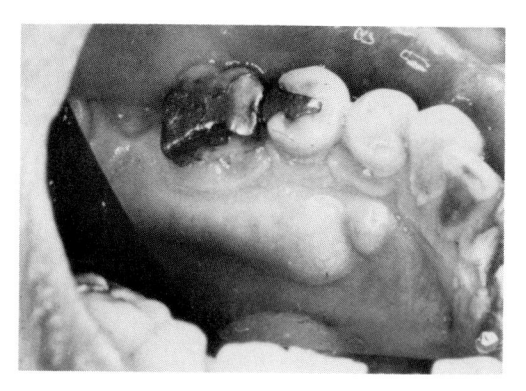

Fig. 6-15. *Torus mandibularis.* Osseous growth above the mylohyoid line.

intraosseous hemorrhage which causes bone destruction and initiates the repair which becomes excessive resulting in further destruction of bone.

The lesion is noted clinically because of expansion of the buccal plates and occasional looseness of the teeth. Radiographic examination demonstrates a multiloculated cyst-like lesion of the jaw with some resorption of roots that project into the radiolucent area. The lesions are slowly progressive and may reach large size, producing considerable facial deformity. Surgical treatment is indicated, and as with peripheral lesions, it must be total to be curative and permanent. Recurrence is frequent because of incomplete removal.

Recurrence of either the peripheral or central lesion may be indicative of initiation by hyperparathyroidism (p. 258). In the patient with a parathyroid adenoma, there is an overproduction of parathormone which mobilizes calcium from the bones. This usually results in the production of fibrocystic lesions in bone, but in a few instances, the same type of overzealous repair initiated by trauma occurs and the lesion is identical with the giant cell granuloma. The hemosiderin imparts a brown color to the lesion; therefore, the lesion is designated "brown tumor" of hyperparathyroidism. This endocrine-produced lesion is not cured by surgery and recurrence is the rule. Therefore, when a giant cell lesion recurs, there is always a suggestion of its being induced by parathyroid dysfunction. Clinical laobratory procedures are indicated to rule out the presence of a "brown tumor" of hyperparathyroidism. The procedures include the evaluation of the serum calcium which will be elevated in hyperparathyroidism.

Torus palatinus is a hard bony lesion arising in the midline of the palate (Fig. 6-14). It may arise in any part of the midpalatal suture as a smooth or lobulated hard lesion covered by normal mucosa. The lesion starts in early life and grows slowly reaching a large size and prevalence by 30 years of

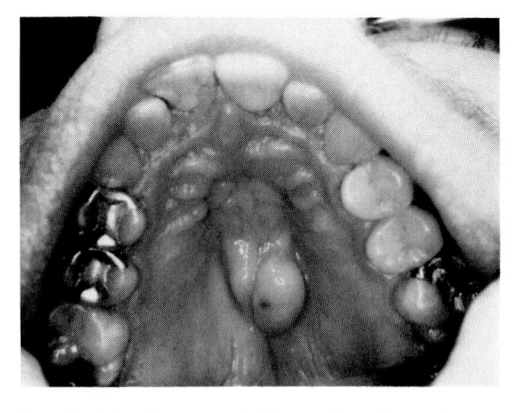

Fig. 6-14. *Torus palatinus.* Reactive change characterized by an increased production of bone along palatal suture. The very thin mucosa over the nodule of bone is subject to frequent trauma and ulceration.

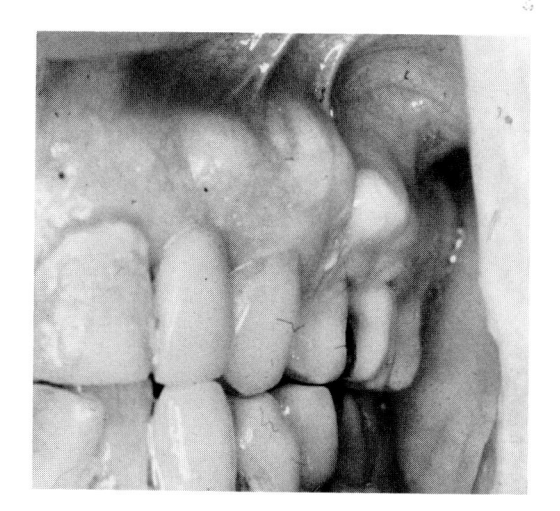

Fig. 6-16. *Exostoses.* These smooth, hard, nodular excrescences over the buccal aspect of the roots of the teeth may result from excess bone production in response to hyperfunction.

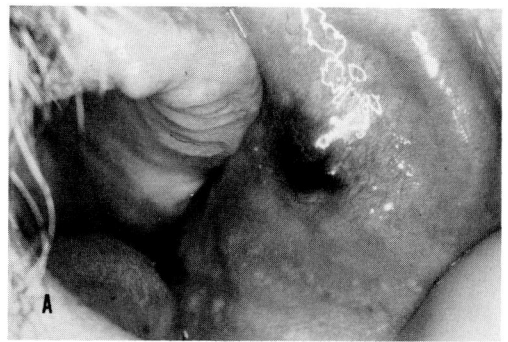

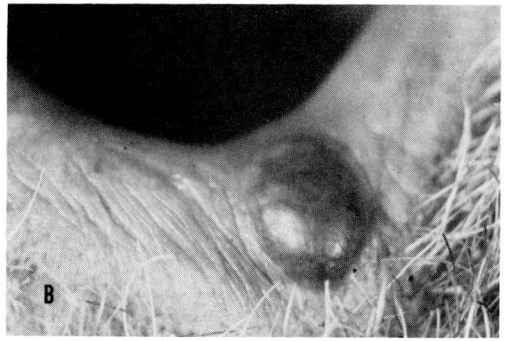

Fig. 6-17. *Traumatic hemangioma. A,* The elevated bluish lesion in the buccal mucosa is soft and blanches on pressure. *B,* The smooth elevated nodule with a broad base is purplish in color, soft to touch, and blanches with pressure. It is produced by mechanical injury.

age. The etiology is not completely understood but may be a proliferation of osseous tissue along the midpalatal suture in response to heavy occlusal stress. The lesion occurs in about 25% of the population. It is twice as common in women as in men.

Torus mandibularis is a nodular growth of osseous tissue on the posterior lingual aspect of the mandible just above the mylohyoid line (Fig. 6-15). It is usually bilateral and may extend from the cuspid to the distal surface of the last molar as a series of discrete or fused nodules 3 to 6 millimeters in size. In some individuals both palatal and mandibular tori may be present. The tori are of concern to the patient who is a denture candidate. Ulcers frequently occur on the summits of the nodules because the mucosa, which is thin over the bone, is injured by hard foods.

Exostosis (Fig. 6-16) occurs as a nodular bony protuberance on the buccal surfaces of the maxilla and mandible. It may accompany palatal and mandibular tori. In most instances the exostosis occurs over teeth positioned towards the labial with very thin labial bone. Exostoses are usually reactive to heavy functional stress and occur as nodules over teeth in heavy function. When all the teeth are in heavy function, the nodules may fuse together to produce a nodular ledge. Like tori, exostoses may be traumatized and become ulcerated.

Amputation neuroma is a proliferation of nervous tissue following the loss of continuity of a nerve owing to trauma. The nerve continues to proliferate and an excess of nerve tissue develops. When near the surface, the lesion is painful on pressure. Lesions arising from the inferior alveolar nerve due to injury during removal of impacted third molars produce pain in the jaw.

Traumatic hemangiomas (varices) are thin-walled, large vascular spaces in the submucosa which produce surface elevation, are purplish in color, are soft and fluctuant in character, and blanch on prolonged pressure (Fig. 6-17). They are several times more common in men than women and, in both sexes, are more common on the lower lip. They may occur on the tongue, especially the inferior surface or the buccal mucosa. They arise in areas of mechanical injury.

BIBLIOGRAPHY

Ake, N., and Landt, H.: Hyperplasia of the oral tissues in denture cases. Acta Odont. Scand., 27:481, 1969.

Blum, T.: Pregnancy tumors: a study of sixteen cases. J. Am. Dent. Assoc., 18:393, 1931.

Hansen, L.S.: Diagnosis of oral keratotic lesions. J. Oral Surg. Anesth. Hosp. Dent. Serv., 17:60, 1959.

Kolas, S., et al.: The occurrence of torus palatinus and torus mandibularis in 2,478 dental patients. Oral Surg., 6:1134, 1953.

Lund, B.A., and Dahlin, D.: Hemangiomas of the mandible and maxilla. J. Oral Surg., 22:234, 1964.

Sapp, J.P.: Ultrastructure and histogenesis of peripheral giant cell reparative granuloma of the jaws. Cancer, 30:1119, 1972.

Sellevold, B.J.: Mandibular torus morphology. Am. J. Phys. Anthropol., 53:569, 1980.

Shklar, G. and Cataldo, E.: The gingival giant cell granuloma. Histochemical Observations. Periodont., 5:303, 1967.

Sist, T.C. (Jr.), and Greene, G.W.: Traumatic neuroma of the oral cavity. Report of thirty-one new cases and review of literature. Oral Surg., 51:394, 1981.

7

AGING, RETROGRESSIVE CHANGES, AND DYSFUNCTION

Aging is a reflection of progressive cellular incapacity and has a genetic basis; however, even though aging may be programmed in relation to a given life span, decreased cellular capacity is accelerated by environmental agents and regulated by neuroendocrine, immune, and humoral factors. To separate aging changes from those due to disease may be difficult, if not impossible. Many disturbances in cells and tissue are not inevitable consequences of aging although the age of the individual may suggest otherwise.

At the present time the etiology of aging must be considered to be multifactorial. However, there are several major areas that receive primary consideration: cells are programmed to cease function, but not at the same time for all cells; major aging phenomena occur in cell populations that have control functions, such as the cells of the central nervous system, neuroendocrine system and the immune system; and aging is a direct result of extracellular factors such as changes in vascular tissues.

Alterations in the structure and functions of cells and tissues considered to be age related include: (1) decreased DNA replication and repair, decreased RNA synthesis, and decreased protein synthesis; (2) cellular and organellar atrophy, with a decrease in size and function and number of cells; (3) vacuoles, inclusions, pigments and other cellular deposits; and (4) abnormal compensatory response such as metaplasia and dysplasia, and occasionally neoplasia (p. 117).

Aging affects all tissues and organs and is predictable, and although it is associated with a decrease in the function of all cells, tissues and organs, the degree of intra- and extracellular alteration is an individual phenomenon and still subject to the human life span. Even though a genetic basis for aging exists, the process can be influenced by a number of environmental factors. In addition to normal physiologic changes that occur with age, many illnesses appear either nonspecifically or atypically in the elderly. For example, the classic symptoms of pneumococcal pneumonia must be modified for the elderly who may fail to muster a febrile response.

AGING AND DISEASE

The separation of the pathology of aging from the consequences of aging is not always possible. The idea that aging is physiologic and not disease is also a concept which is not easy to explain. However, the distinction between aging (chronological versus physiologic, and natural death versus death from disease) and diseases associated with aging (senile dementia and atherosclerosis) are important to make in order to understand aging. The changes seen in aging are also those seen in disease, e.g, there is an age-related decline in glucose tolerance which may be diagnosed as sugar diabetes if not properly evaluated. Another example is hypoproteinemia and hypocalcemia seen with normal aging (Fig. 7-1). Thus the clinician must be aware of how age modifies the textbook description of disease for the elderly may only reflect disease such as hyperthyroidism as little more than cardiac arrhythmia. Also dementia, atherosclerosis, diabetes mellitus, and hypertension are not inevitable consequences of aging. Therefore it seems reasonable that if the broad spectrum of age-related disease were reduced, e.g., all cardiovascular diseases were cured, the average life span would only be increased by 10 years.

Theories of Etiology of Aging

Although there is a trend toward accepting a multifactorial etiology for aging, placing the emphasis on certain areas is not unusual, i.e., on genetic programming, on declining immune, neuroendocrine, and central nervous system control mechanisms, and on extracellular and vascular retrogressive changes. Even though there appears to be an intrinsic "time clock" that regulates the life span for a particular species, it is sometimes suggested that aging reflects the sum of the effects of disease and injury occurring over a lifetime. Obviously the consequence of aging, unlike disease, is 100% mortality.

Evidence for programmed aging includes classic diseases of premature aging such as infantile or adult progeria and juvenile diabetes in which striking aging changes occur without being the consequence of an extrinsic factor disease. Another demonstration is the finding that fibroblasts have a finite number of generations (40 to 60) before cell division and the formation of new cells ceases.

Evidence that changes in the immune system play a dominant role in longevity relates to observations that susceptibility to disease is increased with aging, and that this decline appears to trigger autoimmune, neoplastic, autoimmune, and immune-complex diseases of the blood and blood vessels.

There is evidence that aging is the consequence of injury to blood vessels, for example, the common occurrence of arteriosclerosis in the aged. However, capillaries and venules are not affected by the build-up of fatty material that occurs in the arteries (atherosclerosis) and these smaller vessels account for much of the transport of nutritional substances.

There is no one theory of aging which is able to answer nearly all the questions posed in the clinic or the research laboratory. However, the lack of an acceptable theory about the aging process has not diminished continued inquiry into the decrease in function of cells, tissues, and organs.

Organ Changes

The *skin* of the aging person shows marked changes in the face and neck (Fig. 7-2). It is thin, wrinkled, dry and fragile. Graying of the hair is increasingly frequent. Skin cancer, increased skin pigmentation, and atrophic or deformed fingernails become more common with increasing age.

The *eye* undergoes several structural and functional changes, including decrease of visual acuity, "floating" objects, and an increasing inability to focus on close objects or loss of accommodation (presbyopia). Atrophy of the lacrimal gland may lead to drying of the cornea.

In the *muscles* there is a decline in the size of muscle fibers, muscle mass, and physical strength.

The principal *skeletal* lesions in aging are

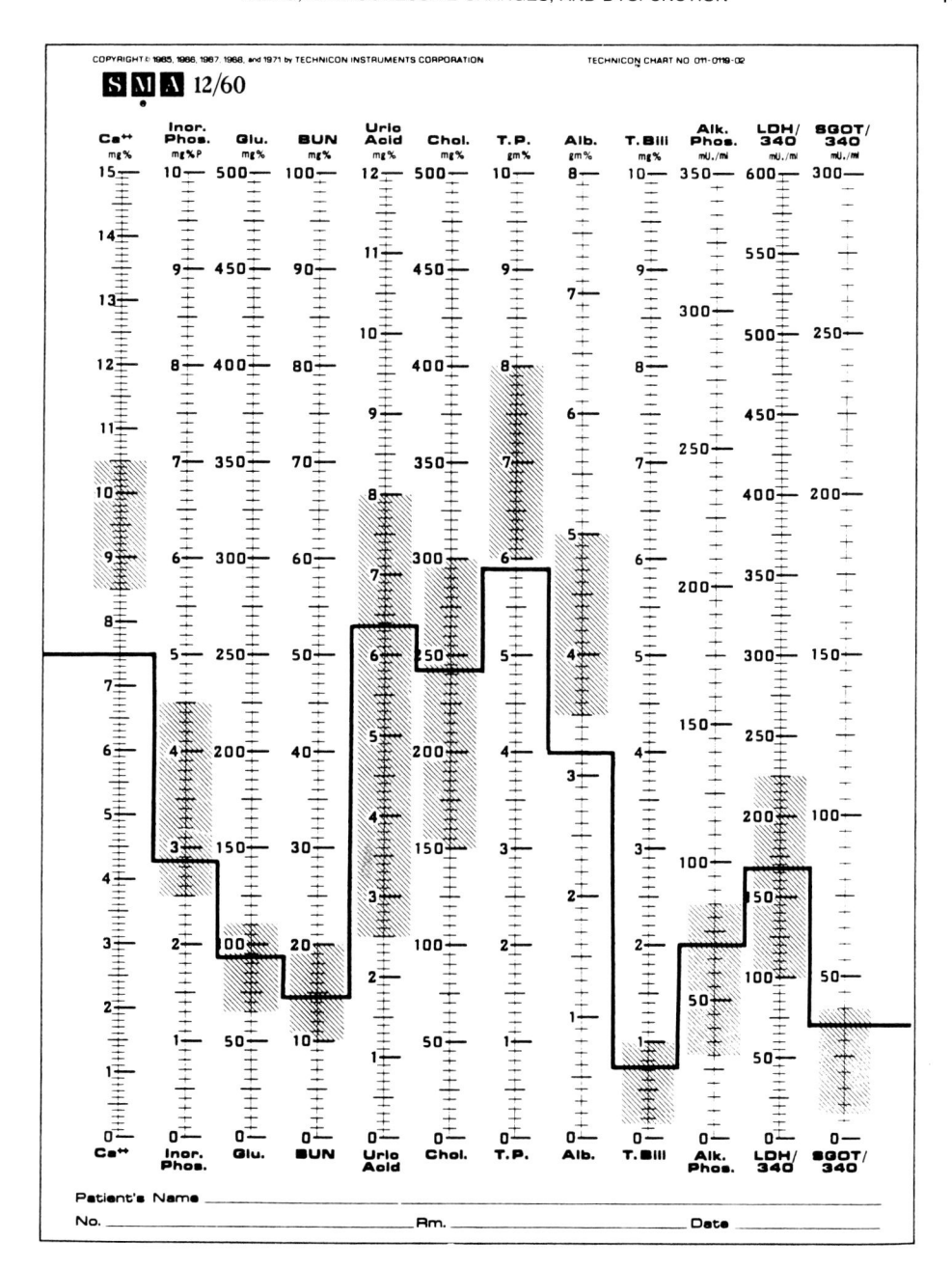

Fig. 7–1. Normal pattern of old age with hypoproteinemia and hypocalcemia.

osteoporosis and osteoarthritis. *Osteoporosis* refers to a reduction in the mass of bone per unit volume. Fractures of the hip and wrists are more common in osteoporotic individuals. *Osteoarthritis* is a degenerative joint disease characterized by a loss of joint cartilage and by hypertrophy of bone. The temporomandibular joint (TMJ) picture is somewhat different because of histologic differences between the TMJ and, for example the knee joint. Osteoarthritis is discussed later in this chapter (p. 107).

The *cardiovascular system* in aging

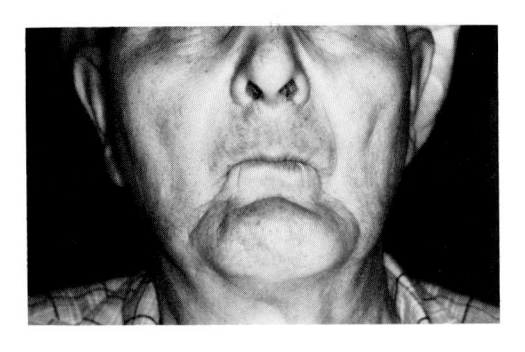

Fig. 7-2. Atrophic changes in skin and muscles associated with aging and loss of teeth.

shows an increase in degenerative changes in the coronary arteries and heart valves. Changes of arteriosclerosis (p. 114) are prominent. Atrophy of heart muscle leads to decreased cardiac output. Arrhythmias, conduction defects, and ischemic (coronary occlusion) heart disease increases with age.

In the *central nervous system*, short term memory and mental agility are diminished, as well as sensory awareness with alteration in position sense, pain perception, and touch.

Changes in the *digestive* tract include a decrease in taste buds, atrophy of gastric mucosa, and decreased production of stomach acids. Root caries, reduced salivary flow, increased periodontal problems and oral cancer, abrasion and erosion, and diseases of the salivary glands require special dental consideration.

Age-related changes in the *kidney* include a reduction in renal blood flood and excretory capacity leading to an increased incidence of kidney disease.

Hearing, sound localization, and sound discrimination become increasingly impaired with increasing age.

AGING AND SPECIFIC DISEASES

Most older people have one or more diseases, and many factors other than age and genetic programming contribute to the involutional changes occurring in older persons. Of particular interest are the changes in the human central nervous system involving *dementia*, i.e., acquired deficits in intellectual and emotional behavior. The most common cause of dementia is referred to as Alzheimer's disease.

Alzheimer's Disease

The term Alzheimer's disease is used to describe senile dementia, i.e., disturbances of recent memory, combined with verbal and nonverbal cognitive deficits such as an inability to translate thought into language (aphasia), inability to perform purposeful movements (apraxia), and abnormalities of space perception. Mild disturbances such as loss of motivation and failure to plan may be seen early in the disease. Only late in the disease does impaired motor function (akinesia) and urinary incontinence become prominent. In the last stages the patient becomes unable to speak or walk and reaches a state of requiring total care. Although Alzheimer's disease usually occurs after age 65, it may occur in the 40s. Thus the early signs of the disease are fading memory, trouble with language or personality changes, and difficulty in performing rote purposeful movements like hair combing. Later the first sign of dementia, difficulty in making appropriate judgments, begins.

The diagnosis of Alzheimer's disease (diffuse cerebral atrophy) can be made by a biopsy of the brain tissue which may disclose the presence of clumps of twisted nerve-cell fibers described by Alzheimer as "neurofibrillary tangles." However, the clinical diagnosis is usually based on less drastic tests and the elimination of other causes of the patient's symptoms.

Although the cause of Alzheimer's disease remains elusive, several lines of research have promise. For example, there may be a lack of an enzyme for synthesizing acetylcholine, a brain chemical necessary for transmitting impulses between nerve cells. Families with an Alzheimer victim are three times more likely to also have a member with Down's syndrome (p. 17). Hopefully the accelerated interest for research in this disease will provide positive help for the some 7% of the 27 million people over 65 in the United States who are severely disabled by Alzheimer's disease.

Osteoarthritis

Degenerative joint disease (osteoarthritis or hypertrophic arthritis) is present in approximately 85% of persons over the age of 70 on the basis of radiologic evidence. Osteoarthritis is characterized by a loss of joint cartilage and hypertrophy of bone. However, degenerative changes in advanced age may be identical to those in young persons when cartilage has been injured. The etiology of osteoarthritis appears to be related to wear-and-tear of the joints especially where heavy stress from a specific occupation or habit has occurred. The cardinal manifestations of osteoarthritis are pain in the joints and bony enlargement of the distal interphalangeal joints of the fingers (Fig. 7–3A). These enlargements (nodes) usually evolve insidiously and without pain. The diagnosis of osteoarthritis is based upon radiographic (Fig. 7–3B) and clinical findings.

Immune Senescence

It is now considered possible and plausible to consider that immune senescence contributes to an age-correlated increase in susceptibility to infections, to autoimmune diseases (p. 88), to an increasing incidence of cancer, and to atherosclerotic vascular disease. Thus with a programmed decline in normal function in aging, a concomitant decline in the immune system occurs, i.e., an age-correlated immunodeficient state in which one or more of the components of the network of regulatory processes is altered leading to immunodeficiency.

Several age-related changes in the immune system are considered to be related to involution of the thymus, some based on animal studies and others conjectural. In normal human aging the thymus declines to 15% of its mass by age 50 and is functionally deficient. There is also a decrease in the concentration of thymus hormones in the blood.

A number of studies indicate that older people are more susceptible to infectious disease than young people, because of impaired immune responsiveness involving delayed hypersensitivity mediated by helper T cells (p. 82), impairment in the ability to develop new hypersensitivity responses, and impaired antibody responses. The immunodeficiency of aging involves a simultaneous decrease in responses to foreign antigens and an increase in autoimmunity. An increase in auto-

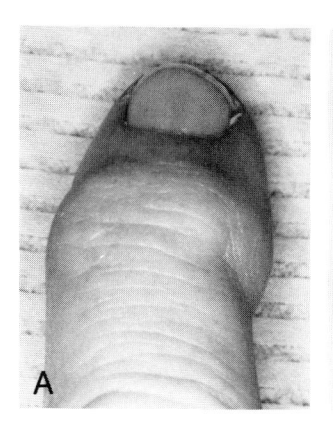

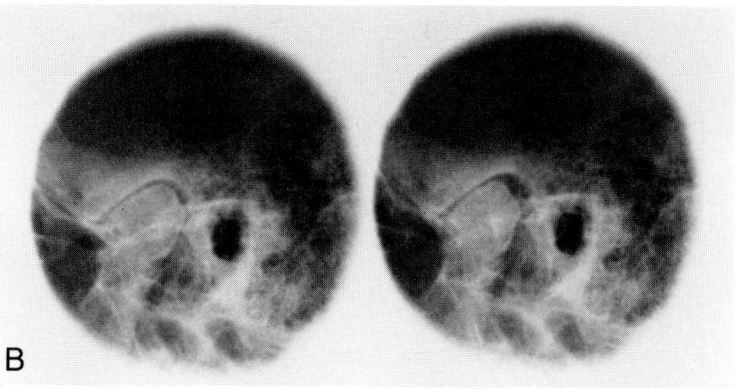

Fig. 7–3. *A*, Bony enlargement of distal interphalangeal joints in osteoarthritis. *B*, Radiographs of temporomandibular joints showing osteoarthritic changes such as loss of joint spaces.

antibodies and immune complexes has been suggested as a possible cause of retrogressive changes of aging, including atherosclerotic cardiovascular disease.

The increased susceptibility to infection and autoimmune disease found in aging is thought to be due to a deficiency of T cells and thus helper T cells, and also a lack of suppressor T cells. The lack of helper T cells leads to enhanced infections, and lack of suppressor T cells leads to increased autoimmune diseases in the aging. Other mechanisms have been hypothesized.

Thymic involution in aging may serve a physiologic role, i.e., protect against autoimmune disease; however, a connection between programmed thymic atrophy and longevity has not been established although immune senescence is important in rising susceptibility to infection and might contribute to an age-related rise in cancer. Thus by premature death from such age-related immune deficiencies, immune senescence may determine the maximum longevity.

RETROGRESSIVE CHANGES

Retrogressive changes involve atrophy, degenerations, infiltrations, concretions, deposits, and "degenerative" changes that impair tissue function. These changes reflect the response of cells to an adverse environment which causes cellular injury. They may also be considered as "wear-and-tear" changes result in a decrease in the functional capacity of cells and a reduction in the efficiency of organs, parts, or the entire organism. When the loss of function is severe enough, the entire organism may be affected to such a degree that continued life is impossible and death results.

Some retrogressive changes start at birth, or before, and progress throughout the lifetime of the individual. The progressive "downward" changes occurring throughout life are also the changes of aging and are significant forms of disease.

Loss of Structure

Attrition is a constant form of retrogressive change seen in teeth. Attrition is the wearing-away of teeth as the result of mastication (Fig. 7–4). It occurs on the occlusal, incisal, and interproximal surfaces. Attrition increases with age and may be influenced by the abrasive quality of the diet and by habits of mastication. In extreme wear the full thickness of the enamel may be worn away to expose dentin, which has a marked tendency to absorb stain from food or tobacco.

Abrasion (Fig. 7–5) refers to the act of abrading—the wear produced by some abnormal mechanical processes. The location and pattern of wear are dependent upon the cause. Notches are seen in the incisal edge of incisors as the result of opening bobby pins, biting thread, and holding tacks or other objects between the teeth. It is also produced in patients who have the habit of grinding their teeth (bruxism). Habits such as chewing tobacco or betal nuts result in intense wear in selected areas. In-

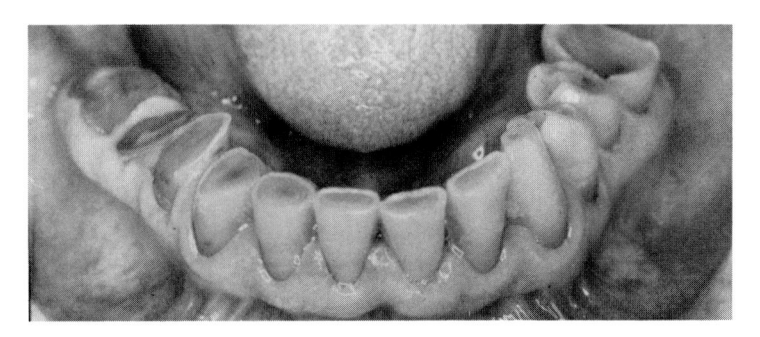

Fig. 7–4. *Attrition.* Excessive occlusal and incisal wear.

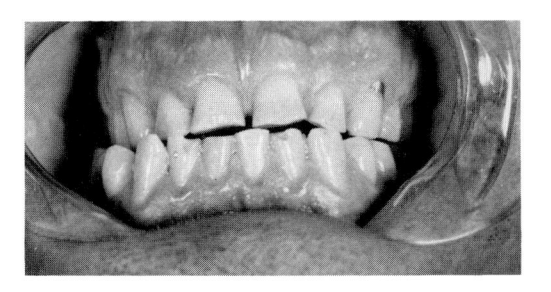

Fig. 7–5. *Occupational abrasion.* Excessive incisal wear associated with glass-blowing.

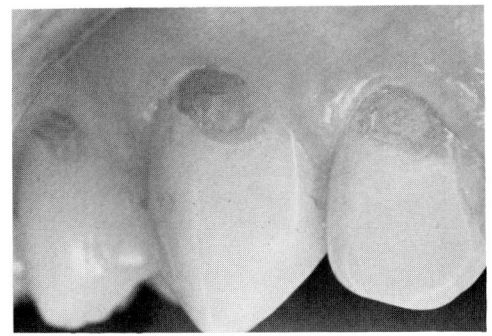

Fig. 7–7. *Erosion.* Extensive loss of enamel due to habitually sucking lemons.

terproximal abrasion may be produced by the incorrect use of toothpicks and dental floss. The wear produced by floss is usually a narrow groove on the mesial and distal surfaces just above the gingival margin. When produced by toothpicks, the wear is a saucer-shaped lesion on the interproximal surface of two adjacent teeth. Abrasion may be produced by the improper brushing of teeth using a hard brush and an abrasive dentifrice (Fig. 7–6). This results when the brushing stroke is horizontal and the abrasion occurs as a notch just above the gingival margin of the buccal and labial surfaces. The process is usually more severe on one side than on the other, depending upon whether the individual is right- or left-handed.

Erosion is a process characterized by the loss of tooth substance through demineralization which occurs on the labial surface of maxillary incisors and the cervical region of bicuspids and molars without apparent cause (idiopathic erosion). It is also produced in other locations from habitually sucking on citrus fruits, ingestion of highly acid medications, habitual regurgitation of stomach contents, or inhalation of acid fumes.

The lesions in idiopathic erosion are trench-like lesions with smooth glistening bases appearing to have been produced by something flowing over the tooth surface. In cases produced by the presence of acid, the changes are loss of enamel and dentin from the surfaces contacted by the acid. The surface is hard and glistening in contrast to caries, in which it is soft and discolored (Fig. 7–7).

Resorption of teeth is a retrogressive change which may occur from within (internal resorption) or it may start on the root surface (external resorption). Resorption of teeth is associated with inflammation, excessive function, and the presence of tumors near the roots of the teeth. The entire root surface may be resorbed and the tooth lost. Internal resorption of the crown produces a pink spot which appears to be in the enamel but is due to the resorption of the underlying dentin (Fig. 7–8A, B, D). The enamel may also be resorbed and the pulp exposed necessitating extraction of the tooth or endodontic therapy.

Atrophy

Atrophy is a retrogressive change characterized by a reduction in the size of cells or a decrease in the total number of cells

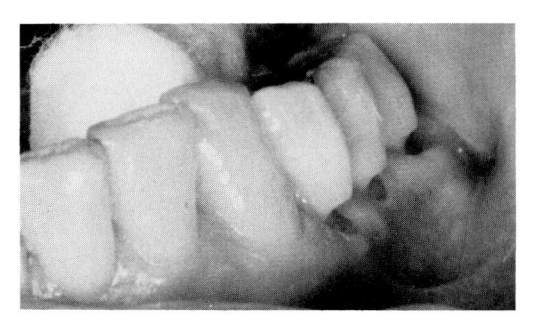

Fig. 7–6. *Abrasion.* Deep cervical notches due to vigorous brushing with a horizontal stroke.

110 AGING, RETROGRESSIVE CHANGES, AND DYSFUNCTION

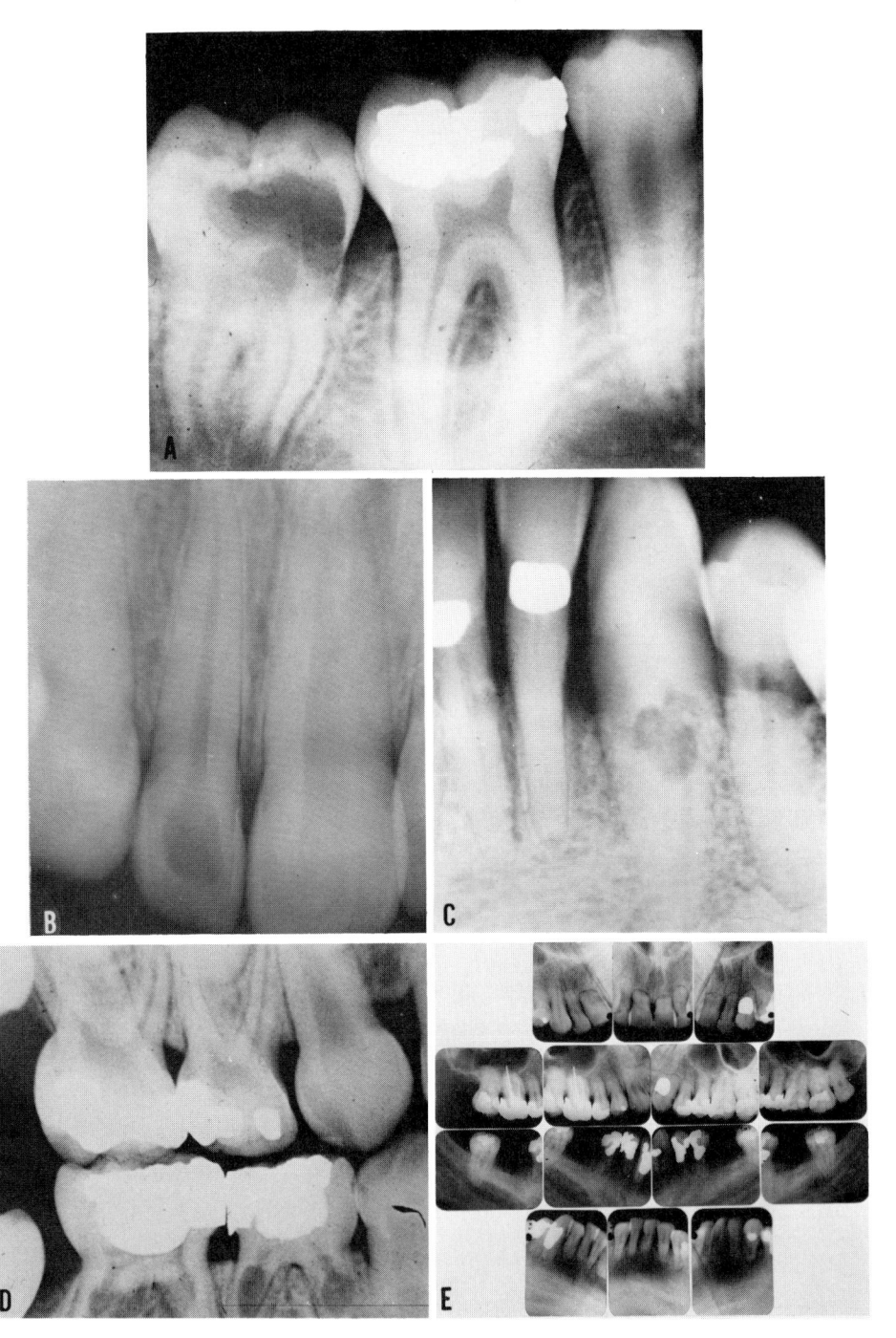

Fig. 7-8. *Internal and external resorption.* A, Internal resorption in the crown of a second molar. B, Marked enlargement of the coronal pulp of a maxillary lateral incisor. Because the vascular pulp shows through the thinned enamel as a pink spot, these teeth are called pink teeth. C, Irregular resorption in mid-root of a mandibular cuspid. In some cases this resorption is initiated externally and in others internally. D, Internal resorption of deciduous molars following pulpotomy. E, Root resorption especially marked in the maxillary incisors.

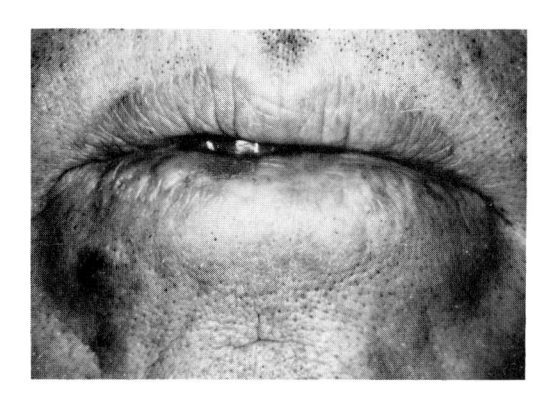

Fig. 7-9. Changes in surface of lips with aging and sunlight.

present in mature tissue or a fully formed organ. Atrophy may be due to disuse of a part, starvation, pressure, toxins, infections, or irradiation.

Atrophy frequently accompanies age, decreased functional demand, and reduced nutrition. Atrophy of the vermilion border of the lip occurs in older individuals due in part to aging and in part to exposure of the lip to sunlight (Fig. 7-9). In this instance the surface epithelium is atrophic and becomes thin and shiny. The lip becomes opaque owing to alteration in keratin metabolism which is also a retrogressive change in squamous epithelium. This condition is called solar or aging cheilitis. Atrophy may occur with age in the tongue and the cheeks. The connective tissue and muscle are reduced in amount and partially replaced by fat. Such a replacement is called fatty atrophy. This results in decrease in size and loss of tissue tone. Atrophy in the salivary glands also occurs with age. The reduced output of saliva produces dryness of the mouth (xerostomia). Xerostomia is not uncommon in elderly patients and is a source of annoyance since it is uncomfortable and makes eating and speaking difficult.

Degenerations, Infiltrations, and Dysfunction

Degeneration refers to those alterations of cells due to the direct action of injurious agents and to secondary changes resulting from an altered intracellular metabolism caused by the injury. Degeneration of many body cells is a daily occurrence due to the "wear and tear" of injury, functional demand, and, to some extent, aging. Degenerative changes may be reversed if alteration of the cells has not progressed too far; otherwise death of the cells occurs.

Cloudy swelling represents subtle cytoplasmic protein changes resulting in granularity and cloudiness of the cytoplasm of the cells. Such changes are most evident in the parenchymal cells, especially of the kidney, heart, and liver, in response to febrile illness, malnutrition, and poisoning.

Hydropic degeneration is a progressive state of cloudy swelling. The degeneration is characterized by the formation of cytoplasmic vacuoles as the result of injury. This type of degeneration is present in liver cells following exposure to certain anesthetics and chemical solvents, such as carbon tetrachloride.

Hyaline degeneration refers to retrogressive changes that result in the cytoplasm taking on a homogeneous translucent, glassy appearance. Hyalinization of the walls of blood vessels is characteristic of certain types of arteriosclerosis and of the vessels of atrophic ovaries and uteri following menopause.

Amyloidosis is the deposition of hyalin-like material between parenchymal cells and in connective tissue and may be a function of aging. It has an amorphous starch-like appearance. There are several forms of amyloidosis but they are usually grouped, for convenience and pathogenesis, into primary and secondary forms. It occurs most often as a primary disease or in association with plasma cell dyscrasias. In primary, the amyloid infiltrates are found primarily in the tongue, heart, skeletal muscle, skin, and gastrointestinal tract. Secondary amyloidosis occurs in relation to other diseases such as chronic suppurative infection or secondary to such diseases as rheumatoid arthritis.

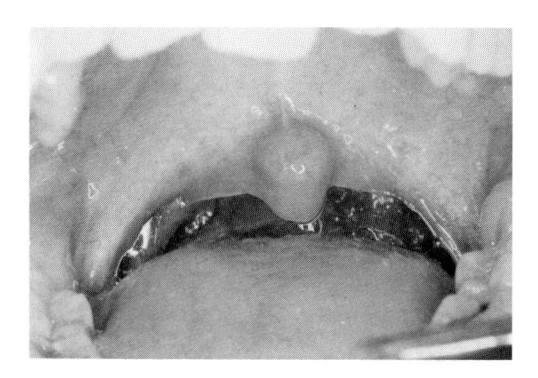

Fig. 7–10. Nodular swelling of soft palate and uvula due to obstruction of mucous gland ducts and retention phenomenon.

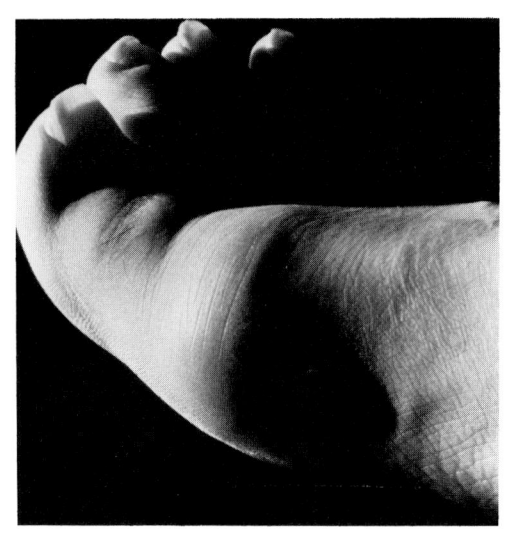

Fig. 7–11. Gouty arthritis of big toe joint (podagra).

Mucinous degeneration is often used to designate the presence of an excess of mucin. Although such an excess is not considered a true degeneration, it is often found interstitially with cellular degeneration. The retention of mucus because of ductal obstruction leads to the formation of mucoceles, viz., retention phenomenon of accessory salivary glands (Fig. 7–10). Myxomas, tumors arising from myxomatous connective tissue, elaborate abundant mucoids. Abnormal accumulations of mucopolysaccharides occur in the *"collagen diseases,"* viz., rheumatic fever, rheumatoid arthritis.

Fatty degeneration refers to an abnormal accumulation of lipids due to cellular damage. For example, alcohol abuse leads to liver damage and to increased fatty acid synthesis, decreased triglyceride synthesis and decreased secretion of lipoprotein from the liver. Nutritional deficiencies in alcoholic subjects may also cause fat to accumulate by upsetting protein synthesis. The accumulation of neutral fat in fatty degeneration is also seen in carbon tetra-chloride poisoning.

The term *infiltration* refers to the accumulation of metabolites within healthy cells due to metabolic derangements of systemic origin. Infiltrations involve lipids and carbohydrates. Infiltration differs from degeneration in the factors which lead up to these regressive changes. The accumulation of metabolites in degeneration follows injury, whereas in infiltration the accumulation of metabolites in healthy or aging cells produces the injury.

Fatty atrophy is the replacement of tissue by fat, especially parenchymal tissue that has undergone marked atrophy. Aging and obesity are important predisposing factors in fatty atrophy of the heart. While the adult fat cells do not reproduce themselves to fill in spaces caused by tissue atrophy, existing mesenchymal tissue accumulates lipids to form adult fat cells. Thus, in obesity, there is an increase in lipids and an increased number of adult fat cells present which store the lipids provided by an excess of food intake over body requirements.

Certain individuals have a limited altered metabolism of uric acid obtained from animal nucleoproteins. The uric acid is deposited in the kidneys and in joint capsules. The deposition in joint capsules and ligaments provides a swollen tender or painful joint due to the accumulation of uric acid crystals in the tissue (Fig. 7–11). The process is designated as gout. Crystals of uric acid may also be deposited in the subcutaneous tissues and produce nodular swellings (tophi).

Necrosis

Necrosis is local cell death due to disease or injury. Cell death is a dynamic process, not an instantaneous occurrence, and involves both nuclear and cytoplasmic changes. The following specific types of necrosis occur: coagulation, liquefaction, caseation, and gangrenous necrosis.

Coagulation necrosis refers to the local death of cells in which the protein elements of the cytoplasm become fixed and opaque by coagulation. A form of this type of necrosis (Fig. 4–8A) is seen in acute necrotizing ulcerative gingivitis. *Liquefaction* necrosis is a type of necrosis in which there is a fairly rapid nonbacterial, enzymatic dissolution and destruction of whole cells. This cellular alteration results in the production of fluid. An example of this type of necrosis is seen in the liquefaction of cells and the formation of pus in a periodontal abscess. *Caseation* necrosis refers to the conversion of dead cells into a soft, friable, cottage cheese-like mass. It is seen with tuberculosis. *Gangrenous* necrosis has all the basic features of infarction plus those changes associated with the infection by putrefactive microorganisms. Gas gangrene is most often seen in the extremities associated with serious wounds contaminated with clostridia, a gas-producing bacteria.

Mineral Metabolism

Mineral infiltration and concretions are primarily concerned with the metabolism and deposition of calcium salts. Pathologic calcification is the presence of abnormal calcific deposits within the soft tissues of the body. The formation of concretions of solid materials in hollow spaces, tubes, or body crevices is termed *lithiasis*. The deposition of calcium in organic matrix gives rise to hard stony calculi. Such calcareous deposits occur primarily in the biliary ducts, collecting system of the kidneys, and ducts of the salivary glands. The formation of sal-

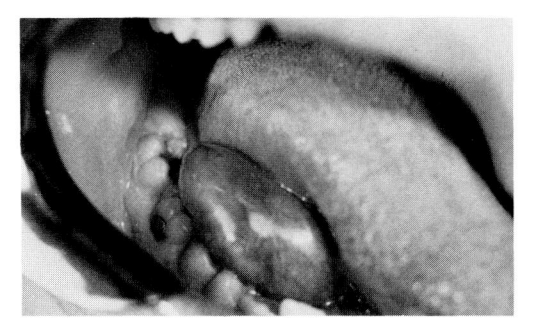

Fig. 7–12. Mucous retention cyst (ranula) of sublingual gland due to an obstruction produced by a sialolith.

ivary calculi (sialoliths) in the ducts of salivary glands is referred to as sialolithiasis. The obstruction of salivary gland ducts by salivary calculi causes dilatation of the duct and chronic inflammation of the entire gland. The obstruction of the duct and the accumulation of saliva give rise to a retention cyst. Such a cyst in the floor of the mouth is often termed a ranula (Fig. 7–12). The formation of gallstones and kidney stones are other examples of the process of lithiasis.

With advancing age, calcium salts are deposited in the dentinal tubules, making the dentin more dense. The process of deposition of calcium salts into a noncalcified tissue, such as a dentinal tubule or blood vessel, is called sclerosis and the involved structure is said to be sclerotic. Sclerosis of dentin is seen in almost all teeth with advancing age and produces a change in the color of teeth. The teeth become more yellow and less translucent. The darkening of teeth with age is often of concern to the patient but cannot be prevented or decreased by any form of treatment.

All teeth undergo regressive changes with age in that calcium salts are deposited in both the radicular and coronal areas of the pulp. In the crown these deposits are spherical in form and are called denticles or *pulp stones* (Fig. 7–13). In the radicular area the calcium is deposited in a diffuse pattern (Fig. 7–14). The spherical masses in the crown can be visualized by x-ray

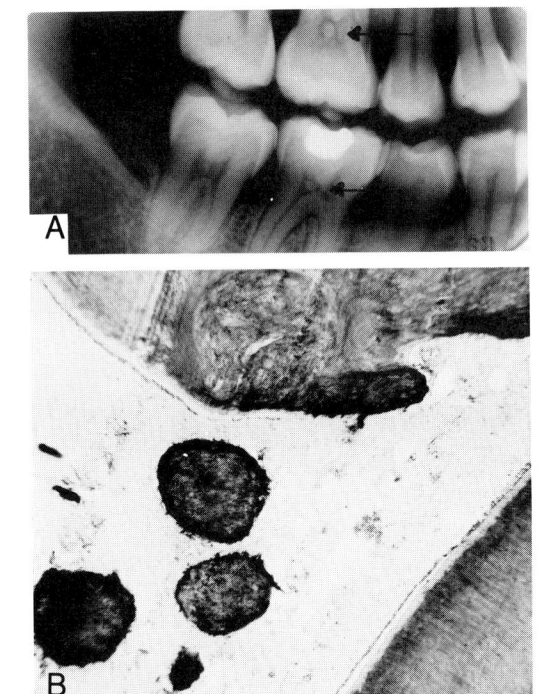

Fig. 7-13. *Denticles (pulp stones).* A, Radiograph of pulp stones in pulp chamber of maxillary first molar. B, Spherical masses in coronal pulp.

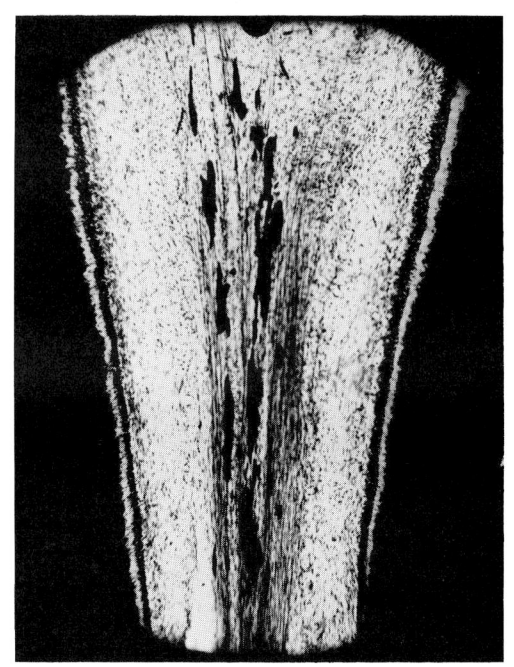

Fig. 7-14. Linear calcification of radicular portion of pulp. Calcium salts deposited in linear masses along path of vessels.

films, but unless extensive the radicular calcification is not readily demonstrated. Accompanying the pulpal calcification there is also a progressive fibrosis or aging of the pulp. Pulp stones rarely produce pain and are of little significance unless root canal procedures are indicated.

Arteriosclerosis

Although the term *arteriosclerosis* actually means hardening of the arteries, it includes several variants which have in common the thickening and loss of elasticity of arterial walls. However, one type, *atherosclerosis,* is a disorder of larger arteries which underlies most coronary artery (heart) disease, aortic aneurysm, and cerebrovascular disease. Atherosclerosis is the leading cause of death in the United States. Atherosclerotic lesions include fibrofatty infiltrates in the intima wall and complex ulcerated lesions that contain hemorrhage, calcium and scar tissue, i.e., fatty streaks, fibrous plaques, and complicated lesions. Fatty streaks are characterized by an accumulation of lipid-filled smooth-muscle cells, macrophages (p. 66) and focal areas of fibrous tissue in the intima of the arteries. Streaks are present in the aorta by age 10 and by age 25 increases to involve as much as 30 to 50% of the aortic surface. The fibrous plaques are firm, elevated and dome-shaped lesions that have a glistening surface. The central core of the lesion contains lipid (mainly cholesterol) and necrotic cellular debris. As the lesion gets more complicated the arterial wall gets progressively weaker leading to rupture aneurysm or hemorrhage. Emboli can form from fragments of plaque breaking away from the vessel wall. Atherosclerosis of the cervical and cerebral arteries, as well as the carotid, basilar, and vertebral arteries, shows a patchy distribution. The internal carotid arteries in the neck appear to be a place of special predilection and the site for emboli to form, leading to cerebral vascular disturbances including transient ischemic attacks (TIAs), apoplexy (stroke), and neurologic defects.

Occlusion of the coronary vessels from atherosclerosis is the immediate cause of myocardial infarction in almost all instances. Ischemic heart disease (IHD) is the cause of death in a sizable portion of nontraumatic sudden deaths. The number who had diabetes or hypertension (diastolic blood pressure greater than 90 mm Hg) is significant. There has been recently a decline in mortality due to coronary atherosclerosis, possibly due to decreased smoking, decreased consumption of animal fats and cholesterol and better control of hypertension. A number of other factors are regarded as possible injurious agents including immune mechanisms.

Risk factors have been established or suspected for a number of agents: *established* factors include high concentrations of blood cholesterol and triglycerides (hyperlipidemia), high blood pressure and cigarette smoking. *Probable risk factors* include diabetes mellitus, family history, contraceptive drugs, and postmenopausal state. *Suspected risk factors* include obesity and physical inactivity.

A decreased incidence of coronary heart disease is seen in patients with high levels of high-density lipoproteins. It is now believed that high-density lipoproteins (HDL) serve as carriers for removing cholesterol from the peripheral tissues. HDL levels are increased in persons who exercise regularly and in persons who consume moderately. The average cholesterol value for Americans is approximately 220 mg (100 m) of blood. Values in excess of 200 are considered to place an individual at increased risk for coronary heart disease. The first step in the treatment of hyperlipidemia involves control of diet, emphasizing decreased intake of saturated fat and cholesterol. If hypertriglyceridemia is present, alcohol should be restricted or eliminated.

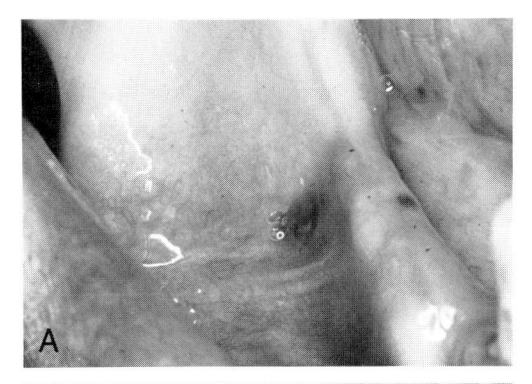

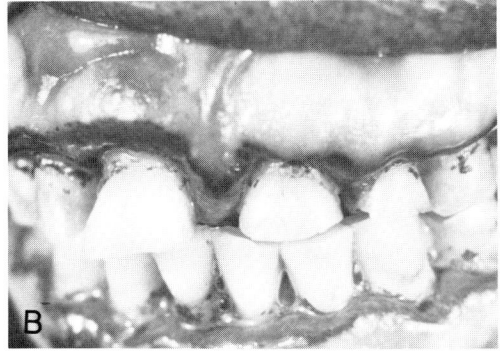

Fig. 7–15. *A,* Argyrosis. Bluish spots on buccal mucosa and alveolar ridge associated with amalgam particles. *B,* Bismuth pigmentation due to ingestion of bismuth.

Control of hypertension, obesity, and diabetes is necessary.

Pigment Metabolism

The term *pigment* refers to a wide variety of chemical deposits formed *within* the body due to abnormal or normal functional activity (endogenous pigments), or their accumulation from *outside* the body due to inhalation or absorption (exogenous pigments). Pigments in general give rise to gross or microscopic discoloration of the tissues involved.

Exogenous pigments include coal dust, metallic silver, and iron dust. The accumulations of coal or iron dusts in the lungs and draining lymphatic tissues in miners are occupational hazards. Silver pigmentation (argyria) gives the skin and mucous membranes a gray-blue discoloration. Localized argyrosis occurs in the gingiva usually from the inadvertent deposition of silver amalgam fragments into alveolar sockets during extraction of teeth (Fig. 7-15).

Endogenous pigments are almost entirely derived from the breakdown of hemoglobin. In conditions where there is an increased destruction of red cells as in the hemolytic anemias, iron pigment may accumulate in certain tissues of the body, especially those of the reticuloendothelial system and in macrophages of the skin and mucous membranes. One pigment not derived from hemoglobin, porphyrin, may occur in excess (rare) and give rise to red deposits in the teeth and other tissues (see Fig. 16-3).

Pigments related to bile, especially bilirubin, are normally excreted in the bile. Bilirubinogenous pigments, when present in excess in the blood plasma, cause *jaundice* (icterus). Icterus may occur as the result of excess hemolysis of red blood cells, liver disease, and obstruction of the bile ducts. Increased pigmentation of skin and oral mucosa occurs in Addison's disease (Fig. 15-3) and of the skin during pregnancy. Melanin pigmentation occurs in the oral cavity in the buccal mucosa and the gingiva (melanosis gingivae) as physiologic pigmentation.

BIBLIOGRAPHY

Anderson, W.A.D. and Kissane, J.M.: *Pathology*, 7th ed., St. Louis, C.V. Mosby Co., 1977.

Bagnara, J.T., et al.: Common origin of pigment cells. Science, 203:410, 1979.

Freimer, E.H., and McCarty, M.: Rheumatic fever. Sci. Amer., 213:66, 1965.

Gambert, S.R.: Aging—an overview. Special Care in Dentistry, 3:147, 1983.

Gorlin, R.J.: Clinical pathologic conference: Sjögren's syndrome. Gerodontic, 1:2, 1985.

Gueft, B., and Ghidoni, J.J.: The site of formation and ultrastructure of amyloid. Amer. J. Path., 43:837, 1963.

Hayflick, L.: The biology of human aging. Adv. Pathobiol., 7:80, 1980.

King, D.W.: Effect of injury on the cell. Fed. Proc., 21:1143, 1962.

King, D.W., et al.: Cell death. Amer. J. Path., 35:369, 1959.

Leevy, C.N.: Fatty liver and a review of the literature. Medicine (Balt.), 41:249, 1962.

Makinodan, T. and Kay, M.B.: Age influence on the immune system. In Kunkel, H.G. and Dixon, F.J. (eds.), *Advances in Immunology*, Series, Vol. 29, New York, Academic Press, 1980.

Ross, R., and Harker, L.: Hyperlipidemia and atherosclerosis. Science, 193:1094, 1976.

Schroeder, H.E.: Melanin containing organelles in cells of the human gingiva I. Epithelial melanocytes. J. Periodont. Res., 4:1, 1969.

Sokoloff, L.: The pathology of gout. Metabolism, 6:230, 1957.

Spain, D.M.: Atherosclerosis. Sci. Amer., 215:48, 1966.

Squier, C.A., and Waterhouse, J.P.: The ultrastructure of the melanocyte in human gingival epithelium. Arch. Oral Biol., 12:119, 1967.

Stamler, J.: Cardiovascular diseases in the United States. Amer. J. Cardiol., 10:319, 1962.

Symposium on Atherogenesis, Acapulco, Mexico, 1975, Ann. N.Y. Acad. Sc., vol. 275, Aug. 27, 1976.

Valenstein, E.: Age-related changes in the human central nervous system. In Beasley, D.S. and Davis, G.A., Aging, *Communication Processes and Disorders*. New York, Grune & Stratton, 1981.

Watanabe, I., et al.: Oral dyskinesia of the aged I. Clinical aspects. Gerodontics, 1:39, 1985.

Weissmann, G. and Rita, G.A.: Molecular basis of gouty inflammation interaction of monosodium urate crystals with lysosomes and liposomes. Nature (New Biol.), 240:167, 1972.

Weksler, M.E.: Senescence in the immune system. In Dixon, F.J. and Fisher, D.W. (eds.), *The Biology of Immunologic Disease*. Sunderland, Mass., Sinauer Assoc., Inc., 1983.

8

NEOPLASIA

DEFINITION

The term neoplasia refers to that formation of abnormal new tissue occurring when the normal regulative processes of cellular differentiation and proliferation have been lost. The subject of neoplasia is a complex but interesting and important one because of the frequency with which neoplastic disease occurs in the population. The lesion that develops in neoplasia is technically called a neoplasm, although the terms *tumor* and *cancer* are used extensively, especially by the laity.

The process of neoplasia is one that takes place within body cells causing them to undergo spontaneous, independent, uncontrolled, and unlimited growth. Without apparent reason, cells responsible for forming mature, functioning tissue lose their normal processes of differentiation and proliferation. They then produce new cells which are quantitatively and qualitatively abnormal and replace the tissue in which the neoplastic process occurs. The area of origin of a neoplasm may be small but may rapidly increase in size to involve an entire organ or part. The neoplasm may remain confined to the site of origin or it may extend to other areas of the body. In many instances neoplasms spread into or replace vital areas and cause the death of the host.

EPIDEMIOLOGY

Neoplastic disease occurs in a large part of the animal kingdom; in humans it involves both sexes of all ages, although it is most common in the older age group. Because there is a high incidence of neoplasms in patients over 50 years of age, this age is sometimes called the "cancer age." Some races show greater tendency for cancer of specific areas than other races. Furthermore, one sex may have a greater incidence of cancer of specific organs than the other sex. Tables 8–1 and 8–2 demonstrate the areas of the body most frequently involved and the incidence of cancer and death according to sex and anatomic location.

In the past 60 years the incidence of neoplastic disease has shown a progressive increase which is in part an actual and in part an apparent increase. During this period cancer has risen from tenth place to second as a cause of death. The *actual* increase in incidence is due to technologic advances (new chemicals, radiation, and other factors) and to our mode of living, which makes it possible to come into contact with carcinogenic agents. For example, with the marked increase in cigarette smoking, there has been an alarming increase in cancer of the lungs owing to inhalation of the combustion products of tobacco. The

Table 8-1. Incidence of Cancer and Death (According to Site and Sex)

Site of Origin	% Incidence of Cancer Male	% Incidence of Cancer Female	% Deaths Due to Cancer Male	% Deaths Due to Cancer Female
Mouth	6.2	2.9	3.3	1.1
Respiratory	12.3	2.5	21.6	4.0
Digestive	33.0	23.3	35.0	33.5
Genital	10.8	24.4	11.2	19.9
Urinary	7.0	3.4	6.0	3.5
Leukemia and Lymphoma	6.3	4.0	10.5	8.6

Table 8-2. Incidence of Cancer in Various Anatomic Sites

Site	Peak Incidence (Years of Age)
Kidney	0-4
Bone	15-25
Brain	40-45
Skin	60-65
Abdominal organs	60-65
Digestive tract	60-80

apparent increase in neoplastic disease is due to public health measures which have increased the life expectancy to above 60 years, so that more people are living to the "cancer age." Because cancer affects all ages of both sexes and stands second as a cause of death, it presents one of our most perplexing health problems.

ETIOLOGY

The cause of neoplasia is unknown. Why a particular cell or group of cells spontaneously undergo unlimited, progressive, independent growth is a perplexing problem which as yet has defied intensive research. However, there are many things known about some of the factors predisposing or influencing the development of neoplasia. These factors are discussed here as hereditary, extrinsic, and developmental factors.

Hereditary Factors

There is considerable evidence that heredity plays a significant role in the development of neoplastic disease. Although neoplasia is not generally considered to be an inheritable disease, some factors of susceptibility or immunity appear to be present. The influence of heredity has been demonstrated in mice; some strains have been developed that are almost 100% susceptible to certain neoplasms and other strains have been bred that are cancer-resistant. In humans the importance of heredity can be demonstrated by the frequency with which identical twins develop identical neoplasms at about the same age even though their environments may have been different. It is also significant that some individuals develop more than one type of neoplasm. There are families in which nearly all members develop neoplasms of the same organ at about the same age. This age is some 10 or more years younger than the average age for such a neoplasm of the same organ in the population at large. Although the familial occurrence of neoplasia is rare, retinoblastoma is a good example of a neoplasm having a familial pattern. There is also a familial tendency for mutiple polyposis which almost invariably leads to carcinoma. All of these and many more observations indicate that heredity plays an important part in susceptibility to neoplastic disease.

Extrinsic Factors

Extrinsic factors are environmental in nature, numerous, and important to the development of neoplastic disease. Examples of various environmental factors will serve to indicate their nature, wide variety, and importance.

MECHANICAL IRRITATION. Clinical observations suggest that chronic mechanical irritation serves as a causal factor in cancer, viz., the development in rare instances of cancer from ill-fitting dentures. Hyperplasia occurs in response to irritation, but, in some instances, the new cells become neoplastic and produce a neoplasm of the alveolar ridge. The new cells in an area of cancer may resemble the normal cells but do not duplicate them, and they proliferate rapidly even though the irritation is removed.

CHEMICALS. Neoplastic causal factors can be demonstrated in a large variety of chemical substances. The first experimental production of a neoplasm in a laboratory was produced by rubbing coal tar on the ear of a rabbit. Today, in high-cancer strains of laboratory animals, neoplasms can be produced by many substances refined from coal tar. These chemicals and many others that influence the development of cancer are called *carcinogens*. Hormonal factors may be important in the development of cancers of the breast, uterus, and prostate. Important carcinogens are those in our foods, e.g., food dyes, nitrates, and nitrosamines. Attempts are being made to limit exposure to these agents by the U.S. Food and Drug Administration.

IRRADIATION. Irradiation by x rays, radioactive material, and sunlight all play an important part in the production of cancer. X-ray irradiation in a single massive dose or in repeated small doses predisposes the skin to the development of cancer. This was evidenced by the frequency with which dentists and technicians developed cancer of the hands from holding x-ray films in patients' mouths for exposure. The repeated small quantity of x ray received was cumulative, and after a period of years the individual develops an x-ray dermatitis which progressed to cancer (Fig. 8–1). With massive doses of x ray producing tissue destruction (the so-called x-ray burn), healing is delayed sometimes for years, and cancer develops at the site of attempted repair.

Small doses of radioactive material ingested or introduced into the body may also produce cancer; this occurred in watch-dial

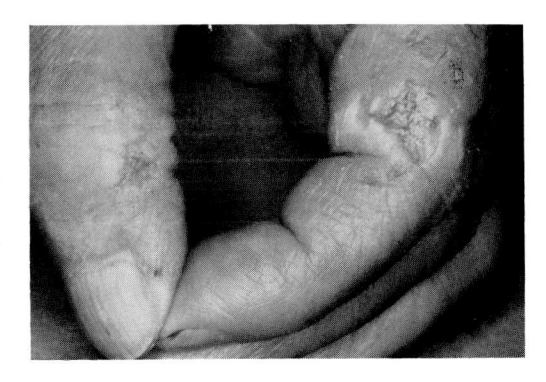

Fig. 8–1. *X-ray dermatitis*. X-ray burns on thumb and forefinger from frequently holding x-ray films in patients' mouths. Squamous cell carcinoma (skin cancer) often develops in these areas.

painters in the 1920s. In making luminous watch dials, women employees applied paint with a fine brush which they pointed with their lips. Unfortunately, by this maneuver, small quantities of radioactive material in the form of radium salts were ingested. The radium salts united with calcium and became stored in the bones. After less than a year of this practice, nearly all of the women developed cancer of the bone.

SUNLIGHT. Sunlight is a potent factor in producing cancer of the skin, especially in individuals who have little natural pigment for protection. Over a period of years, repeated exposure of the skin to ultraviolet rays conditions the skin so that later in life numerous small skin cancers may develop on the face or other exposed parts. The face is the most common site and the cancers are of a specific type—basal cell carcinoma.

There also is a definite relationship between cancer of the lip and exposure to sunlight. Individuals, usually males who have light skin and spend much time out of doors, develop solar cheilitis which predisposes to cancer of the lip. The lip changes in solar cheilitis occur slowly over a period of years. The first change is the loss of definition between the vermilion portion of the

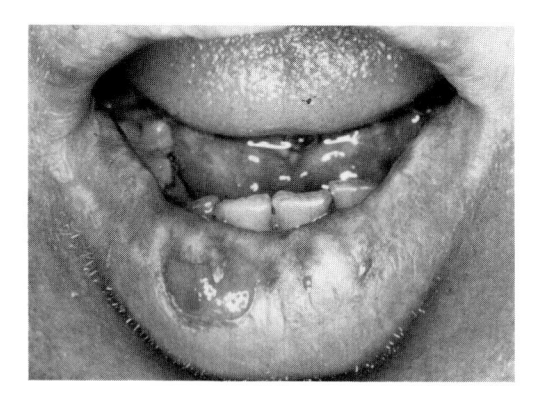

Fig. 8-2. *Solar cheilitis*. The vermilion border is thin, smooth, opaque, and ulcerated from prolonged exposure to sun and wind.

lip and the adjacent skin. The lip takes on a smooth shiny parchment-like quality to the epithelium of the exposed vermilion border. As the process progresses, the epithelium shows increased cornification and imparts a bluish-gray opacity to the lip. In limited areas small whitish plalques may develop. There is a tendency for small flakes of keratin to occur on the surface along with small cracks or ulcers (Fig. 8-2). In the more advanced stages periodic ulceration occurs, especially with continued exposure to sunlight. Such changes predispose to cancer of the lip. However, if the predisposing changes are recognized early, the patient can prevent cancer by protecting his lips from exposure to sunlight.

Viruses

Oncogenic viruses are those capable of causing cancer. Although these viruses have been demonstrated as a cause of neoplasia in animals, oncogenic viruses have not been demonstrated in humans except for the common wart caused by a DNA virus (a papovavirus), the herpesvirus genitalis (herpes simplex 2) is suspected of being oncogenic in women.

Immunologic Defects

It has been suggested that cancer may be associated with a decline or impairment of the surveillance capacity of the immune system. However, patients with grossly impaired immunity are no more likely to develop cancer than others. The exception to this rule is lymphoma which is much more common in immunodeficient subjects, either those born with the defect or artifically depressed. Thus, with the exception of lymphomas, human malignant tumors appear more likely to be due to chemical carcinogens than to oncogenic viruses.

Developmental Factors

Developmental factors are inherent forces of growth and differentiation responsible for the proper development of a tissue or organ. These forces may be disturbed during the development of a tissue or part so that the cells lose their ability to continue differentiation while at the same time they retain or accentuate their growth potential. When a developng tissue undergoes independent proliferation at some stage of differentiation short of final maturity, a neoplasm is produced. An excellent example of a developmental neoplasm is the ameloblastoma arising from the developing enamel organ.

GENERAL CHARACTERISTICS

Neoplasia occurs in any tissue of the body and exhibits a variety of characteristics distinctive for each neoplasm in each type of tissue. For this reason it is necessary to describe and to label each type of neoplasm so that it can be distinguished and placed in its proper position in the large field of neoplasia. Two large divisions of neoplasms are designated—*benign* and *malignant*.

Benign Neoplasms

The benign neoplasm arises in any area of the body from any type of tissue and presents specific features which give it a somewhat predictable behavior. The benign neoplasm generally grows slowly because of a limited ability for proliferation, but it has a high degree of ability for differen-

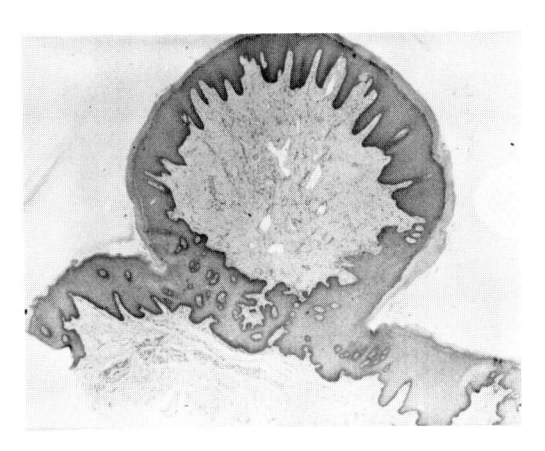

Fig. 8-3. *Fibroepithelial papilloma.* A benign lesion of papillomatous character demonstrating expansile growth.

tiation. The cells making up a benign neoplasm duplicate well the parent type of cell and resemble normal cells. Cells of a benign neoplasm have a level of differentiation high enough in some instances to retain normal but independent functional activity. Benign neoplastic cells divide with a nearly typical mitotic pattern resulting in an expansile lesion which does not invade other tissues but does produce pressure atrophy of surrounding tissue as its bulk slowly increases (Fig. 8-3). With expansile growth there frequently is compression of the stroma surrounding the developing mass giving the neoplasm the appearance of being surrounded by a fibrous capsule. Because of its slow growth, high level of differentiation, limited ability to invade, and somewhat limited potential for growth, the benign neoplasm is of local significance and can be totally removed by surgical procedure and a cure accomplished. These factors are characteristic of a benign neoplasm and for that reason it is referred to as a tumor by the lay person.

Malignant Neoplasms

In contrast to the benign neoplasm is the malignant neoplasm. The malignant neoplasm also arises from any type of tissue in any part of the body, but it exhibits a rapid rate of proliferation and a poor level of differentiation (so poor that it may be impossible to recognize the type of tissue from which the neoplasm arises). Because of rapid growth and poor differentiation, malignant cells develop bizarre mitotic figures and grow by infiltration rather than expansion. In infiltrative growth the surrounding tissue is replaced completely and no distinct boundaries or capsule develops (Fig. 8-4). Absence of a tissue boundary and extension by growth between various tissue structures result in widespread and extensive invasion resulting in difficulty of localization and removal. The invasion occurs in any area, often in vascular channels. When vascular spaces are invaded, the invading cells find a favorable habitat for growth, and they proliferate extensively within the lumen of a blood vessel or lymphatic. The loosely arranged new cells may propagate along the lumens of vessels and spread the neoplasm for some distance; or, they may be broken away from the main mass and be carried by blood or lymph to some distant area where they become lodged and set up a second foci of growth. This discontinuous spread from one area to another is called *metastasis,* a feature of malignant neoplasms. A neoplasm with a low level of differentiation, rapid invasive growth, and discontinuous spread is called a malignant neoplasm and is generally known to the lay person as cancer. Cancer, like tumor, is a term understood by laity and may be used to inform a patient that he has a malignant neoplasm, but it does not designate the type of neoplasm. Thus, to the patient, the term cancer means that he has a new growth which is difficult to remove, will spread to other areas of his body, and, if not entirely removed, will continue to grow and ultimately will cause his death.

This summary (Table 8-3) is only general and does not include specific and detailed clinical and microscopic differences, which are necessary to make the diagnosis of a specific neoplasm.

CLASSIFICATION

Neoplasms of both benign and malignant types may arise from either epithelial or con-

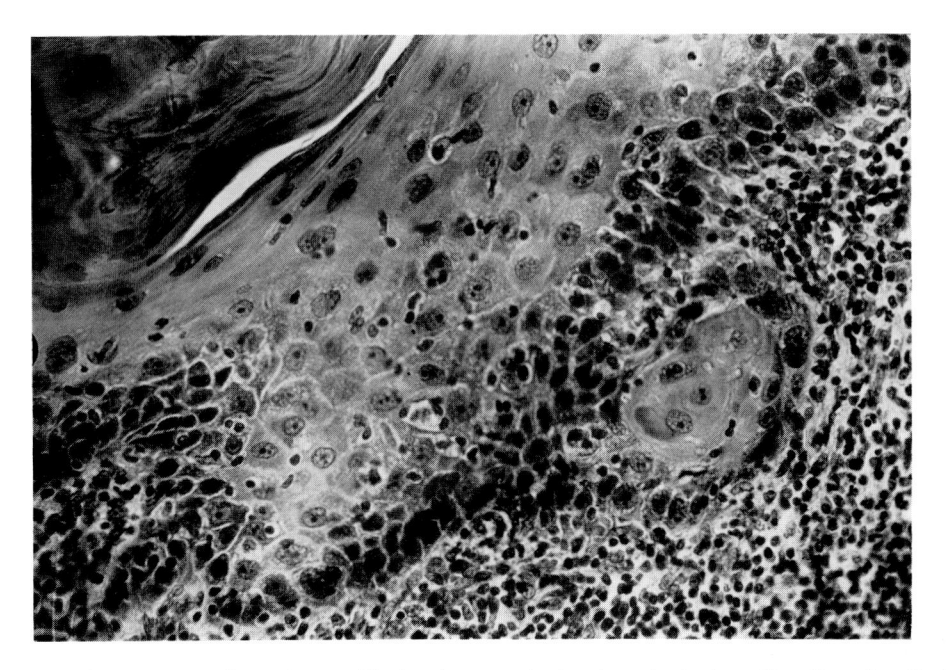

Fig. 8–4. *Squamous cell carcinoma.* Photomicrograph showing atypical proliferation of epithelium with small islands below the basal layer demonstrating invasive growth of a malignant neoplasm.

nective tissue, or both, and may be named according to the type of tissue from which they originate as well as according to their nature. The suffix, -*oma,* is a nonspecific term which usually implies a neoplasm; however, it should be pointed out that the suffix, -*oma,* is sometimes used to designate malignant neoplasms. The term cancer refers to a malignant neoplasm which can be classified on the basis of tissue origin (histogenesis) into: *carcinomas,* which arise in epithelium; *sarcomas,* arising in mesenchymal tissues; and *leukemias* and lymphomas, which arise in the blood-forming cells of the bone marrow and lymph nodes. Table 8–4 indicates the variety of neoplasms which may occur in the body. It is a simplified classification based upon histogenesis.

Neoplasms of Epithelial Origin

Papilloma is a benign neoplasm arising from squamous epithelium and occurring with some frequency in the oral cavity (Fig. 8–5). It occurs in the gingiva, palate, tongue, floor of mouth, and lip as a lobulated or filiform elevation 2 to 5 millimeters in diameter. It is white and has a firmer consistency than the normal mucosa. Growth is slow and the lesions rarely reach a centimeter in diameter. Complete surgical removal provides a cure.

Basal cell carcinoma is a neoplasm arising from squamous epithelium which du-

Table 8–3. Summary of Differences between Benign and Malignant Cancers

Characteristics	Benign	Malignant
Metastases	Never	Almost always
Recurrence	Rare	Frequent
Mitosis	Almost normal	Rapid, atypical
Growth	Expansile, slow	Invasive, rapid
Character of cells	Nearly normal	Poorly differentiated
Limitation	Often encapsulated	Not encapsulated

Table 8-4. Classification of Neoplasms

Cell Origin	Benign	Malignant
Epithelial		
Squamous cell	Papilloma	Squamous cell carcinoma
Glandular cell	Adenoma	Adenocarcinoma
Ameloblasts	Ameloblastoma	
Mesenchymal		
Fibroblast	Fibroma	Fibrosarcoma
Nerve cell	Neuroma	Neurosarcoma
Fat cell	Lipoma	Liposarcoma
Bone cells	Osteoma	Osteogenic sarcoma
Cartilage cells	Chondroma	Chondrosarcoma
Endothelial cell	Angioma	Angiosarcoma
Melanoblasts	Nevus (melanotic)	Malignant melanoma
Hemopoietic, lymphoid and recticuloendothelial cells		Leukemia
		Lymphoma
		Myeloma
Odontogenic cells	Odontogenic fibroma	
	Odontogenic myxoma	

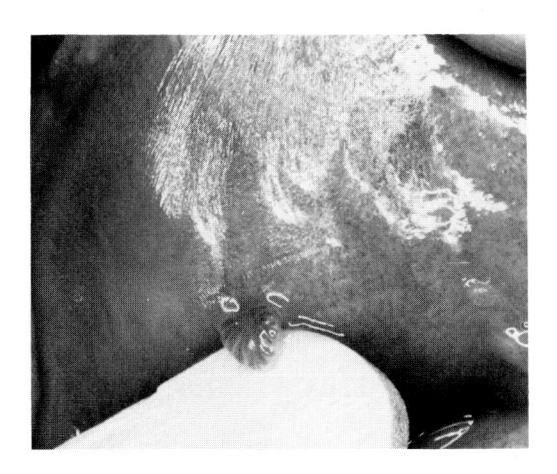

Fig. 8-5. *Papilloma.* Filiform lesion on the buccal mucosa.

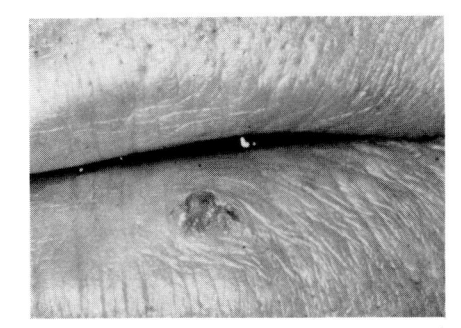

Fig. 8-6. *Early squamous cell carcinoma.* Small, slightly elevated hyperkeratotic lesion in the mid-vermilion of the left lip.

plicates the pattern of the cells of the basal layer of the epithelium. Basal cell carcinoma occurs most often on the face of older people, especially men who have had prolonged exposure to intense sunlight or people with light complexions who have little resistance to actinic radiation. A basal cell carcinoma may be a flat or slightly elevated lesion 3 to 10 millimeters in size. The early lesions are usually scaly, whereas the older lesions are ulcerated. As the lesion grows, the border becomes slightly elevated and pearly white, while the ulcerated center becomes larger and deeper. Basal cell carcinoma has a tendency to invade tissue locally but rarely metastasizes. Lesions may be destroyed by x-ray irradiation or removed by surgical procedure. Type of treatment indicated depends on location, size, and changes present in the skin.

Squamous cell carcinoma is the most common malignant neoplasm of the oral region. It is most common on the lip but also occurs on the tongue, alveolar ridge, floor of mouth, palate, and in the buccal mucosa. Squamous cell carcinoma occurs predominately on the lower lip of older males. Carcinoma of the lip may present a variety of appearances depending upon the degree

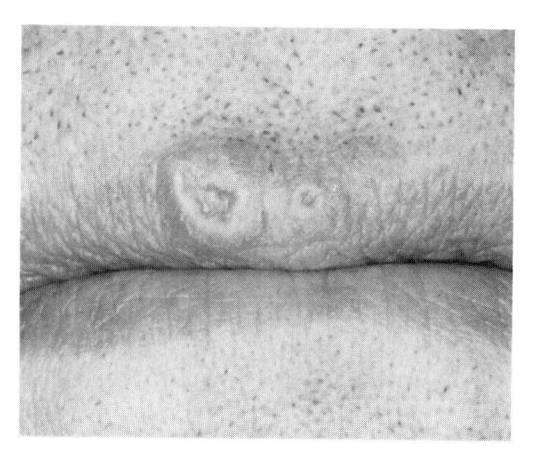

Fig. 8-7. *Carcinoma of the upper lip.* Early cancer showing typically depressed center with a whitish elevated periphery. The depressed center is due to early ulceration.

of advancement. The early lesion may be a slightly elevated plaque firmer than the surrounding vermilion and whitish or grayish in color. It may be a keratinized plaque (Fig. 8-6) or a superficial ulcer (Fig. 8-7). As the lesion advances it becomes elevated and ulcerated (Fig. 8-8). The border is rolled and grayish. Large lesions may be either fungating or destructive. Carcinoma of the lip metastasizes late to the regional lymph nodes and, therefore, offers a good prognosis when treated early. Advanced carcinoma of the lip has a guarded prognosis even with extensive treatment. Carcinoma of the lip may be treated with either x-ray irradiation or surgery. Both methods provide a cure and satisfactory cosmetic results.

Carcinoma of the tongue usually starts on the lateral border either as an elevated white lesion or as an ulcer (Fig. 8-9). It may invade the under surface of the tongue and extend into the floor of the mouth. The patient frequently states that the lesion was initiated by biting his tongue, and the acceptance of this statement causes the true nature of the lesion to be overlooked. In most instances, the patient bit the tongue because the neoplasm was present but had not been recognized. Carcinoma of the tongue metastasizes early. The more posterior the lesion, the poorer the prognosis. Even with radical treatment early carcinoma of the tongue offers a poor prognosis. Carcinoma of the tongue may be treated by surgery or x-ray irradiation, or by surgery with postoperative irradiation.

Carcinoma of the alveolar ridge is usually associated with using chewing tobacco or snuff. This variety of carcinoma usually starts as an ulcer, which enlarges and becomes elevated at the periphery, or it may start as an area of hyperkeratinization. Carcinoma of the alveolar ridge metastasizes late, but may still have a poor prognosis because of its proximity to bone which it invades making treatment difficult. Treatment of carcinoma of the alveolar ridge is usually surgical excision and is severely mutilating because of the required resection of the jaw.

Adenoma and *adenocarcinoma* arise in the oral region from the accessory or major salivary glands, but these neoplasms are not common. Because they arise in the substance of the gland, they are clinically manifest only as swellings in the areas of origin (Fig. 8-10). The most common neoplasms of the salivary glands are the mixed salivary gland tumors (pleomorphic adenomas), which, as the name indicates, should be both epithelial and mesenchymal in origin. Actually these neoplasms are derived from salivary gland ducts and are therefore only epithelial in origin. Changes in the mesen-

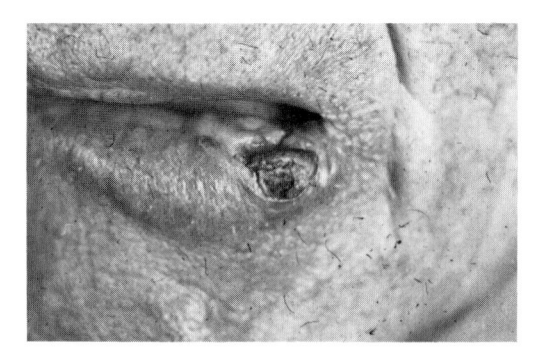

Fig. 8-8. *Advanced carcinoma of the lip.* Ulcerated lesion with elevation at the border and thickening of the lip. This is characteristic location for lip cancer.

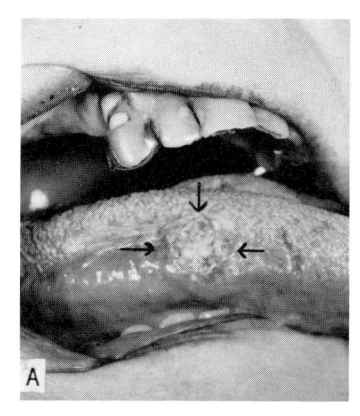

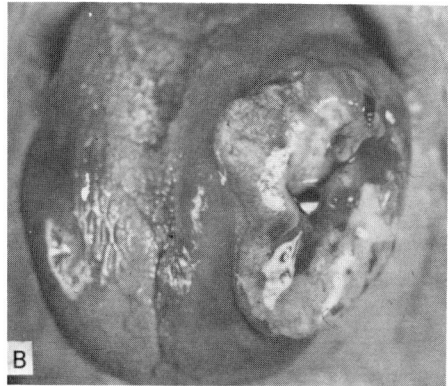

Fig. 8-9. *A, Early carcinoma of the tongue.* The extent of this early lesion is indicated by the arrows. The lesion followed irritation from a broken partial denture clasp. *B, Fungating lesion with central necrosis.* The patient stated this lesion started from biting his tongue.

chyme are induced by the epithelial cells. Treatment is usually surgical removal as these neoplasms are not radiosensitive. Approximately one-fourth of the major salivary gland neoplasms are malignant, whereas one-half of the intra-oral accessory gland neoplasms are malignant. In the benign variety the prognosis is good, whereas in the malignant variety the prognosis is poor.

Ameloblastoma is one of the special epithelial neoplasms arising in the oral region (Fig. 8-11). Ameloblastoma arises from epithelial elements of the enamel organ and because of this origin it is sometimes designated a developmental neoplasm. In most instances, it develops within the jaw, most often in the third molar region of the mandible of patients about 40 years of age. It has been reported as early as three years of age and as late as 70 years, but the average age of occurrence is 40 years.

Ameloblastoma grows in proliferating buds resembling the enamel organ or dental lamina so that it has a tendency to extend

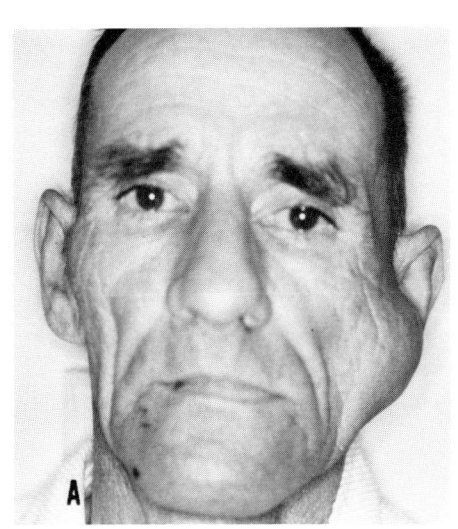

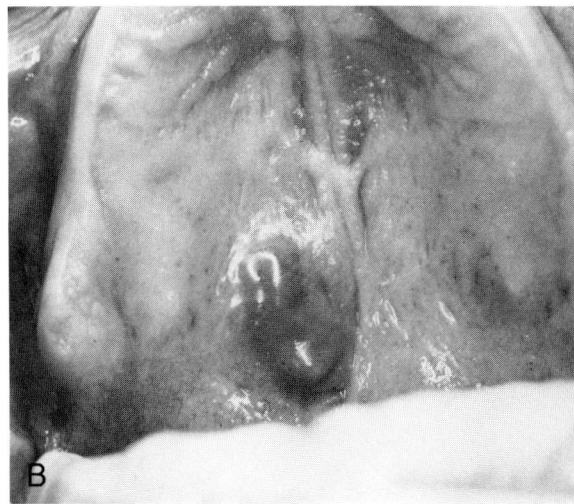

Fig. 8-10. *Tumors, A,* Swelling of midlateral face is typical of parotid gland tumor. *B,* Tumor involving the small glands of the palate.

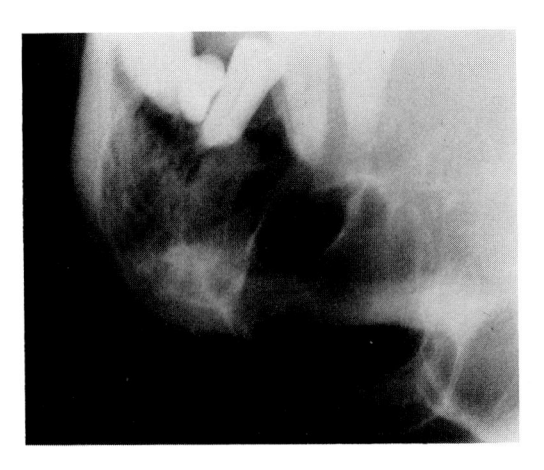

Fig. 8–11. *Ameloblastoma.* Large radiolucent, well defined lesion at the angle of the jaw is typical of ameloblastoma.

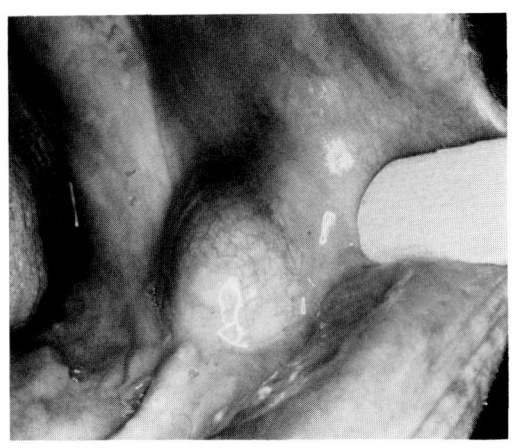

Fig. 8–12. *Lipoma.* Smooth nodular mass in the buccal mucosa is yellowish in color. The tortuous capillaries are evident on the surface because the mucosa is stretched. The mass is poorly circumscribed and easily compressible on palpation.

through the marrow spaces. It also has a strong tendency to become cystic causing it to be expansile. With the development of a cystic pattern, it produces local swelling and deformity of the face, which in advanced cases may be extensive. Although the neoplasm has some tendency to invade locally, it remains well differentiated and usually does not metastasize. Some reports of metastasis appear in the literature, but most of these are to the lung in patients who have undergone repeated incomplete surgical removal. They probably represent spread by aspiration rather than true metastasis.

Ameloblastoma is treated by surgical procedure as the neoplasm is not radiosensitive. Its pattern of growth necessitates wide surgical excision and sometimes resection of the jaw. Because of its tendency to extend through the marrow spaces and sometimes its incomplete removal, the neoplasm frequently recurs and may have to be removed several times. In spite of repeated recurrences, the neoplasm rarely kills the patient even when there is evidence that it has spread to the lungs.

Neoplasms of Mesenchymal Origin

The mesenchymal neoplasms, with the exception of odontomas, are rare in the oral region, and even odontomas are not too common. Benign mesenchymal tumors occur more frequently than the malignant ones. This finding is fortunate, because sarcomas of the head and neck region have a poor prognosis; in fact, they are rarely cured.

Lipoma is a tumor composed of adipose tissue and occurs in all parts of the body

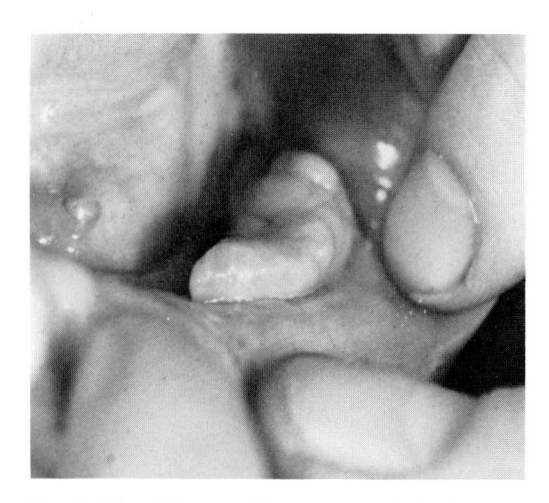

Fig. 8–13. *Fibroma.* The crescentric lesion extending from the lower alveolar ridge is slightly lighter than the normal mucosa. It is firm in consistency and solidly fixed to the mandible.

where there is fat (Fig. 8–12). It is, therefore, a tumor which occurs in many anatomic locations. In the oral region it occurs in the buccal fat pads of the cheek and the floor of the mouth as an indistinct, smooth, soft swelling. Lipomas grow slowly, remain benign, and are easily treated surgically.

Fibromas are composed of fibrous connective tissue and may occur in the lips, tongue, palate, gingiva, and jaws (Fig. 8–13). They are usually slow-growing nodular lesions which become pedunculated when near the surface. Fibromas are easily cured by complete local excision.

Tumors arising from *nervous* tissue are rarely pure tumors, but are composed of nerve tissue and fibrous tissue. Either tissue may predominate and any element of the nerve may be present. When the nerve elements grow as nerve fibers in fibrous tissue, they are called cirsoid *neurofibromas,* the most common variety seen in the oral region. Neurofibromas occur in the lips, buccal mucosa, tongue, and occasionally in the jaw. They produce a nodular swelling, which may cause pain because the nerve fibers are functional. Other tumors of nervous tissue origin may arise from the elements of the nerve sheath which become intermingled with the fibrous tissue. Such tumors are called neurilemmomas or Schwannomas. Both types of tumors grow slowly and produce limited symptoms other than local deformity. All types of neural neoplasms are treated by surgery and the results are excellent, except in congenital neurofibroma which holds a poor prognosis when the whole tongue is involved or when the neoplasm extends into the neck.

Hemangioma and *lymphangioma* (angiomas) occur in the oral cavity; the former are by far the more frequent. Angiomas occur in the lips, buccal mucosa, tongue, and occasionally in the substance of the jaw (Fig. 8–14A, B, C). The tumors are composed of vascular structures varying in size from a capillary to large endothelial-lined spaces. The appearance of the lesion is dependent upon the size of the vascular spaces. Those composed of numerous capillaries are slightly elevated, bright-red lesions of small size, usually not more than a centimeter in diameter. Those composed of large vascular spaces are elevated, nodular, bluish masses, which may be from a centimeter to several inches in area. The large tumors are soft, and pulsations may be felt on palpation if they are closely associated with an artery.

Angiomas of the tongue are sometimes congenital and produce marked macroglossia. The congenital angiomas of the tongue may extend into the neck and involve it extensively. Angiomas of varying color and size may involve the skin of the face and lip and extend through the full thickness of the lips and cheeks. On the skin they are called "birthmarks" or "port wine stains." Small angiomas may be cured by surgical excision, but removal of large ones is difficult and may necessitate skin grafts to repair the defect.

Odontogenic neoplasms arise from tooth-forming elements, either from mesenchymal or from both epithelial and mesenchymal elements. Those arising from only the epithelial elements have already been discussed under ameloblastomas. Odontogenic neoplasms of mesenchymal origin are the *odontogenic myxomas* which arise from the dental papilla and the *odontogenic fibromas* which arise from the dental sac. The odontogenic myxoma and odontogenic fibroma are rare benign tumors arising in the portion of the jaw where a tooth is missing. They grow slowly and expand the jaw but usually present no other symptoms. The tumors are treated successfully by surgical removal.

The majority of the odontogenic tumors are derived from both epithelial and mesenchymal elements with varying proportions of both tissues being represented in different tumors. In some odontogenic tumors the epithelial elements predominate, whereas in others the epithelium is sparse. Some of these tumors form calcified enamel and dentin and are called hard or calcified

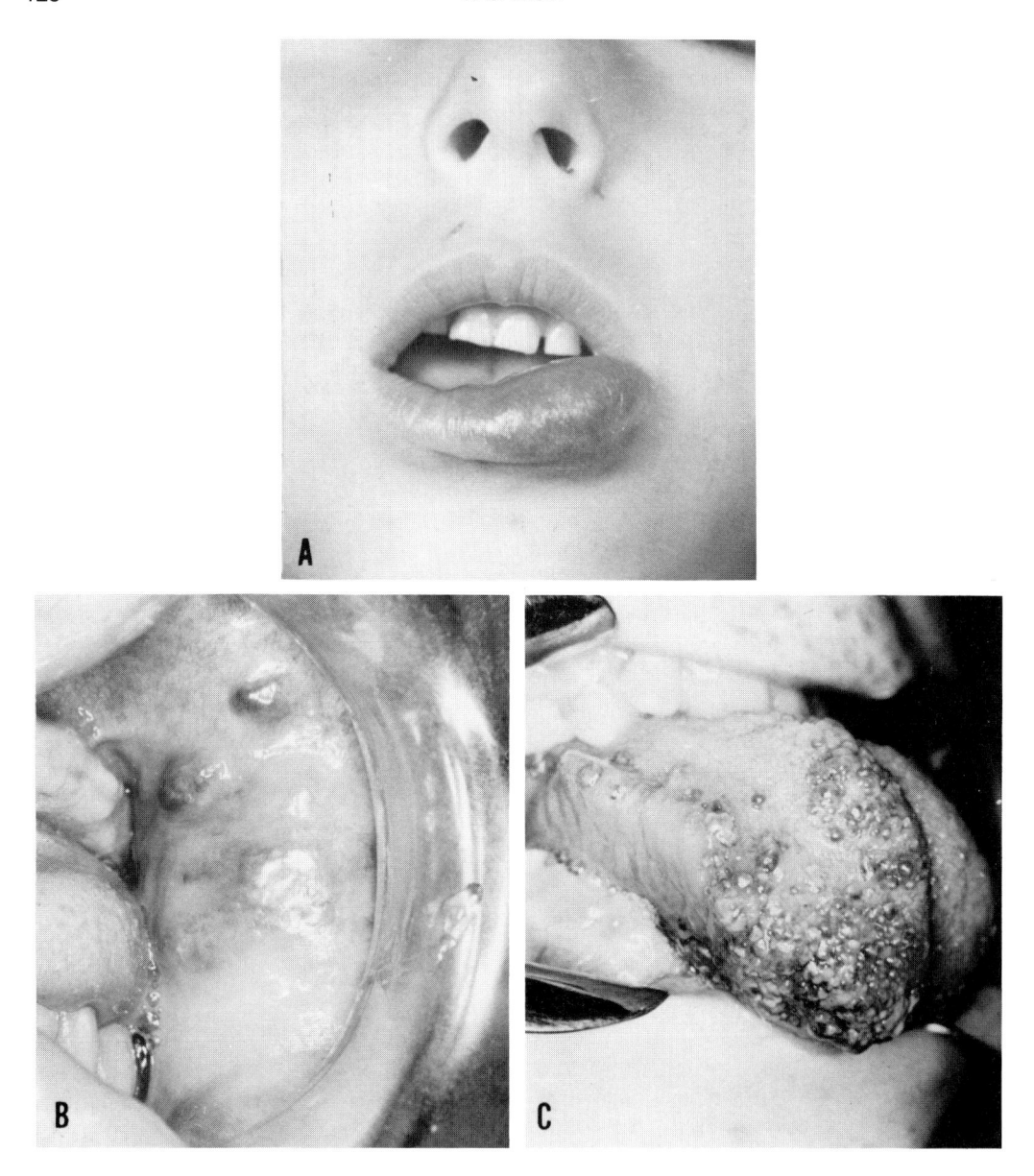

Fig. 8-14. *Hemangioma.* A, The smooth dark swelling of the left half of the lower lip is a hemangioma of the type often present in children. B, Numerous dark nodules of buccal mucosa are due to cavernous hemangioma. C, Numerous small nodules on dorsum and lateral tongue present one pattern of lymphangioma of the tongue.

mixed odontogenic tumors. In contrast to those which are not differentiated to such a level that they can produce calcifiable enamel or dentin are the soft or noncalcified mixed odontogenic tumors. Some of the calcified tumors are composed almost entirely of enamel and dentin in varied proportions and arrangement. Both the soft and calcified mixed odontogenic tumors are benign, slow-growing, and can be successfully treated surgically.

Odontogenic tumors composed almost entirely of calcified tissue are called *odontomas*. When the tumor tissue exhibits only

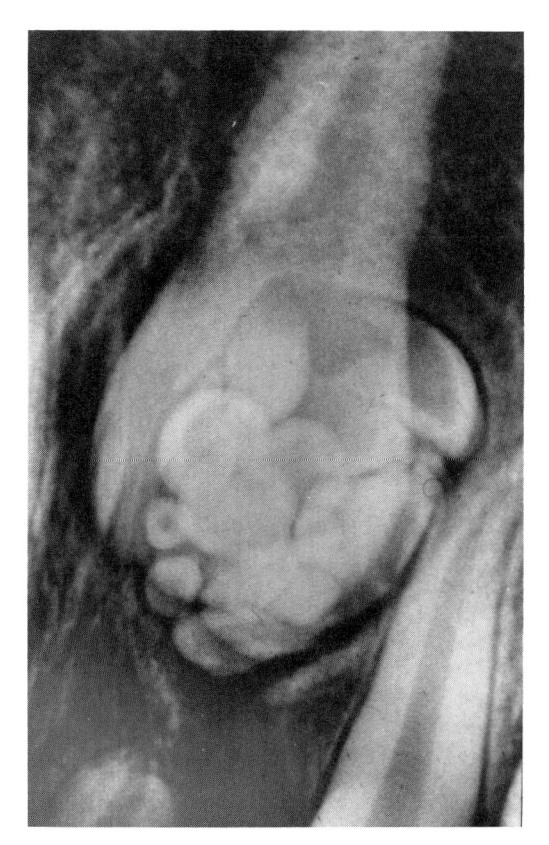

Fig. 8–15. *Compound odontoma.* Several small calcified structures representative of miniature teeth are contained in a radiolucent area surrounded by a connective tissue membrane.

histodifferentiation and the enamel and dentin do not simulate the arrangement of a tooth, it is called a *complex odontoma*. When the tumor exhibits both histo- and morphodifferentiation and the enamel and dentin have the arrangement of miniature teeth, the tumor is designated a *compound odontoma* (Fig. 8–15). Both of these types of odontoma are benign, slow-growing tumors which can be treated successfully surgically.

Malignant mesenchymal neoplasms of all types may involve the jaw, but the incidence is low for all types. The fibrosarcoma and osteogenic sarcomas are the most frequent primary malignant mesenchymal neoplasms of the oral region, while the neoplasms of lymphoid tissue origin are the most common variety which are primary in the neck. All of the malignant mesenchymal neoplasms in the head and neck region have a grave prognosis because they present difficult treatment problems in that they are usually not radiosensitive and are difficult to remove completely by surgical procedure. The malignant mesenchymal tumors have a decided tendency to metastasize by the hematogenous route, and, therefore, the metastatic lesions are more remote and extensive.

Metastatic neoplasms of both epithelial and mesenchymal origin may involve the oral region, especially the jaws. The most common metastatic neoplasm found in the jaws is carcinoma of the breast, which has a marked tendency to metastasize to bone, and often the jaw is the site of metastasis. Carcinoma of the thyroid and prostate likewise metastasize to bone and may occur in the jaw. Metastatic tumors of the jaw have a poor prognosis since the primary neoplasm is elsewhere, and even though the lesion of the jaw is eliminated, the patient is not free of the disease and may ultimately be killed by the primary neoplasm.

Leukemias and Lymphomas

Leukemias are a group of neoplastic diseases involving the blood-forming cells and lymph nodes. There are several types based on the type of cell involved and the degree of differentation that the cell has reached. Acute leukemia is characterized by the presence of primitive leukocyte precursors, i.e., myeloblasts or lymphoblasts. In chronic leukemia the cells that predominate are differentiated to the point that they appear to be structurally similar to normal cells. In acute leukemia the blast cells progressively replace normal bone marrow, migrate and invade other tissues. Anemia, infection, and hemorrhage are general complications of acute leukemia because the bone marrow no longer produces normal red blood cells, granulocytes, and platelets. Leukemias are discussed further in Chapter 16, Hematologic and Hematopoietic Diseases.

Lymphomas are a group of malignant neoplasms which arise from lymphocytes, histiocytes (monocytes that have migrated into the tissues), or primitive precursor cells of the immune system, i.e., malignant diseases of lymphoreticular origin (lymphoid components of the immune system). Thus the lymphomas arise in the lymph nodes or lymphoid tissues of the skin, lung, gut, etc. The presence of cell surface markers (p. 76) using immunologic techniques may indicate the class of cancer cell from which the cell originates and the stage of differentiation.

On the basis of immunologic characterization of lymphoreticular neoplasms, lymphomas may be categorized as being of B cell origin, T cell origin, or of histiocyte origin. Almost all non-Hodgkin's lymphomas appear to be derived from B cells or have no distinctive cell markers. Lymphoreticular neoplasms are often described in terms of "Hodgkin's disease and other lymphomas," as well as in terms of "Hodgkin's disease and non-Hodgkin's lymphoma." Ninety percent of all cases of Hodgkin's disease originate in lymph nodes whereas only 60% of non-Hodgkin lymphomas originate in the nodes. The diagnosis of Hodgkin's disease is made on the basis of lymph node biopsy and the presence of distinctive giant tumor cells (Reed-Sternberg cells). The node enlargement is usually asymptomatic and often only noticed on routine examination; however, a patient may have undiagnosed fever, weight loss, night sweats and sometimes pruritus (itching) of the skin over the enlarged lymph node. The cause of Hodgkin's disease is unknown, although investigators have searched for infective agents because its clinical and histologic features suggest a granulomatous inflammation (p. 71) as well as neoplasia. In many cases long-term disease control can be achieved by combined radiotherapy and chemotherapy.

Non-Hodgkin's lymphomas (NHL) refers

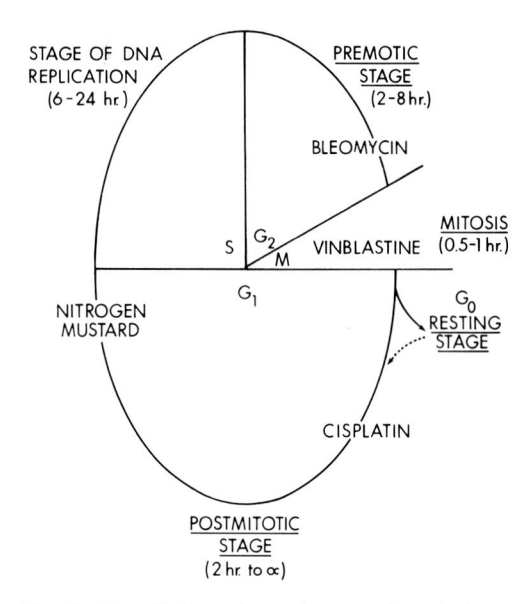

Fig. 8–16. Cell cycle and examples of drugs which are used for most effective site of action. Other drugs include hydroxyurea or alkeran which are effective in early G, phase (normal DNA), and methotrexate in the 5 phase (DNA synthesis).

to a wide variety of lymphoreticular disorders including lymphocytic, histiocytic, pleomorphic, and lymphoblastic lymphomas, and Burkitt's tumor. The etiology of NHL is unknown, but a viral factor has been suggested. NHL accounts for 3% of all new cases of neoplasia. The most common clinical manifestation of NHL is painless enlargement of lymph nodes. In 40% of the cases NHL arises in the lymphoid tissues of extranodal origin, i.e., parenchymal organs such as the gut, skin, and lung. The diagnosis is made by histologic examination of material from lymph nodes. Various forms of malignant lymphoma occur in the oral cavity, although their incidence is rare. However, these lesions should be included in any review of neoplasia because of the impact that immunologic techniques have had on identifyng the cells of origin of the various subtypes of lymphomas. Such identification of these cells helps in determining the different courses that these subtypes may take and the most appropriate treatment developed.

CANCER THERAPY AND COMPLICATIONS

The principles of cancer therapy are in part related to the fact that different types of cells renew (marrow, germ cells), others expand (kidney, liver), and others remain static (neurons, striated muscle). In terms of ionizing radiation it is necessary to deliver a therapeutic dose to the neoplasm and minimize damage to the surrounding tissues. To some extent ionization is damaging to all cells, but more so to proliferating cells especially during the early phase of DNA synthesis and during the mitotic phase of the cell cycle (Fig. 8-16). In this aspect some lymphomas are highly sensitive to radiation in contrast to a radioresistant sarcoma of skeletal muscle. Thus radiotherapy of cancer is likely to be least beneficial in tumors which contain only a small fraction of actively dividing cells. However, a number of other considerations such as radioresponsiveness and radiocurability must be taken into account, as well as the complications or radiation reactions that occur in normal tissues.

Complications following radiation therapy include xerostomia (dry mouth), loss of taste, and dental caries (Fig. 2-4). Major complications include osteoradionecrosis and soft tissue ulcerations that are difficult to heal. Preventive periodontal and dental caries treatment should be instituted prior to radiotherapy. All teeth that are potential sources of postradiation necrosis should be extracted if they cannot be treated effectively prior to radiotherapy. Soft tissues should cover all extraction sites before irradiation is started.

Cancer *chemotherapy* involves the use of a variety of drugs which exploit the biologic differences between cancer cells and normal cells. Since both are susceptible to the cytotoxic effects of most of the agents being used, the effectiveness of chemotherapy is often related to subtle cell growth kinetics, pharmacokinetics, the action of the drugs, and their toxicity in man. For example, tumor growth is initially rapid but slows with an increase in tumor size. On the other hand, normal tissues such as the bone marrow grow faster than solid tumors. Therefore, agents which are cytotoxic to rapidly growing normal cells (e.g., bone marrow, gastrointestinal mucosa or hair follicles) may be more damaging to these cells than to the tumor cells which are in a slow growth stage. This kind of problem requires careful attention to drug selectivity, scheduling and proper combination of drugs. With a combination of drugs (nitrogen mustard, vincristine, prednisone and procarbazine) the cure rate for Hodgkin's disease is significantly improved. The relationship of drug selection to the cell cycle is illustrated in Figure 8-16. Cancer cells may become resistant to the toxicity of drugs, whereas normal cells rarely do. The use of new drugs after effective use of the drugs which are initially effective may minimize the emergence of resistant clones of cells.

Cancer chemotherapy agents include: *Antimetabolites,* folic acid analogs (e.g., Methotrexate); *Alkylating agents,* nitrogen mustards (e.g., mechlorethamine); *Antibiotics* (e.g., Bleomycin); Vinca alkyloids (e.g., vincristine); platinum (e.g., cisplatin); and *hormones,* adrenal steroids (e.g., prednisone, estrogens).

A number of side effects occur with chemotherapy and may limit the use of an agent. Nausea and vomiting, bone marrow depression, loss of hair (alopecia), impairment of kidney function, heart damage, and pulmonary fibrosis occur selectively with one or more agents being used. As with all forms of cancer therapy knowledge of the extent (staging) of the malignant disease is essential to plan effective treatment.

Immunotherapy utilizes immunologic reactions to destroy tumor cells, i.e., augmentation of the immunity of the host to tumor cells. Unlike cytotoxic chemotherapy, irradiation, and surgery which inherently produce damage to normal tissues, immunotherapy attempts to enhance immunologic competence that has been progressively impaired with tumor growth. The specificity of the immune response and lack of toxicity offer promise for immunotherapy but as yet it has not been significantly effective for human cancer.

BIBLIOGRAPHY

Anderson, D.L.: Cause and prevention of lip cancer. J. Can. Dent. Assoc., 37:138, 1971.

Baserga, R.: The cell cycle. N. Engl. J. Med., 304:453, 1981.

Becker, F.F. (ed.): Cancer. A comprehensive treatise. Vol.6, *Radiotherapy, Surgery and Immunotherapy*. New York, Plenum Press, 1977.

Blum, H.F.: Sunlight as a causal factor in cancer of the skin of man. J. Nat. Cancer Inst., 9:247, 1948.

Cairns, J.: *Cancer, Science, and Society*. San Francisco, Freeman, 1978.

DeVita, V.T., Jr., et al.: The consequences of chemotherapy of Hodgkin's disease. Cancer, 47:1, 1981.

Dorn, H.F., and Cutler, S.J.: *Morbidity from Cancer in the United States*. Public Health Monograph No. 29, U.S. Public Health Service, pt. 2, 1955.

Drew, S.I.: Immunologic surveillance against neoplasia: an immunologic quandry. Hum. Pathol., 10:5, 1979.

Dulbecco, R.: The turning point in cancer research: sequencing the human genome. Science, 231:1055, 1986.

Fine, G., Marshall, R.B., and Horn, R.C.: Tumors of minor salivary glands. Cancer, 13:653, 1963.

Foote, F.W., and Frazell, E.H.: Tumors of major salivary glands. Cancer, 6:1065, 1953.

Green, I., Cohen, S., McClusky, R.T.: *Mechanisms of Tumor Immunity*. New York, John Wiley and Son, 1977.

Heidelberger, C.: Chemical carcinogens. Cancer, 40:430, 1977.

Kerr, D.A.: Keratotic lesions of the oral cavity. J. Dent. Med., 13:92, 1958.

Lijinsky, W.: Nitrosamines and nitrosamides in the etiology of gastrointestinal cancer. Cancer, 40:2446, 1977.

Marshall, J., et al.: Diet in the epidemiology of oral cancer. Nutr. Cancer, 3:145, 1982.

Mehta, F.S., Gupta, P.C. and Pindborg, J.J.: Chewing and smoking habits in relation to precancer and oral cancer. J. Cancer Res. Clin. Oncol., 99:35, 1981.

Potdar, G.G., and Paymaster, J.C.: Tumors of minor salivary glands. Oral Surg., 28:310, 1969.

Regezi, J.A., Courtney, R.M., and Kerr, D.A.: Dental management of patients irradiated for oral cancer. Cancer, 38:994, 1976.

Shklar, G.: *Oral Cancer*. Philadelphia, W.B. Saunders Co., 1984.

Smith, C.J.: Global epidemiology and aetiology of oral cancer. Int. Dent. J., 23:82, 1974.

Smith, J.F.: Salivary gland lesions—variations and predictability. Oral Surg., 27:499, 1969.

Spouge, J.D.: Odontogenic tumors. Oral Surg., 24:392, 1967.

Wynder, E.L., Mushinski, M.H., and Spivak, J.C.: Tobacco and alcohol consumption in relation to the development of multiple primary cancers. Cancer, 40:1972, 1977.

9

NUTRITIONAL DISTURBANCES

Although the prevalence of classical nutritional deficiencies has been significantly reduced in the United States and most other industrialized countries, there are some overt as well as subclinical remaining problems related to inadequate intake of nutrients and to metabolic imbalance. Even though the body consists of a large number of organic molecules, most do not come via dietary intake and are nonessential insofar as the diet is concerned. Thus, the vast majority of the organic food molecules do not enter into the problem of dietary deficiencies.

The requirements for health include 9 essential amino acids, 1 or 2 fatty acids, and 13 vitamins. The nutritionally essential inorganic elements include calcium, chloride, chrome, cobalt, copper, iodine, iron, magnesium, zinc, chromium, phosphorus, manganese, molybdenum, and selenium. The recommended daily allowance (RDA) is set two standard deviations above the mean requirement and provides a margin of safety for 90 to 95% of the population. However, subjects receiving less than the RDA are not necessarily malnourished, nor are subjects who receive the RDA necessarily adequately nourished. Genetic and environmental factors may significantly influence nutrient thresholds.

Tables of recommended dietary allowances (Recommended Dietary Allowances, Washington, D.C., National Academy of Sciences, 1980) do not take into account those additional needs which may arise during infectious diseases, malignancies, disorders of the gastrointestinal tract, metabolic disease (p. 263), and traumatic injury. Also such tables do not consider growth, exercise, pregnancy, lactation, or composition of diet (metabolic availability may vary widely). Dietary fiber is a nonessential substance but appears to have some physiologic effects, although yet unclarified.

An excess of essential or nonessential nutrients can lead to reversible or irreversible disturbances. What may be considered to be an excess is uncertain for most nutrients; however, the effects of excessive use of some nutrients has not been well established.

NECESSARY NUTRIENTS

Maintenance of cellular activity and growth requires an amount of *energy* furnished in the diet that equals the sum of daily expenditures incurred by an individual, respective of age, sex, physical activity, environmental temperature, and size. The total daily requirement is usually expressed as the sum of the basal metabolic rate (energy expended at rest without food), energy expended in daily physical activities, and the specific dynamic action of food (calories produced during the ingestion and metabolism of food). The assessment and management of macronutrient deficiencies involves some knowledge of protein and caloric requirements.

Protein

Dietary *protein* supplies the body with amino acids for cellular protein synthesis and for a source of energy. In addition to the nine essential amino acids required, nitrogen along with nonessential amino acids is needed because of the energy required for incorporation into protein, i.e., energy consumed in the metabolic process (specific dynamic action). Thus protein requirements include sufficient amounts and proportions of essential amino acids and adequate nitrogen. The exact amount of extra calories to produce positive nitrogen balance and to avoid *protein-calorie* malnutrition depends on a number of factors, including the ratio of energy to protein sources in food. To prevent protein-calorie malnutrition in children for every kilocalorie provided by protein, 19 kcal of nonprotein energy is needed. For a 70-kg person the estimated energy requirement is approximately 50 kcal from nonprotein sources per gram of protein, or about 300 kcal per gram of nitrogen. The average protein requirement is about 0.5 g/kg/day (range of 0.33 to 0.8) for adults and up to 2.0 g/kg/day for young children.

Protein-calorie deficiencies seen in the United States are usually mild or subclinical except in patients hospitalized for other diseases. However, in developing countries, in patients with infectious diseases, during growth, and in deficient or marginal diets, gross protein-calorie deficient states occur, including *marasmus* in which the child is reduced to "skin and bones," and *kwashiorkor* in which the child has edema, muscle wasting, skin lesions, thin, brittle straight hair, extended abdomen, and extreme apathy. Similar changes may occur in adults. In systemic amino acid deficiencies caused by starvation or malnutrition, amino acids from the plasma proteins and muscle are directed to the liver and heart to ensure continued nutrition; when this compensatory regulatory mechanism fails, as in *kwashiorkor,* the patient dies. Protein-calorie deficiencies may occur because high-calorie, low-protein foods are used, including alcohol and snack foods. These high carbohydrate diets, or use of only glucose in intravenous feeding, prevents the reduction of insulin secretion. If insulin secretion is not reduced, adipose tissue is preserved and mobilization and redistribution of amino acids from skeletal muscle to the heart fails and fatty infiltration of the liver commonly occurs. Protein-calorie deficiencies are generally associated with a loss of minerals, including a shift of potassium and magnesium from muscle to plasma in exchange for sodium.

Carbohydrates

Carbohydrates are the major source of energy for the body, and the major carbohydrate is glucose, a product of the breakdown of such polysaccharides as starch. Glucose is usually stored as glycogen in the liver. There is no fixed requirement. Various genetic diseases produce an accumulation of glycogen due to a deficiency of enzymes in the glucose-glycogen pathway (e.g., glycogen-storage disease). Hyperglycemia and hyperglycosuria occur in patients with diabetes mellitus (p. 263) unable to transport and to use glucose normally in cells.

Fats and Lipids

Fats or *lipids* also serve as a principal source of energy. The essential fatty acids are linoleic and arachadonic acids. Cholesterol and triglycerides (neutral fats) are associated with increased levels of lipoproteins in the blood stream and deposits of fat in the heart, liver, and muscle. As already indicated, cholesterol and other fats are attached to lipoproteins in the blood, but one class of lipoproteins, a low density lipoprotein (LDL), deposits cholesterol in the blood vessels, and a high density lipoprotein does not. Rather, the high density lipoprotein (HDL) actually removes excess cholesterol from cells (p. 114).

Americans consume 37% of their energy as fats although the American Heart Association recommends that no more than 25 to 30% of calories be derived from fat. Exercise increases high density lipoprotein cholesterol. Over the last two decades there has been a 26% reduction in the death rate from coronary heart disease (CHD), e.g., atherosclerosis, while consumption of cholesterol and saturated fat went down. A very low density lipoprotein (VLDL) contains only a little cholesterol but a lot of triglyceride, the basic type of fat used for energy storage.

As the total cholesterol (HDL + LDL + VLDL) increases above 150 mg/dl, the risk of coronary heart (artery) disease increases. And if the person with a cholesterol level of greater than 200 mg/dl also has high blood pressure, smokes cigarettes, or is a diabetic, the risk factor is dramatically increased. Defects in lipid metabolism may arise from excess activation of normal pathways of lipid metabolism, defects in the elimination of end products, and problems in nutrition.

Minerals

Minerals that are important in human nutrition include those which are present in large quantities in body store (Na, K, Ca, Mg, P) and those which are trace elements (Fe, Zn, Cu, I, Se and Cr). A number of other trace minerals are important for animals but their role in humans has not been clarified.

The minimal *sodium* needs for normal persons in Western societies is met through the addition of salt (NaCl) to food. The amount of salt added in processing is considerable. The normal requirement will vary with increased sweating but obligatory sodium losses in the urine are small compared to body stores. Abnormal retention of sodium usually involves disturbances in which there is edema. A deficiency of sodium is usually related to severe losses of extracellular fluid volume as in severe diarrhea.

The requirements for *potassium* are not clearly defined. However, the recommended intake is probably below the usual dietary intake, but unlike sodium, some obligatory losses of potassium occur. The major causes of deficiency include increased renal exertion and losses from the intestinal tract. A deficiency in the dietary intake is uncommon.

The principal causes of potassium deficiency are the use of diuretics, pulmonary disease, and diseases which lead to edema. To prevent potassium deficiency or hypokalemia in diuretic-treated hypertensive (diastolic blood pressure greater than 90 mm Hg) patients, potassium supplementation or potassium-sparing agents have been advocated. However, serious arguments have been made against the idea that potassium deficiency might be unhealthy because it might induce carbohydrate intolerance, hypercholesterolemia (p. 114), and irregularities of heartbeat in hypertensive patients. More recent ideas have been that potassium has hypotensive value, i.e., it reduces hypertension. However, there are a number of potential risks in raising the potassium of the diet (and lowering its sodium content). Diabetics, the elderly, and patients receiving such drugs as beta-adrenergic blocking agents, nonsteroidal anti-inflammatory agents, and captopril, and those patients with renal insufficiency, are susceptible to an excess of potassium.

Calcium is a major element of bone and is needed in increased amounts during periods of growth. Because absorption is not efficient the amount of ingested calcium must exceed the requirement. Any deficiency of calcium must be evaluated in relation to vitamin D deficiency. A calcium deficiency may be a factor in some instances of osteoporosis, but not the sole or major cause in idiopathic, aging, or postmenopausal osteoporosis. Oral calcium increases calcium retention in some patients with osteoporosis, but both estrogen deficiency and aging have been implicated in the pathogenesis of osteoporosis in postmenopausal women. However, as with the use of calcium, the use of estrogen tends to arrest rather than "cure" osteoporosis. The administration of estrogen is associated with serious side effects. Patients treated with large amounts of heparin develop symptomatic osteoporosis. *Hypercalcemia* may occur in patients with several granulomatous diseases (p. 71) including tuberculosis and sarcoidosis, which can be accompanied by augmented intestinal calcium absorption, the classical biologic effect of vitamin D. Most patients with increased blood serum calcium in granulomatous diseases have impaired kidney function.

TRACE MINERALS. A deficiency of the *trace mineral* iron (Fe) results in *anemia* (p. 268) which in an adult or adolescent male or in a postmenopausal woman often indicates blood loss, usually from the intestinal tract. Not all bleeding from the colon is an ulcer or a cancer. In the older person intestinal bleeding may arise from a cluster of blood vessels just beneath the lining of the bowel. These small clusters about 4 to 5 mm in diameter are usually a deformity of the blood vessels (angiodysplasia) and are located at the beginning of the colon, not far from the site of the appendix. Iron stores are not regulated by increased or decreased excretion, but intestinal absorption does increase with an iron deficiency. Total daily losses for the male is 0.9 to 1.4 mg per day and an additional 0.5 to 1.0 mg/day for menstrual losses for women. The mg/Fe needed/kg body weight varies from 0.16 at age 6 months to 0.01 in adult males, 19 to 51 years of age. An excess of iron may occur with excessive iron ingestion or when abnormal amounts of iron are absorbed. An overload of iron in the body can lead to hemochromatosis and clinical manifestations related to the accumulation of iron in the parenchymal tissues. Symptoms may be bronzing of the skin, diabetes mellitus, cardiac failure, hepatic dysfunction, and evidence of hypogonadism.

Zinc deficiency is associated with several symptoms including skin lesions, loss of hair, loss of taste, and possible altered taste. Zinc is relatively nontoxic but ingestion of more than 150 mg/day of zinc may interfere with copper or iron metabolism.

Copper is necessary for the formation of hemoglobin, but except for possible severe anemia following extensive duodenal surgery, a deficiency is uncommon inasmuch as the usual diet contains 2 to 4 mg/day. An excess of copper in the liver and tissues occurs in a rare disease (Wilson's) because of a defect in the excretion of copper. Other diseases may cause an increase in hepatic copper but not free tissue copper and do not demonstrate the degenerative changes that are seen in Wilson's disease. About 1 µg/kg of *iodine* is necessary to prevent goiter (enlargement of thyroid gland) in the adult. The recommended allowance is 150 µg/day because goitrogens such as fluoride decrease thyroid uptake of iodine. As with any anionic trace elements (e.g., iodine, fluoride, selenium), the place where it is grown may be more important than the type of food. Nonseacoastal areas generally require the use of iodized salt. Patients who are on low sodium ("salt-free") diets may require another source of iodine. Dietary iodine may be supplemented by iodized table salt which contains 75 µg of iodine/gram of salt. A deficiency of iodine can lead to delayed growth and weakness, fatigue, and mental confusion. Toxic intake of iodine will occur when the intake exceeds 2000 µg/day and is therefore unusual. Excessive iodine therapy may induce thyrotoxicosis (hyperthyroidism) with a number of clinical manifestations (p. 258).

A deficiency of *fluoride* does not occur in humans because of its adequate presence in food and water. However, its protective effect on the teeth against dental caries (p. 191) has led to the addition of sodium fluoride to the drinking water in nonfluoridated areas. In the absence of fluoridated communal water supplies the addition of 1 to 2 mg/day of sodium fluoride in the diet has been suggested as an appropriate anticaries supplement. In children an excess of over 8 parts per million (8 ppm) of fluoride in the drinking water may result in mottling of the enamel (p. 56). An excess of fluoride sufficient to cause systemic fluorosis with skeletal deformities occurs in some areas of the world where intake of fluoride reaches 20 to 80 mg/day for years.

A deficiency of *magnesium* is seen clinically most frequently in alcoholism and accompanying malabsorption syndromes. Hypomagnesemia rarely occurs as a single deficiency and therefore the signs and symptoms of an associated deficiency may be more apparent. The consequences of magnesium deficiency include neuromuscular and gastrointestinal disturbances. An excess of magnesium is rarely seen because of the ability to excrete magnesium. The excessive use of magnesium-containing antacids by patients with renal insufficiency may cause hypermagnesemia which produces depressive effects on the central nervous system and cardiovascular system.

Other trace elements, such as chromium, cobalt, molybdenum, and selenium, require further evidence of their essentialness in human nutrition. *Chromium* may be required for carbohydrate metabolism. *Cobalt* is a part of vitamin B_{12} but a human deficiency of the element is unknown. Although *manganese* is an essential element needed for bone and is required in several enzyme systems, a human deficiency has not been established. *Molybdenum* and *selenium* may function nutritionally in man, but there is insufficient data to recommend a dietary allowance. All of the elements if given in sufficiently high levels can cause injury.

Vitamins

Vitamins may be classified as fat-soluble (A, D, E, K) or water-soluble (B_1, B_2, B_6, B_{12}, C, folic acid, and nicotinic acid). A deficiency of some vitamins has never been clearly established, perhaps because they are so ubiquitous in the diet or efficiently conserved by the body that a deficiency is not readily seen. Although vitamins are used to supplement the diet frequently in the United States, toxicity is limited principally to the fat-soluble vitamins A and D. Alcoholism is the principal disturbance from which vitamin deficiencies develop. A number of factors influence vitamin deficiency other than dietary intake.

VITAMIN A. Vitamin A is a term which includes active substances other than carotenoids that exhibit qualitatively the activities of retinol. Retinoids is a generic term that includes both naturally occurring compounds with vitamin A activity and synthetic analogues of retinol, with or without biologic activity. An international unit of vitamin A is defined in terms of retinol. The major sources of dietary vitamin A are from certain plants and animal tissues. The only unequivocal clinical signs of deficiency in humans relate to changes in the eye: poor dark adaptation (night blindness); dryness of the conjunctiva with lesions called Bitot's spots; ulceration of the cornea. Only night blindness is usually seen in the United States and most often associated with alcoholism. The recommended dietary allowance of 5000 IU/day assumes an intake of half retinol and half beta-carotene. Therefore, 5000 IU of retinol is excessive.

Vitamin A toxicity may occur if the intake is over 2000 IU/kg/day and can easily be reached by the use of vitamin supplement capsules of 50,000 IU. Nonspecific changes from chronic toxicity include hair loss, skin dryness, bone and joint pain, and weight loss. Vitamin A or retinoids taken in therapeutic doses has been shown to be teratogenic (p. 19) in humans. The risk in taking vitamin A in the form of isotretinion (e.g., Accutane) of spontaneous abortion or congenital malformations may be as high as 100% when taken therapeutically into the second month of gestation. Fetal malformations also occur in retinoid (vitamin A) deficiency.

VITAMIN D. Vitamin D_3 (cholecalciferol) is formed in the skin by the action of sunlight. It has been suggested that vitamin D is a hormone, not a vitamin. Vitamin D together with parathyroid hormone and calcitonin regulates the intestinal absorption of calcium and remodeling of bone. Inadequate production of D_3 in the skin, insufficient dietary supplementation, and/or defective absorption of vitamin D from the small intestine can cause hypovitaminosis D.

A deficiency of vitamin D may result in defects in the skeleton such as *rickets* in children (bowing of long bones, i.e., bowing of legs, retarded growth and developmental anomalies of the teeth, delayed eruption of the teeth, and deformities of skull and chest, or other problems related to decreased calcification of cartilage), and *osteomalacia* (adult rickets, pelvic pain, softening of skeletal bones and pelvic bones and a tendency to fracture due to inadequate calcium and insufficient exposure to sunlight). Prevention and treatment is vitamin D and calcium supplementation (see also osteoporosis).

Vitamin D-resistant rickets is characterized by hypophosphatemia (low serum phosphate) and hyperphosphaturia (increased phosphate in the urine) associated with kidney dysfunction, familial occurrence, normal blood serum calcium, diminished calcium and phosphate absorption, decreased growth with short stature, and disturbances in the development of the teeth. The teeth are prone to pulpal exposure and periapical involvement. Abnormal cementum and supporting bone have been reported. Another disturbance hypophosphatasia has many aspects similar to vitamin D-resistant rickets, and is transmitted as a recessive autosomal characteristic (p. 16). The principal defect is a deficiency of the enzyme alkaline phosphatase. There is premature exfoliation of the deciduous teeth due to the apparent absence of cementum. Vitamin D therapy is not effective.

Vitamin D toxicity is a rare occurrence in adults, but in some instances calcification of soft tissues has been described mainly in the kidneys and arteries.

VITAMIN E. Vitamin E has the generic name of tocopherol and has antioxidant properties. The main function of this vitamin is to prevent peroxidation of polyunsaturated fatty acids, e.g., destroy peroxides and singlet oxygen and prevent damage from free radicals. Deficiency status is rare in the absence of malabsorption; however, an increased intake has been suggested for pregnant and lactating women and for premature infants with hemolytic anemia. Possible side effects of high doses include the potentiation of the anticoagulant effect of the anticoagulant warfarin used for coronary heart disease and impairment of leukocyte functions.

VITAMIN K. Vitamin K occurs in one form naturally in plants and in another form in bacteria in the colon. The dietary requirements are uncertain because of the amount produced by bacterial synthesis. Vitamin K stimulates the production of clotting factors II, VII, IX and X (p. 69) in the liver. Subjects at risk for a deficiency of vitamin K include newborn infants and patients with malabsorption disturbances and liver disease and those receiving broad-spectrum antibiotics. Hemolytic anemia and liver damage have been reported with high doses of vitamin K_3 (Menadione). The minimum daily dietary requirement of vitamin K is met in the "normal mixed diet" found in the United States. Abnormal prothrombin circulates in the blood of patients with vitamin K deficiency, patients with hepatic dysfunction and those treated with coumarin anticoagulants. Abnormal prothrombin is a serum antigen not found in normal persons but can be detected in vitamin K-deficient persons with normal prothrombin times (p. 70), and can serve as a marker for early vitamin K deficiency and certain forms of carcinoma of the liver.

VITAMIN B GROUP. The vitamin B group includes thiamin (B_1), riboflavin (B_2), niacin, pyridoxine (B_6), cobalamin (B_{12}), and folacin, as well as pantothenic acid, choline,

NUTRITIONAL DISTURBANCES

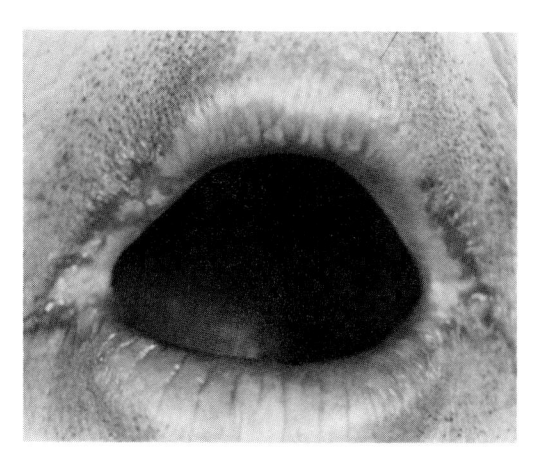

Fig. 9–1. *Vitamin B deficiency.* Angular cheilitis of the type seen in severe riboflavin deficiency.

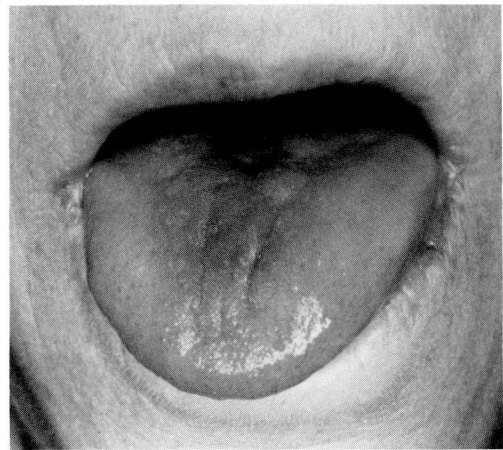

Fig. 9–2. *Vitamin B deficiency.* The smooth, dark red tongue is typical of the change seen in pellagra as a part of niacin deficiency.

and inositol. Most B complex vitamins, except for nicotinic acid and choline, are not synthesized by the body and must be absorbed from the intestinal tract either as a consequence of their presence in ingested food or from bacteria of the intestinal tract.

Vitamin B_1 (thiamin) sufficient for daily requirements is supplied by rather small quantities of food. It plays an important role in carbohydrate metabolism. A deficiency is most commonly seen with chronic alcoholism, nausea and vomiting of pregnancy, and with malabsorption syndromes. Multiple deficiencies may be present to modify the clinical symptoms. In man the deficiency leads to beriberi, a disease with multiple symptoms that include cardiac failure, generalized edema, and disturbances involving the peripheral nervous system (neuropathy) and decreased muscle strength. With requirements in excess of 1 mg/day, the deficiency can develop rapidly in a period of weeks.

Riboflavin (B_2) is involved in biological oxidations which are linked to protein and energy intake, and the requirement to avoid deficiency symptoms is probably at a level of 0.4 to 0.5 mg/1000 kcal. For older patients with a low caloric intake the minimum requirement is 1.2 mg/day. The recommended dietary allowance for lactating women reaches 2.0 mg/day. The average Western diet contains about 2.7 mg/day in excess of the recommended daily allowance (RDA). The initial symptoms of riboflavin deficiency are soreness and burning sensations of the mouth, lips, and tongue, as well as eye symptoms such as tearing, burning, itching and sensitivity to light (photophobia). The filiform papillae of the tongue become atrophic, but the fungiform papillae remain the same or enlarged. In severe cases the tongue is smooth and takes on a magenta color. Angular cheilosis evidenced by fissuring of the angles of the mouth becomes prominent (Fig. 9–1). The differential diagnosis includes smoking, iron deficiency, anemia, antibiotic therapy, sensitivity to topical agents (dentifrices, mouthwashes, lipsticks), and pellagra. There appears to be no toxic effects from the use of riboflavin.

Niacin (nicotinic acid, nicotinamide) is an essential component of the mitochondrial transport system. Nicotinic acid (but not the amide) has an effect on peripheral vasodilatation and cholesterol lowering. A deficiency of niacin is often compounded by a deficiency of vitamin B_6. The classic deficiency syndrome of *pellagra* is characterized by the triad of dementia, diarrhea, and dermatitis. Other gastrointestinal symptoms

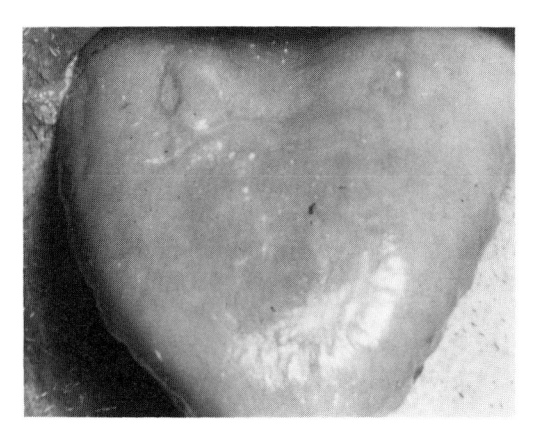

Fig. 9-3. *Vitamin B deficiency.* A smooth atrophic pale tongue with superficial chronic ulcers is the type of change seen in severe deficiencies of riboflavin. A smooth tongue of this type is also seen in folic acid and B_{12} deficiencies.

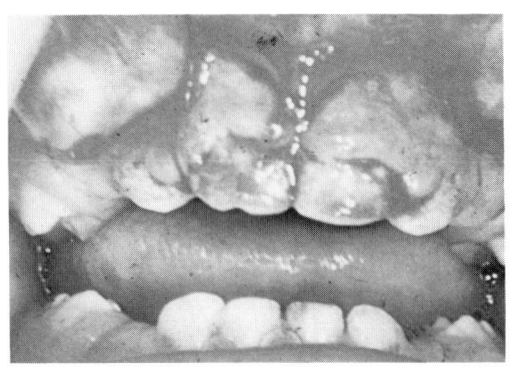

Fig. 9-4. *Scurvy. Vitamin C deficiency in a young child.* Enlarged gingiva with extensive hemorrhage is the typical change of scorbutic gingivitis.

include "burning" tongue (Figs. 9-2 and 9-3) and mucous membrane. Nicotinic acid in corn is not absorbable and a basic diet of corn and pork led to pellagra as a widespread problem in the southeastern United States at one time. The recommended dietary allowance for niacin equivalents (i.e., 1 mg niacin or 60 mg of tryptophan) in humans is 8 mg/day for infants up to the age of 6 months and 16 to 18 mg/day for adult men. Isoniazid therapy can lead to pellagra. With large doses (greater than 3 g/day), nausea, vomiting, diarrhea, and arrhythmias may occur.

A deficiency of *vitamin B_6* (pyridoxine) is rarely related to a dietary restriction. A deficiency usually arises in relation to malabsorption syndromes and treatment with vitamin B_6 antagonists, the latter producing glossitis, cheilosis, peripheral neuropathy, and lesions about the mouth, nose, and eyes. The RDA for vitamin B_6 for adults with a protein intake of 100 g/day is 2 mg/day, and 2.5 mg/day for lactating women. Megavitaminosis (over 2 g/day) has been reported to produce progressive sensory ataxia, and neurologic dysfunction has been reported with much smaller doses (500 mg/daily) with prolonged use.

Folacin is a generic term for compounds having structures and functions similar to folic acid (PGA). The RDA for folacin is 400 μg/day for adults and 800 μg/day for pregnant women. The diet in the United States contains on the average about 700 μg of folacin. Acute symptoms of folate deficiency have been observed after the use of antagonists and include nausea, hair loss, diarrhea, glossitis, and thrombocytopenia (p. 273). The toxic symptoms are seen following aminopterin therapy for leukemia.

Vitamin B_{12} (cobalamin) is a cobalt-containing biologically active substance which is found in animal tissues and synthesized in the colon by bacteria but not absorbed. Thus strict vegetarians (on a holovegetarian diet) develop a cobalamin deficiency. The average diet in the United States provides 5 to 15 μg/day and the RDA for adults is 3 μg/day. A deficiency occurs with low intake in the diet, with gastrointestinal disease, with pancreatic disease, and if a carrier protein (called transcobalamin II) is lacking. Symptoms of a deficiency relate to anemia and include weakness, dyspnea, sore tongue (Fig. 9-3), diarrhea, and memory disturbances. Toxic effects do not appear to be a problem.

VITAMIN C. Vitamin C (ascorbic acid) is necessary for a number of biological functions but is best known for its relationship to scurvy. Many of the symptoms of scurvy are related to disturbances in the development of intracellular ground substances in bone and other connective tissues, including the dentin and periodontal ligament. The inflammatory response of the periodontal tissues is proportional to the degree of local irritants present. Loss of attachment and supporting bone leads loosening of the teeth. Periosteal, skin, gingival (Fig. 9–4), and gastrointestinal hemorrhage occur. Scurvy is a rare disorder in the United States. No deficiency state other than scurvy has been documented with vitamin C deficiency. Vitamin C therapy has not been substantiated for the common cold nor for the treatment of cancer. Toxicity has been reported with doses of 1 g or more, but higher doses are more likely to produce diarrhea, dry mouth, and kidney stones. A dietary allowance of 60 mg/day is recommended for adults. The normal body pool of vitamin C contains sufficient reserves for 30 to 45 days.

There is no reason to believe that any benefits occur if vitamin supplementation is increased once the optimal level has been reached, although that level may not be obvious, especially with parenteral therapy. Many unfounded claims have been made for the effects of vitamins on so-called subclinical deficiency diseases. Such unfounded claims must be considered carefully but do not void the necessity for the proper use of vitamins in infants, growing children, and pregnant women and in chronic gastrointestinal disturbances where vitamin, protein, and other deficiencies may occur.

CLINICAL CONSIDERATIONS

Although a well-balanced diet requires certain minimal amounts of each of the three basic foods—carbohydrates, fats, and proteins—the transformation of proteins into carbohydrates and fats makes the distinction between these basic foods less sharp than once thought. There is no absolute value for different foods, since requirements vary according to the needs of the individual. Pathologic changes secondary to malnutrition are variable. Combined deficiencies are the rule even in studies apparently designed to be pure deficiencies. For example, the patient with pellagra does not selectively eliminate only those foods containing niacin, but refuses to eat most foods, and what is eaten is lost because of diarrhea, so the effect is generalized.

It is apparent, from experimental studies where animals have reached a terminus, that observations attributed to any single deficiency are most often pathologic changes brought about by multiple deficiencies and quite probably endocrine disturbances also. These observations point out the possibility of a wide variety of changes that may occur in the periodontium in deprived animals, especially when such conditioning or modifying factors as growth or local irritants are present.

The presence of osteoporosis, degeneration of the principal fibers, loss of alveolar bone support, and widening of the periodontal membrane cannot be considered as occurring in healthy individuals clinically, but only in patients with severe deprivation states. More important, such changes do not represent chronic destructive periodontal disease with the presence of periodontal pockets. It is quite possible such changes can accelerate the progress of periodontal disease initiated by local factors, especially where deprivation is continued; however, any specific assessment as to degree of deficiency necessary to modify the progress of periodontal disease is purely hypothetical. Because of the adaptive capacity of most organisms and the absence of pure deprivation or the absence of such changes as are generally attributed to such states, it appears quite unlikely that clinical vitamin or protein deficiencies have any great bearing on the progress of periodontal disease. In such instances where the effect of a nutritional element is more specific to the periodontium, such as vitamin C, the progress of periodontal disease is accelerated and the tissues respond more unfavorably than normal to local irritants. Even so, there is no evidence to support the hypothesis that vitamin C is a significant factor in the progress of periodontal disease, unless the deficiency is absolute for long periods of time and other manifestations of scurvy are present.

From a practical clinical standpoint one might consider the nutritional status of a patient as having a bearing on periodontal disease when his clinical manifestations and history suggest the possibility. Clinical manifestations refer here to general manifestations; not a poor response to removal of local factors, unless all local irritants are definitely removed. Even with a nutritional disturbance, systemic treatment of periodontal disease is not the objective; the goal is the establishment of a good tissue response so that removal of local irritants will be most effective.

BIBLIOGRAPHY

Alfano, M.C., Miller, S.A., and Drummond, J.F.: Effect of ascorbic acid deficiency on the permeability and collagen biosynthesis of oral mucosal epithelium. Ann. N.Y. Acad. Sc., 258:253, 1975.

Alpers, D.H., et al.: *Manual of Nutritional Therapeutics*. Boston, Little, Brown & Company, 1983.

Bruckner, R.J., et al.: Hypophosphatasia with premature shedding of teeth and aplasia of cementum. Oral Surg., 4:623, 1951.

Cannon, P.R.: *Some Pathologic Consequences of Protein and Amino Acid Deficiencies*. Springfield, Charles C Thomas, 1948.

Chawla, T.N., and Glickman, I.: Protein deprivation and the periodontal structures of the albino rat. Oral Surg., 4:578, 1951.

Dreizen, S.: Oral manifestations of nutritional anemias. Arch. Environ. Health, 5:66, 1962.

Eaton, S.B. and Konner, M.: Paleolithic nutrition: a consideration of its nature and current implications. N. Engl. J. Med., 312:283, 1985 (see also 312:1458, 1985).

Goodman, D.W.: Vitamin A and retenoids in health and disease. N. Engl. J. Med., 310:1023, 1984.

Judd, J.L., et al.: Estrogen replacement therapy: indications and complications. (UCLA Conference). Ann. Intern. Med., 98:195, 1983.

Kassirer, J.P. and Harrington, J.T.: Fending off potassium pushers. N. Engl. J. Med., 312:785, 1985.

Kreitzman, S.N.: Enzymes and dietary factors in caries. J. Dent. Res., 53:218, 1974.

LeMann, J. and Gray, R.W.: Calcitrol, calcium, and granulomatous disease. N. Engl. J. Med., 311:1115, 1984.

Levine, A.S., et al.: Food technology: A primer for physicians. N. Engl. J. Med., 312:628, 1985.

Mellanby, M.: Dental research with special reference to parodontal disease produced experimentally in animals. Dent. Pract., 59:227, 1939.

Moertel, C.G.: High dose vitamin C versus placebo in the treatment of patients with advanced cancer who have had no prior chemotherapy. N. Engl. J. Med., 312:137, 1985.

Newman, R.G., and Martin, S.: The national nutrition survey in New York City. Trans. N.Y. Acad. Sc., 33:(Series II), 316, 1971.

Nizel, A.E.: Guidelines for dental nutrition counselling. Int. Dent. J., 23:420, 1973.

Ralli, E.P., and Sherry, S.: Adult scurvy and the metabolism of vitamin C. Medicine (Balt.), 20:251, 1941.

Richelson, L.S., et al.: Relative contributions of aging and estrogen deficiency to postmenopausal bone loss. N. Engl. J. Med., 311:1273, 1984.

Rosa, R.W.: Teratogenicity of isotretinoin. Lancet, 2:513, 1983.

Russell, A.L.: International nutrition surveys: A summary of preliminary findings. J. Dent. Res., 42:232, 1963.

Schaumburg, H., et al.: Sensory neuropathy from pyridoxine abuse: a new megavitamin syndrome. N. Engl. J. Med., 309:445, 1983.

Sebrell, W.H. and Bufler, R.E.: Riboflavin deficiency in man (ariboflavinosis). Public Health Rep., 54:2121, 1939.

Slade, E.W., Bartuska, D., Rose, L.F., Cohen, D.W.: Vitamin E and periodontal disease. J. Periodontol., 47:352, 1976.

Slade, E.W.: Vitamin E in clinical medicine. Lancet, 1:18, 1974.

Snively, W.D.: The tiny giants. Bull. Path., 8:305, 1967.

Waerhaug, J.: Epidemiology of periodontal disease—review of the literature. In, *World Workshop on Periodontal Disease*. S.P. Ramfjord, D.A. Kerr, and M.M. Ash, Eds. Ann Arbor, Mich., The University of Michigan Press, 1966.

Wilson, C.W.M.: Clinical pharmacological aspects of ascorbic acid. Ann. N.Y. Acad. Sc., 258:355, 1974.

Wolbach, S.B., and Bessey, O.A.: Tissue changes in vitamin deficiencies. Physiol. Rev., 22:233, 1942.

Wolblach, S.B., and Howe, P.R.: The incisor teeth of albino rats and guinea pigs in vitamin deficiency and repair. Amer. J. Path., 9:275, 1933.

10

DENTAL PLAQUE, MICROBIOTA, CALCULUS, STAINS AND DISEASE

When oral hygiene procedures are inadequate, masses of bacteria imbedded in an amorphous matrix accumulate on the teeth. The matrix consists of macromolecules synthesized by proliferating bacteria, as well as constituents derived from the saliva and crevicular fluid. Such bacterial accumulations are referred to as *dental plaque* (Fig. 10–1).

Plaque is a highly organized ecologic unit consisting of relatively characteristic collections of bacteria. Differences in the composition of plaque have been related to different sites on the teeth and to different diseases, e.g., caries and gingivitis. The pathogenic characteristics of plaque relate to virulence factors possessed by bacteria, including (1) the capacity to colonize (attach and grow) at specific sites, (2) the ability to evade the host's defenses, and (3) the capacity to cause injury to the tissues.

Whether or not disease occurs at the site of plaque formation depends on the types of bacteria present, how the organized bacterial ecologic unit functions, and the defenses of the host. In effect one or more members of the plaque microflora may provide the necessary growth factors for a pathogen which would otherwise not be capable of maintaining an infection. Such bacterial synergism, as well as bacterial antagonism, may explain localized patterns of disease. Thus in addition to the requirement that bacteria be able to adhere to a surface to avoid being washed away by the flow of secretions, bacterial colonization parameters which affect bacterial growth and virulence must be considered, including nutritional, metabolic, and cooperative versus antagonist interactions between bacteria and between bacteria and host constituents, as well as immune and nonspecific defense mechanisms in the saliva.

The microorganisms which characteristically dwell on the internal and external surfaces of the body make up what is known as the normal or *indigenous microflora*. In general, the association of host and indigenous microbiota remains in balance and is relatively innocuous, even beneficial in many instances. It is probable that indigenous microflora may be a deterrent to the establishment of pathogens when the opportunity presents itself. The development of the indigenous microflora begins at the time of birth with the passage of the fetus

DENTAL PLAQUE, MICROBIOTA, CALCULUS, STAINS AND DISEASE

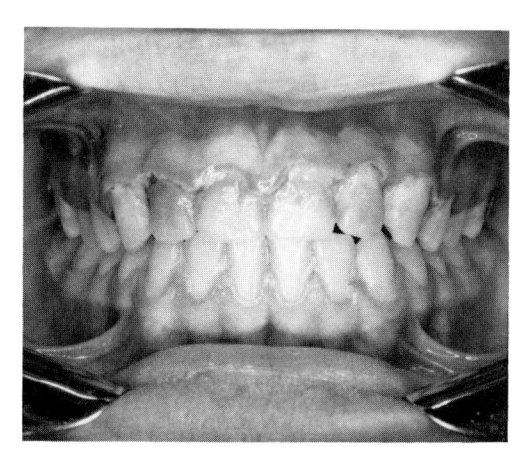

Fig. 10–1. *Dental plaque.* Heavy accumulation of plaque associated with acute necrotizing ulcerative gingivitis.

Table 10–1. Predominant Genera of Subgingival Bacterial Flora in Periodontitis

Gram-positive cocci	—Streptococcus
Gram-positive rods	—Actinomyces
Gram-negative cocci	—Veillonella
Gram-negative rods	—Bacteroides
	—Fusobacterium
	—Capnocytophagia
	—Eikenella
	—Actinobacillus
	—Selenomonas
Spirochetes	—Treponema

through the maternal birth canal and continues in accordance with the general principles which govern ecologic processes elsewhere. Some organisms require teeth for oral colonization. For example, Streptococcus mutans are not found in the mouths of infants prior to the eruption of teeth nor after the loss of all teeth. Direct contact with the mother seems to be important ecologically for S. mutans, which is considered one of the primary pathogens in dental decay.

In bacterial studies of plaque, microbiologists usually concentrate on those bacteria which constitute a large proportion of the flora, i.e., the predominant cultivable flora. Bacteria constituting small proportions of flora may not be represented and actual data on quantities of microorganisms are not generally available. A number of the bacteria present are not readily cultured in vitro, including some of the more invasive forms of spirochetes. When the predominance of certain bacteria in various periodontal diseases are stressed (Table 10–1), it must be remembered that the microflora is a complex range of normally resident bacteria, and the identification of the etiologic agent difficult. An important pathogen could be insignificant in relation to the total microbial population.

The specific ability of bacteria to attach to a tooth and/or to other microorganisms plays an important role in the colonization of an oral surface by indigenous bacteria. Although plaques can be characterized by their location, microbial composition, metabolic activities, and pathogenic potential, common to all is the characteristic of *adherence*. This characteristic by which bacteria attach to tissues or to each other is not a feature of *materia alba,* an adventitious, creamy-white loose accumulation of microorganisms, cell debris and food residues which can be removed with a stream of water. However, the distinction between plaque and materia alba has little clinical significance at this time.

The importance of bacterial adherence relates to the potential for developing therapeutic approaches that interfere with the specificity of target pathogens to attach to host tissues and to each other. The importance of the initial attachment process of bacteria in the development of dental plaque relates to the idea that plaque-mediated diseases, such as caries and gingivitis, can be controlled by limiting bacterial colonization utilizing methods similar to those that occur naturally, i.e., blocking adherence specifically.

From these introductory remarks it is obvious that oral microbial ecology reflects complex dynamic ecosystems in which potent selective forces regulate bacterial colonization of the oral tissues. The following discussion briefly summarizes some of the concepts of the composition and formation of plaque.

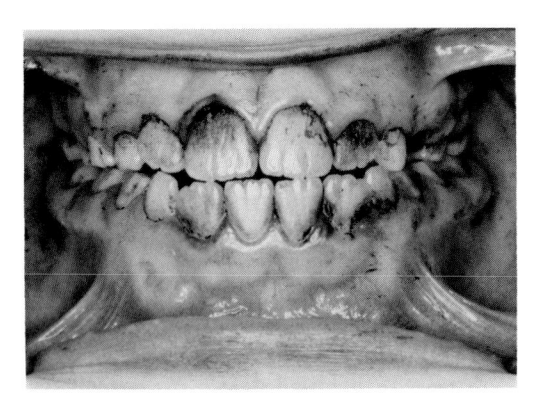

Fig. 10–2. Disclosing solution indicating area of plaque.

CLINICAL ASPECTS OF PLAQUE

Dental plaque can be seen most easily by the use of disclosing solutions (dyes) applied to the teeth (Fig. 10–2). Because there is some mechanical cleansing action by the tongue and buccal mucosa and by the action of foods, and because of determined and effective use of such home care aids as the toothbrush and dental floss, plaque forms most rapidly in protected interproximal areas and in pits and fissures. However, when oral hygiene is poor, plaque may accumulate over all the surfaces of the teeth. There is some basis for the opinion that mastication of fibrous foods is somewhat of a limiting factor for plaque on incisal and occlusal surfaces. However, effective plaque control is essentially based on the use of a toothbrush and interdental and sulcular cleaning aids. Good home care procedures and periodic professional care is necessary for the control of dental plaque, especially subgingival and interproximal plaque.

Although such measures can be highly successful for gingival health, evidence that the same degree of plaque control would be as successful for control of caries has not been clearly established. In contrast to the concept of the elimination of all plaque to control periodontal disease and dental caries, is the concept of using methods of prevention which require less emphasis on mechanical methods of plaque removal and more emphasis on control of specific microorganisms presumably responsible for caries and certain kinds of periodontal disease. However, no single putative causative microorganism has been found for caries or specific types of periodontal disease.

Considering that some kind of plaque is common to both caries and gingivitis, another factor associated with caries and not found in gingivitis is the unfavorable sucrose consumption pattern required for caries to develop into a major problem. There is no question that cariogenic bacteria (plaque) are required to cause dental caries, and that other bacteria (plaque) may be potential causative agents in some forms of periodontal disease. And although it is sometimes suggested that there is an inverse relationship between caries and periodontal disease, there is little acceptable evidence to demonstrate a positive or negative correlation in the prevalence of caries and periodontal disease in the same subjects.

The possibility of controlling dental caries and some forms of periodontal disease has been directed toward the use of mechanical, chemical or immunologic methods. To a certain extent the objectives of a particular method are based upon the acceptance of a specific etiology for caries or for periodontal diseases.

ECOLOGIC DETERMINANTS OF PLAQUE

An important ecologic determinant for some bacteria is oxygen or oxygen products (Fig. 10–3). Some microorganisms are killed at low levels of oxygen, whereas others grow only in the presence of oxygen. Microorganisms that do not grow on the surface of blood agar in the presence of air are referred to as *anaerobic* bacteria; those that grow only in the presence of air are called *aerobic* bacteria. *Facultatively anaerobic* microorganisms grow almost as

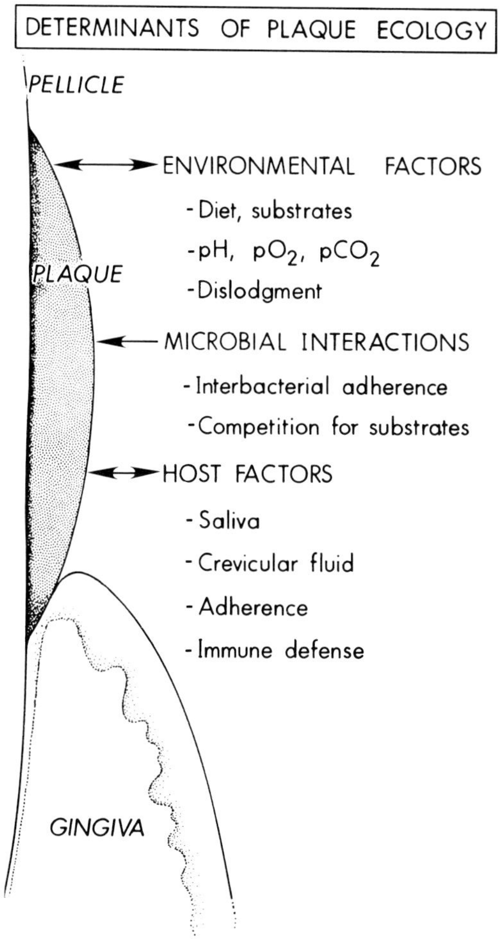

```
DETERMINANTS OF PLAQUE ECOLOGY

PELLICLE

PLAQUE ←——→ ENVIRONMENTAL FACTORS
            - Diet, substrates
            - pH, pO₂, pCO₂
            - Dislodgment

       ←—— MICROBIAL INTERACTIONS
            - Interbacterial adherence
            - Competition for substrates

       ←——→ HOST FACTORS
            - Saliva
            - Crevicular fluid
            - Adherence
            - Immune defense

GINGIVA
```

Fig. 10-3. Determinants of ecology.

well under either condition. The extremely sensitive obligate anaerobes grow in gingival or periodontal pockets where the oxygen level is especially low.

Some of the bacterial nutrients on the surface of a tooth are provided by the saliva, some by the crevicular fluid, and still others by commensal relationships that arise from the production of metabolites in the ecosystem. It has been reported that the nutritional value of saliva is low compared to the source of nutrients in the gingival pocket where a number of bacteria are capable of producing hydrolytic enzymes that break down macromolecules into simple molecules which can be utilized as nutrients. In some instances the food chain involves synergistic relationships where certain species of bacteria may have very specific nutritional requirements. For example, Streptococcus mutans requires p-amino benzoate which is produced by S. sanguis. Also some black pigmented Bacteroides require vitamin K and hemin which are furnished by other bacteria. Hemin may also come from bleeding into the gingival pocket. Some bacteria called "capnophilic" bacteria will not survive in the absence of carbon dioxide.

Although the oral environment supports rapid growth, the increasing thickness of plaque becomes limited by a number of ecologic determinants as well as mechanical and washing actions in the mouth. The different nutrients which make up the substrate used by the bacteria to grow may not be adequate and competition for substrate will become an important limiting ecologic determinant. The availability of certain substrates may be too low to support the growth of certain bacteria, e.g., sugar may be a limiting substrate for S. mutans.

Substrates (organic starting materials), which enable bacteria in the plaque ecosystem to grow, are derived from the saliva, crevicular fluid, and the host's diet. The coexistence of a wide variety of microorganisms in a plaque is dependent upon the limitations of a mixed substrate to provide the required needs of competing bacteria. In terms of substrate limitation a given organism may have an ecologic advantage if one of the substrates of a mixture of substrates is lost to competing bacteria.

Hypothetically the coexistence of streptococci and actinomyces in plaque may be related to simultaneous utilization of carbon and energy sources and competition for available carbohydrates. There is an inverse relationship between S. mutans and S. sanguis which depends upon dietary carbohydrate. In a normal diet they coexist but in the absence of carbohydrate, which has been replaced by protein, S. sanguis has an advantage and S. mutans is lost from the plaque. These findings and many others suggest that bacterial substrate can be a major ecologic factor in plaque formation.

FORMATION OF PLAQUE

Plaque is an organized bacterial mass on the surfaces of the teeth that is initiated by specific species of bacteria and which matures by a generally ordered succession of microbial inhabitants. The ecologic complexity and properties of the plaque are determined by bacterial commensalism, competition, antagonism, factors affecting bacterial adherence and interbacterial aggregations, and immune and nonspecific defense mechanisms in saliva. Potent selective forces regulate bacterial attachment and colonization in the mouth and suggest why different sites in the mouth are colonized by certain populations of bacteria more than others. Some types of bacteria can attach and colonize certain surfaces, e.g., the tongue or teeth, whereas others cannot do so or compete in those sites.

The formation of dental plaque reflects the accumulation of bacteria already present in the oral cavity. Bacterial colonization is thought to be relatively independent of normal variations in salivation, malocclusion, type of food eaten, and mastication, but highly dependent on specific attachment mechanisms. Therefore, importantly, the development of dental plaque is related to: (1) the ability of various bacteria to adhere specifically to a pellicle, a structureless, non-mineralized thin film that begins to form within minutes after a tooth erupts or has been cleaned, and (2) the ability of bacteria to adhere to each other. Bacterial accumulation in plaque occurs when surface components of organisms interact and bind to those of other bacterial cells, including the same or different species of bacteria.

The eventual composition of plaque depends upon a number of known and unknown environmental and intermicrobial interactions, especially those involving early colonizers of enamel pellicle. The amorphous matrix of plaque consists of polymers synthesized by bacteria and components derived from the saliva and also from crevicular fluid (i.e., serum transudate) which comes into the mouth between the gingiva and teeth, i.e., through the gingival sulcus.

Intraoral Pellicles

Within a short time after a tooth has been cleaned and polished, specific salivary proteins coat the exposed surface of a tooth. This film or pellicle is 1 to 3 μm in thickness, but when less than 1 μm in thickness it is sometimes described as a cuticle. Similarly when bacteria enter the mouth, they are immediately coated with salivary constituents. Probably all oral surfaces are coated with specific salivary proteins and considered as intraoral pellicles, e.g., enamel, cementum, mucosal and bacterial pellicles. However, the term pellicle most often refers to the pellicle covering the enamel. Some of the proteins promote specific colonization and maintenance of indigenous oral flora, whereas others function as antimicrobial factors. The organic composition of pellicles is varied, but generally enamel pellicle contains proteins, glycoproteins (mucins), and a substantial amount of lipids.

Bacterial Colonization

The colonization of the pellicle begins mainly with Gram-positive cocci and rods, but soon other bacteria aggregate to the first colonizers and then they all proliferate to form scattered colonies and then large coherent masses of plaque. In "superclean" subjects a relatively simple microbial flora is present on the teeth. The sparse microflora consists almost exclusively of Gram-positive cocci, mainly S. sanguis, although Gram-positive rods (mainly Actinomyces) may be present.

In experimental gingivitis, initiated by having subjects refrain from practicing any oral hygiene measures, the indigenous Gram-positive flora proliferate and an increasing number of Gram-negative cocci and rods appear during the first two days of plaque formation. The cocci and rods which are important in the early development of plaque are streptococci and actinomyces, mainly S. mitior, S. sanguis, A. viscosus, and A. naeslundii.

In the next phase at two to four days there is proliferation of fusobacterium and filamentous bacteria, as well as other bacteria already present. During the third phase at four to nine days, vibrio-like organisms and spirochetes appear in larger numbers in the plaque. After two weeks of no oral hygiene the bacterial flora has changed to a complex flora with the greatest relative increase occurring in Actinomyces species.

During the following weeks of mechanically undisturbed plaque formation the relative proportion of various types of bacteria continues to change with an increasing, but limited, thickness of plaque. Anaerobic microorganisms are favored and increasing numbers of Gram-negative rods appear. The shift to the more complex flora and further development of plaque is ascribed to specific adherence, bacterial aggregation, and changes in growth conditions such as anaerobiosis and nutritional interaction between plaque bacteria.

The initiation of clinical gingivitis is seen when the complex flora is established, although subclinical inflammation as indicated by the flow of gingival exudate begins much earlier. Studies of the development of experimental gingivitis have not clearly defined: (1) that a specific profile (group) of bacteria, or a specific organism, is responsible for gingivitis; (2) that the amount of plaque specifically initiates gingivitis; (3) that in time all plaque produces gingivitis; (4) that a non-gingivitis producing plaque does exist; (5) that still unidentified bacteria may be responsible for periodontal disease; (6) that the observed microbial population in a gingival pocket is fortuitous or causative. Of course no experimental periodontitis study has been done in man.

Subgingival Dental Plaque

Subgingival plaque (Fig. 10–4) is characterized by a predominance of facultative anaerobic Streptococcus and Actinomyces species in addition to other bacteria including a variety of Gram-negative rods (Table 10–1). The initial colonization of the subgingival area is by Bacteroides gingivalis which attach to the tissues and Gram-positive bacteria such as Actinomyces species in existing plaque.

Subgingival plaque has been described as consisting of two zones: an innermost zone which is adherent to the tooth and continuous with supragingival plaque, and an outer zone which is loosely attached or even unattached. The inner zone consists of a complex mixture of Gram-positive and Gram-negative bacteria, whereas the outer zone consists predominately of spirochetes and Gram-negative rods, many of which are motile in deep pockets. The complexity of spirochetal flora in the oral cavity increases in association with gingival disease. Most of the spirochetes have not been cultivated successfully and taxonomic diversity is extensive. Most appear to be treponemes and a large number of the species remain to be named and described.

Although spirochetes are reported to be among the predominant microorganisms of subgingival plaque from patients with advanced destructive periodontitis, it is not known whether these organisms are involved in the initiation of chronic gingivitis-adult periodontitis complex or are present as an associated phenomenon. Spirochetes and other motile organisms have been reported to be found more frequently and in higher proportions in gingivitis and in adult and juvenile periodontitis and to be correlated with pocket depth.

In summary, the percentage distribution of various groups of cultivable bacteria in the gingival sulci of patients with a healthy gingiva reflect about 40% streptococci, 40% Actinomycetes, and somewhat less than 20% anaerobic Gram-negative rods. In moderate gingivitis there are approximately 25% Streptococci, 25% Actinomycetes, and 25% Gram-negative anaerobic rods in subgingival plaque. In advanced

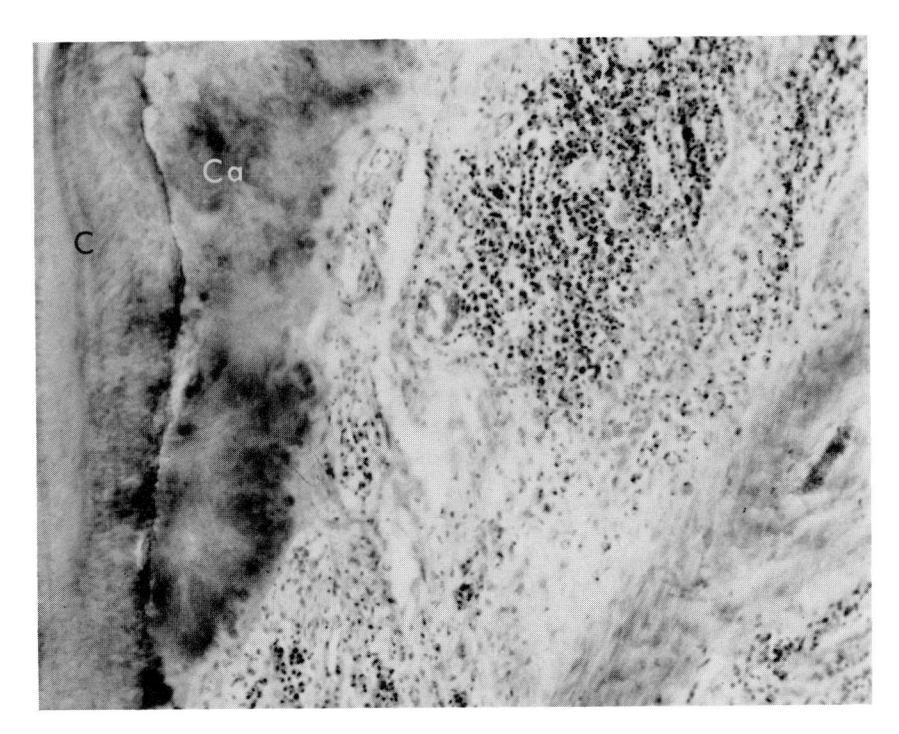

Fig. 10-4. Subgingival plaque and calculus (Ca) on the surface of cementum (C).

marginal periodontitis the percentage predominantly cultivable bacteria in periodontal pockets is about 5% Streptococci, 15% Actinomycetes, and 80% Gram-negative anaerobic rods. Thus from health to an increasing severity of periodontal disease the proportion of Gram-positive cocci and rods decreases, while the Gram-negative rods greatly increase. The predominant genera in periodontitis is shown in Table 10-1.

Colonization by Streptococcus Mutans

Streptococcus mutans preferentially colonizes areas of the retentive areas of the teeth such as pits and fissures. These organisms have the ability to form large bacterial masses and live in high concentrations of acids from dietary sugars. By the enzymatic action of the enzyme glucosyltransferase (GTase) most cariogenic organisms are able to synthesize polysaccharides from dietary sugars. These polysaccharides (glucans) make up the interbacterial matrix of plaque. Such extracellular polymers are sticky, gelatinous substances which promote cohesion between streptococcal cells and foster an accumulation of greater masses of S. mutans on the teeth than would be expected from the number of S. mutans cells that initially attach to the pellicle. Glucan synthesis does not appear to be required for the initial attachment of S. mutans cells to the teeth, but is important for the accumulation of S. mutans. The composition of plaque varies from tooth to tooth, from mouth to mouth, and even from site to site on a tooth. Such variations may help explain regional variations in the pathogenicity of plaque.

Mechanisms of Colonization

A number of bacterial interactions contribute to microbial colonization of tooth surfaces, including direct attachment of microorganisms to pellicle, aggregation of bacteria by salivary agglutinating factors, and specific interbacterial adherence or coaggregation.

It has become increasingly clear that microbial adherence, colonization, and initiation of gingivitis or caries are dependent upon interactions of surface structures on bacteria with those on oral tissues and other bacteria. Bacteria attach to various hosts and tissues with a remarkable degree of specificity. Such specificity suggests the presence of a complex recognition system, perhaps analogous to the mechanisms involved in antigen-antibody reactions, i.e., "lock and key" mechanisms.

The adherence of bacteria is a specific interaction in which macromolecules (adhesions) on the surface of bacteria bind to complimentary structures (ligands) on the surfaces of the host's tissues. The adhesions, which are often present in filamentous surface appendages (such as pili or fimbriae), are thought to involve lectin-like and/or hydrophobic ligands. Thus bacteria express on their surface a carbohydrate-binding protein, akin to lectin, which serves as the adhesion that binds the organisms to a corresponding glycoconjugate on the host's tissue surface. The site to which the bacterial cell attaches is called a *binding site* and the molecules on the host with which the adhesions interact are called *receptors*. The adhesion of indigenous oral bacteria appears to involve specific lectin-like interactions between complementary surface components and physicochemical forces such as hydrophobic and electrostatic interactions.

Once the initial layer of bacteria has become attached to the pellicle by adhesion-ligand mechanisms, the subsequent accumulation of bacteria may be the result of aggregation of bacteria mediated by glucans (polysaccharides produced by bacteria) or the result of bacteria being held together by salivary constituents which comprise part of the matrix of plaque. In addition, interbacterial binding of specific pairs of different species of organisms which benefit from each other's presence are formed. Such intergeneric bacterial aggregation (coaggregation) is seen with the binding together of dissimilar pairs of organisms like cocci (Veillonella parvula) and rods (Actinomyces viscosus). The cell-cell interaction in the organization of microbial communities is demonstrated in the distinct "corncob" appearance of the surface of an established four-day supragingival plaque as seen by scanning electron microscopy. The frequent coaggregation between actinomyces and Gram-negative organisms such as Bacteroides suggests that actinomyces may be an important marker in the transition from a Gram-positive plaque flora to one in which various Gram-negative species predominate.

Adverse Influences

Several factors appear to negatively influence bacterial adherence and thus alter colonization of oral tissues. Salivary components which are thought to interfere with adherence include salivary glycoproteins, lysozyme, mucins, and secretory IgA antibodies. Such salivary components bind with bacteria causing agglutination and interferences with attachment mechanisms. The bacteria are clumped into aggregates which are more easily washed from oral surfaces. The bacterium-aggregating glycoprotein active in the prevention of bacterial adhesion is generally a large glycoprotein rich in carbohydrates.

Dietary lectins may bind to bacteria and cause their aggregation. For example, human milk contains free oligosaccharides with receptor activity that may inhibit the attachment of pneumococci and pneumococci and pneumococcal infection. The development of therapy interfering with adherence has not been clarified, but lectin-like components in bananas and other foods could mask or cover binding sites on pellicle binding sites for S. mutans and other oral streptococci.

Such ecologic factors as lactoferrin, lysozyme, and bacteriocidins have been reported to influence bacteria adversely. Lactoferrin is a glycoprotein present in milk, saliva, tears and neutrophils. Although antibacterial, its significance in plaque ecology is unclear. Lysozyme is a protein found in saliva, tears and neutrophils that can bind to microorganisms and display antibacterial activity. Its significance to plaque has not been established. Bacteriocidins is a protein produced by bacteria that have the capacity to inhibit the growth of some strong strains of bacteria and thus possibly the microbial ecology of dental plaque.

PATHOGENICITY AND VIRULENCE OF PLAQUE AND MICROBIOTA

The establishment of a normal indigenous flora on body surfaces may result in one or more outcomes. The growth of microbes on the surface may be considered one form of infection even though there is no damage to the host. Generally, however, infection is considered to be present when bacteria results in injury or elicits a reaction that damages the tissues. Thus the outcome of the microbial colonization and growth of microbes related to plaque is disease, i.e., dental caries and gingivitis. Many microbes establish a commensal relationship with the host, even prevent the establishment of more dangerous pathogenic microbes.

Although colonization of oral tissues is an early feature of the newborn, an elaborate defense system makes oral disease relatively infrequent except for caries and periodontal disease which are the most common causes for loss of teeth. The microbes involved in these diseases must possess certain characteristics in order to produce such destructive effects in spite of potentially effective host defense systems. These characteristics are spoken of generally as microbial *pathogenicity* (or ability to cause disease). The degree of pathogenicity is reflected in the term *virulence* which is an expression of how easily the microbe overcomes the defenses of the host, establishes infection, and the severity of damage which results.

Virulence Factors

As already indicated the attachment of microbes to the host tissues is an important factor in virulence. Several characteristics of pathogenic bacteria enable them to colonize specific oral tissues and prevent elimination from the mouth. Surface structures related to attachment mechanisms include pili, capsule, long fibers, vesicles, and lipopolysaccharides. Most of these bacterial cell surface structures are found on several suspected periodontal pathogens, including Bacteroides gingivalis, Bacteroides intermedius, Actinobacillus actinomycetemcometans, and Capnocytophaga sputigena. Several growth stimulating and growth-inhibiting factors derived from the host or bacteria influence virulence. For example, the necessary growth factors for the pathogenic black pigmented Bacteroides include naphtoquinone which is provided by other oral bacteria, especially Bacteroides oralis and Veillonella parvula which are non-infective.

Potential Bacterial Mechanisms for Evading Host Defenses

Several potential factors may enable bacteria to avoid the defenses of the host, including the inhibition of polymorphonuclear leukocytes, resistance to complement mediated killing, elaboration of enzymes which cleave immunoglobulins, elaboration of leukotoxin, production of fibrinolysin which prevents the formation of a fibrin barrier around infecting bacteria, the production of potent endotoxins, and elaboration of products that block chemotaxis. In effect these factors represent mechanisms of evading normal host defense systems. Black pigmented Bacteroides, in particular B. gingivalis and B. intermedius, as well as Capnocytophaga and A. actinomycetemcomitans, appear to be significant bacteria in human periodontal disease and exhibit many of the bacterial factors of importances in the evasion of host defense systems. These bacteria also have the potential for tissue destruction of periodontal tissues.

Potential Bacterial Mechanisms for Destruction of Periodontal Tissues

The bacterial factors which have been reported as possible agents in the destruction of gingival tissue and periodontal attachment include enzymes such as collagenase, toxic agents such as epitheliotoxin, and polyclonal B-cell activators. Thus the destructive action of bacteria may be caused directly by enzymes and toxins, and indirectly by activation of the immune system. Although these factors are potentially capable of the destructive aspects of periodontal disease, their actual role in destructive periodontal disease has yet to be determined.

Virulence Mechanisms of S. Mutans

Streptococcus mutans have been implicated in the initiation as well as the progression of carious lesion, but there are limited data on the microbial determinants of carious lesions. Of particular interest are the abilities of these microorganisms to colonize the teeth and to effectively compete and persist on the teeth. These abilities relate to a number of traits of S. mutans implicated in its virulence. Such traits include the ability to adhere to teeth and form plaque, to make certain glucans, to engage in agglutination (aggregation), to make extracellular dextranases, to grow at a low environmental pH (aciduric), to produce acids (acidogenic) rapidly from carbohydrate, to use intracellular and extracellular polysaccharides for acid production when no food is taken into the mouth, to transport carbohydrates (sucrose), and to be able to attach to the teeth independent of a sucrose substrate. Such traits are important for the attachment, accumulation and survival of S. mutans in the host's dental ecology.

The reduction of caries by dietary restriction of sugar is well established, but other approaches to directly block these traits of virulence have not been fully developed, although the use of chlorhexidine demonstrates marked antiplaque properties and the chemical control of plaque is possible. One aspect of such control is that chlorhexidine often produces atypically thick and stained pellicles which are extensively calcified. Although the rapid evolution of genetic variants resistant to antibiotics has been used as a caution against the widespread use of antibiotics for the control of bacteria involved in diseases related to the presence of plaque, the development of selective resistance to the action of chlorhexidine does not appear to be a significant factor in its use.

Microbial Resistance

Bacteria have responded to the introduction of antibiotics for treating disease by producing genetic variants resistant to one or more of the antibiotics. After the introduction of each new antibiotic it is only a matter of time before resistant bacteria emerge. The development of multiply resistant strains occurred in the early sixties and was found to be related to genes found on extrachromosomal elements called *plasmids*. These plasmids without the resistant genes were present before the introduction of antibiotics. The kind of plasmid, which contains genes that convert drug-sensitive bacteria to antibiotic-resistant bacteria, can be transferred by conjugation from one bacterial cell to another. *Conjugation* is the process by which some bacteria attach to other bacteria and transfer genetic material. Externally the donor differs from the recipient by the presence of at least one sex pilus extending from its surface to the recipient cell during conjugation. All species of bacteria seem to participate in at least some degree of conjugation. S. mutans and S. sanguis appear to utilize the mechanism of *transformation,* which is based on the release and uptake of DNA that has been released into the medium surrounding the bacterium. An important factor for gene transfer not involving the conjugative element is the close contact necessary for an interaction to occur. Such close contact may be facilitated by growth of bacteria in dental plaque and gingival crevices.

There are examples of transferable drug resistance where no plasmid is evident but relate to conjugative transposons. Many of the genes specifying antibiotic resistance are found on *transposons*. These moveable elements of DNA can be copied and transferred to any other DNA molecule. Thus mechanisms of antibiotic resistance must be considered in relation to the plasmids which carry the resistance traits and the resistance genes as well.

The transfer of antibiotic resistance by plasmids has conferred resistance to many commonly used chemotherapeutic agents including tetracyclines, chloramphenicol, streptomycin, kanamycin, neomycin, sulfanilamide, and penicillin. Such resistant bacteria are also more resistant to many disinfectants that contain mercury, cobalt and nickel.

Host Responses to Plaque Components and Microorganisms

The surface of the tooth and the gingiva is the interface of both local salivary and systemic immune mechanisms. The salivary domain is largely dependent upon the function of secretory IgA, and the gingival domain is controlled mostly by the immune components of the blood. In order for plaque to induce an immune response or cause direct toxic effects it must penetrate the intracellular spaces of the junctional epithelium (p. 210). The presence of Gram-positive and Gram-negative bacteria and their products in plaque enable a variety of immunologic responses to be activated. Such bacterial by-products in plaque as polyclonal B-cell mitogens, including lipopolysaccharides (LPS), levans, and dextrans, are potentially capable of activating complement pathways, stimulating lymphocytes, inducing the release of lymphokines and activation of macrophages (Chapter 5). Mitogens are substances that stimulate lymphocytes to proliferate independent of any specific antigen. Whether the host response is harmful or beneficial in periodontal disease and caries has not been clarified although there exists evidence to support both the beneficial and harmful effects of immune responses. For example, immunopotentiation by plaque antigens may have a protective immune effect on dental caries and a damaging effect on gingival disease. Other mechanisms by which microorganisms combat host defenses include the anti-opsonic properties of staphylococcal protein A, formation of histolytic enzymes, secretion of endotoxins, formation of exotoxins, and neutrophil receptor modulation.

Immune Responses to Plaque

The immune systems common to bacterial infections are: (1) secretory-mucosal immune system, (2) neutrophil-antibody-complement system, (3) lymphocyte-macrophage system, and (4) immune regulation. Responses of these systems may interfere with bacterial attachment and the killing of bacteria. The immune responses to the components of dental plaque include antibodies, complement activation, polymorpholeukocyte killing, activation of macrophages, and release of lymphokines by plaque sensitized lymphocytes (both T- and B-cells). The components of dental plaque that are associated with these responses are cariogenic bacteria (S. mutans, Actinomycis viscosus, Lactobacilli), periodontopathic microorganisms (Actinomyces, Actinobacillus, Veillonella, Bacteroides, Capnocytophagia, Eikenella, and Spirochetes), and potentiating and immunosuppressive agents (LPS, levans, dextrans and lipoteichoic acid).

Saliva

Secretory IgA (sIgA) is the predominant immunolgobulin in saliva and has been reported to inhibit the adherence of oral bacteria to epithelial cells of the buccal mucosa. The generation of protective sIgA responses in the mouth by local stimulation alone is dependent upon the presence of

(1) *affector* lymphoid tissue where antigen is processed and presented to IgA cell precursors (with appropriate T-cell regulation), and (2) *effector* sites where IgA is produced and secreted. Although the oral cavity is relatively deficient in lymphoid tissue functions required for effective mucosal IgA responses to local antigen, there exists a common mucosal immune system whereby cells originating in one mucosal tissue can disseminate to other mucosal sites.

Precursors of intestinal IgA producing cells, which arise in Peyer's patches in the intestine in response to intestinal immunization, migrate via lymph to the thoracic duct and blood stream, then to the lamina propria of the gut epithelium where they extravasate as IgA plasma cells. These precursors have the ability to extravasate at other mucosal sites including the salivary glands. Thus the gut-associated lymphoid tissue (GALT) insures maximum local immune responses at sites deficient in primary mucosal-associated lymphoid tissue such as the oral cavity. IgA then appears to be secreted by salivary gland plasma cells, the B-cell precursors of which may come to the salivary glands from GALT.

The potential of antibodies to combine with microorganisms and prevent their initial adherence and hence colonization has been studied in humans in relation to S. mutans. There is the possibility that antibody directed toward lectins of bacteria can inhibit bacterium to bacterium interaction (coaggregation) in the subgingival area. The secretory IgA in saliva may protect the oral mucosa and tooth surfaces from uncontrolled bacterial colonization.

Crevicular Fluid

The response of the gingiva to very little plaque consists of a cellular infiltrate in which lymphocytes predominate. But with the development of gingivitis there is a change to plasma cells. This lymphoid infiltration may be cells originating in the regional lymph nodes in response to antigenic stimulation to produce blasts cells and which come to and proliferate in the gingiva. The immunoglobulins formed by the plasma cells in the gingiva may be to a certain extent non-specific. These humoral as well as cellular components of the blood can reach the tooth surface via the passage of crevicular fluid into the gingival sulcus. The fluid and cells of the crevicular fluid function in the sulcus and plaque in a way analogous to the ways the cells and fluid function in the blood and tissues.

The junctional epithelium (p. 210) is used as a pathway for crevicular fluid and transmigrating cells. The features of the junctional epithelium, both intercellular and renewal time, suggest a permeable tissue through which potentially a variety of substances, cells and fluid from the connective tissue pass to the oral cavity and from the oral cavity to the connective tissues. The pathway for bacterial substances is provided by the intercellular spaces of the junctional epithelium. It has been reported that the junctional epithelium is permeable to substances up to a molecular weight of 700,000. Recently bacteria have been reported to be found in the connective tissue in severe periodontal disease (p. 207).

Immunoglobulin IgA, IgG and IgM, as well as C_3, C_4, C_5 and C_3 proactivactor, have been detected in crevicular fluid, suggesting that the classical and alternate complement pathways (p. 80) may be activated in the gingival crevice. The primary functions of immunoglobulins are defensive, although the potential for damaging surrounding tissues is present. A number of enzymes are present in the fluid also, but their activity in the gingival crevice and their source (bacteria, saliva, cells, etc.) have yet to be fully determined.

The cellular components of crevicular fluid are largely neutrophils (92%). Other viable cells are macrophages, T-cells and B-cells. Dental plaque contains chemotactic substances which enhance migration of neutrophils to the gingival crevice where they are capable of phagocytosis of microorganisms. Although the capacity for opsonization is slightly reduced, the killing capacity of crevicular neutrophils is not affected.

Systemic and Local Responses to Plaque

The responses of the gingiva to plaque irritants, antigens, or mitogens is inflammation. The general aspects of the vascular and cellular responses of inflammation have been discussed in Chapter 4 and the immune responses in Chapter 5. Of special interest is the junction between soft and hard tissues (gingiva-tooth) via a specialized junctional epithelium that is to a certain extent permeable yet prevents the penetration of bacteria through the epithelium to underlying supporting tissues. This junction, which is continually at risk to bacteria and antigenic molecules but not easily penetrated by bacteria except in severe periodontal disease, is the site of access to the immune system. Whereas the immune mechanism of the saliva is provided chiefly by the function of sIgA, that of the gingiva probably reflects all of the immune components of the blood.

When plaque is allowed to accumulate on the teeth, there is an associated gingival inflammation and a diffusion of some serum-derived immunoglobulins into the gingival sulcus. During inflammation immunoglobulin formation occurs with IgG-producing immunocytes predominating. The formation of antibodies locally (gingiva) and in distant sites (lymph nodes, Payer's patches, etc.) provides a protective mechanism for binding noxious agents (antigens, mitogens) to form immune complexes (antigen-antibody) which neutralize the biological effects of the antigens at the site of access to the immune system.

The presence of antibodies in the blood (serum) of patients with periodontal disease has been documented specifically with strains of Bacteroides gingivalis which comprise one antigenic type. It has been reported that patients with adult periodontitis have levels of IgG antibodies to Bacteroides gingivalis which are on average five times higher than that found in the serum of normal subjects.

The classic pathway of the complement system (p. 80) is activated by immune complexes (Ag–Ab) formed from plaque antigens (Ag) in the presence of antibodies (Ab). The alternate pathway can also be activated by plaque components, including lipopolysaccharides (endotoxin) and some species of bacteria. It can be mobilized before antibodies have appeared. Periodopathic microorganisms, which are coated with antibody and thereby activate the complement system, will be opsonized for phagocytosis by polymorphonuclear leukocytes (PMNs) and macrophages (Mø). Both PMNs and Møs have receptors on their surfaces for the activated third component (C_3b) of complement and for the Fc fragment (p. 79) of the IgG class of immunoglobulin. PMNs have an Fc receptor for the IgA class of immunoglobulin.

Killing of bacteria may occur by complement-dependent cytolysis, by complement-antibody mediated cytolysis, by opsonization, antibody and complement action, or by direct action of phagocytes. These mechanisms involve the potential for antibody, complement and neutrophils to act in concert to kill potential periodopathic organisms. Antibody and complement-mediated phagocytosis and killing are important mechanisms for dealing with Gram-positive bacteria, whereas complement-dependent lysis without phagocytosis is important for dealing with Gram-negative organisms. The precise in vivo function of neutrophils in periodontal disease has yet to be clarified, although humans with depressed neutrophil function (e.g., cyclic neutropenia) often have severe loss of supporting bone and attachment (p. 228).

The variety of other lymphokines released from stimulated lymphocytes includes a factor which inhibits the migration of macrophages (MIF), a leukocyte inhibiting factor (LIF), macrophage activating factor (MAF), a lymphocyte mitogenic factor

(LMF), and a lymphotoxin which is cytotoxic to other cells (fibroblasts, etc.). Monocytes are all potentially protective and destructive. The lymphoproliferative response which occurs locally in periodontal tissues in response to mitogens or antigens and produces these various lymphokines, may play a role in periodontal destruction. Macrophages which are activated by MAF may produce tissue damage via collagenase. Other lymphokines which may act as effector molecules include alpha-lymphotoxin, which may cause the death of adjacent cells and OAF which may stimulate osteoclastic activity.

Macrophages also produce monokines (soluble, hormone-like proteins) which amplify immune responses, and via a lymphocyte activating factor (LAF) or Interleukin I (Il 1) influences lymphocyte reactivity to mitogens and antigens. Fibronectin is a monokine which directs fibroblast migration and acts as a chemotactic factor for fibroblast migration. It also acts as a modulator of bacterial ecology in that it increases the adherence of some cells. Fibronectin is found in saliva and the extracellular matrix of many tissues.

Lymphocytes can also influence fibroblast function by the production of a chemotactic factor for fibroblasts. Both lymphocytes and macrophage produce factors which influence fibroblasts in inflammation and have significance for healing of connective tissue via replacement by collagen.

The regulation of the immune response requires a vast network of communicating processes that range from enhancement to suppression signals. Immunosuppressive agents in plaque, including lipopolysaccharides (LPS), lipoteichoic acid (LTA), levan and dextran, prevent the immune-inflammatory reactions from getting out of hand. For example, LPS can depress cellular immune responses and LTA can depress antibody responses.

Regulatory interactions are complex multicellular processes with a variety of feedback and feedforward circuits. The T lymphocyte regulation of the immune system can be seen, for example, in systemic lupus erythematosus where there is a deficiency in suppression T-cell systems. The major histocompatibility region (p. 77) may be associated with genetic restrictions physiologic T-cell and B-cell interactions as well as with other immune regulation.

Summary of Host Responses

In summary of host responses to dental plaque, it is not clear how the mechanism by which plaque-induced gingivitis, whether related to specific or nonspecific bacteria, results in destruction of supporting structures of the teeth. One possibility is that neutrophil-mediated tissue destruction occurs in periodontal disease as well as other diseases such as arthritis. Certainly the patient with compromised neutrophil function presumably permits the initiation of severe periodontal breakdown. And although the microorganisms associated with precocious periodontal disease, e.g., localized juvenile periodontitis (LJP), differ from those associated with adult periodontitis, the linkage of PMN dysfunction with decreased periodontal resistance is not clear. A number of reasons have been advanced to explain the cellular, host-response features in LJP especially as a model of bacterial interactions with the neutrophil-antibody-complement system.

The mechanism of neutrophil dysfunction is related to defective chemotaxis and its modulation by serum factors and bacteria. The defect is characterized by a decrease in the rate of cell migration. Nondiseased siblings also exhibit abnormal neutrophil chemotaxis and absence of disease. This finding suggests hereditary factors play a role in LJP.

It has been proposed that several factors may inhibit the chemotactic responsiveness of PMNs by interfering with the binding of chemotactic factors to their receptors. It has also been reported that several microorganisms, including the putative etiologic pathogen actinobacillus actinomycetemcommitans, can inhibit neutrophil chemotaxis by blocking ligand-receptor binding for chemotactic factors on the neutrophil surface. The number of receptors for chemotactic factors is less in LJP than in normal subjects but the receptors are normal. Thus bacteria which can take advantage of an intrinsic neutrophil chemotactic defect by impeding the chemotactic response would have a seclective advantage in colonizing the host. However, the host responds by producing antibodies which opsonize the organism for ingestion and killing by phagocytosis. Although migration is delayed, the activation of its antibacterial effector mechanism is not. Presumably the neutrophil in its protective role releases a sufficient amount of extracellular histolytic substances (e.g., acid hydrolases, neutral proteases) to cause tissue damage in a localized area until localization and resolution of the infection occurs.

PLAQUE AND DISEASE

There is some evidence to suggest that several types of periodontal disease and degrees of severity of chronic gingivitis adult periodontitis complex are associated with different combinations of bacterial pathogens. No single strain or combination of bacteria has yet been found to determine susceptibility to chronic adult periodontitis. Conversely there is general recognition that Streptococcus mutans is a major pathogen in the development of smooth coronal surface caries. However, it is not the only cariogenic organism associated with dental decay. Strains of lactobacilli and actinomycetes are also involved in yet incompletely understood ways.

Nonspecific vs Specific Plaque Hypotheses

Some investigators believe that several bacterial species contribute to periodontal disease; others believe that it will be possible to identify one or a few key pathogens which are responsible for progressive periodontal disease.

The concept that some, if not all, forms of periodontal disease are related to the presence or overgrowth of one or more types of bacterial types in subgingival plaque is based on comparisons of the bacterial flora of teeth with and without periodontal disease. The identification of plaque flora is determined by two general approaches. Representative plaque samples are cultured and many taxonomic tests are done to designate a genus or species for all or representative isolates from a given plaque sample. Only a few plaque samples can be thoroughly analyzed and there is the chance of overlooking a previously unknown microorganism. Another approach has been to evaluate a large number of plaques for more conspicuous organisms, including Bacteroides, spirochetes, Capnocytophagia, Fusobacterium, Actinomyces viscosus, and Actinobacillus actinomycetemcomitans. The latter approach is useful for evaluating a larger sample of patients than is the first approach. Using such an approach the bacterial profile for plaque from patients with adult periodontitis was found to be about 45% spirochetes. The profile for successfully treated and maintained patients showed significantly higher proportions of Streptococcus sanguis, Actinomyces viscosus, A. odontolyticus, and S. mutans compared to that of some categories of untreated disease where there were significantly lower proportions of B. gingivalis and spirochetes. This profile of a combination of elevated proportions of facultative, plaque-forming bacteria and decreased proportions of anaerobic bacteria and spirochetes for nondisease-associated plaque has been suggested to support the specific plaque hypothesis.

Although it has been reported that the presence of such a profile of spirochetes and various Gram-negative rods might be used as a diagnostic criterion of actively progressing disease and their disappear-

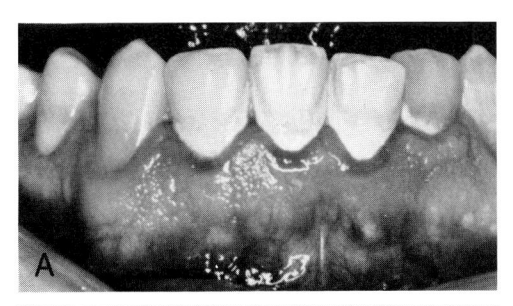

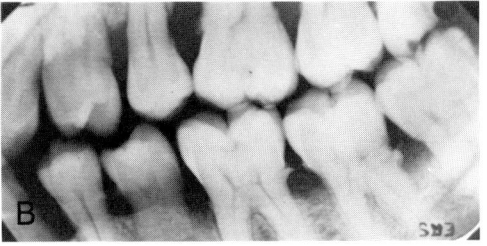

Fig. 10–5. *A,* Calculus on the facial surfaces of mandibular incisors. *B,* Subgingival calculus seen on posterior bitewing radiographs.

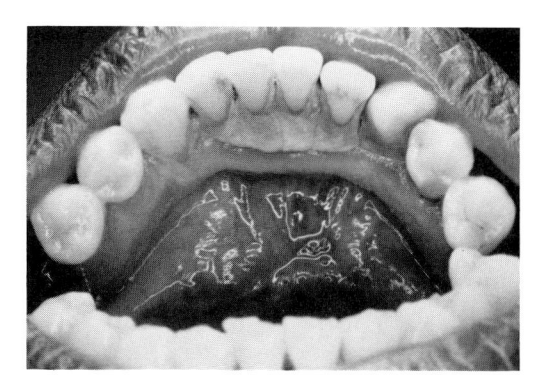

Fig. 10–6. Heavy deposits of calculus adjacent to orifices of salivary glands beneath the tongue.

ance as an indicator of effective treatment, such diagnostic profiling has yet to be accepted generally.

CALCULUS

Calculus or tartar on the teeth is generally considered to be calcified plaque (Fig. 10–5A and B), although such calcareous deposits are found on the teeth of germ-free animals. Even so in most people if bacterial plaque is left undisturbed, calcification occurs in a matter of weeks or months. The quantity and distribution of calculus varies among individuals, but generally more calculus is formed adjacent to the openings of the major salivary glands than elsewhere in the mouth (e.g., buccal surfaces of the maxillary molars and lingual surfaces of the mandibular incisors (Fig. 10–6). Clinically calculus is classified as supra- and subgingival calculus.

Composition of Calculus

The constituents of dental calculus include a number of different phosphates, including hydroxyapatite ($Ca_{10}(OH)_2(PO_4)_6$), octacalcium phosphate ($Ca_4H(PO_4)_3 2H_2O)_3$, whitlockite ($Ca_3(PO_4)_2$, and brushite ($CaHPO_4 2H_2O$). More simply the main constituents of calculus are a carbonate containing apatite, a Mg and Zn containing whitlockite, and octacalcium phosphate. When the pH of saliva is low enough, dicalcium phosphate dihydrate is also present in dental calculus. Whitlockite (WH) is abundant in subgingival calculus and brushite is found only in supragingival calculus attached to mandibular anterior teeth. It has been reported that octacalcium phosphate (OCP) is found most abundantly and hydroxyapatite (OHA) least frequently in posterior supragingival calculus.

The composition of supragingival calculus appears to vary somewhat with the layer or zonal structure. The supraficial layer attached to the gingiva or gingival pocket is a homogenous, highly calcified layer in which WH is the most common component. Whitlockite is the most common component of subgingival calculus.

Calculus is studied in a number of ways, including ground sections (Fig. 10–7) and decalcified specimens. Ground sections may appear to be layered with varying degrees of calcification. The surface of plaque is often covered by a layer of unmineralized plaque (Fig. 10–8).

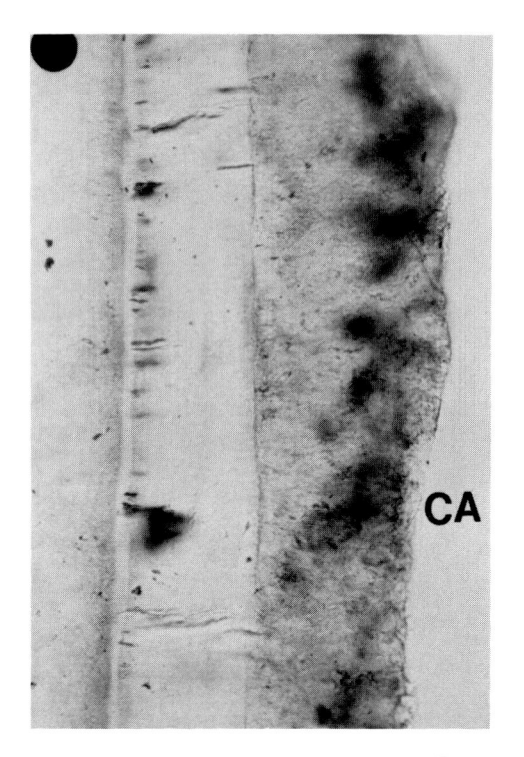

Fig. 10–7. Ground section of calculus (CA) on coronal surface.

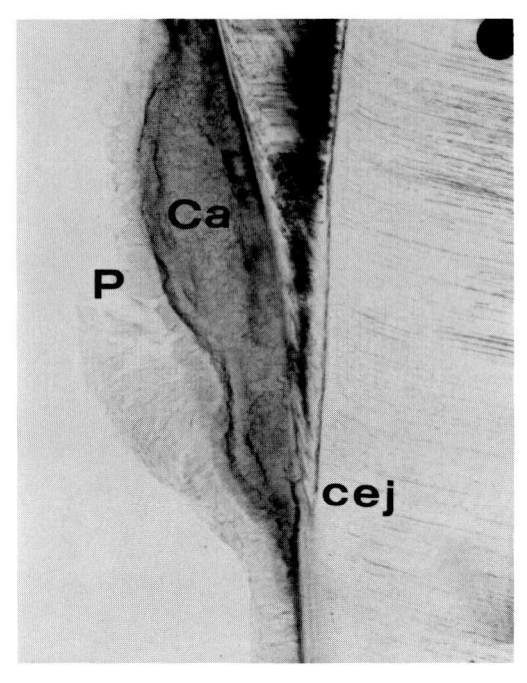

Fig. 10–8. Plaque (P) on surface of calculus (Ca) at the cemento-enamel junction (cej)

Saliva and Calculus

The role of saliva in the formation of calculus relates to its physicochemical properties. The major inorganic components of saliva include calcium, phosphate, sodium, potassium, magnesium, chloride, carbon dioxide, as well as trace elements. However, saliva is saturated or supersaturated with respect to hydroxyapatite. Also, resting saliva is undersaturated and stimulated saliva is saturated with respect to brushite and octacalcium phosphate. A prerequisite for calcification of dental plaque is that it is more alkaline than saliva and/or crevicular fluid. The level of salivary pH is related to the components of the calculus; the organic materials which form the matrix include components from both bacteria and saliva. Lipids in the matrix are considered to be important for the mineralization of plaque.

Mechanisms of Calculus Formation

A number of hypotheses have been advanced to explain the mechanism by which dental calculus forms. It has been that octacalcium phosphate or brushite form during the initial phase of calcification of bacterial plaque and is then gradually hydrolyzed into hydroxyapatite (OHA) and/or whitlockite (WH). Thus the bacteria and matrix of supragingival plaque are calcified with OCP forming first and then transformed into OHA. If the pH is low and the Ca/P ratio is high, brushite is formed initially and transformed into OHA or WH in an early stage of calcification which is related to the presence of NH_4 produced by plaque bacteria. Under anaerobic conditions and in the presence of $Mg,^{2+}$ $Zn,^{2+}$ and Co_3^{2-} and tissue fluid, whitlockite is formed and is the main component of subgingival calculus.

Mineralization of Plaque

The formation of calculus is a process of plaque mineralization involving intra- and extracellular calcification. The initial calcification (extracellular) originates in the interbacterial matrix. Intracellular calcification begins as crystals in Gram-positive and Gram-negative bacteria with calcification of bacterial walls occurring subsequently.

As already indicated, saliva may be supersaturated with respect to the calcium phosphates (e.g., apatite), and precipitation occurs spontaneously when metastable saliva is seeded by the presence of crystals on which new crystals can form. Although such seeding crystallites are present in enamel, the pellicle acts as a barrier to its availability. However, compounds having a different chemical composition than apatite could act as seeding agents. When such compounds nucleate crystallization, the process is called epitaxis. It has been suggested that the matrix of plaque and bacterial compounds could by epitactic mechanisms initiate mineralization of plaque.

It has been suggested that the reason more calculus is found near the exits of major salivary glands is the loss of carbon dioxide and rise in pH that occurs when the saliva leaves the salivary ducts. The increase in pH (more alkaline) would then, according to the carbon dioxide theory, lead to spontaneous precipitation of calcium and phosphates from the saliva.

Attachment of Calculus

Calculus forms in surface irregularities and calcification may involve the pellicle, so that attachment may involve crystal interaction between calculus and enamel or between the crystals of calculus and cementum. The formation of calculus in surface irregularities accounts for the greater difficulty of removing calculus from cementum than from smooth enamel surfaces.

Significance of Calculus

Calculus is calcified plaque and contains in some respect all of the same endotoxins, antigens, and mitogens as the bacterial plaque which is being mineralized. Also, calculus is always covered by plaque which is more adherent to rough than smooth surfaces. Calculus is a reflection of poor oral hygiene and its presence must be considered as important in the pathogenesis of periodontal disease. Calculus surface roughness per se does not appear to be a significant factor in the initiation of gingivitis, but rather the toxic products in its porous surface and the plaque on its surface.

STAINS

Staining of teeth may result from pigments or colored substances taken into the mouth, such as tobacco, medicines, dentifrices, and foods, from the action of chromogenic bacteria, or from the deposition of pigments in the structure of the tooth itself as the result of systemic disease or disease of the pulp. Stains derived from substances in the mouth are designated exogenous stains; those derived from blood-borne pigments associated with systemic disease or as a result of disease of the pulp are designated endogenous stains. Exogenous stains may be further subdivided into those of metallic composition and those of nonmetallic composition. Exogenous stains are deposited in films and plaques on teeth and in rough, pitted and porous surfaces of teeth. Exogenous staining of teeth is usually indicative of poor oral hygiene; endogenous staining is most often indicative of pulpal death.

Exogenous Stains

METALLIC STAINS. Metallic staining of teeth is generally associated with the occupational hazards of metal workers or with the use of medicines containing metals or their salts. Metallic dust, associated with the fabrication of metal products, may lead to inhalation and accumulation of metals in plaques and films present on the teeth. A bluish-green stain may occur on the surfaces of the teeth of workers in copper, brass, or bronze. This stain may be removed by polishing if it has not penetrated into the tooth structure. Brown stains may

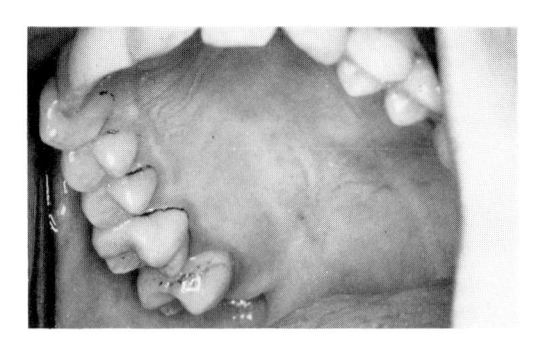

Fig. 10-9. *"Mesenteric line"*. Black stain at the free gingival margin.

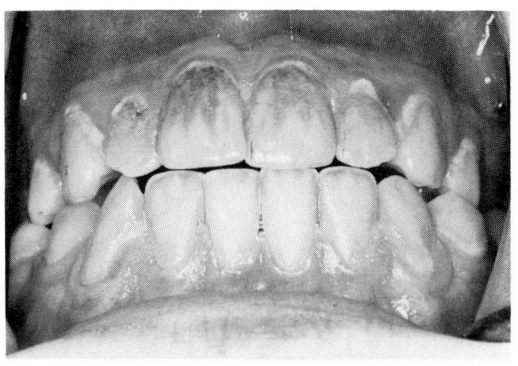

Fig. 10-10. Green stain, plaque and materia alba on the teeth of a patient with inadequate oral hygiene.

result from the use of drugs containing iron or from the industrial inhalation of iron-containing metals. Iron stains may be brown to black and similar to tobacco stains. Silver staining most often occurs as the result of the use of silver nitrate on the teeth by the dentist. Mercury and manganese give rise to black stains, and nickel to green stains.

NONMETALLIC STAINS. Nonmetallic stains may be associated with the incorporation of pigmented substances into plaques and accretions on teeth, rough, pitted and decalcified surfaces of teeth, and remnants of the enamel cuticle. It may be impossible to remove stains which have penetrated pits, fissures, and porous areas of teeth.

BLACK STAIN. Two variations of black stain of nonmetallic origin may occur on the teeth. They include the black stains caused by the products of tobacco combustion and the more or less characteristic "metabolic" stain. Tobacco stains are dark brown or black and discolor the teeth diffusely in areas where there are adherent mucinous plaques present. Tobacco stains are present most often on the lingual surfaces of the teeth, especially in those areas where pipes, cigars, or cigarettes are held. A black stain in the form of a fine line adjacent to the free gingival margin, which is not related to smoking, has been called metabolic stain and "mesenteric line." This stain may occur as a broad or thin black line following the contour of the free gingival margin onto the interproximal surfaces of the teeth. (Fig. 10-9). The cause of this stain is probably related to bacteria. Such black stains may be removed with some difficulty by polishing agents but tend to recur promptly in many instances. Removal is sometimes more difficult because of pitting of the underlying enamel.

GREEN STAIN. A green stain frequently occurs on the teeth of children, especially on the cervical third of the labial surfaces of the maxillary incisors (Fig. 10-10). This stain may or may not be associated with the remains of the enamel cuticle. Not infrequently the enamel beneath this stain is roughened and predisposes to the formation of mucinous plaques and the recurrence of the stain.

ORANGE STAIN. Orange and red stains may be present on the teeth in various locations but more especially on the cervical third of the teeth. Such stains are related to soft plaques on the teeth and probably the action of bacteria. They are easily removed by polishing agents and may be effectively prevented by proper tooth-brushing.

Endogenous Stains

Internal discoloration of the teeth may occur as the result of decomposition of blood pigments associated with the death of the pulp. Such pigments give the tooth a grayish or blue-black discoloration. The teeth occasionally may be discolored by blood-borne pigments associated with severe systemic diseases or inborn errors of pigment metabolism such as congenital porphyria.

Discoloration of the teeth may also occur as the result of hereditary and developmental disturbances such as mottled enamel, amelogenesis imperfecta, dentinogenesis imperfecta, and the use of tetracycline during pregnancy (Chapter 3).

SUMMARY

Dental plaque is an accumulation of bacteria, bacterial products, proteins from saliva and crevicular fluid, and lectins from ingested foods. Although it may appear only to be an amorphous mass of debris on the teeth, it is a highly organized bacterial ecologic unit.

Dental plaque is initiated by various indigenous oral bacteria that are able to adhere specifically to selected oral surfaces. The basis of adherence is a specific interaction mediated by cell surface macromolecules (adhesions) which combine with complementary structures (receptors) on tissue surfaces. For example, some bacteria are capable of attaching to a tooth covered by a film (pellicle) of selectively absorbed salivary proteins and glycoproteins. The initiation of plaque begins with the formation of the pellicle which itself begins within a matter of minutes after tooth eruption or tooth cleaning. Thus plaque begins by selective attachment of bacteria to the pellicle. Within a few hours additional organisms of the indigenous oral flora attach and further multiplication of the original colonizers occurs.

The adhesive interactions which contribute to the microbial colonization of tooth surfaces include direct attachment of bacteria to the pellicle, the aggregation of bacteria by soluble and insoluble glucans, salivary macromolecules, and specific interbacterial adherence by coaggregation of one bacterium with another. Specific adherence to the salivary pellicle is important for early colonizers such as Gram-positive Streptococcus and Actinomyces species. It has been postulated that certain Gram-negative microorganisms preferentially colonize Gram-positive bacteria in plaque and thus promote their colonization. Such interspecies coaggregation could establish beneficial relationships between filamentous and coccal bacteria in mature dental plaque.

Further colonization of the tooth surface occurs via several concurrent processes, including the attachment of new organisms to extracellular materials produced by the original colonizers, attachment of new organisms to previously attached or original colonizers, and the multiplication of original and subsequent colonists. After a few days a mature plaque has developed that has a composition which is dependent upon a multiplicity of environmental and intermicrobial interactions of the early colonizers. The multilayered colonization of the surface of a tooth is limited by abrasive and washing forces, although the specificity of cohesive interactions between bacteria and their synthesized surface polymers (aggregation) and between cells of different bacterial genera (intergeneric coaggregation) has been reported to be significant for the sequence of microbial colonization.

With increasing bacterial accumulation there is a shift from a predominantly Gram-positive coccal form to a complex population of filamentous organisms, Gram-negative cocci, vibrios and spirochetes. Closely associated with the accumulation is the development of gingivitis. Also the accumulation of plaque adjacent to the gingiva has been correlated with some immune responses. Unlike the large body of information that suggests that Streptococcus mutans is a plaque-forming bacterium capable of producing dental caries in humans, the evidence for the role of specific microorganisms in periodontal diseases is less convincing. Although evidence does not support the existence of a single microorganism which causes a specific periodontal disease, an increased number of different organisms can generally be found with one or several appearing to dominate. Whether a profile of specific bacteria indicates active disease or a person at risk for periodontal disease remains to be determined.

Changes in the nature and amount of food or major environmental changes may upset the balance of the ecosystem and result in the emergence of opportunistic pathogens. A pertinent example is the change in dental plaque composition from one of predominantly Gram-positive cocci and rods to one of increased colonization of non-retentive tooth surfaces by S. mutans as a result of excess sucrose consumption by the host. The establishment of S. mutans results in the fermentation of dietary sugars (sucrose) and formation and accumulation of acids which cause decalcification of enamel.

A number of epidemiologic, clinical and animal studies demonstrate a close relationship between dental plaque and periodontal diseases. The microorganisms which form plaque on teeth contain or release substances which induce or mediate inflammatory responses in the gingiva. The shift from gingivitis without loss of connective tissue and supporting bone to periodontitis with loss of attachment and alveolar bone has not been demonstrated in human disease. However, long term clinical studies indicate that the removal and prevention of dental plaque and calculus on the teeth by proper home care and professional dental care leads to the elimination of gingival inflammation and prevention of further loss of supporting structures in patients with advanced periodontal disease. Although supporting evidence has not yet established a cause and effect relationship between accumulated plaque and a progression of disease from human gingivitis to periodontitis, the clinical response (e.g., elimination of overt inflammation and maintenance of supporting structures) following the elimination of bacterial plaque clearly indicates the importance of the inflammatory response in plaque associated periodontal diseases.

The net effect of the inflammatory responses is protective, i.e., humoral and cellular responses are defense mechanisms for dealing with bacteria and their products. However, because the virulence of plaque has yet to be clarified, the mechanisms by which destruction of the periodontal tissues occurs are thought to involve direct cytotoxic effects of bacterial enzymes (proteases, collagenase, hyaluronidase, etc.) and endotoxins, and/or the indirect consequences of plaque antigens or mitogens which elicit a local and systemic immune reaction that may also cause damage in addition to the protection provided. Patients with immunodeficient disease of the lymphocyte-macrophage system do not appear to be more susceptible to periodontal disease than normal subjects. However, patients with neutrophil disorders (e.g., cyclic neutropenia, drug-induced agranulocytosis, etc.) where there are less numbers of neutrophilia and where there is reduced neutrophil function (e.g., diabetes mellitus, Down's syndrome, etc.) are susceptible to periodontal disease. The protective role of neutrophils in periodontal disease is seen in localized juvenile periodontitis where most patients have depressed neutrophil chemotaxis and phagocytosis and severe periodontal disease.

BIBLIOGRAPHY

Ainamo, J., et al.: The prevalence of caries and periodontal disease in the same subjects. In Lehner, T. and Cimasoni, G. (eds.) *The Borderland between Caries and Periodontal Disease II*, 2nd Ed., New York, Grune & Stratton, 1980.

Bodmer, J. and Bodmer, W.: Histocompatibility 1984. Immunology Today, 5:251, 1984.

Driessens, F.C.M., et al.: On the physiochemistry of plaque calcification and the phase composition of dental calculus. J. Periodont. Res., 20:329, 1985.

Genco, R.J. and Slots, J.: Host responses in periodontal diseases. J. Dent. Res., 63:441, 1984.

Gibbons, R.J.: Adherent interactions which may affect microbial ecology in the mouth. J. Dent. Res., 63:378, 1984.

Gibbons, R.J.: Adhesions of bacteria to the surface of the mouth. In R.C.W. Berkeley et al. (eds). *Microbial Adhesion to Surfaces*. Society of Chemical Industry, London, Chichester, Ellis Horwood Ltd., 1980.

Holm-Pedersen, P., et al.: Experimental gingivitis in young and elderly individuals. J. Clin. Periodont., 2:14, 1975.

Husband, A.J., et al.: Induction and delivery of mucosal immune responses. J. Dent. Res., 63:465, 1984.

Kani, T., et al.: Microbeam X-ray diffraction analysis of dental calculus. J. Dent. Res., 62:92, 1983.

Lin, E.C.C., et al.: *Bacteria, Plasmids, and Phages*. An Introduction to Molecular Biology. Cambridge, Harvard University Press, 1984.

Listgarten, M.A.: Structure of the microbial flora associated with periodontal disease and health in man. A light and electron microscopic study. J. Periodont., 47:1, 1976.

Loe, H., et al.: Experimental gingivitis in man. J. Periodont., 36:177, 1965.

Loe, H.: The specific etiology of periodontal disease and its application to prevention. In Carranza, F.A. (Jr.) and Kenney, E.B. (eds.) *Prevention of Periodontal Disease*, Chicago, Quintessence Publ. Co., 1981.

Loesche, W.J., et al.: Bacterial profiles of subgingival plaques in periodontitis. J. Periodontal., 56:447, 1985.

Loesche, W.J.: Chemotherapy of dental plaque infections. Oral Sci Rev., 9:63, 1976.

Pittard, A.J.: Contribution of molecular biology to the understanding and control of microbial infections. J. Dent. Res., 63:374, 1984.

Ramfjord, S.P. and Ash, M.M.: *Periodontology and Periodontics*, Philadelphia, W.B. Saunders Co., 1979.

Ruzicka, F.: Structure of sub- and supragingival dental calculus in human periodontitis. J. Periodont. Res., 19:317, 1984.

Schroeder, H.E.: *Formation and Inhibition of Dental Calculus*, Berne, Switzerland, Hans Huber, 1969.

Theilade, E. and Theilade, J.: Role of plaque in the etiology of periodontal disease and caries. Oral Sciences Rev., 9:23, 1976.

Unanue, E.R. and Benacerraf, B.: *Textbook of Immunology* (2nd ed.). Baltimore, Williams & Wilkins, 1984.

11

THE DENTIN-PULP COMPLEX AND DISEASE

The dental pulp is a loose connective tissue located anatomically within the calcified tissues of the tooth, i.e., within the dentin (Fig. 11–1). Although its primary function is to form, nurture and repair the dentin, the role of neural and vascular components of the pulp in controlling the functions of the masticatory system has yet to be fully clarified. The formative role of the pulp in dentinogenesis is mediated by the odontoblast (i.e., forming the organic matrix of dentin and then controlling its mineralization). The mature odontoblast lies at the edge of calcified tissue and has a cytoplasmic process that extends directly into tubules in the dentin (Fig. 11–2). The extent to which these processes traverse the dentin has yet to be determined, as evidence can be cited to both support and refute the observation that processes extend throughout the full length of the tubule under normal conditions. The odontoblast process appears to be a secretory site for dentin collagen and other components of the organic matrix of dentin.

The cells and extracellular matrices of the dental pulp and dentin constitute a dentin-pulpal complex which has clinical importance in relation to inflammatory reactions (pulpitis), the formation of reparative dentin, and intratubular changes in the dentin whereby its permeability is affected.

DENTIN-PULP COMPLEX

The extracellular components of the dental pulp are largely responsible for the physiological properties of this tissue. The composition of the pulpal extracellular matrix of the mature tooth includes certain types of collagen, fibronectin, and proteoglycans. Traditionally extracellular components of connective tissue are referred to as ground substance and fibrous components. In this respect certain proteoglycans are responsible for the gelatinous character of the ground substance, whereas other glycoproteins relate to cell surface components. Noncollagenous proteins have not been studied extensively. The glycoprotein fibronectin has been suggested to be a mediator of cell adhesion, both to extracellular components and other cells. The principal fibrous components of the dental pulp are interstitial collagens (i.e., they form fibrillar structures in the intercellular spaces). Fibronectin, as well as the type of collagen found in most soft connective tissues, is not found in dentin.

Innervation

The nerves entering the teeth into the pulp have been identified histologically as myelinated (A-fibers) and unmyelinated

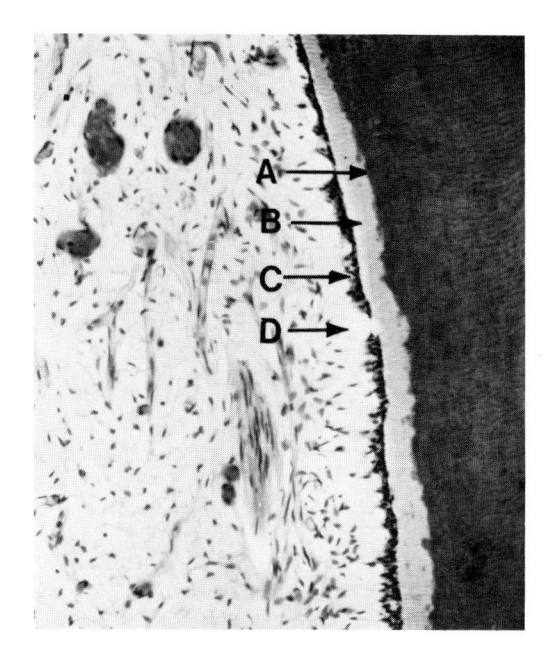

Fig. 11-1. *Dentin-pulp complex.* A, Primary dentin; B, predentin; C, odontoblast layer; D, cell free layer. Nerves and vessels are scattered throughout the pulp. The cells of the odontoblast have a variable morphology in the mature tooth.

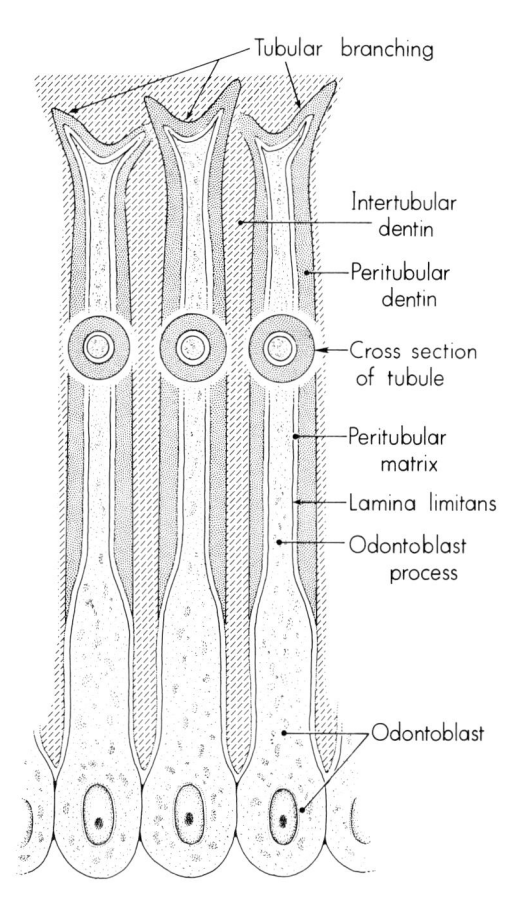

Fig. 11-2. Diagrammatic representation of odontoblasts and processes extending the full width of the dentin. Represented are the intertubular dentin (ID), peritubular dentin (P), lamina limitans (LL), and peritubular matrix space (PMS).

(C-fibers) nerves. Both have pain sensory functions whereas the unmyelinated fibers have been shown to have a sympathetic function. There is limited terminal branching of the nerves entering the apical foramen until the coronal portion of the pulp is reached. There the nerve bundles diverge, fan out, and form a plexus in the subodontoblastic region. Extension of unmyelinated fibers into the dentin is usually limited to a few micrometers. It has been suggested that A-fibers are responsible for dentin sensitivity and associated with sharp pain, whereas C-fibers are associated with dull, poorly localized or "burning pain." Both may be activated by injury to the pulp tissues. The variation in painful sensations perceived by the same or different individuals may be related to the activation of different types and numbers of pulp nerves or to different patterns of action potentials in individual nerves. Such variations in sensation may make rendering a diagnosis of specific pulp changes difficult.

The mechanism of pain transmission across the dentin has not been determined although the hydrodynamic theory has been generally accepted as a working hypothesis. According to the theory, when a stimulus is applied to the surface of a tooth (e.g., exposed cervical dentin), fluid in the dental tubules hydrodynamically distorts nerve receptors in the region of the pulp-dentin interface. The appeal of the hypothesis relates to present interest in changing the permeability of the tubules and reduction of the hydraulic conductance of dentin.

Fluid flow in the tubules has not been measured in vivo and the hypothesis remains unsubstantiated.

Burnishing (smearing) of the dentin, use of fluorides, as well as other forms of treatment that attempt to block or seal the dentin tubule aperatures, have been the most successful forms of palliative therapy for cervical hypersensitivity (Fig. 11–3).

Several local factors may alter sensory activity and influence the pain experienced by patients. For example, the diagnostic value of pain may be confounded if nerve fiber function is changed by local changes in the environment. These environmental changes may or may not be associated with inflammation of the pulp. They may be related to caries, dentin exposure (cervical abrasion, cavity preparation), application of dental materials to cut dentin, or changes in the microcirculation of the pulp. Also, small diameter pain fibers contain vasoactive substances which can initiate and maintain inflammatory-like responses and alter sensory activity of pain fibers.

Pulp Circulation

The blood vessels of the pulp consist of a network of feeding arterioles, capillaries, and collecting venules, as well as arteriovenous anastomoses (shunts). The arterioles enter the pulp at the apical foramen and pass without extensive branching to a capillary network terminating beneath the odontoblastic layer in the coronal portion of the tooth. This dense network of terminal capillaries is not present in the center of the pulp. Although blood flow to the teeth may be controlled by external mechanisms, vessels in the pulp which have alpha- and beta-adrenergic receptors can alter blood flow. Stimulation of alpha receptors causes a decrease in pulpal blood flow, and activation of beta receptors causes a reduction of pulpal blood flow. The latter response is paradoxical, inasmuch as beta receptor acti-

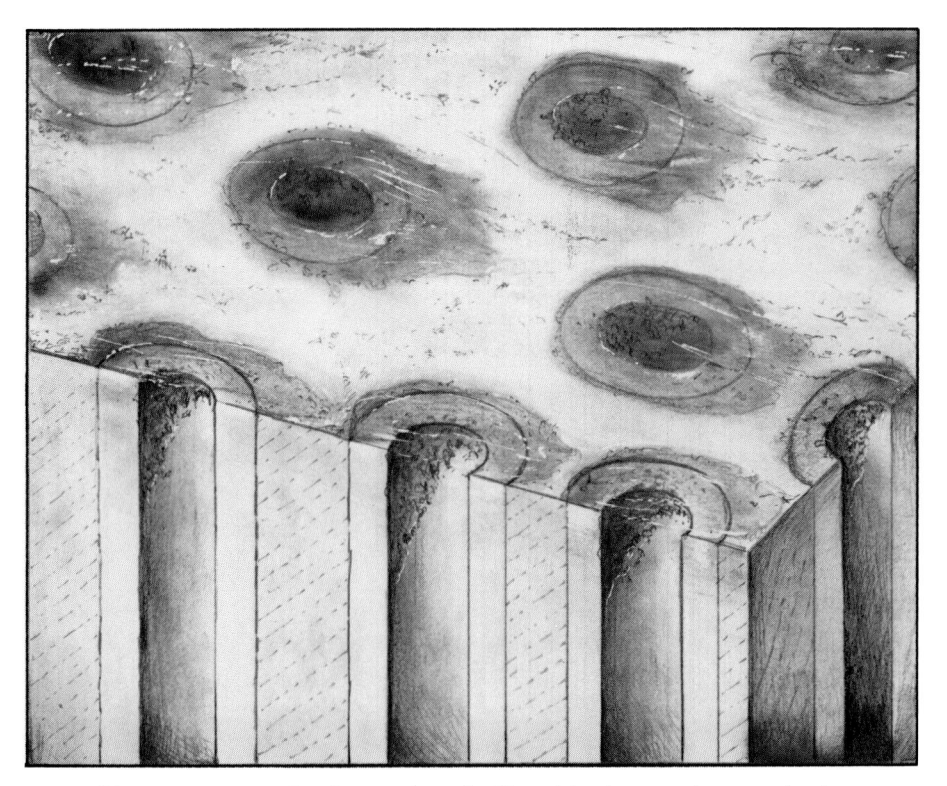

Fig. 11–3. Diagram representing "smear layer" of burnished, ground or cut dentin.

vation generally leads to increased blood flow in sites other than the pulp. The reason for this response is possibly related to passive compression of the venules secondary to an increased blood flow in the tissue confining pulp chamber where tissue compliance is low.

Tissue pressure in the pulp, or interstitial pressure, refers to the hydrostatic pressure exerted by the interstitial fluid in the extravascular tissues. An increase in pulp tissue pressure tends to compress the walls of venules and thereby reduce blood flow. The vasodilation and increased capillary permeability which occurs in inflammation (pulpitis) results in an increase in local tissue pressure. As this tissue pressure increases, the venous side of the microcirculation becomes strangled and results in ischemia and necrosis. Such a vicious cycle is generally controlled by increased lymph flow as well as other edema-preventing mechanisms, but pulp necrosis may occur by compression of blood vessels when large areas of the pulp become ischemic. Pulp necrosis can occur also through the direct action of bacterial toxins.

Vasodilation and local edema may occur when pulpal nerves are stimulated and release a polypeptide mediator (P substance). This mediator is able to impair the microcirculation and cause an increased vascular permeability without structural damage ("neurogenic inflammation").

Dentin

Dentin is the mineralized portion of the dentin-pulp complex. It is characterized by the presence of tubules and odontoblast processes which appear to extend throughout the thickness of the dentin. The presence of gap junctions between nerve-like fibers and odontoblasts have been reported and suggest the possibility of a connection between nerves and odontoblasts and their processes.

Dental tubules are formed at the time of deposition and mineralization of the predentin matrix around the odontoblast process (Fig. 11–2). At the dento-enamel junction the odontoblast processes are highly branched as are the tubules. Such branching does not appear to be present in the pulpal third of the dentin. The number of tubules decreases from the pulpal surface to the DEJ and has been shown to be more permeable at the pulpal side of the dentin. This difference in permeability may have significance for restorative procedures and protection of the pulp.

The dental tubules are lined with peritubular dentin which is more mineralized than intertubular dentin and is thicker toward the dento-enamel junction. The separation between the odontoblast process and the tubule wall is called the periodontoblastic space. A sheet-like structure, called the lamina limitans (Fig. 11–2), lines the length of dental tubules and corresponds to the inner hypomineralized layer of peritubular dentin. Several investigators have reported that the odontoblast process is limited to the pulpal third of the dentin and that the lamina limitans is what is seen extending throughout the thickness of the dentin.

The fluid present in the dental tubules is similar to extracellular fluid in that it is low in K^+, high in Na^+ and saturated with respect to Ca^{2+} and PO_4^{3-}. It contains a number of proteins similar to those found in plasma. The flow of the fluid from the pulp to the surface occurs slowly as long as the perispheral ends of the tubules remain closed. If the ends are opened, as occurs in cavity preparation, there is bulk fluid movement from the pulp to the surface of the cut dentin. Even though there is leakage of the fluid from the tubules at the cut surface, the concentration of the substances in the fluid remains the same. During the process of cutting dentin the tubule openings may be smeared over or plugged, leaving a "smear layer" which decreases the permeability of the dentin (Fig. 11–3). A "smear layer" is composed of grinding debris mixed with saliva and/or water and/or liquid components from the dentin. Thus,

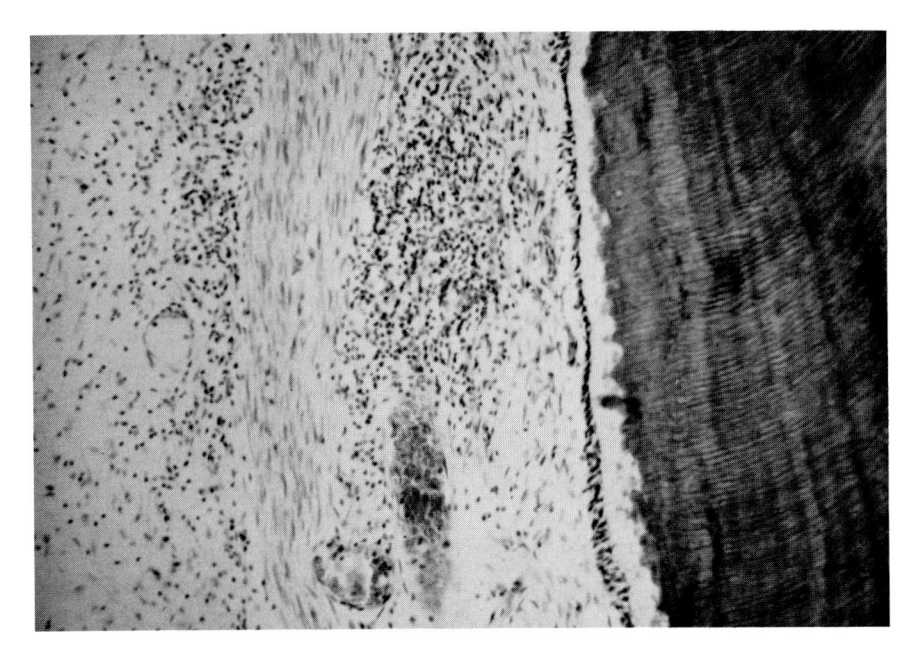

Fig. 11–6. Pulpitis with inflammatory cell infiltration adjacent to a nerve and just above a small blood vessel. Although the response is histologically mild, the clinical symptom was acute pain.

puration and abscess formation, or to liquefaction and necrosis of the entire pulp. Extirpation of the pulp and endodontic therapy is usually the required treatment.

Chronic Pulpitis

The clinical diagnosis of chronic pulpitis can be made on the basis of recurring episodes of pain, usually so mild and intermittent that the patient has not sought relief. Such mild clinical symptoms may reflect serious involvement of the pulp irrespective of the degree of destruction of the hard tissues.

The histologic features of chronic pulpitis may have little correlation with clinical symptoms. However, the histologic diagnosis is based primarily on the microscopic features present, although the history of the disturbance may be useful information. The histologic features of chronic pulpitis include infiltration of the pulp tissues with lymphocytes and plasma cells and replacement of the loose connective tissue with prominent capillaries and fibroblast activity. The entire pulp or only a small area adjacent to a carious lesion may be involved.

Chronic hyperplastic pulpitis is a clinical diagnosis reserved for an exposed and enlarged pulp that protrudes from the pulp chamber of a tooth that has little or no occlusal surfaces present (Fig. 11–7). This type of pulpitis is usually seen in primary molars or first permanent molars of young adults. The exposed pulp is usually a pink mass of soft tissue which is seldom sensitive to manipulation. The histologic feature is granulation tissue, often epithelized. This is an inflammatory process and is treated by extirpation and endodontic therapy or extraction of the tooth.

SEQUELAE OF PULP DISEASE

The sequelae of untreated pulp disease are periapical lesions which reflect different tissue reactions either because of the type of organism involved in the spread of infection or the anatomic sites involved. Thus differences in the lesions may be related more to the uniqueness of the periapical vation generally leads to increased blood flow in sites other than the pulp. The reason for this response is possibly related to passive compression of the venules secondary to an increased blood flow in the tissue confining pulp chamber where tissue compliance is low.

Tissue pressure in the pulp, or interstitial pressure, refers to the hydrostatic pressure exerted by the interstitial fluid in the extravascular tissues. An increase in pulp tissue pressure tends to compress the walls of venules and thereby reduce blood flow. The vasodilation and increased capillary permeability which occurs in inflammation (pulpitis) results in an increase in local tissue pressure. As this tissue pressure increases, the venous side of the microcirculation becomes strangled and results in ischemia and necrosis. Such a vicious cycle is generally controlled by increased lymph flow as well as other edema-preventing mechanisms, but pulp necrosis may occur by compression of blood vessels when large areas of the pulp become ischemic. Pulp necrosis can occur also through the direct action of bacterial toxins.

Vasodilation and local edema may occur when pulpal nerves are stimulated and release a polypeptide mediator (P substance). This mediator is able to impair the microcirculation and cause an increased vascular permeability without structural damage ("neurogenic inflammation").

Dentin

Dentin is the mineralized portion of the dentin-pulp complex. It is characterized by the presence of tubules and odontoblast processes which appear to extend throughout the thickness of the dentin. The presence of gap junctions between nerve-like fibers and odontoblasts have been reported and suggest the possibility of a connection between nerves and odontoblasts and their processes.

Dental tubules are formed at the time of deposition and mineralization of the predentin matrix around the odontoblast process (Fig. 11–2). At the dento-enamel junction the odontoblast processes are highly branched as are the tubules. Such branching does not appear to be present in the pulpal third of the dentin. The number of tubules decreases from the pulpal surface to the DEJ and has been shown to be more permeable at the pulpal side of the dentin. This difference in permeability may have significance for restorative procedures and protection of the pulp.

The dental tubules are lined with peritubular dentin which is more mineralized than intertubular dentin and is thicker toward the dento-enamel junction. The separation between the odontoblast process and the tubule wall is called the periodontoblastic space. A sheet-like structure, called the lamina limitans (Fig. 11–2), lines the length of dental tubules and corresponds to the inner hypomineralized layer of peritubular dentin. Several investigators have reported that the odontoblast process is limited to the pulpal third of the dentin and that the lamina limitans is what is seen extending throughout the thickness of the dentin.

The fluid present in the dental tubules is similar to extracellular fluid in that it is low in K^+, high in Na^+ and saturated with respect to Ca^{2+} and PO_4^{3-}. It contains a number of proteins similar to those found in plasma. The flow of the fluid from the pulp to the surface occurs slowly as long as the perispheral ends of the tubules remain closed. If the ends are opened, as occurs in cavity preparation, there is bulk fluid movement from the pulp to the surface of the cut dentin. Even though there is leakage of the fluid from the tubules at the cut surface, the concentration of the substances in the fluid remains the same. During the process of cutting dentin the tubule openings may be smeared over or plugged, leaving a "smear layer" which decreases the permeability of the dentin (Fig. 11–3). A "smear layer" is composed of grinding debris mixed with saliva and/or water and/or liquid components from the dentin. Thus, the smear layer has a protective effect and increases resistance to fluid flow.

The transport of plasma proteins through dentin is dependent upon pulpal tissue pressure, dentinal tubule resistance, and the permeability of pulpal capillaries and venules. Plasma proteins leaking from pulpal vessels in response to cavity preparation and/or "neurogenic inflammation" have been reported to enter the tubules and decrease dentin permeability. Several mediators of inflammation (e.g., histamine, substance P, prostaglandins, etc.) present in the pulp could cause leakage of plasma proteins into the interstitial fluid adjacent to the dentin where they could be transported into the tubules. Interestingly, plasma proteins are found histologically in carious dentin. Presumably, fluid movement in the tubules is responsible for the presence of antibodies to Streptococcus mutans found in carious dentin.

Demineralization of dentin as a result of caries or erosion causes resorption of the peritubular dentin and increases the width of the tubules. Dental procedures may also widen the tubules and increase the permeability of tubules. Conversely, decreases in tubule permeability may be related to growth of peritubular dentin but not necessarily related to aging. Also, precipitation of mineral salts within the tubules may occur and is referred to as dentin sclerosis or "dead tracts" (Fig. 11–4).

Reactive or irregular secondary dentin (Fig. 11–5) is found subjacent to caries and restorations and can be a response to the carious process, to the trauma of cavity preparation, and/or to the irritating aspects of the material used in the restoration. The interface between primary dentin at the base of the cavity preparation and the irregular secondary dentin may lack tubules, be less permeable, and therefore be protective of the pulp.

PULP DISEASE

From the foregoing discussion it is evident that disorders of primary dentin are concerned with intratubular changes and that disorders of the pulp are generally related to inflammation of the pulp. In either case the pathologic changes in the dentin and/or pulp may be caused by trauma and fracture of teeth, exposure of dentin, operative procedures, chemicals, and bacteria. The response of the dentin-pulp complex to iatrogenic damage and disease is not always predictable, and the relationship between clinical symptoms, especially pain, and the state of the dentin-pulp complex is based largely on clinical judgment.

Although pulpitis may be categorized on the basis of operative procedures, chemical irritants, mechanical and thermal injury, and microbial irritants, such divisions do not reflect consistent responses of the dentin-complex to various forms of irritation. Much the same can be said for histologic clas-

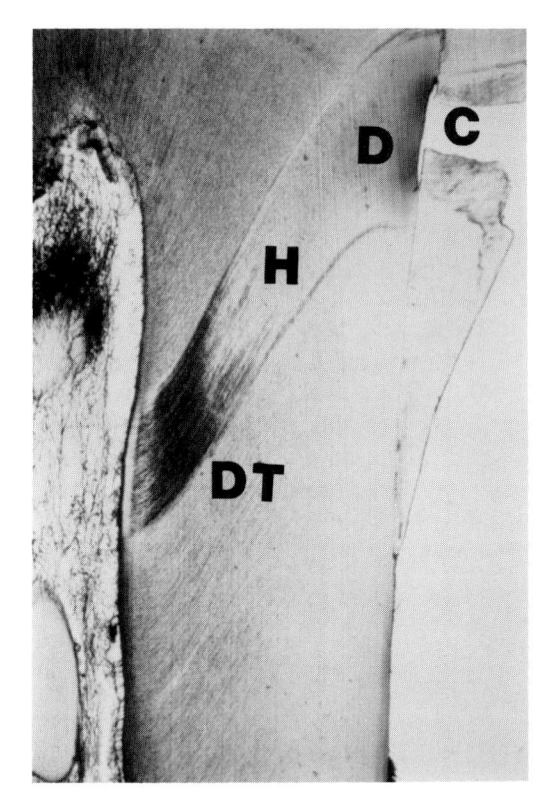

Fig. 11–4. Response of dentin to carious process (C), demineralized area (D), hyalinized zone (H), and "dead tracts" (DT).

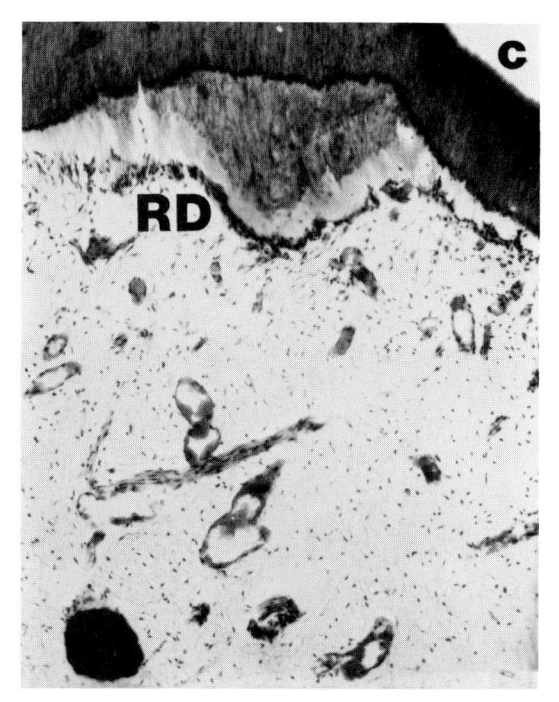

Fig. 11–5. Response of dentin-pulp complex with irregular secondary or reactive dentin (RD) in relationship to cavity preparation (C). The dentin formed is irregular and tubular structure abnormal.

sifications of pulp disease inasmuch as the histologic finding must wait for the tooth to be extracted or the pulp extirpated to formulate the diagnosis. Even so there is little assurance that the clinical symptoms will reflect accurately the histologic findings. The following classification of pulp disease reflects clinical convenience and the need to have a provisional clinical diagnosis in order to render even palliative treatment.

Pulpitis

Pulpitis may be classified clinically as acute or chronic, depending on the duration and severity of the symptoms (Fig. 11–6). It should not be assumed that pain reflects the presence of pulpitis or that the most severe histologic changes can always be related to the severity of pain. The reason for this disparity has already been discussed in relation to the innervations of the dentin-pulp complex, including so-called "neurogenic inflammation" of the pulp.

The persistent symptoms of pain which occur in relation to a carious lesion and ingestion of sweets may reflect a pathologic change in the dentin and a direct algogenic property of hyperosmotic sugar solutions rather than histologic changes of pulpitis. Although increased nerve sensitivity associated with inflammation may occur in such instances, it is possible that the sugar has a direct excitatory effect. Thus a brief burst of pain following the ingestion of sugar may be the initial symptom of pathologic changes in the hard tissues and reflect the activation of hydrodynamic pain via hyperosmotic sugar stimuli. A number of stimuli may evoke painful sensations in relation to hydrodynamic mechanisms.

Acute Pulpitis

The clinical diagnosis of acute pulpitis may be made when the complaint is constant, severe pain. The radiographic extent of the lesion may not reflect the severity of the symptom. It must be kept in mind that pain has an affective component which may not correlate with the clinical findings. When the tooth is exquisitely tender to touch, the patient may have difficulty in swallowing and eating. If severe pain is relieved only by cold or ice, pulpal necrosis is likely to be present. And where multiple canals are present, one root may have vital tissue and the other necrotic pulp tissue. In general, if pain is not constant but persists after being induced by either heat or cold, pulpitis is usually present.

The principal characteristic of acute pulpitis is constant, severe pain, which may or may not be relieved by heat or cold, and evidence of a carious lesion approaching the pulp tissue. Severe pain which is elicited by, and persists after, cold stimulation usually reflects an irreversible acute pulpitis.

The histologic diagnosis of acute pulpitis is made on the basis of the inflammatory changes present. These may range from focal accumulations of neutrophils to sup-

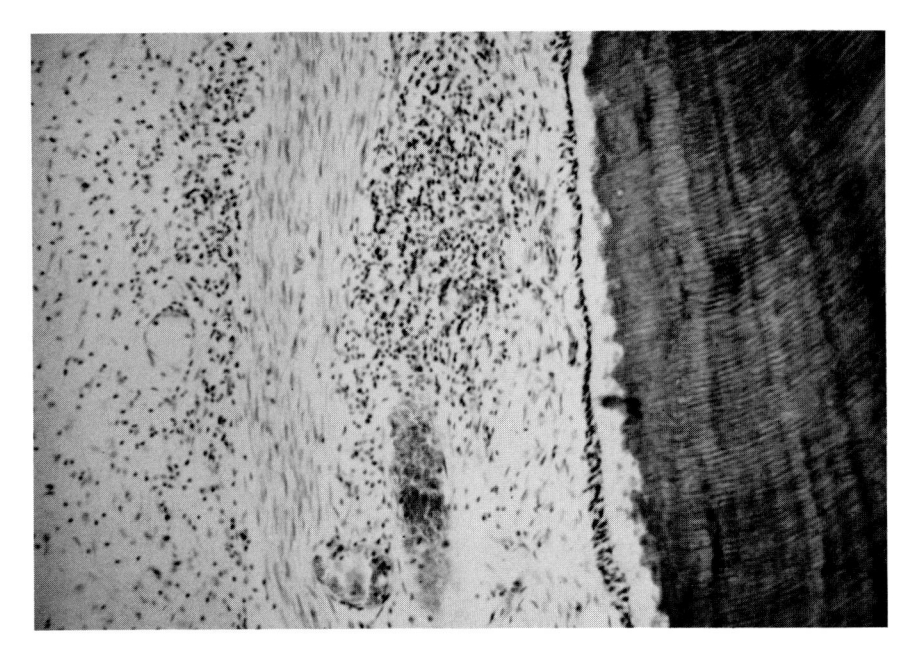

Fig. 11-6. Pulpitis with inflammatory cell infiltration adjacent to a nerve and just above a small blood vessel. Although the response is histologically mild, the clinical symptom was acute pain.

puration and abscess formation, or to liquefaction and necrosis of the entire pulp. Extirpation of the pulp and endodontic therapy is usually the required treatment.

Chronic Pulpitis

The clinical diagnosis of chronic pulpitis can be made on the basis of recurring episodes of pain, usually so mild and intermittent that the patient has not sought relief. Such mild clinical symptoms may reflect serious involvement of the pulp irrespective of the degree of destruction of the hard tissues.

The histologic features of chronic pulpitis may have little correlation with clinical symptoms. However, the histologic diagnosis is based primarily on the microscopic features present, although the history of the disturbance may be useful information. The histologic features of chronic pulpitis include infiltration of the pulp tissues with lymphocytes and plasma cells and replacement of the loose connective tissue with prominent capillaries and fibroblast activity. The entire pulp or only a small area adjacent to a carious lesion may be involved.

Chronic hyperplastic pulpitis is a clinical diagnosis reserved for an exposed and enlarged pulp that protrudes from the pulp chamber of a tooth that has little or no occlusal surfaces present (Fig. 11-7). This type of pulpitis is usually seen in primary molars or first permanent molars of young adults. The exposed pulp is usually a pink mass of soft tissue which is seldom sensitive to manipulation. The histologic feature is granulation tissue, often epithelized. This is an inflammatory process and is treated by extirpation and endodontic therapy or extraction of the tooth.

SEQUELAE OF PULP DISEASE

The sequelae of untreated pulp disease are periapical lesions which reflect different tissue reactions either because of the type of organism involved in the spread of infection or the anatomic sites involved. Thus differences in the lesions may be related more to the uniqueness of the periapical

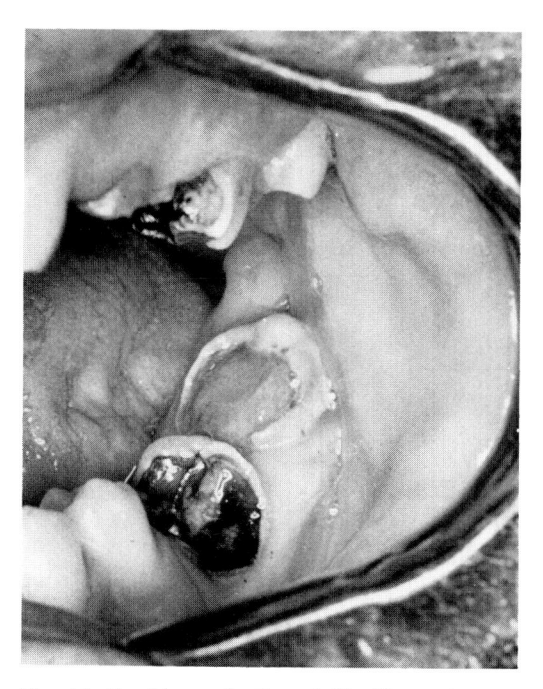

Fig. 11–7. *Hyperplastic pulpitis.* Mass of granulation tissue arising from pulp tissue after carious process has destroyed coronal covering of pulp chamber.

tissues than to the nonspecific reactive processes.

Periapical Granuloma

The periapical granuloma is a mass of granulation tissue at the end of a root and reflects a response of the periapical tissues to injurious agents involved in the pulpitis. The natural history of the periapical granuloma is obscure, although a number of suggestions demonstrate a transition from pulpitis to the periapical granuloma.

Although the clinical symptoms of a fully developed granuloma are often mild or absent, the symptoms associated with the preceding pulpitis may have been severe. These lesions may be asymptomatic for long periods of time but may undergo an acute exacerbation.

Radiographically a fully developed chronic granuloma is well-circumscribed and may be outlined by a thin radiopaque line or band of sclerotic bone.

The histologic appearance of the periapical granuloma has a number of features which are not necessarily present in a single lesion. The typical granuloma consists of fibroblastic proliferation and an infiltration with lymphocytes and plasma cells. In some instances macrophages filled with lipoid material are present as well as cholesterol slits. Generally the granulation tissue is surrounded by a "capsule" of dense connective tissue. In most periapical granulomas epithelium can be observed if enough of the lesion is sectioned for review.

The bacteriologic profile for the periapical granuloma is obscure, with conflicting evidence ranging from sterility to microorganisms which might have difficulty surviving under anaerobic conditions.

The treatment of periapical granuloma is based on clinical judgment. Extraction may depend upon the state of the canals and access to the apex with endodontic instrumentation. When instrumentation to remove all the pulp tissue is not possible, extraction may be necessary. Entry to the periapical area through the alveolar bone to remove the granuloma and root tip may be done. In some instances it is likely that the lesion transforms into a periapical (radicular) cyst.

Periapical Cyst (Radicular Cyst)

These cysts arise in long-standing periapical granulomas when there are epithelial rests in the periapical area. Bacteria or bacterial products stimulate proliferation of the epithelial rests in the periapical area and, as they grow, surround the apex of the root or cover the surface of granulation tissue adjacent to the root. This results in an epithelial-lined space at the apex which is called a periapical cyst (Fig. 11–8). Like the granulomas, they may remain present without symptoms for long periods of time. They gradually increase in size due to accumulation of fluid in the cyst space and produce destruction of the surrounding bone. In exceptional cases they may produce expansion of the jaw. Radicular cysts frequently undergo exacerbation of the inflammatory

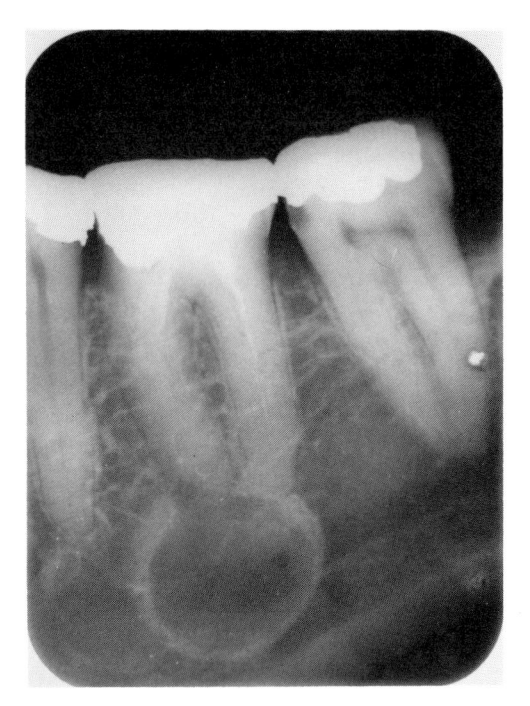

Fig. 11-8. Periapical or radicular cyst and associated incomplete endodontic therapy. The border of the cyst is well defined with a zone of dense reactive bone.

process and produce swelling and pain in the jaw. Radiographically the radicular cyst is identical in most cases to the periapical granuloma. Histologically the radicular cyst is lined by squamous epithelium covering connective tissue infiltrated with lymphocytes and plasma cells. Except for the lumen present, the histologic features are the same as the periapical granuloma and treatment the same.

Cellulitis

Cellulitis is a diffuse inflammation of the soft tissues surrounding the jaws produced by the spread of an acute periapical inflammation outside the jaw. In some cases, the periapical inflammation is severe and the body is unable to localize it to the periapical area. The infection spreads into the surrounding tissues, especially facial spaces, resulting in marked swelling, intense pain, and general malaise with elevation of temperature. Cellulitis is a severe process and may be life threatening.

Periapical Abscess

The periapical abscess is a suppurative process which usually results from pulpal infection. The clinical symptoms reflect an acute inflammation of the periapical tissues. If the acute reactive process is confined to the periapical region, the systemic manifestations are generally limited to regional lymphadenopathy and fever. The tooth is extremely sensitive to touch and is somewhat extruded so that occlusal contact may give rise to muscle spasms and pain. A chronic periapical abscess may present no clinical symptoms.

The histologic feature (Fig. 11-9) of a periapical abscess is a central area of suppuration composed of lysed polymorphonuclear leukocytes or frank pus. The chronic abscess may develop in a periapical granuloma.

Parulis, Fistula, Gum Boil

These terms are used to indicate the spontaneous drainage of a periapical abscess. In children the roots of the deciduous teeth are close to the surface of the jaw and the cortical bone is thin, so that periapical abscesses easily rupture to the exterior of the jaw. The pus accumulates beneath the mucosa, producing a localized swelling that ruptures, allowing pus to escape into the mouth. The elevated area with an opening from which pus escapes is called a parulis or gum boil (Fig. 11-10). Once drainage is established, symptoms subside and the drainage is persistent until the tooth is treated or extracted. On some occasions the pus makes it through the jaw apical to the mucobuccal fold and migrates through the tissue to the skin. It ruptures through the skin and the pus escapes to the exterior (Fig. 11-11). The drainage tract is termed a fistula or sinus tract (Fig. 11-12). A draining sinus persists until the involved tooth is treated or extracted.

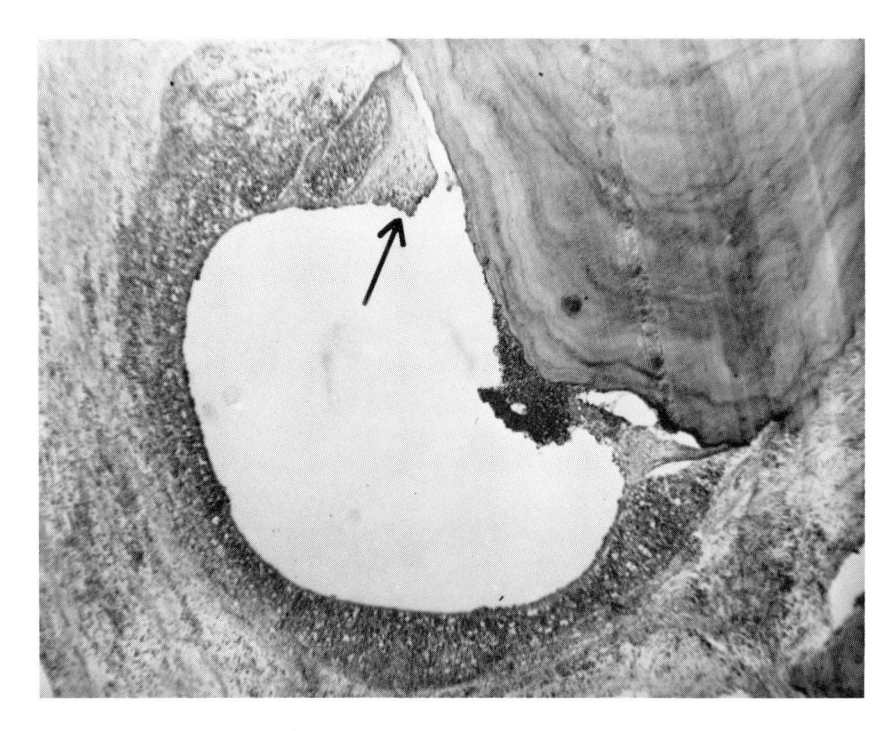

Fig. 11-9. *Periapical abscess.* Space adjacent to tooth lined with granulation tissue except for early epithelial proliferation indicated by arrow. The central area may be filled with pus if not lost during processing of specimen.

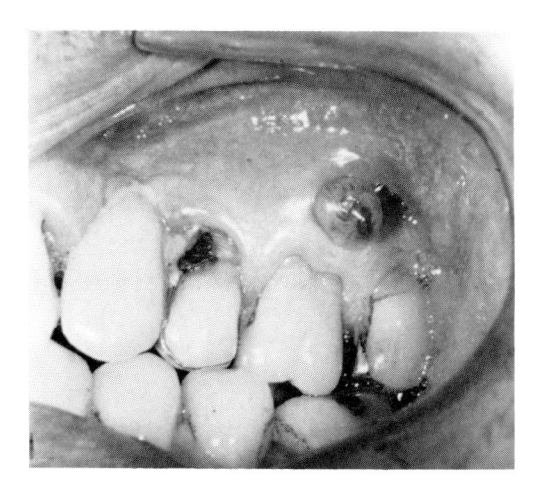

Fig. 11-10. Parulus or "gum boil" above the first molar root.

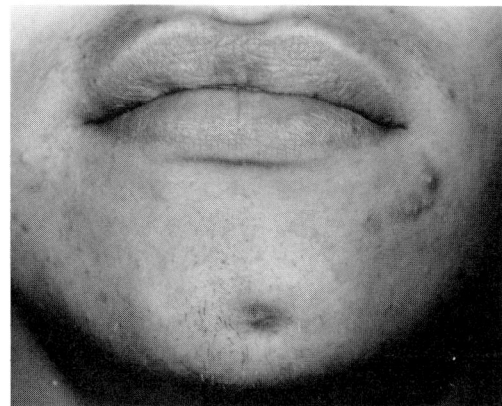

Fig. 11-11. Drainage site on the skin from a mandibular central incisor.

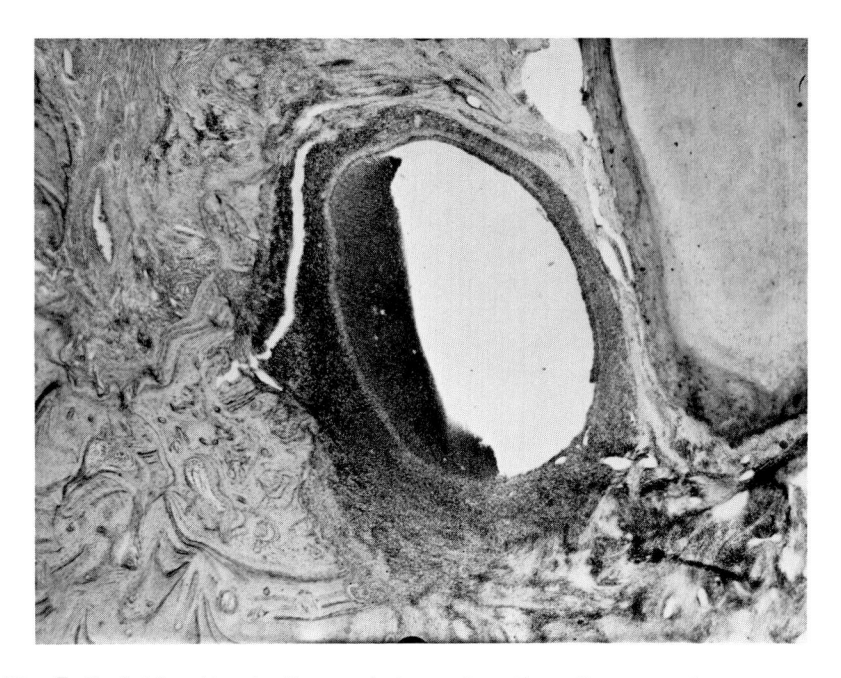

Fig. 11–12. Epithelial lined tract with pus drainage from the adjacent tooth.

Osteomyelitis

If an infection spreads to the marrow spaces of bone the process is designated as osteomyelitis. When drainage cannot be established naturally through the cortex of bone, the infection and pus may spread into the marrow spaces. The bone may undergo localized necrosis attended by pain and swelling of the area. The patient has malaise and an elevation of temperature. The dead bone, which is separated from the living bone, is called a sequestrum.

Treatment for osteomyelitis is dependent upon the causative organisms and the appropriate antibiotic therapy.

SUMMARY

The dentin-pulp complex, and especially the predentin-dentin complex, has become the site of renewed interest because of new ideas about the permeability characteristics of dentin. Changes in permeability of dentin, including those caused by reactive or irregular dentin, obturation of the dental tubules by growth of the peritubular dentin, permeation of plasma proteins into the tubules, and formation of a "smear layer," are potentially important for the success of restorative treatment. Thus, treatment procedures and restorative materials may play a significant role in shaping beneficial changes in the dentin.

The response of the pulp to the process of caries is inflammation. Because the pulp tissues are enclosed in calcified tissue, the microvascular circulation and tissue pressure may cause greater problems than those occurring in tissues where tissue compliance (expansion) is possible. The response of the pulp is also determined by the nature of the bacteria present. Diagnostically the relationship between painful symptoms and the actual status of the pulp is often obscure. Therefore a clinical classification of pulpitis may only be acute or chronic pulpitis.

BIBLIOGRAPHY

Aison, E.L.: Osteomyelitis of the jaw. J. Am. Dent. Assoc., 25:1261, 1938.
Bourgoyne, J.R., and Quinn, J.H.: The periapical abscess. J. Oral Surg., 7:320, 1949.

Buchanan, J.C.: Oral abscesses and granuloma. Dent. Cosmos, 72:605, 1930.

Cook, T.J.: Dental granuloma. J. Am. Dent. Assoc., 14:2231, 1927.

Durbeck, W.E.: Mandibular osteomyelitis: its diagnosis and treatment. J. Oral Surg., 4:33, 1946.

Eisenbud, L., and Klatell, J.: Acute alveolar abscess; a review of 300 hospitalized cases. Oral Surg., 4:208, 1951.

Freeman, N.: Histopathological investigations of the dental granuloma. J. Dent. Res., 11:175, 1931.

Heyeraas, K.J.: Pulpa, microvascular and tissue pressure. J. Dent. Res., 64 (Spec. Iss.):585, 1985.

Holland, G.R.: The odontoblast process: form and function. J. Dent. Res., 64 (Spec. Iss.):499, 1985.

Kim, S.: Regulation of pulpal blood flow. J. Dent. Res., 64 (Spec. Iss.):590, 1985.

Linde, A.: The extracellular matrix of the dental pulp and dentin. J. Dent. Res., 64 (Spec. Iss.):523, 1985.

Lundy, T. and Stanley, H.R.: Correlation of pulpal histopathology and clinical symptoms in human teeth subjected to experimental irritation. Oral Surg., 27:187, 1969.

McConnell, G.: The histopathology of dental granuloma. J. Am. Dent. Assoc., 8:390, 1921.

Mjör, I.A.: Dentin-predentix and its permeability: pathology and treatment overview. J. Dent. Res., 64 (Spec. Iss.):621, 1985.

Olgart, L.M.: The role of local factors in dentin and pulp in intradental pain mechanisms. J. Dent. Res., 64 (Spec. Iss.):572, 1985.

Padgett, E.C.: Osteomyelitis of jaws: analysis of 59 patients. Surgery, 8:821, 1940.

Pashley, D.H.: Dentin-predentin complex and its permeability: physiologic overview. J. Dent. Res., 64 (Spec. Iss.):613, 1985.

Seltzer, S. and Bender, I.B.: *The Dental Pulp*, 3rd ed. Philadelphia: J.B. Lippincott Co., 1984.

Shafer, W.G.: Chronic sclerosing osteomyelitis. J. Oral Surg., 15:138, 1957.

Shear, M.: Cholesterol in dental cysts. Oral Surg., 16:1465, 1963.

Stephan, R.M.: Correlation of clinical tests with microscopic pathology of the dental pulp. J. Dent. Res., 16:267, 1937.

Ten Cate, A.R.: *Oral Histology: Development, Structure and Function*. St. Louis: C.V. Mosby Co., 1980.

12

DENTAL CARIES

Dental caries (decay) is a disease of dental hard tissues initiated by acid producing bacteria in plaque on the surface of the teeth. The carious process is characterized by an initial softening or partial demineralization of enamel and then, unless the process is arrested or reversed, by a progressive solubilization of the tooth mineral and total destruction of the organic portions of the enamel, dentin and cementum. The initiation and progression of events in the disease depend upon dietary, bacterial, environmental, and genetic factors. Even though dental decay has been recorded in the teeth of fossil jaws and associated with toothache in the earliest written chronicles, the significance of dietary and bacterial factors involved in the disease has only recently begun to be understood. The mechanism of tooth decay involves bacterial acid production, regulated by the nature and frequency of sugar intake, and by factors in the saliva and on the tooth which neutralize the acids. In effect, dental caries is a multifactorial disease requiring cariogenic microorganisms, nutrients for the bacteria, a suitable ecologic niche, and a susceptible host.

The mere presence of bacteria capable of forming demineralizing acids is not sufficient evidence to establish that acidogenic bacteria alone are the cause of human dental decay, nor that dental caries is a human infectious process. In order for bacteria to cause dental decay they must have the ability to adhere to, as well as colonize, one or more susceptible surfaces of the teeth, the ability to live in an acid environment, the ability to live during periods when no nutrients are available, and the ability to evade the defenses of the host. Also required for bacteria to cause dental decay is the presence of dietary nutrients, viz., sugars and starches. Streptococcus mutans and some strains of lactobacilli and actinomycetes are cariogenic in man.

Even the presence of cariogenic bacteria and dietary sugar may not lead progressively to loss of tooth structure and cavitation or cavities. Remineralization may take place before a cavity forms if the acid formation is curtailed before demineralization has had time to occur completely. In this respect the presence of fluoride and the mineralization potential of saliva and plaque can be major factors in the process of remineralization. The biochemistry of dental plaque is of central importance for bacterial metabolism and for inorganic components in the plaque which can influence the mineral content of the tooth. The essential role of bacteria and dietary carbohydrates (e.g., sucrose) in the cause and initiation of caries has been developed on the basis of epidemiologic, clinical, laboratory and animal studies.

EPIDEMIOLOGY

In order to describe the incidence or prevalance of dental caries, an index is used called the DMF index. This index refers to the number of Decayed-Missing-Filled teeth present in an individual over time. The phrase DMF prevalence can be used as a measure of the occurrence of decayed teeth in a population at a given time. If a population is measured twice (e.g., 1982 and 1987), an increase or decrease in the DMF scores is referred to as the incidence of decayed-missing-filled teeth in that population. Of course, the DMF index has a number of limitations for the permanent dentition where loss of teeth may occur from diseases other than caries. Even so, the DMF (permanent dentition) or dmf (primary dentition) is widely used for recording the degree and intensity of the carious attack. The term DMFS refers to decayed, missing and filled surfaces.

PREVALENCE OF CARIES

Prior to this century, the prevalence of dental caries was low—less than 3 DMF teeth per 12 year old—in the rapidly industrializing countries of Western Europe, Canada, the U.S., Australia and New Zealand. However, because of the "Western diet," which includes high quantities of sugar, by the 7th decade of the 20th century the disease levels had reached 6 to 12 DMF teeth per 12-year-old child, and 19 to 25 DMF teeth per 35- to 44-year-old adult. But then the sum total effect of fluorides, better oral hygiene, and dietary control led to a reduction of the DMF rate in the 12 year old to 2 to 4 DMF and 13 to 19 DMF in the 35 to 44-year-old adult. This phenomenon appears to be in the process of repeating itself in the developing countries where DMF rates which are now low are beginning to rise.

SITES OF CARIES

Streptococcus mutans appears to be the predominant cariogenic bacteria colonizing

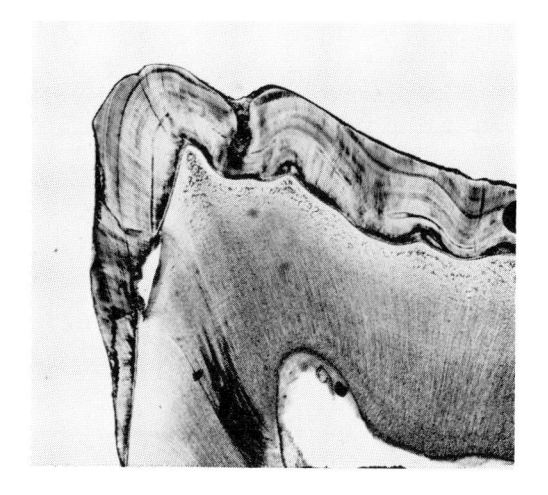

Fig. 12-1. Smooth surface caries with shrinkage of decalcified enamel and formation of a space at the dentoenamel junction.

the smooth surfaces (Fig. 12-1) of the teeth (proximal, facial, lingual surfaces), whereas S. mutans and lactobacilli are the predominant organisms that colonize the pit and fissures (Fig. 12-2) of occlusal surfaces. The latter account for 50% of all carious lesions. When the root surface is exposed, as with gingival recession, cariogenic bacteria may cause root caries because of gingival recession secondary to periodontal disease. The predominant bacteria in plaque or root surfaces are Actinomyces viscosus and naeslundii. Root surface caries appears to be more common in non-Western societies.

The results of longitudinal studies indicate that 60 to 80% of the occlusal surfaces of molars have carious lesions only a few years after eruption, and that once in dentin the disease progresses rapidly. In contrast, carious lesions of proximal and smooth surfaces tended to develop slowly or even reverse with rehardening of previously softened areas. Several studies have reported that many proximal enamel lesions diagnosed radiographically at 7 to 9 years of age did not in the following 7 to 8 years progress into the dentin. In some short term studies as many as 50% of the lesions followed did not progress and many reflected

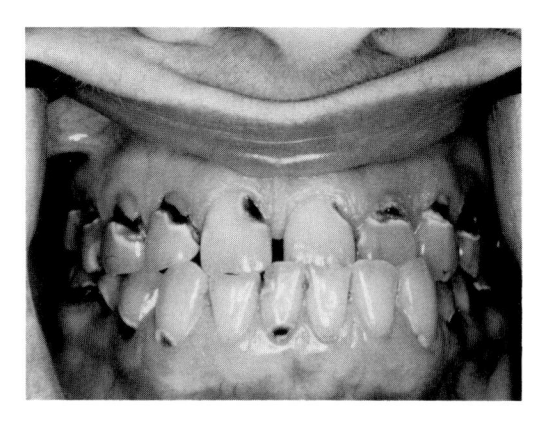

Fig. 12-3. Rampant decay in young adult who was a heavy user of "soft drink" beverages.

after eruption of the teeth and that the natural remineralization process should in some way be enhanced in order to reverse incipient proximal and smooth surface lesions.

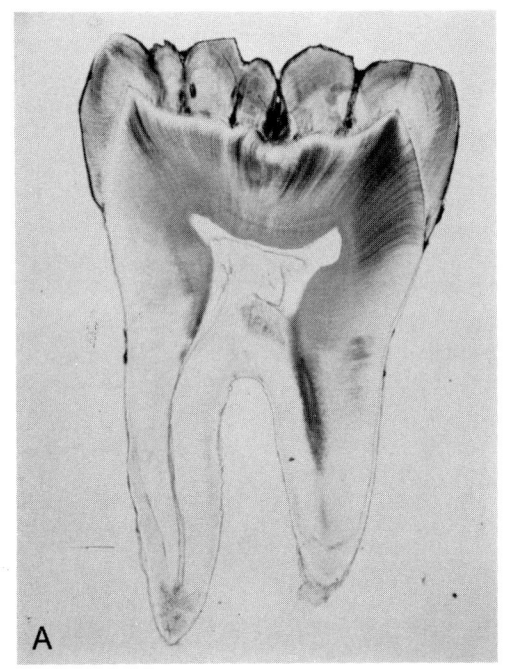

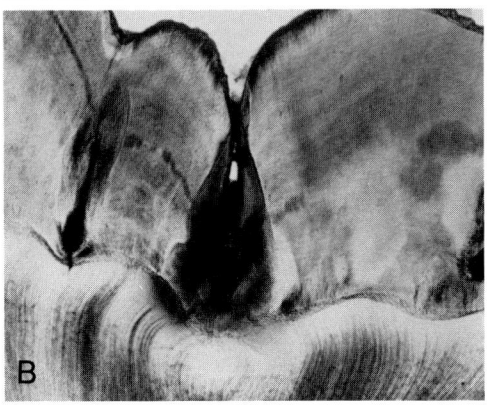

Fig. 12-2. *Occlusal surface caries. A,* Ground section photographed with transmitted light. *B,* Carious lesion of developmental groove.

reversals to rehardened enamel. In dental students the percentage of no change in early carious lesions may reach as high as 70 to 90%.

Data from longitudinal studies suggest that the rate of progression of initial proximal lesions is generally quite low and that caries arrest may be greater in smooth surface lesions than proximal lesions. These data also suggest that preventive treatment for pit and fissure lesions should begin soon

TARGET POPULATIONS

Populations at risk for dental caries include infants who go to sleep with night or naptime-bottles containing beverages with significant cariogenic potential. If an individual drinks a "soft drink" beverage before going to sleep, the pH on the tooth surface may go to less than 4.0 and persist for long periods of time because of reduced flow of saliva and less of buffering action of the saliva. As a consequence of the prolonged contact of acid and sugar in "soft drinks" or prolonged contact of sugar solutions with the surfaces of teeth, so-called "nursing bottle caries" can develop. The mandibular incisors are not involved.

When there is a reduction of saliva due to radiation therapy, use of certain drugs, and old age, an increased dental caries activity occurs (p. 27).

Individuals who frequently drink sugar beverages between meals and snack on sugar-containing foods between meals are especially susceptible to dental caries (Fig. 12-3). Handicapped patients and institutionalized patients who are not able to maintain oral hygiene are also susceptible populations, especially when there is frequent ingestion of foodstuffs containing sugar between meals.

There does not appear to be a target population based on genetic differences between caries-free and caries-susceptible subjects. However, several non-immune antibacterial mechanisms involving host defenses, which cause clumping of bacteria to facilitate salivary clearance, may be genetically determined. It is difficult to ascertain whether a familial pattern of caries experience over several generations is due to true genetic inheritance. Bacterial transmission from mother to child and the perpetuation of similar diets may be the primary factors involved rather than inherited factors for dental caries.

Several reports have suggested that environmental factors may play a secondary role in dental caries. Except for the presence of fluoride, which may occur naturally in the drinking water and diet, environmental factors have not been demonstrated to be as important in dental caries as bacterial factors. There is no accepted theoretical basis for believing that purely climatic variations are significant factors in determining the prevalence of dental caries.

There appear to be no real differences between men and women in their dental caries experience, although certainly cultural differences may be of clinical importance, e.g., attitudes toward dental care. Racial differences are difficult to assess because of such environmental variables as social and cultural factors. Where marked differences between DMF scores persist even after being standardized for income and education, social and cultural factors appear to outweigh any real differences that may exist between races.

DIET AND DENTAL CARIES

Several epidemiologic studies have demonstrated that dental caries is a sucrose-dependent disease or that sucrose is a major contributor to human dental decay. A classic long-term study occurred at the time of World War II in Norway where, throughout much of the war, carbohydrate consumption was reduced. Caries was dramatically reduced between 1941 and 1946, but increased dramatically by 1949 when food rationing was eliminated.

A prospective, long-term study was done at the Vipeholm Mental Hospital in Sweden where inmates of the institution were divided into groups on the basis of the degree of access (on a 24-hour per day basis) to refined sugar (sticky toffees). Although the study is unlikely to be repeated on an ethical basis, the results are fundamental to the relationship between caries and diet. The variation in the incidence of caries related to differences in sugar consumption was dramatic. The data from the study showed that the frequency of sucrose consumption and the form of sucrose were more important than sucrose consumption per se. The conclusions reported were: (1) sugar intake increases caries activity; (2) the sticky form of the fermentable carbohydrate is as important as its chemical composition; (3) the risk of caries is greatest if the sucrose is taken between meals; (4) the increase in caries activity decreases with withdrawal of the sticky sweets from the diet; (5) there is great individual variation in the increase in dental caries activity as a result of increased sugar consumption; and (6) dental caries can occur in the absence of total dietary carbohydrates, including natural as well as refined sugars.

It should be concluded, on the basis of these as well as other studies, that any pattern of ingestion of sucrose which maximizes the availability of this carbohydrate for use by acidogenic and aciduric bacteria in plaque should be considered as an important contributing factor in dental caries attack. However, it should be pointed out that it is also important to remove bacteria (plaque) because bacteria can make and store intracellular polysaccharides and use them as substrates for acid production in periods when no sugar is taken into the mouth. Clearly the attachment of sticky sugar substances of the teeth for extended periods of time should also be avoided.

MICROBIOLOGY OF DENTAL CARIES

The relationship between bacteria and plaque has been discussed earlier and therefore only microorganisms associated with dental caries will be discussed.

It was shown that germ-free rats of a caries-susceptible line did not develop caries even when fed a high sucrose diet. But, when certain bacteria were introduced into these animals, caries developed. Many strains of bacteria, reflecting a number of species, have been tested for their cariogenic potential in such test animals. Most of the gnotobiotic (germ-free and subsequently mono-infected) animal studies have been designed to test the cariogenicity of specific bacteria, especially streptococci. Many of these studies relate to Streptococcus mutans but a few report the induction of caries by other genera of bacteria.

It should not be concluded that the results of animal studies can be applied directly to man, for the conditions under which the research is accomplished are highly artificial; e.g., the diet contains over 50% sucrose, and generally only a single strain of organism is used (mono-infected). In some studies it has been shown that, when certain other strains of bacteria (Veillonella) are introduced along with S. mutans, there is a reduction in caries. Thus, other organisms may exert a protective effect. The use of animal caries-models has obvious limitations for elucidating the specific role of carious microorganisms in human caries.

After it was reported that S. mutans was able to produce caries in animals, several epidemiologic studies have since reported correlations between dental caries index scores and the number of S. mutans present. The number of S. mutans colonies observed is often expressed as a percentage of the presumptive total streptococcal count on a selective growth medium which favors those particular streptococci which can readily be recognized. Other flora may exist in higher numbers but are ignored when using high-sucrose media.

The presumptive cause and effect relationship that exists between caries and S. mutans can be resolved by longitudinal studies which show that S. mutans colonization precedes caries. It would also require that the elimination of S. mutans on specific surfaces would result in less carious lesions. Although S. mutans is considered the chief putative causative agent in coronal caries, other bacteria show greater site selectivity. For example, members of actinomyces and lactobacillus genera may be significant pathogens in pit and fissure caries, whereas streptococcal species, such as S. sanguis and S. salivarius, are also present. Actinomyces are implicated in root caries and lactobacilli and filamentous rods in deep dentin caries.

Although longitudinal studies tend to support a correlation between caries and S. mutans, some teeth which are highly colonized with S. mutans do not develop carious lesions, while others develop lesions without S. mutans being present. It is presumed that other bacteria contribute to the carious process; i.e., the cariogenic potential of various plaque bacteria may be as relevant as the presence or absence of one specific species of bacteria.

ETIOLOGY OF CARIES

Theories for the cause of dental caries are the "acidogenic theory," the "proteolytic theory," and the more recent "proteolysis-chelation," "sucrose-chelation," and "autoimmunity" theories. The acidogenic or chemico-parasitic theory was proposed by W.D. Miller in 1890 and reflects a relationship between oral microorganisms that produce acid, dietary carbohydrates, dental plaque and dental decay. A majority of investigators have accepted the acidogenic theory although other theories may also be combined with the concept.

The proteolytic theory suggests that proteolytic enzymes produced by oral bacteria cause destruction of the organic matrix of enamel leading to collapse of the enamel. The concept does incorporate to a certain extent acid formation. Although proteolysis does occur, especially in the destruction of cementum and dentin, the concept of proteolysis must be coupled with the acidogenic theory in order to be reconciled with the known mechanisms of dental decay.

The proteolysis-chelation theory proposes that the products of bacterial proteolysis act as chelating agents to remove calcium ions from the tooth. The concept does not account adequately for the relationship between increased caries with increased sugar consumption nor the reduction of caries with fluorides. However, the concept does provide a mechanism for the destruction of both organic and inorganic elements simultaneously and interdependently.

The sucrose-chelating theory proposes that sucrose in high concentrations forms complexes with calcium (Ca-saccharides) which require that inorganic phosphate be removed from the enamel. However, it does not appear likely that calcium saccharates can form in the pH range normally found.

The auto-immunity theory suggests that some odontoblasts at certain sites in some teeth are damaged by an auto-immune process. Because of such damage the overlying dentin and enamel is compromised, leaving the site vulnerable to caries. No histologic evidence for such damage has been presented.

These concepts of the etiology of dental caries are not necessarily mutually exclusive. However, the acidogenic concept has the most convincing support, although some proteolysis and chelation would seem to be necessary to explain the complex process of a progressive carious lesion.

ACID PRODUCTION IN PLAQUE

Dental plaque contains bacteria capable of using carbohydrates as substrates (organic starting materials) for their energy requirements. In the catabolic process of degrading these substrates, a number of metabolites or end-products are formed, including acids such as lactic acid. The catabolism of substrates by anaerobic microorganisms without the use of oxygen results in the transformation of carbohydrates to lactic acid. This process is called fermentation and is shown in the following equation:

$$C_6H_{12}O_6 \xrightarrow{\text{(Energy)}} 2CH_3CHOH \cdot CO_2H$$
glucose   lactic acid

It is possible for carbohydrate fermentation to occur in plaque most of the time inasmuch as many oral bacteria store glycogen, and carbohydrate is potentially available from salivary glycoproteins. However, the greatest production of acid occurs when fermentable carbohydrate (e.g., sugar) is ingested; the pH of plaque falls in a matter of a few minutes to 4.0 to 4.5 (pH 7 is neutral) and may take 10 to 30 minutes to return to its original value. At a pH of 7 both saliva and plaque are supersaturated with calcium and phosphate and dissolution of enamel is prevented. However, at about pH 5 or less the saturation is overcome and demineralization occurs.

In addition to low-molecular-weight carbohydrates such as glucose and sucrose, other low-molecular weight substances such as xylitol and sorbitol diffuse into dental plaque but do not ferment rapidly, and therefore do not produce a significant drop in pH. High-molecular-weight polysaccharides such as starch do not penetrate into plaque. Considerable concentrations of acids other than lactic acid may occur in plaque when fermentable carbohydrates are not available.

Of particular interest is the utilization of the catabolic end-products from one strain of bacteria by another for growth and as a source of energy. One such strain is Veillonella, which uses lactic acid as an energy source for growth. In effect, Veillonella is dependent upon the substrate (lactic acid) produced by lactic acid bacteria. Lactic acid is metabolized by Veillonella to two weaker acids and thus removes lactic acid from the plaque.

In addition to antibacterial factors in the saliva and crevicular fluid such as agglutinating agents, enzymes and antibodies, and the washing action of saliva, the buffering systems of the saliva and plaque have been related to reducing the effect of acids produced by the plaque bacteria. However, these buffer systems are not effective when sufficient sugar is ingested and enough acid is produced to defeat the plaque and salivary buffering systems. The acid accumulation is slowly neutralized as the acid diffuses into the saliva and the salivary buffer diffuses into the plaque to reach a state of equilibrium. As the pH returns to neutrality the flux of calcium and phosphate from the tooth is balanced by the diffusion of these ions into the tooth from the plaque and saliva which are supersaturated with respect to calcium and phosphate. When plaque acid production does not occur, there is a diffusion of calcium and phosphate ions into the tooth and remineralization occurs. Thus the events in dental decay involve demineralization, equilibrium, and remineralization.

The demineralization-remineralization of enamel hydroxyapatite (calcium) phosphate arranged in a crystalline structure may be viewed according to the equation:

$$8H^+ + Ca_{10}(PO_4)_6OH_2 \underset{\text{Remineralize}}{\overset{\text{Demineralize}}{\rightleftarrows}} 6(HPO_4)^{2-} + 10Ca^{2+} + 2H_2O$$

Acid — Hydroxyapatite — Phosphate — Calcium — Water

The physical-chemical considerations involved in such acid/hydroxyapatite interactions are extensive, and extend beyond this discussion. But, in brief, the acids produced in plaque diffuse into the enamel where they react with the calcium phosphate to form soluble phosphate and the calcium and lactate products. These end-products of demineralization diffuse out of the enamel and create a porous subsurface enamel. However, an outer layer of enamel which is relatively smooth and intact is seen in incipient carious lesions. The foregoing equation cannot explain all the complex events in the carious processes. Also, it should be recognized that enamel is not made completely of pure hydroxyapatite, which is quite unreactive. Rather, enamel crystals consist primarily of carbonated apatite, which is very reactive. Enamel solubilization begins with diffusion of acid between the enamel crystals, followed by their dissolution. As shown in the equation, calcium and phosphate are removed from the enamel. Thus, the acids produced by the bacteria diffuse through the water-protein-lipid matrix surrounding the enamel crystals, initiating the carious process.

CARIOUS LESIONS

Carious lesions vary in their macroscopic, microscopic, and radiographic appearance according to the location of caries and the pattern of progress of the lesion. However, the destruction of tooth structure takes place in a characteristic way, especially the initial carious lesion.

Initial Enamel Lesion

The earliest evidence of enamel caries that can be seen by the unaided eye may be seen on an extracted tooth (Fig. 12–4A) as an opaque white spot on an approximal surface (supergingivally) and on facial and lingual surfaces (Fig. 12–4B). An incipient carious lesion of enamel is characterized by subsurface demineralization and a narrow band of relatively unaffected surface enamel (Fig. 12–5). The surface layer has a high fluoride content and may resist dif-

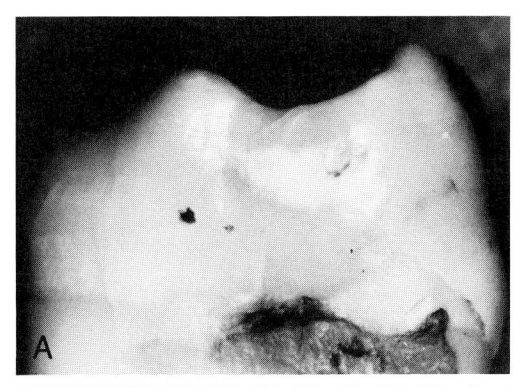

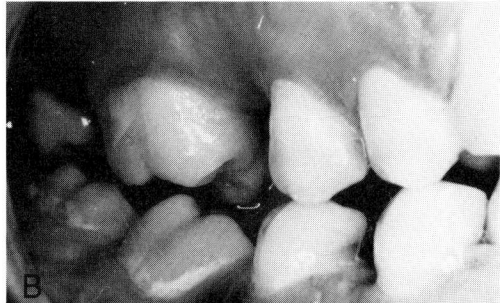

Fig. 12–4. *A*, Early proximal subsurface lesion ("white spot"), *B*, Cervical lesion adjacent to gingival margin.

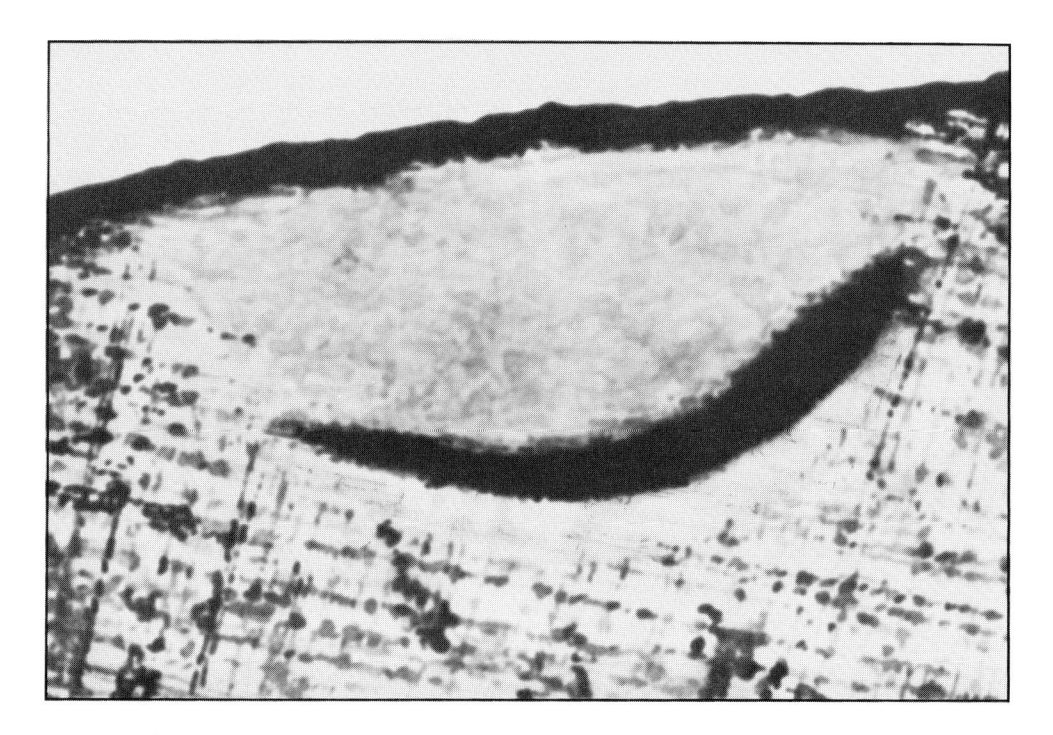

Fig. 12–5. Histologic features of an early proximal smooth surface lesion.

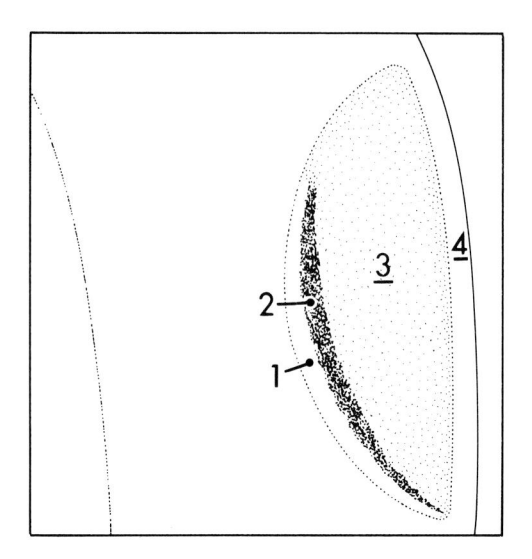

Fig. 12–6. *Illustration of an early enamel lesion.* Zone 1 is a translucent layer which is seen when a ground section is examined in quinoline. Zone 2 is a dark layer also seen in quinoline. Zone 3 is the body of the lesion which is seen when the section is transferred to water. Zone 4 is the surface layer seen in water. Zones 1 and 3 are sites of demineralization, and zones 2 and 4 are zones of remineralization.

fusion away from the site of calcium and phosphate ions released during demineralization.

When a small, smooth surface lesion is examined using ground sections and polarized light, at least four histologically distinct layers or zones can be seen: two zones can be seen when the ground sections are examined in quinoline and two zones when placed in water (Fig. 12–6). Zones 1 and 3 are areas of demineralization where the enamel crystals are relatively small and the enamel is porous. Zones 2 and 4 are remineralized regions.

Zone 1, which is the translucent zone, is not present in all lesions, but, when present, may extend to the dentin. This zone lies at the advancing front of the lesion. It has been reported that magnesium and carbonate have been preferentially removed. *Zone 2*, which is the *dark zone*, is usually found just superficial to the advancing front of the lesion. It is made up of 2 to 4% small spaces of pores. *Zone 3*, which is the *body of the lesion*, constitutes the largest proportion of the lesion. This zone corresponds with the radiolucency region on a microradiograph. *Zone 4*, which is the *surface zone*, is relatively unaffected by the carious attack in the initial carious lesion. It is radiopaque and approximately 30 μm in depth. Normal enamel consists of about 0.1% spaces or pores, whereas the pore volume of the surface zone is 1 to 5%.

Up to this point the enamel surface has remained intact and presumably the cariogenic bacteria are confied to the surface of the enamel. However, some studies report the presence of bacteria in subsurface enamel in connection with initial caries. The pulp and dentin respond in a number of ways to early enamel caries (see chapter 11) without the presence of bacteria. The most significant response is the formation of peritubular dentin (sclerosis), histologically called translucent dentin. The progress of bacteria into dentin is delayed by this zone. Also, the pulp responds by forming reactive or secondary dentin at the dento-pulpal junction.

In summary, the early enamel lesion ("white spot") has been characterized as subsurface demineralization with a narrow zone of sound surface enamel. However, entry of the carious attack through a relatively unaffected enamel surface is puzzling. Recent evidence suggests that, since carious lesions are the result of acids reacting with individual crystals, the most important pathways for diffusion of ions in and out of the enamel are the intercrystalline spaces. It has been demonstrated that initial carious surface dissolution precedes the classical "white spot lesion." Furthermore, it has been suggested that the well-defined surface layer overlying the demineralized subsurface layer represents a relatively late state in the development of the "white spot lesion." The relative maintenance of the surface zone may be related to inhibitors acting at the enamel/plaque interface such as fluoride and salivary proteins, and/or calcium and phosphate present in plaque, and/or redeposition of mineral removed from the interior of the enamel. The high content of fluoride in the surface enamel, which is released at the time of demineralization, also favors remineralization at the surface of the enamel.

Remineralization Phenomena

The concept of healing small caries through the process of remineralization has recently become a goal of preventive dentistry. Rehardening of acid-softened enamel by saliva has been established in experimental studies. There is little doubt that calcium salts deposit on enamel surfaces and within tissues softened by caries.

In terms of caries control, the fluoride ion accelerates rehardening and remineralization of a lesion and is one of the main cariostatic mechanisms of fluoride (Fig. 12–7). Partially demineralized enamel takes up fluoride preferentially relative to sound enamel. Thus small lesions, not diagnosable by conventional methods of clinical examination and radiography, take up fluoride and act as fluoride-ion reserves (Fig. 12–8). It has been suggested that, when conditions favor demineralization, fluoride is released in addition to calcium and phosphate ions and minerals are redeposited into the lesion. This remineralization is the basis for "arrested decay" and rehardening of softened enamel. As already indicated, smooth surface carious lesions progress slowly, requiring perhaps up to 4 years to reach the dentin. Therefore, lesions can be remineralized provided loss of mineral from enamel does not exceed certain limits. It is unlikely that carious cavitated enamel can be repaired by the remineralization phenomena. There is evidence which demonstrates that low concentrations of fluoride ions significantly influence the degree of mineralization. Apparently low levels are more effective than high fluoride levels in respect to fluoride in the enamel and caries susceptibility.

MECHANISM OF FLUORIDE ACTION: REMINERALIZATION

```
┌─────────────────┐
│  SOUND ENAMEL   │
└─────────────────┘
  -Slow fluoride absorption
          ↓
┌─────────────────────┐
│ CARIOGENIC CHALLENGE│
└─────────────────────┘
          ↓
┌─────────────────┐
│ DEMINERALIZATION│
└─────────────────┘
  -Histologic carious lesion
  -Rapid fluoride absorption
  -Fluoride reservoir
          ↓
┌──────────────────────┐
│ REMINERALIZATION SYSTEM│
└──────────────────────┘
  -Free calcium and phosphate
     in saliva
         +
  -Fluoride ions
         +
  -Demineralized tissue
         +
  -Crystal deposition
          ↓
┌────────────────────────┐
│ REMINERALIZED HARD TISSUE│
└────────────────────────┘
  -More resistant enamel
```

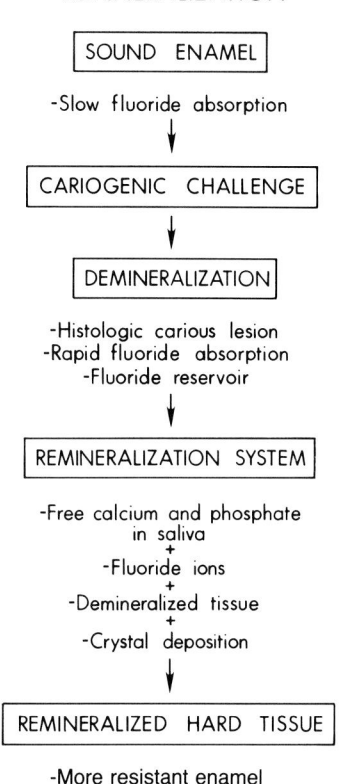

Fig. 12–7. *Mechanism of fluoride action-remineralization.*

Advancing Carious Lesion

When the demineralization process overrides the remineralizing process for a sufficient period of time, enamel cavitation occurs (Fig. 12–9). A carious lesion is usually present beneath the enamel surface for 3 to 4 years before it is detected clinically, especially in proximal surfaces, and not at all if the lesion has remineralized before cavitation occurs. It would not be until the lesion reaches the dentin and spreads laterally that the carious process can be seen with bite-wing radiography (Fig. 12–10). The destruction of the mineral and organic matrix of dentin produces transverse clefts (Fig. 12–12), and aggregations of bacteria and necrotic tissue form liquefaction foci. As the carious process progresses laterally and deeper into the dentin (Fig. 12–11),

188　　　　　　　　　　　　　　　　DENTAL CARIES

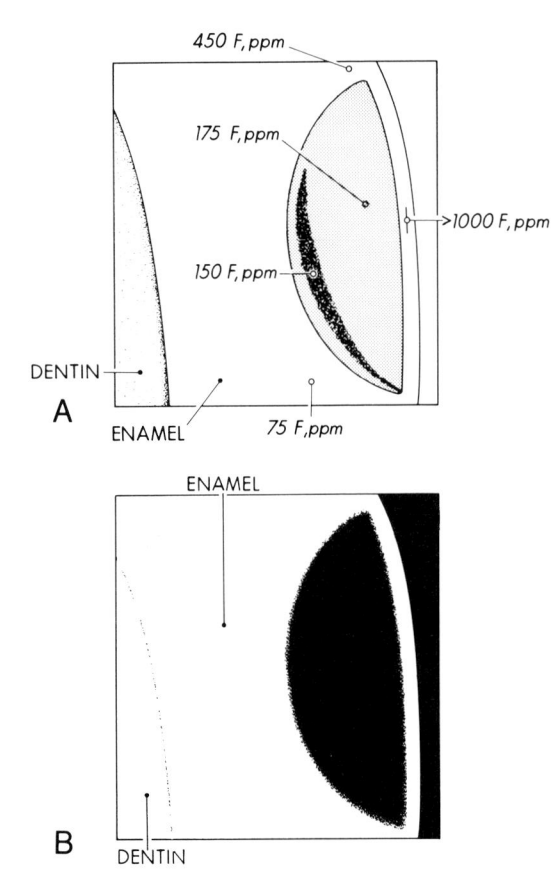

Fig. 12-8. *A*, Illustrated areas of fluoride distribution in and around a "white spot" (after Wheatherall et al.). *B*, Simulated microradiograph showing that a subsurface radiolucent area (decalcified) forms the body of the lesion and a radiopaque, relatively unaffected surface enamel.

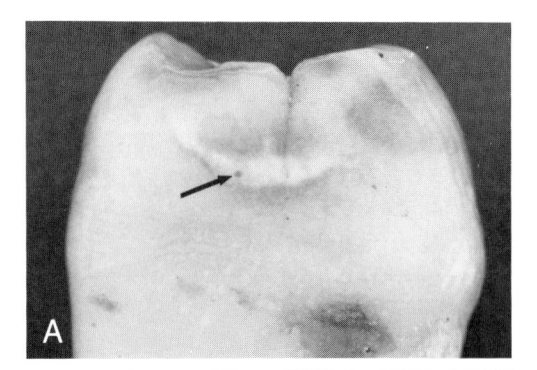

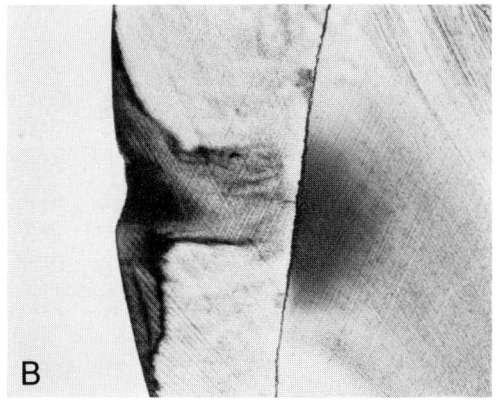

Fig. 12-9. *A*, Early loss of enamel surface at the periphery of the "white spot" lesion. *B*, Histologic section of lesion just penetrating to the dentin.

cavitation and undermining of the occlusal surface occurs and the extent of the demineralization of dentin is seen on the radiographs. Inflammation of the pulp does not occur ordinarily until the organisms are within 0.3 to 0.8 mm of the pulp, but the pulp responds initially to bacterial toxins.

Microorganisms

Initially the bacteria at the enamel-plaque interface are primarily acidogenic, but as the enamel is demineralized and cavitation occurs the buffering potential of the saliva and plaque is diminished. A lower pH favors organisms which can survive in an acid en-

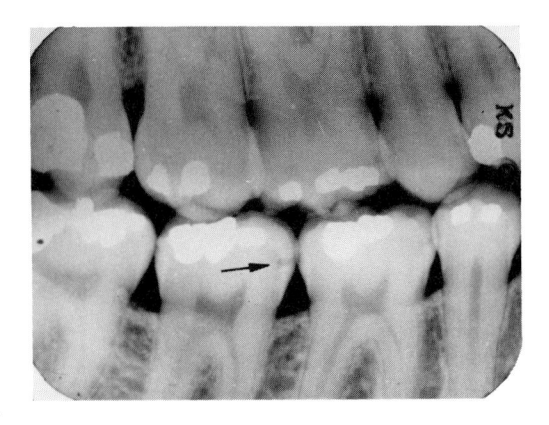

Fig. 12-10. Bite-wing radiograph showing proximal carious lesion involving the dentin.

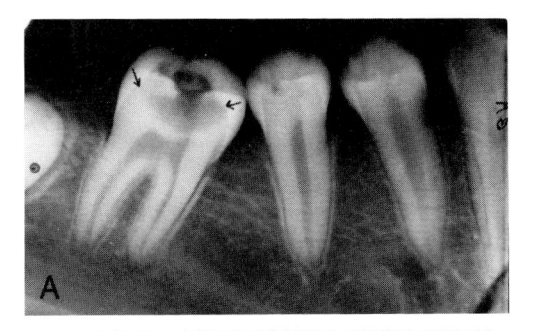

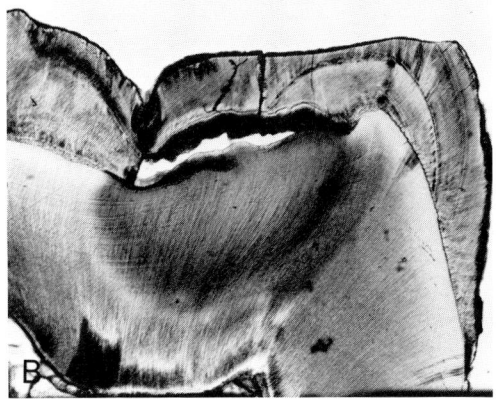

Fig. 12–11. *A,* Radiograph of carious lesion which started in the occlusal surface. *B,* Histologic section showing undermined enamel and involvement of dentin.

vironment and can utilize the denatured collagen, i.e., the scaffold remaining after the dentin is demineralized. The flora becomes mixed with several types of bacteria that produce acid, as well as those that produce proteolytic and hydrolytic enzymes.

The types of organisms present in carious dentin are considered to be anaerobic, both facultative and obligate anaerobes, including Lactobacillus and Actinomyces. It is apparent that the flora may vary from site to site on the tooth, and from tooth to tooth, but generally the microbes tend to be obligate anaerobes in the deep layers of carious dentin. Streptococcus mutans constitute a minor, if any, part of the microbial flora of deep carious dentin although they have been found in superficial layers. Thus there appears to be no specific pathogenic bacteria or group of organisms in established dentin caries. The presence of a large number of microorganisms may reflect more favorable growth conditions for those particular organisms than the primary course of caries in dentin.

Root Surface Caries

Reports of the prevalence of root surface caries are essentially based on cross-sectional studies and uncertain indices for comparative purposes. Some general conclusions can be drawn, but must be viewed with caution until baseline and incidence data of longitudinal studies are available. It has generally been accepted that the incidence of root surface caries increases with advancing age, presumably correlating with gingival recession, periodontal surgery or other reasons for exposure of root surfaces. Several studies indicate that the mean number of lesions ranges from less than one to three, but in isolated tribes living under primative conditions and hospitalized patients the rate is much higher.

It has been suggested that root surface caries are likely to be found in human populations that have poor oral hygiene and subsist on starch diets, and therefore the plaque would be selective for A. viscosus. Although it is generally thought that the composition of bacterial plaque on cemental surfaces is likely to be different from that of coronal plaque, there is no accepted body of evidence to demonstrate that a specific organism is the cause of root caries. The nature of the bacteria of the advancing front of the dentinal lesion of root caries has not been established.

The incipient lesion of root caries has not been studied to the same extent as early enamel caries, although there is some data available which suggests that the mechanisms are similar, if not the same. Thus, there appears to be subsurface demineralization and a relatively intact surface layer in the early root surface lesion.

CONTROL OF DENTAL CARIES

The prevention of dental decay involves plaque control by mechanical and chemical

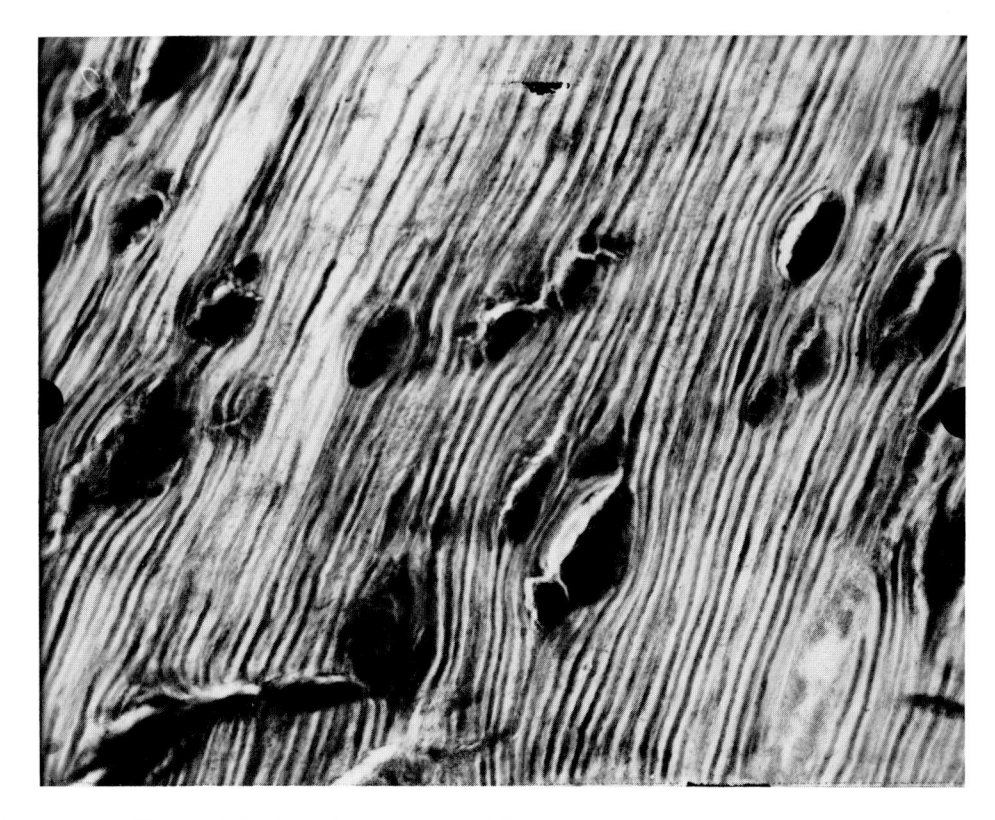

Fig. 12-12. Caries of dentin with transverse clefts and liquefaction foci.

methods, dietary modification, immunization, and increasing the resistance of the tooth with fluorides, and pit and fissure sealants.

Mechanical and Chemical Control of Plaque

The mechanical elimination or reduction of plaque by tooth-brushing and use of dental floss, as well as professional prophylaxis, has been demonstrated to prevent or reduce the incidence of caries and prevalence of gingivitis. Motivation to undertake such meticulous care and cost effectiveness have been suggested as factors which may be difficult to ensure on a practical community-wide basis.

The use of antimicrobial agents such as vancomycin and kanamycin have been suggested, but their use, especially on a long-term basis, has not been encouraged because of alterations of flora elsewhere in the body and development of resistant strains of bacteria. The use of such antibiotics as penicillin does not appear to be a correct approach to the prevention of dental caries even though caries reduction may occur.

Chlorhexidine is a chemical agent which is active against a wide range of bacteria, and is capable of inhibiting plaque formation. Chlorhexidine-resistant streptococci have been reported to occur with the use of chlorhexidine. There has been no convincing evidence reported from long-term clinical trials that chlorhexidine reduces the incidence of dental caries.

Dietary Control of Sugars

Several ways of reducing dietary risks in dental decay have been considered. There is little doubt that the elimination of sugars and cooked starches from the diet would eliminate cariogenic bacteria. However, such an extreme modification of the diet is not an acceptable proposal. Alternative approaches to dietary control involve attempts to reduce the cariogenicity of foods. For example, replacement of the sucrose content of foods by noncariogenic sugars such as xylitol and sorbital. However, the small intestine cannot utilize large amounts of these polyols and diarrhea does occur with extensive use. Sugarless gum utilizes sorbitol. A variety of sugar substitutes are in various stages of development and clinical testing.

Immunization

Systemic immunization to control diseases in which there is bacterial colonization of systemic tissues is often possible, but systemic immunization against dental caries has not been successful in humans. Local injection of S. mutans into the oral tissues has had limited success and other strategies are being developed. The safety of immunization is a primary question inasmuch as there is the possibility of any streptococcal vaccine's inducing antibodies that cross-react with heart tissue antigens. In order for the immune response to be effective, antibodies or sensitized cells would have to reach the enamel-plaque interface via the saliva or crevicular fluid. Vaccination has been successful in animals and therefore the possibility for human immunization remains.

Replacement Therapy

The purposeful colonization of a susceptible host with a nonvirulent organism in order to prevent infection by a resident pathogen such as S. mutans has been tried as a means of preventing dental caries in humans. A mutant strain of S. mutans has been isolated which produces a bacteriocin that can kill virtually all other strains of S. mutans. Efficient replacement therapy is difficult because the vast majority of people are infected with S. mutans at an early age.

Natural Defense Mechanisms

In addition to the remineralizing mechanism of defense involving the saliva and plaque, the clearing action (agglutination of bacteria) of saliva, and the presence of enzymes or proteins in the saliva (lysozyme, lactoferrin, etc.) which can inhibit bacteria, immune responses have been suggested to play a role in protecting against caries. However, there is little evidence that IgA antibodies provide significant protection against caries in humans.

It has been thought for some time that individuals vary in susceptibility to dental decay, and recently differences have been found between caries-resistant and caries-susceptible individuals. Caries-resistant individuals have lower proportions of S. mutans and lactobacilli and higher proportions of S. sanguis and veillonella in plaque than caries-susceptible individuals. Also, it has been reported that saliva-mediated bacterial agglutinating ability in caries-resistant individuals is twice that of caries-susceptible individuals. In addition, it has been found that the time needed for plaque pH to return to the resting level following cariogenic challenge is significally longer in caries-susceptible individuals.

Cariostatic Mechanisms of Fluoride

The use of fluoride for the control of dental caries stems from the observation that the percentage of caries-free children in communities where water supplies contained high concentrations of fluoride was higher than the percentage of caries-free children in communities with low concentrations of fluoride in the drinking water. The topical application of fluoride also has been shown to be effective in reducing dental caries in children. At low concentrations fluoride will exchange with hydroxyl ions in apatite, the calcium phosphate complex that is the basic mineral constituent of enamel. The presence of fluoride reduces the solubility of enamel by promoting the precipitation of hydroxyapatite and preventing the formation of more soluble calcium phosphate.

$$Ca_{10}(PO_4)_6(OH)_2 + 2F^- \longrightarrow Ca_{10}(PO_4)_6F_2 + 2OH^-$$
$$\text{Hydroxyapatite} \qquad\qquad \text{Fluorapatite}$$

The amount of fluoride in the enamel correlates positively with reduced solubility, but it has not been established that the same degree of correlation exists between the incidence of caries and enamel solubility. This observation does not detract from the correlation between the presence of fluoride in the drinking water and the reduced incidence of dental caries. The importance of fluoride in stimulating the remineralization process has already been discussed.

The effect of fluoride on microbes depends upon its concentration. A high level, such as found in a fluoride gel where the concentration reaches 12,000 parts per million (ppm), is bactericidal. Fluorides in dentifrices (1000 ppm) and mouth rinses (250 ppm) are low concentrations which do not suppress colonization of plaque by S. mutans or lactobacilli. However, low-level concentrations of fluoride do reduce dental caries, possibly by inhibiting bacterial enzymes and thereby reducing the production of acid, and hence suppressing caries activity. The caries reduction produced by fluoride-containing dentifrices is about 20% less DMF surfaces (DMFS).

Morphologic changes in teeth associated with fluoride areas are inconsistently related to reduced caries activity. However, there is some agreement that fluoride results in an increase in prevalence in atypically shallow pits and fissures. A reduction in the depth of pit and fissure sites might reduce plaque retention and reduce dental decay.

Fissure Sealants

The greatest reduction of caries from fluoridated water accrues to proximal surfaces and the least to occlusal surfaces because the latter surfaces retain bacteria and food in pits and fissures. For this reason adhesive sealants were developed to exclude bacteria and food constituents. The application of sealants requires etching the tooth surface with acid. Thus acid etching is an essential prerequisite for bonding of resins to the tooth structure. When a lesion is small or there is doubt as to its presence, the use of fissure sealant is an appropriate solution even though the long-term outcome may remain uncertain for some time.

PREDICTION OF CARIES

There are several laboratory tests which have been advocated to determine caries activity, but the two most widely used tests are the Snyder colorimetric test and the lactobacillus count. In the Snyder test saliva is innoculated into a semisolid culture medium containing a pH indicator. If growth of aciduric organisms occurs, the color of the medium changes from green to yellow. The rapidity of the color change is indicative of caries activity. The lactobacillus count is done by an elaborate procedure of growing and counting colonies of lactobacillus on a highly selective media. Although correlations between lactobacillus count and past caries experience is reasonable, the ability to predict future caries increments is poor. Thus the reliability of using the number of aciduric bacteria in the saliva to identify the high-caries-risk patient prior to clinical caries has not been demonstrated.

The salivary levels of S. mutans have been reported to correlate with tooth levels of S. mutans, with the number of carious lesions and with DMFS scores. However, further experimental work is required to confirm such correlations.

SUMMARY

Dental caries is a progressive destruction of tooth structure initiated by bacteria in dental plaque. It is a multifactorial disease in that its initiation and progress is determined by a number of factors, including dietary, bacterial, environmental and genetic. Dental caries is also a dynamic process in that the carious process has periods of progression and regression, i.e., demineralization, equilibrium, remineralization.

The process of dental decay begins with the production of acids by acidogenic and aciduric bacteria present within dental plaque on the surfaces of teeth. This lesion begins before it can be detected by any currently available diagnostic methods. By the time a carious lesion is detectable clinically or radiographically, it may have been present below the surface of the tooth for several years.

Acids produced by acidogenic bacteria such as S. mutans diffuse from the enamel surface to the enamel crystals inside the enamel structure. Thus acids diffuse through the surface of a tooth and initiate a lesion in the subsurface enamel. It is at this time that the process may be arrested or even reversed, especially with fluoride stimulation. Fluoride not only acts to enhance remineralization, but may also exert an antimicrobial effect in both high and low concentrations (e.g., applied fluoride gels or fluoride dentifrices). The carious lesion absorbs fluoride and acts as a fluoride reservoir.

The presence of fluoride in drinking water reduces the incidence of caries. The primary action is local, even though the fluoride is incorporated into developing structures, i.e., fluoride is released locally at the site of dissolution of enamel containing fluoride. The amount of fluoride in enamel corresponds with reduced enamel solubility. When the minerals of enamel are dissolved, they are replaced by a more insoluble mineral and more resistant to decay. In effect, dissolved enamel crystals are replaced by fewer but larger fluoride containing enamel crystals which are more resistant to dissolution. Thus fluoride favors the formation of fluoridated hydroxyapatite crystals in the presence of calcium and phosphate. The production of acid by acidogenic bacteria is related to dietary sugars. When sugar is not present and bacteria stop the formation of acid, the pH rises and crystal deposition occurs. The presence of calcium and phosphate in the saliva plus low levels of fluoride locally provides an efficient remineralizing system, a mechanism for repairing the effects of the carious process.

The prevention of dental decay involves reduction of dietary sugars which act as a substrate for acid producing bacteria, the use of fluoridated drinking water, topical applications of fluorides, prevention of plaque, and use of adhesive sealants. Proposed methods include a caries vaccine, replacement with mutant bacteria defective in some aspect of caries virulence, and reduction of the cariogenicity of foods.

Changing patterns of dental caries reflect a dramatic decrease in this disease in industrialized countries, presumably because of fluorides, plaque control, and dietary substitutes for sugar. In contrast, developing countries appear to be entering a rapid rise in caries incidence because of the introduction of cariogenic foods. The incidence of root surface caries is related to exposure of the root surfaces because of periodontal disease and age related gingival recession, as well as to dietary considerations. Prevention, rather than repair of dental decay, is the future trend of dental practice.

BIBLIOGRAPHY

Abbott, F.: Caries of human teeth. Dent. Cosmos, *21*:113, 177, 184, 1879.

Anderson, B.G.: Clinical study of arresting dental caries. J. Dent. Res., *17*:443, 1938.

Axelsson, P. and Lindhe, L.: Effect of controlled oral hygiene procedures on caries and periodontal disease in adults. Results after 6 years. J. Clin. Periodontal., *8*:239, 1981.

Backer-Dirks, O.: Posteruptive changes in dental enamel. J. Dent. Res., *45*:503, 1966.

Barmes, D.E.: How to bridge the gap. In Angelopoulus, A.P. (ed.) Proceedings of the Ninth Annual Meeting of the Association for Dental Education in Europe, 1–3 September, 1983, Delphi, Greece, Athens, Greece, "Beta" Medical Publishers, 1984.

Banting, D.W., et al.: A longitudinal study of root caries: Baseline and incidence data. J. Dent. Res., *64*:1141, 1985.

Besic, F.C.: The fate of bacteria sealed in dental cavities. J. Dent. Res., *22*:349, 1943.

Bibby, B., et al.: A critique of three theories of caries attack. Int. Dent. J., *8*:685, 1968.

Bibby, B.G. and Shern, R.J. (eds.): Proceedings, "Methods of Caries Prediction." Sp. Supp. Microbial Abstracts, 1978.

Black, G.V.: Susceptibility and immunity to dental caries. Dent. Cosmos, *41*:826, 1899.

Bowen, W.H.: Nature of Plaque. Oral Sci. Rev., *9*:3, 1976.

Brooks, J.D., et al.: A comparative study of two pit and fissure sealants: three-year results in Augusta, Georgia. J. Am. Dent. Assoc., *99*:42, 1979.

Brunelle, J.A., and Carlos, J.P.: Changes in the prevalence of dental caries in U.S. schoolchildren, 1961–1980. J. Dent. Res., *61*:1346, 1982.

Cheyne, V.D., and Horne, E.V.: The value of the roentgenograph in the detection of carious lesions. J. Dent. Res., *27*:50, 1948.

Cook, S.R.: A longitudinal radiographic study of caries progression in dental students. Aust. Dent. J., *29*:315, 1984.

Darling, A.I.: Studies of the early lesion of enamel caries with transmitted light, polarized light, and microradiography. Its nature, mode of spread, points of entry, and its relation to enamel structure. Br. Dent. J., *105*:119, 1958.

Dean, H.T.: Endemic fluorosis and its relation to dental caries. Publ. Hlth. Rep., Washington, *53*:1443, 1938.

Dean, H.T.: Fluorine and dental caries. Am. J. Orthod. Oral Surg., *33*:49, 1947.

Edwardsson, S.: Bacteriological studies on deep areas of carious dentine. Odontologist., Revy. 25 (Suppl. 32), 1974.

Featherstone, J.D.B., et al.: Chemical and histological changes during development of artificial caries. Caries Res., *19*:1, 1985.

Frisbie, H.E.: Caries of the dentin. J. Dent. Res., *24*:195, 1945.

Frisbie, H.E., and Nuckolls, J.: Caries of the enamel. J. Dent. Res., *26*:181, 1947.

Glass, R.L. (ed.): The first international conference on the declining prevalence of dental caries. J. Dent. Res., *61*:1303, 1982.

Granath, L., et al.: Progression of proximal caries in early teens related to caries. Acta Odontica Scandinavic, *38*:247, 1980.

Gustafsson, B.E., et al.: The Vipeholm dental caries study. The effect of different levels of carbohydrate intake on caries activity in 436 individuals observed for five years. Acta Odontica Scandinavic, *11*:232, 1954.

Hardie, J.M., et al.: A longitudinal epidemiological study on dental plaque and the development of caries-interim result after two years. J. Dent. Res., *56*:90, 1977.

Hazen, S.P., et al.: The problem of root caries. I. Literature review and clinical description. J. Am. Dent. Assoc., *86*:137, 1973.

Head, J.A.: A study of saliva and its action on tooth enamel in reference to its hardening and softening. J. Am. Med. A., *59*:2118, 1912.

Hillman, J.D., et al.: Colonization of human oral cavity by a strain of streptococcus mutans. J. Dent. Res., *64*:1272, 1985.

Holmen, L., et al.: A polarized light microscopic study of progressive stages of enamel caries in vivo. Caries Res., *19*:354, 1985.

Hoshino, E.: Predominant obligate anaerobes in human carious dentin. J. Dent. Res., *64*:1195, 1985.

Jordan, H.U. and Sumney, D.I.: Root surface caries; review of literature and significance of the problem. J. Periodont. Res., *44*:158, 1973.

Katz, R.V., et al.: Prevalence and distribution of root caries in an adult population. Caries Res., *16*:265, 1982.

Klein, H., et al.: Studies on dental caries I. Dental status and dental needs of elementary school children. Public Health Reports, *53*:751, 1938.

Koulorides, T. and Cameron, B.: Enamel remineralization as a factor in the pathogenesis of dental caries. J. Oral Path., *9*:255, 1980.

Krasse, B. and Carlsson, J.: Various types of streptococci and experimental caries in hamsters. Arch. Oral Biol., *15*:25, 1970.

Löe, H., et al.: Inhibition of experimental caries by plaque prevention. The effect of chlorhexidine mouthrinses. Scand. J. Dent. Res., *80*:1, 1972.

Loesche, W.J.: *Dental Caries: A treatable infection.* Springfield, Charles C Thomas, Publisher, 1982.

Loesche, W.J.: Chemotherapy of dental plaque infections. Oral Sci. Rev., *9*:65, 1976.

Loesche, W.J., et al.: Association of Streptococcus mutans with human dental decay. Infection and Immunity, *11*:1252, 1975.

Marthaler, T.M. and Wiesner, V.: Rapidity of penetration of radiolucent areas through mesial enamel of first permanent molars. Helv. Odontol. Acta, *17*:19, 1973.

McHugh, W.D. (ed.): *Dental Plaque.* Edinburgh and London, E. & S. Livingstone Ltd., 1970.

McKay, F.S.: The relation of mottled enamel to caries. J. Am. Dent. Assoc., *15*:1429, 1928.

Mergenhagen, S.E. and Rosan, B. (eds.): Molecular Basis of Oral Microbial Adhesion. Proc. of a workshop held in Philadelphia, Pennsylvania, 5–8 June, 1984. American Society for Microbiology, Washington, D.C., 1985.

Miller, W.D.: Die Mikroorganismen des Mundhohle., Leipzig, 1889.

Miller, W.D.: *Microorganisms of the Human*

Mouth. Philadelphia: S.S. White Publishing Co., 1890.

Schamschula, R.G., et al.: Root surface caries in Lufa, New Guinea, I. clinical observations. J. Am. Dent. A., 85:603, 1972.

Scott, D.B.: A study of the bilateral incidence of carious lesions. J. Dent. Res., 23:105, 1944.

Seppä, L., et al.: A scanning electronic microscopic study of bacterial penetration of human enamel in incipient caries. Arch. Oral Biol., 30:595, 1985.

Silverstone, L.M.: Remineralization phenomena. Caries Res., 11 (Suppl. 1):59, 1977.

Silverstone, L.M.: Structure of carious enamel, including the early lesion. Oral Sci. Rev., 3:100, 1973.

Silverstone, L.M.: The effect of fluoride in the remineralization of enamel caries and caries-like lesions in vitro. J. Pub. Health Dent., 42:42, 1982.

Silverstone, L.M.: Structure of carious enamel including the early lesion. In Melcher, A.H. and Zarb, G.A. (Eds.), Oral Sciences Reviews: No. 3 Dental Enamel. Copenhagen, Munksgaard, 1973.

Sumney, D.L. and Jordan, H.L.: Characterization of bacteria isolated from human root surface carious lesions. J. Dent. Res., 53:343, 1974.

Theilade, S., and Theilade, J.: Role of plaque in the etiology of periodontal disease and caries. Oral Sci. Rev., 9:23, 1976.

Thylstrup, A., et al.: Surface morphology and dynamics of early enamel caries development. In Leach, D. (ed.), *Demineralization and Remineralization of the Teeth*. London, IRL Press, 1983.

U.S. Department of Health, Education and Welfare; Public Health Service. Decayed, Missing and Filled Teeth in Adults, Series II, No. 106, National Center for Health Statistics, Washington, D.C., 1967.

Weatherell, J.A., et al.: Assimilation of fluoride by enamel throughout the life of the tooth. Caries Res., II (Suppl. I): 85, 1977.

Westbrook, J.L., et al.: Root surface caries: a clinical, histopathologic and microbiographic investigation. Caries Res., 8:249, 1974.

Wright, C.Z., et al.: The Dorchester dental flossing study: final report. Clin. Prev. Dent., 1:23, 1979.

Zamir, T., et al.: A longitudinal radiographic study of the rate of spread of human approximal dental caries. Arch. Oral Biol., 21:523, 1976.

Zander, H.A. and Bibby, B.G.: Penicillin and caries activity. J. Dent. Res., 26:365, 1947.

13

PERIODONTAL DISEASES

Periodontal diseases are disturbances of the investing and supporting structures of the teeth that occur primarily as the result of bacterial dental plaque on the teeth. These inflammatory diseases are clinically recognized as gingivitis and periodontitis and affect to varying degrees all individuals in all populations of the world. Collectively, periodontal diseases are the primary cause of tooth loss after age 35. And although most periodontal diseases can be prevented by intensive control of bacterial plaque, a number of challenging questions remain to be answered about the histology, epidemiology, histopathology, etiology, pathogenesis, and treatment of these diseases. Most of the material relative to bacterial plaque is found in Chapter 10.

Basic processes such as inflammation are not unique to the periodontium. However, because the periodontium is rather unique in function and structure, pathologic processes involving the investing and supporting structures of the teeth give rise to the need for special terminology. Therefore, in order to facilitate the study of periodontal diseases, a brief review of the periodontal structures is presented.

PERIODONTIUM

The periodontium consists of the investing and supporting structures of the teeth and includes the periodontal ligament, the gingiva, the alveolar bone, and the cementum. These structures are arranged as a functional unit for the maintenance of the dentition.

Gingiva

The gingiva is a specialized portion of the mucous membranes of the mouth that surrounds the cervical region of the teeth and covers the alveolar processes (Fig. 13–1). It is divided clinically into the free gingival margin, the attached gingiva, and the interdental papilla.

The *marginal gingiva* extends from the cemento-enamel junction and the attached gingiva to the coronal edge of the gingiva, i.e., to the free gingival margin (Fig. 13–2). The *gingival crevice* is a clinical term used to describe the separation created between the tooth surface and the marginal gingiva with a periodontal probe (Fig. 13–7). There is some semantic confusion about the difference between the terms sulcus and crevice. The gingival sulcus is a shallow groove between the tooth and healthy normal gingiva (Fig. 13–2). It extends from the free surface of the junctional epithelium to the free gingival margin. Its existence and depth are not determined by clinical periodontal probing. It is a histologic and anatomic configuration of tissues (p. 210). The marginal gingiva is usually referred to as

PERIODONTAL DISEASES 197

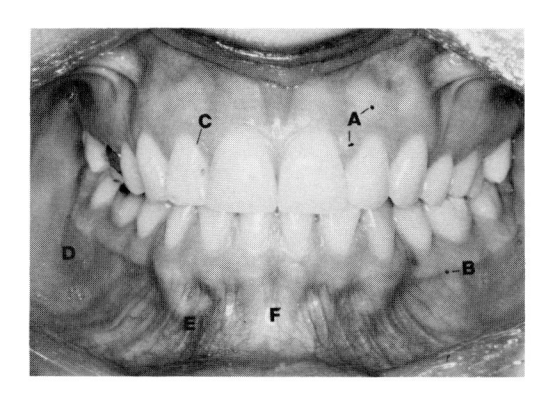

Fig. 13–1. *Normal gingiva.* A, attached gingiva (upper), interdental papilla (lower point); B, mucogingival junction; C, free gingival margin; D, mucobuccal reflection of mucosa; E, mucolabial (fold) reflection of mucosa; F, frenum.

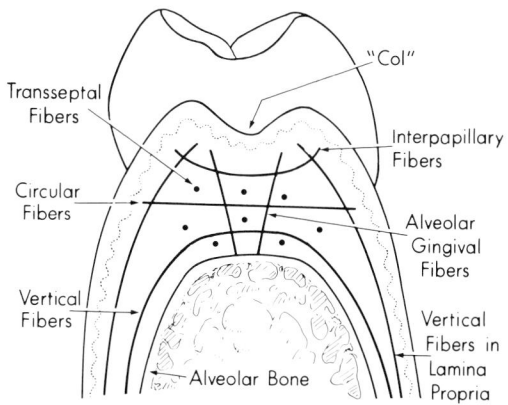

Fig. 13–3. Schematic representation of the "col" and principal fibers of the interdental gingivae.

the "unattached" or "free" gingiva due to an apparent lack of attachment to the enamel surface because there is generally present, even on careful probing, a space produced between the tooth surface and the gingiva. Also, the marginal gingiva is not attached to the cementum and hence "free" of attachment in this sense.

The *attached gingiva* is that part of the gingiva attached to the underlying cementus and the alveolar bone (Fig. 13–2). It extends from the free gingival groove to the mucogingival junction.

The *interdental papilla* is that portion of the gingiva which fills the interproximal space. The facial and lingual heights of contour of the papillae are often more coronal than the area between the approximating contact areas. This dip in the interproximal contour is called a "col" (Fig. 13–3). It is the "borderland" between caries and periodontal disease.

The free or marginal gingiva contains dense collagen fibers referred to as free

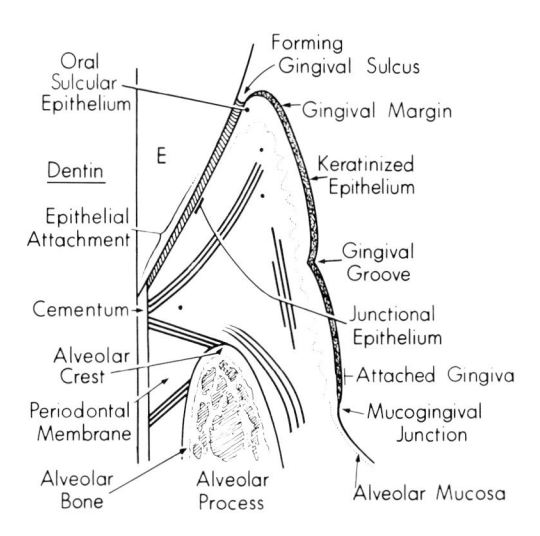

Fig. 13–2. Schematic illustration of gingival sulcus (groove) in a clinically healthy gingiva. E = enamel space.

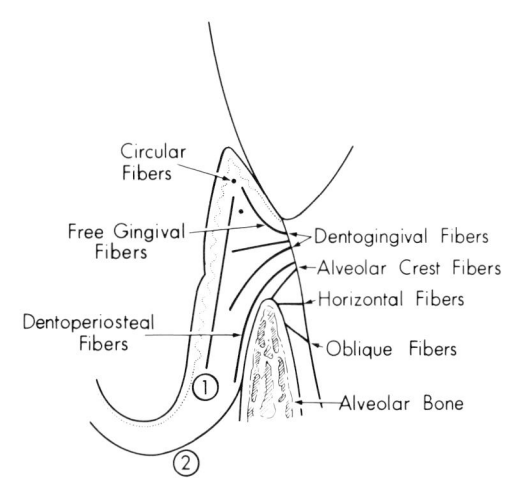

Fig. 13–4. Schematic illustration of periodontal fibers using a labial-lingual section. (1) Termination of attached gingiva. (2) Mucolabial fold.

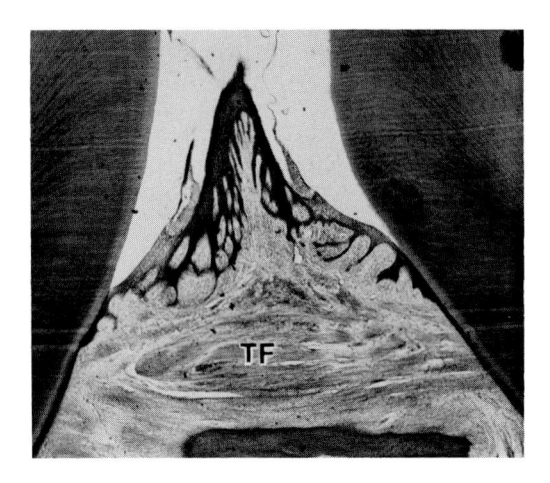

Fig. 13-5. Photomicrograph showing transseptal fibers between teeth.

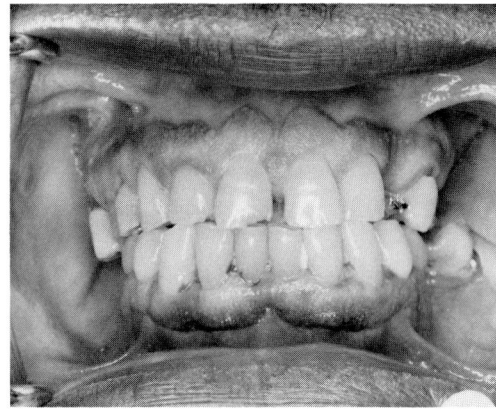

Fig. 13-6. *Normal pigmentation of the gingiva.* Note also stippling.

gingival, circular fibers, dentogingival fibers, and dentoperiosteal fibers (Fig. 13-4). These fiber groups are considered by some histologists to be a gingival ligament. A group of fibers located on mesial and distal sides of the teeth and running from the cementum of approximate teeth over the alveolar crest are called transseptal fibers and collectively the *interdental ligament* (Fig. 13-5). This ligament is considered to be important as a barrier to the progress of periodontal disease.

Clinical Evaluation—an evaluation of the gingiva is based upon color, form, crevice depth, tendency to bleed on probing and level of attachment. An evaluation of the gingival/crevicular fluid may also be used.

A healthy, normal gingiva is uniformly pale pink in color, although physiologic (normal) pigmentation may alter its color (Fig. 13-6). The color of the gingiva is dependent upon its vascularity, keratinization, and the presence or absence of inflammation. In areas of chronic inflammation the tissue has a slight bluish cast. With loss of keratinization, the color is bright red.

The form of the gingiva is related to the form of the crowns of the teeth, the spacing of the teeth, the form of the alveolar processes, the contour of the roots of the teeth, and to the presence of disease. To be considered normal, the free gingival margin should be closely adapted to the surfaces of the teeth (Fig. 13-1). In chronic gingivitis the tissues may increase in size (Fig. 13-31), and the normal relationship of the gingiva to the tooth is changed, e.g., increase in depth of the gingival crevice and thickening of the free gingival margin.

On careful periodontal probing of the gingival crevice, there should be no bleeding (Fig. 13-7). When bleeding is present, the amount of bleeding can be clinically correlated in a nominal way with the severity of gingivitis.

The depth of the gingival crevice should not exceed 1 to 2 mm on lingual and facial surfaces and 2 to 3 mm on the proximal surfaces of the teeth. Even with careful probing (<lg) some penetration of epithelium occurs. In the presence of subgingival plaque, a gingival pocket develops and the probing depth of the crevice increases, but gingivitis may not be clinically evident.

When there is gingivitis present, a serum exudate known as gingival or crevicular fluid flows from around the teeth. However, in a clinically heathy gingiva, little or no fluid can be collected from the gingival sulcus. With the development of gingivitis there is an increase in the rate of flow of gingival fluid. Several methods are used for measuring the flow of gingival fluid, several using

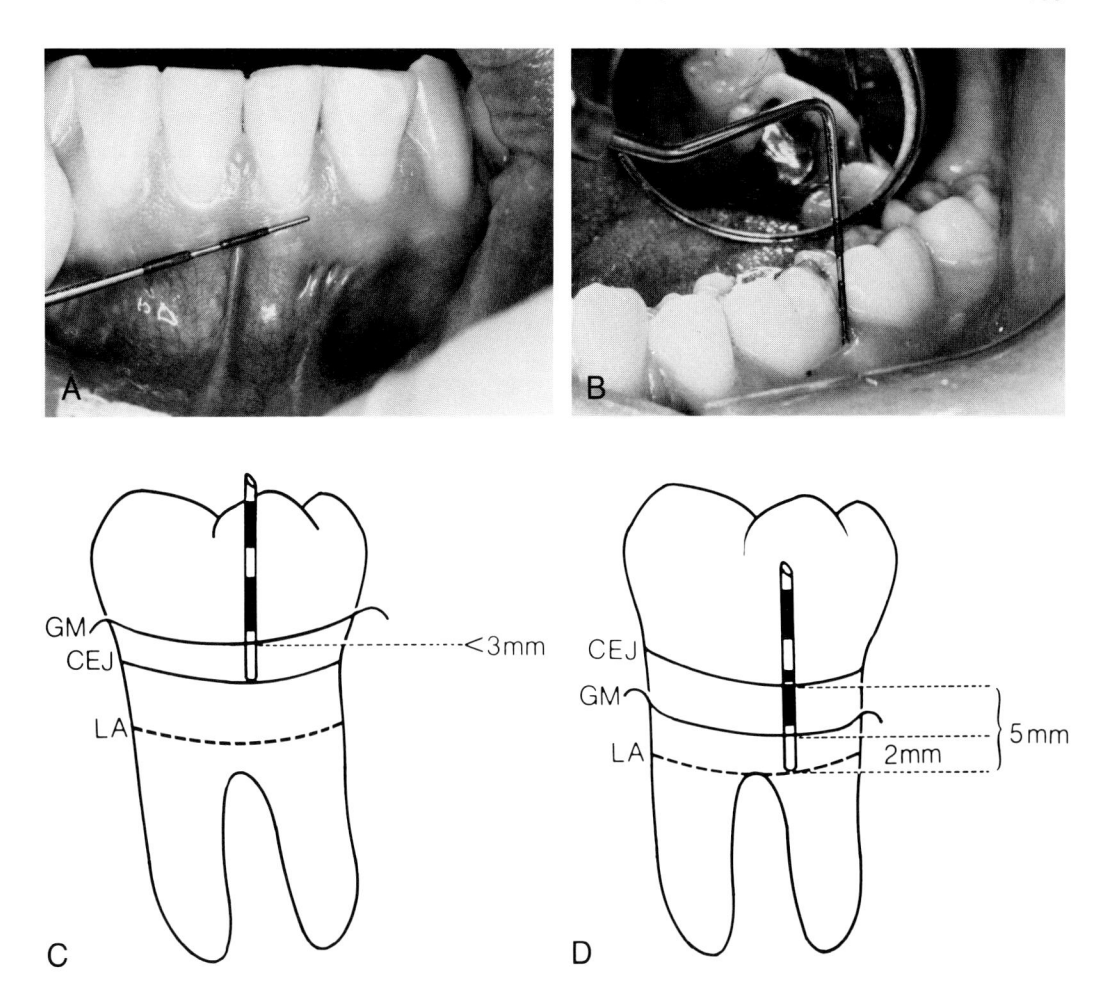

Fig. 13-7. *Periodontal probing.* A, Probe showing markings at 3, 6 and 8 mm. B, Probe in position. C, Probe to CEJ (cementoenamel junction) showing relationship of free gingival margin (GM) to CEJ. D, Probe to attachment level (LA). Depth of pocket is 5 mm.

filter paper strips. Most recently, a device called a Periotron has been utilized to measure quickly the amount of gingival fluid absorbed on paper strips. This method has been used clinically to determine indirectly the degree of gingival inflammation. The gingival fluid contains functional components, including low levels of antibodies which are specific to plaque antigens.

The level of attachment in a normal periodontium is coronal to the cementoenamel function. The method of determining the attachment level is illustrated in Fig. 13-7. The presence of an attachment on the cementum is an indication of past or active loss of support and periodontitis.

Periodontal Ligament

The periodontal ligament is the specialized connective tissue surrounding the roots of the teeth and is responsible for the support of the teeth (Fig. 13-8).

The parts of the principal fibers which are inserted into the cementum and bone are called Sharpey's fibers. The periodontal ligament varies in width depending upon the amount the tooth is used, the age of the individual, and the area of the root involved. The width of the periodontal ligament is greatest when there is hypermobility of the teeth. The average width of the periodontal ligament is about 0.25 mm. Clinically, the

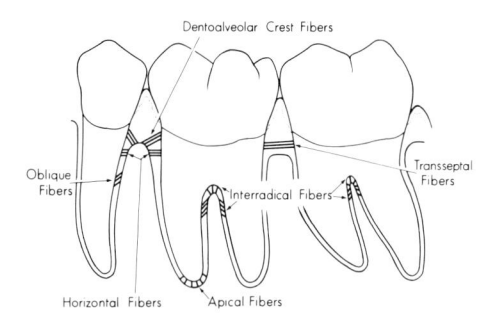

Fig. 13-8. Illustration of principal periodontal fibers.

width of the periodontal ligament can only be visualized as the periodontal ligament space on the proximal surfaces of the teeth using radiographs.

Alveolar Bone

The *alveolar bone* (alveolar bone proper) is that bone which forms the walls of the sockets of the teeth into which the principal fibers of the periodontal ligament are attached. The *alveolar process* is the bone of the mandible and maxilla which supports the teeth. Radiographically, it is the finger-like projection of cancellous bone seen between the teeth that supports the alveolar bone proper and the alveolar crest (Fig. 13-9). The term lamina dura is used to describe the radiographic appearance of the thin radiopaque border of alveolar bone proper which is adjacent to the periodontal ligament and extends over the crest of the alveolar process interproximally.

When a tooth is moved orthodontically or because of occlusal trauma, pressure and tension are transmitted to the alveolar bone proper causing its formation or resorption (Fig. 13-10).

A radiographic examination should show that in the normal individual the lamina dura is continuous; when there is a lack of continuity, periodontal or pulpal disease is most often the cause. The height of the alveolar crest should be within 1 to 1½ mm of the cementoenamel junction. A loss of alveolar crest is most often related to chronic destructive periodontal disease. Root resorption is often associated with pulp disease and periapical sequelae and trauma from occlusion.

Cementum

Dental cementum is a highly specialized type of connective tissue which is deposited throughout the life of the teeth. Continuous deposition is necessary for reattachment of the principal fibers to accommodate for movement of the teeth and to repair injury. Cementum is not resorbed under normal conditions except in association with the resorption of the roots of the primary dentition.

EPIDEMIOLOGY

The occurrence of disease is spoken of as incidence or prevalence. *Incidence* refers to the number of people having a disease in a given period of time per unit of population, e.g., 50 cases of measles per 10,000 children in 1 year. *Prevalence* refers to the number of people with a disease at a particular time in a unit of population, e.g., one infant with cleft palate/1,000 newborn. Obviously, where a disease has a vague or insidious onset and no definite termination, incidence data might be difficult to determine. Usually data on chronic forms of per-

Fig. 13-9. Radiograph showing lamina dura alveolar process, and alveolar crest.

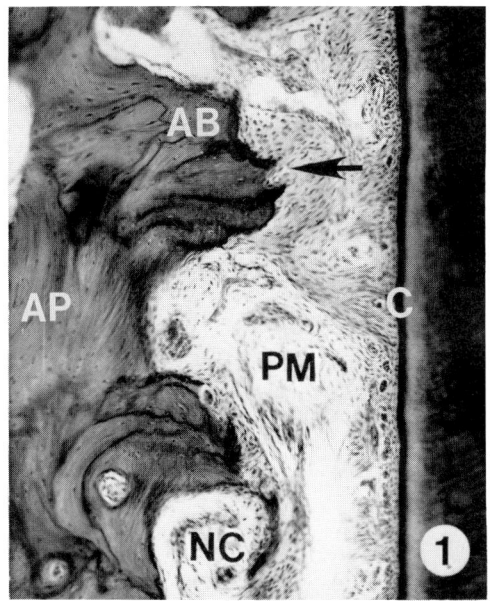

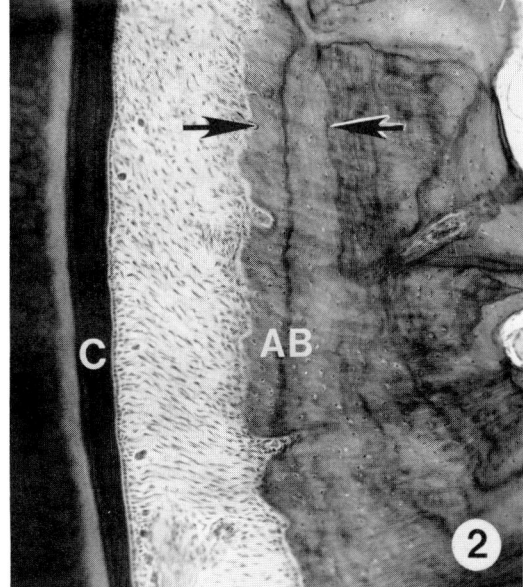

Fig. 13–10. *Periodontal changes with movement of teeth.* Photomicrographs showing mesial movement of a tooth. (1) Pressure side of alveolar bone showing resorption at arrow. PM, periodontal ligament; NC, nutrient channel undergoing fibrosis; AB, alveolar bone; C, cementum; AP, alveolar process; (2) Apposition of bone between arrows on tension side.

iodontal disease are given in terms of prevalence.

Measurement of Periodontal Disease

Methods for assessing periodontal health and disease include indices for scoring plaque and gingivitis, measurement of crevicular fluid flow, bleeding tendency, and measurement of the level of attachment. Some of the indices are simple observations of the degree of inflammation of the gingiva, e.g., number of inflamed papillae (P), gingival margins (M), and the attached gingiva (A) of the labial gingiva of the anterior teeth. Thus, the PMA index is a measure of the severity of gingivitis of the anterior teeth, but gives no insight into the status of the level of attachment, i.e., loss of supporting structures. Following the introduction of this simple index, a number of indices have been developed, including the Periodontal Index (PI) which provides a score for each tooth based upon: 0—no inflammation, 1—gingivitis around part of the tooth, 2—gingivitis encircling the tooth, 6—pocket formation, and 8—excess tooth mobility.

Another index, the periodontal disease index (PDI), uses a scoring system based on scores of 0 to 3 for various degrees of gingivitis and measurement of attachment level relative to the cemento-enamel junction. When the attachment level is apical to the cemento-enamel junction, but not more than 3 mm, a score of 4 is given; when greater than 3 mm, but not more than 6 mm, a score of 5 is given; and when the attachment is more than 6 mm, apical to the cementoenamel junction, a score of 6 is given. Thus, the PDI score, like the PI score, is a composite index of gingivitis and periodontitis. More recently, indices of gingivitis are used separately from attachment level data. Thus, in clinical trials actual attachment level data are used to assess periodontal status and gingivitis scores are reported separately. Much of the early information on the nature of periodontal disease was developed from the use of such indices in epidemiologic studies.

A widely used clinical index of gingivitis is the Gingival Index (GI). A score of 0 reflects minimal or no inflammation with no bleeding on probing; a score of 2 indicates moderate inflammation with bleeding on probing; and a score of 3 indicates severe inflammation, ulceration, and a tendency for spontaneous bleeding. A number of other gingival disease indices have been proposed and have been reviewed recently (see Ramfjord and Ash, 1979).

Several indices for plaque, calculus and oral hygiene have been used in clinical studies. Plaque and calculus studies have been used to relate oral hygiene status to the severity of periodontal disease. A widely used index of plaque deposits is the Plaque Index (Pl. I.) which assesses plaque on the basis of a scale of 0 to 3. A score of 0 indicates that no plaque is present; a score of 1 indicates that plaque adheres to the free gingival margin and adjacent tooth surface and is detected when a probe is passed across the tooth surface; a score of 2 indicates a moderate accumulation, both supra- and subgingivally; and a score of 3 indicates an abundance of plaque, both supra- and subgingivally.

ETIOLOGY OF PERIODONTAL DISEASES

Periodontal diseases must be considered to have multifactorial causes whether due to nonspecific or specific bacterial plaque (Fig. 13–11). Considering that most periodontal diseases reflect inflammatory and immune responses to bacteria and/or their metabolites, differences in their severity, time of onset, selective involvement of sites in the mouth, and clinical appearance suggest the presence of factors which modify the defenses of the host to the injurious agents, provide selective advantage for some of the indigenous flora residing in the mouth, or interfere with the repairative phase of the inflammatory process. Such a division of etiologic factors in periodontal diseases is given in Table 13–1.

Initiating Factors

The role of bacterial plaque in the etiology of periodontal diseases, changes in bacterial flora which occur with the development of gingivitis in association with the formation of supragingival plaque, and the changes in bacterial flora that occur with the development of subgingival plaque and the development of periodontal pockets have been considered in Chapter 10, and will only briefly be considered here. However, the histopathology and pathogenesis of plaque-induced gingivitis and periodontitis will be discussed in this chapter.

Generally the gingival sulcus in a healthy gingival state contains only a relatively few gram-positive streptococcal and facultative *Actinomyces* species. With the development of gingivitis, gram-negative organisms are found in increasing numbers, including *Bacteroides* and *Fusobacterium* species. Spirochetes and motile rods are seen as well. With advanced adult periodontitis, the cultivable organisms consist predominantly of gram-negative rods. On phase contrast microscopy about 50% of the organisms have been reported to be spirochetes and motile rods.

The gram-negative microorganisms which have been implicated in periodontal diseases include: *Bacteroides intermedius* and intermediate-sized spirochetes in acute necrotizing ulcerative gingivitis; *Bacteroides gingivalis* in adult periodontitis; *Actinobacillus actinomycetemcomitans* (A.a.) in localized juvenile periodontitis; *Capnocytophaga* species in advanced periodontitis in juvenile diabetes mellitus, in granulocytopenia, and in patients with compromised immune states; and *Bacteroides intermedius* in pregnancy gingivitis. The suggested periodontopathic potentials of these organisms appear sufficient to account for much of the destructive effects of periodontal diseases. However, the role of microorganisms in periodontal disease is

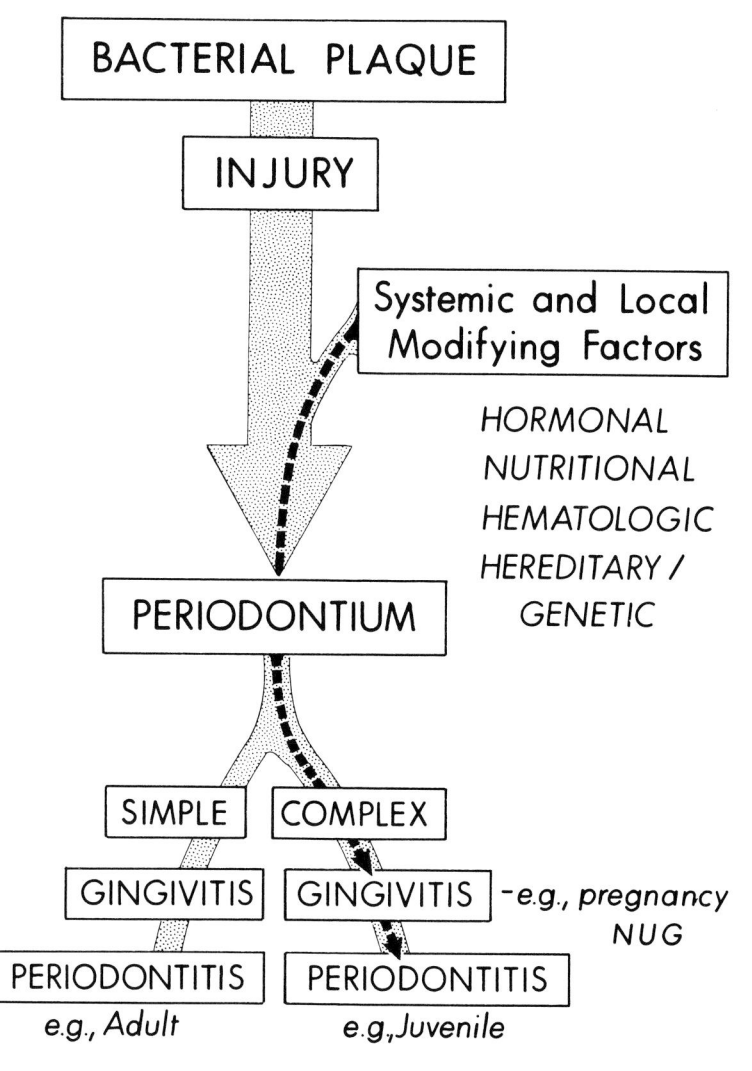

Fig. 13–11. *Pathogenesis of periodontal diseases.* Initiating bacterial plaque and systemic/local factors which modify the immuno-inflammatory response.

complex and far from being completely understood.

Modifying Factors

Several systemic factors may alter inflammatory and immune responses so that the host's defenses against bacteria or their metabolites are compromised. An outline of systemic factors which may influence the way in which the initiating causes are handled is given in Table 13–2. The question arises of course as to whether periodontal disease will occur in the absence of bacterial plaque even though severe systemic modifying factors are present. Considerable control of periodontal disease can be obtained by rigorous home care procedures and professional care, including chemical plaque control with chlorhexidine and prescribed use of antibiotics.

Several recent investigations suggest that localized juvenile periodontitis, which has been linked by association to a gram-negative organism (A.a.) based on recovery of the organism in high numbers and on significantly increased levels of serum and

Table 13-1 Etiologic Factors in Inflammatory Periodontal Disease

A. *Initiating Factors*
   Bacterial plaque, calculus

B. *Modifying Factors*
   Systemic
      Hormonal
      Nutritional
      Drug therapy
      Hematologic
      Hereditary/Genetic
   Local
      Trauma from occlusion
      Food impaction
      Impinging overbite
      Mouthbreathing
      Faulty restorations

gingival fluid antibodies to A.a., can be successfully controlled by conventional periodontal treatment combined with antibiotic therapy. Individuals with aberrant neutrophil production or behavior often have early-onset, severe forms of gingivitis/periodontitis, including localized juvenile periodontitis. Thus systemic factors are classed as modifying rather than initiating factors.

The principal host resistance factor against bacteria is the neutrophil, which migrates to sites of bacteria in response to chemotactic substances released by bacteria as well as other exogenous substances including lymphokines, tissue degradation products, prostaglandins and complement activation products. Neutrophils accumulate in the junctional epithelium and periodontal pockets as a line of defense. The neutrophil is an important cellular component in acute non-infectious inflammation, in inflammation mediated by pyogenic bacteria, and in reactions involving antigen-antibody complexes. Neutrophils can kill some kinds of bacteria, but antibody and complement are required for ingestion by the leukocytes.

Inasmuch as the neutrophil has a key defensive role against invasive and potentially pathogenic bacteria, defects in the production or function of the neutrophil are often associated with early-onset (12 to 30 years), severe forms of periodontitis. Patients with Down's syndrome, drug induced agranulocytosis, cyclic neutropenia, Chédiak-Higashi syndrome, and Papillon-LeFèvre syndrome (p. 228) often demonstrate increased susceptibility to severe gingivitis and periodontitis because of disturbances in number and/or function of neutrophils. Thus, the ability of the antibody-complement-neutrophil system to cope with bacteria or their metabolites is a significant modifying factor in the etiology of periodontal disease.

Resistance to microorganisms is also mediated by lymphocytes (and the lymphokines they produce) and macrophages. This lymphocyte-macrophage system has been implicated also in tissue destruction in periodontal disease. The immunopathic (destructive) potential of the cell mediated immunity system is supported to a limited extent by studies of patients with immunodeficiencies (e.g., hypo- or agammaglobulinemia) and deficient lymphocyte function. These patients were reported to have less gingivitis than normal subjects. The protective and potentially destructive roles of the lymphocyte-macrophage system as modifying factors in periodontal disease has yet to be clarified.

Another systemic factor which contributes to gingivitis is pregnancy. It has been suggested that pregnancy gingivitis is an exaggerated inflammatory response which may be due to hormonal changes, especially during the second to ninth month of

Table 13-2 Systemic Modifying Factors in Periodontal Diseases

Hormonal	—Pregnancy, puberty
Nutritional	—Vitamin C deficiency
Therapy	—Dilantin
Hematologic	—Leukemia Cyclic neutropenia Diabetes mellitus Immune disorders
Hereditary/ Genetic	—Down's syndrome Papillon-LeFèvre syndrome Chédiak-Higashi syndrome Localized juvenile periodontitis Hypophosphatasia

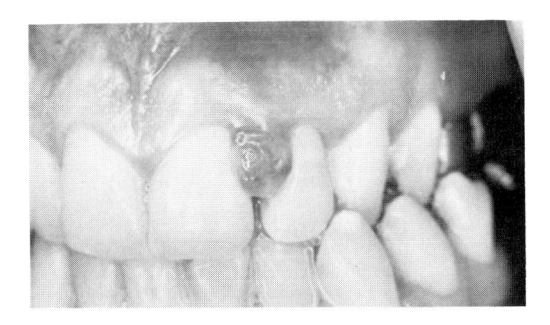

Fig. 13–12. *Granuloma pyogenicum* ("pregnancy tumor").

pregnancy when there is a definite decrease in the level of gingivitis. The occurrence of the "pregnancy" granuloma (Fig. 13–12) has already been considered (p. 96). Of particular interest is the incidence (1 in 450) of a deficiency of serum IgA in pregnant women. The significance of immuglobulin A deficiency to gingivitis in pregnancy has not been determined. The role of increased *Bacteroides intermedius* in pregnancy gingivitis has yet to be determined. There appears to be agreement generally that during pregnancy complex factors appear to modify the normal response of the gingiva to the presence of bacterial plaque.

The role of vitamin C deficiency in the development of periodontal disease has been established. And in the presence of frank scurvy and bacterial plaque on the teeth, the historical record of "gum disease and tooth loss" before knowledge of a relationship to fresh fruits speaks for itself. Classical human studies demonstrate the difficulty of producing gingivitis-periodontitis changes when oral hygiene is reasonably effective. Depletion of vitamin C is difficult to demonstrate in the diet of industrialized countries and the significance of a so-called "subclinical deficiency" has yet to be determined.

Therapeutic use of drugs may alter the inflammatory response of the host as in drug induced agranulocytosis with severe periodontitis, hyperplasia associated with the use of the anticonvulsant drug, diphenylhydantoin (Dilantin sodium), and increased gingivitis with long-term use of oral contraceptives.

Local modifying factors that contribute to the progress of plaque induced periodontal disease include trauma from occlusion which, when it is not self-limiting, tends to accelerate pocket formation and bone loss. However, trauma from occlusion probably plays a minor role, if any, in the pathogenesis of early to moderate periodontitis. Long-term progressive trauma from occlusion, often related to bruxism (gnashing and grinding of teeth) and faulty dental restorations, is especially significant in patients with advanced loss of periodontal support. Thus the role of trauma from occlusion appears to increase with a decrease in the remaining support for the teeth, especially with untreated periodontal pockets.

Food impaction may occur when proximal contacts are inadequate and/or when the occlusion causes distal molars (3^d molars absent) to be forced distally. Plunger cusps, usually the distal lingual cusp of the maxillary first molar, force food into the interproximal area between the mandibular first and second molars. An impinging overbite occurs when the mandibular incisors do not make normal occlusal contacts on the lingual surfaces of the maxillary central incisors (Fig. 13–13). In such instances the incisal edges of the mandibular teeth impact on and traumatize the palatal gingival tissues.

Mouthbreathing and continued exposure and drying of the facial gingiva of the maxillary anterior teeth often lead to mouthbreather's gingivitis (Fig. 13–14). The hyperplastic gingivitis associated with such chronic irritation tends to follow the line of the upper lip. In some instances, the effects of mouthbreathing may involve the palatal gingiva.

Faulty restorations with overhanging margins may also adversely influence the response of the tissues to treatment (Fig. 13–15). Such margins trap bacteria and

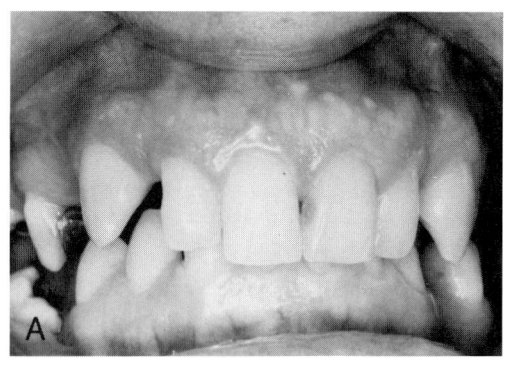

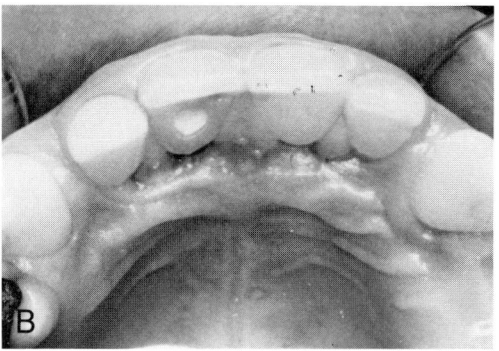

Fig. 13–13. *Traumatic gingivitis.* A, impinging overbite; B, indentations of mandibular teeth.

prevent proper elimination of the local initiating factors.

PATHOGENESIS OF PERIODONTAL DISEASES

The mechanism involved in the development of destructive periodontal disease from gingivitis is not entirely clear, although it is generally accepted that the gingivitis–adult periodontitis axis is a response to injury from bacterial plaque on the teeth. Therefore, the most common forms of periodontal disease reflect plaque induced inflammatory changes in the periodontium. It is the mechanism by which destruction of these unique structures occurs that presents most of the questions about the pathogenesis of chronic destructive periodontal disease. Several answers have been suggested: destruction is caused by the direct action of substances produced by bacteria in subgingival plaque, invasion of the gin-

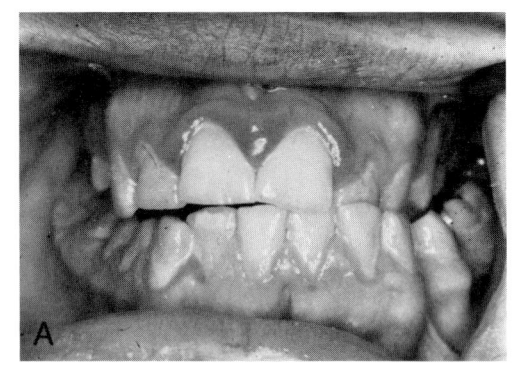

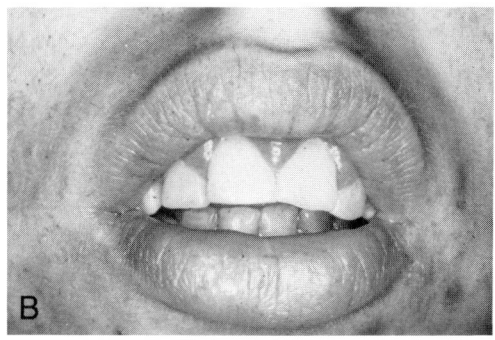

Fig. 13–14. *Mouthbreather's gingivitis.* A, Hyperplastic gingiva of anterior teeth associated with mouthbreathing and plaque on the teeth. B, Note lip line and exposed gingiva.

giva by specific or nonspecific pathogenic bacteria, and/or the consequences of aberrant immune responses.

Pathogens

Much of the recent research on the pathogenesis of periodontal disease relates to

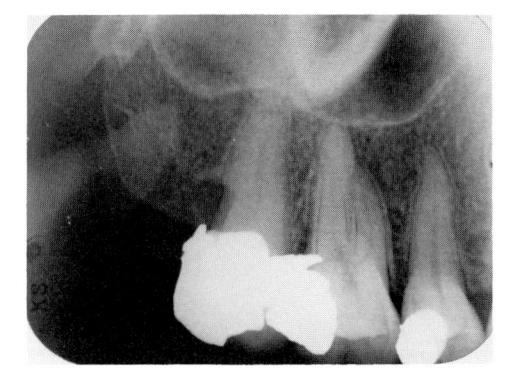

Fig. 13–15. Overhanging margin of restoration and loss of bone on distal of second molar.

conditions under which periodontal disease occurs and a search for specific pathogens. Findings from these lines of research have lead to the concept that certain specific microbes are unique to a type of periodontal disease or appear in proportionally higher numbers in that disease. Retrospective sampling of bacteria in established disease and association of organisms with the clinical status of the periodontium have not provided answers to what changes plaque into a disease-producing plaque and whether the population of bacteria present is causative or fortuitous. If the changes occurring in bacterial plaque (described in Chapter 10) during the passage from health to disease are causative, then evidence to this effect should be demonstrable through prospective bacteriologic studies, including a consistent relationship of the specific bacteria with the disease syndrome, and tissue-invasive capability of the specific organisms. However, the evidence provided so far does not demonstrate a simple one-to-one correspondence between specific pathogens and periodontal disease. Nor does it appear that microbial pathogenicity is solely related to numbers of organisms inasmuch as a highly virulent microorganism may have more destructive potential even though present in relatively fewer numbers than a less virulent organism present in significantly larger numbers.

The possibility that certain forms of periodontal disease reflect an "opportunistic" bacterial disease has been proposed. For example, periodontal disease might develop when a selective increase in one or more bacteria occurs in subgingival plaque as a result of an environmental "opportunity." An ecologic shift due to local factors such as changes in oral hygiene and/or changes in immune mechanism or neutrophil function could favor one and then another potential pathogen to overgrow or express its virulence. Thus, under favorable conditions for some potential pathogens, which already exist in a balance of indigenous flora, an "opportunity" is presented that leads to disease. Such opportunities may be transient, and chronic progressive periodontal disease reflects a number of periods of lowered states of the host's resistance. There are no clinically useful tests of disease activity. Studies that depend on longitudinal studies and demonstration of bone loss tend to support the concept of "bursts" of active disease rather than an unchanging downward progression of supporting tissue loss.

That changes in the host's defense mechanisms can favor differential bacterial proliferation and/or increased virulence of indigenous oral flora and lead to a loss of supporting structures, points to the need to view periodontal disease as something more than localized infections. The complex relationship between the host's defenses and pathogens at systemic as well as local levels requires further clarification. Of particular interest in the pathogenesis of periodontal disease and pocket formation is the way that bacteria overcome the defenses of the host and directly or indirectly cause tissue damage.

Bacterial Invasion

Although it has been accepted for some time that spirochetes invade gingival tissues in necrotizing ulcerative gingivitis, and reported since early in the 20th century that bacterial invasion occurs in periodontal disease, it has only been recently demonstrated that bacteria are present in the tissues in the late stage of adult periodontitis and in localized juvenile periodontitis. Because bacteria are found in tissues as the result of tissue manipulation and occur as a part of transient bacteremia, reports of the presence of bacteria in the tissues require careful evaluation. However, there appears to be somewhat more published evidence for bacterial invasion than against. Bacteria reported to have invasive capacity include *Bacteroides* species, A. *actinomycetemcomitans,* and *Capnocytophaga.*

In order for bacteria to invade the tissues, bacteria must utilize some of the following:

the ability to attach and multiply on tissues and cell surfaces (p. 145); the ability to resist phagocytosis (e.g., produce surface slime—a polysaccharide capsule to avoid opsonization); the ability to avoid digestion and inhibit lysosomal fusion when engulfed by phagocytes (p. 66); the ability to inhibit the chemotactic movement of neutrophils; the ability to kill phagocytes by producing toxins; and the facility for some form of locomotion.

Pocket Formation

The question of bacterial invasion may also be related to mechanisms underlying the development of gingival and periodontal pockets. One concept of periodontal pocket formation suggests that apical migration of the junctional epithelium is preceded by destruction of the underlying connective tissue attachment and then subgingival plaque forms on the surface of the tooth secondary to the loss of attachment. This mechanism would support the concept of "cementopathia" (attachment loss related to inherent defect in cementum), the idea of a "negative bone factor", and a connective tissue defect (e.g., vitamin C deficiency, etc.). Another broad concept suggests that loss of attachment is the consequence of destructive mechanisms involved directly with bacterial penetration and separation of the attachment from the tooth. In this concept the pocket follows the formation of plaque. Evidence for these concepts or similar concepts is limited. It is possible to relate hypophosphatasia to cementopathia; loss of fibers to collagenase, a specific metalloprotease produced by fibroblasts, polymorphonuclear leukocytes, and macrophages; and bone loss to prostaglandins. However, such relationships have not been developed at the clinical level. The mechanism of pocket formation and bone loss has yet to be fully clarified, although the potential for destructive effects of bacterial plaque and aberrant protective mechanisms of the host appears to be clear.

Host Defenses

The defenses of the body to bacteria and their products involve surface barriers (gingiva and dentogingival junction); nonspecific components of the saliva, such as lysozyme and transferrin, which are capable of disposing of or killing bacteria; and so-called "innate" immunity provided by "broad-spectrum antibiotics" that are produced by the normal bacterial flora and that provide some measure of control over potential periodontopathic bacteria. In addition to these natural barriers, potential pathogenic plaque bacteria are subjected to complement, phagocytic cells (neutrophils, macrophages), antibodies, and cell-mediated immunity involving lymphocytes.

The defenses of the host against periodontopathic bacteria begin with blocking of their attachment and thus colonization of the tooth. Aside from mechanical/chemical methods of preventing colonization, it is reasonable to assume (on the basis of the small amount of direct evidence available) that antibodies produced by the host interfere with adherence mechanisms and thus with colonization (p. 145). The antibodies involved, both secretory IgA (saliva) and gingival fluid (serum) antibodies, have the potential for inhibiting bacterial adherence and co-aggregation of plaque bacteria.

Neutrophils function to protect the host against bacteria. They accumulate at the tissue-plaque interface and below the junctional epithelium to form a "barrier" against microbial invasion. Neutrophils play a primary role in the pathogenesis of periodontal disease. Although antibodies (Ab) and complement (C) are often sufficient to kill bacteria (Ag), neutrophils may act in concert with Ab and C to facilitate the killing of periodontopathic bacteria, especially prior to and during the early invasive process. How well these bacteria are able to invade the tissues is related to their ability to circumvent the defenses of the neutrophil.

Immune Mechanisms in Periodontal Disease

Ordinarily a complex network of immune defenses are present to destroy or neutralize bacteria and their products. However, considerable attention has focused on immune factors that may be subverted to tissue destruction. Concepts of the mechanism of plaque-induced periodontal disease not only suggest the direct cytotoxic and proteolytic effects of bacterial plaque, especially subgingival plaque, but also implicate the indirect effects of the responses of the host's immune system to the continued presence of dental plaque. Thus, immunologic phenomena have been considered in the etiology of periodontal disease, either as a result of immunologic deficiency or hypersensitivity phenomenon. In effect, immune responses may exert destructive as well as protective effects in periodontal disease.

The basis for the concept that immune mechanisms may be responsible for the destructive effects of periodontal disease comes from evidence demonstrating that bacteria, bacterial parts, chemotactic factors, and other plaque products penetrate the junctional epithelium and induce host sensitization. Chronic penetration is thought to lead to immediate and delayed hypersensitivity (p. 87).

The activation of cell-mediated immunity (delayed hypersensitivity), which involves the lymphocyte-macrophage system, stimulates the proliferation of lymphocytes (T- and B-lymphocytes). In an established lesion, which may persist for years without pocket formation, there is a localized infiltration of plasma cells. Cell-mediated immune responses have the potential via T cells to influence bone loss by stimulating or suppressing T- and/or B-lymphocyte effector cells that produce lymphokines, including an osteoclast activating factor, that are potentially destructive to the periodontal tissues.

It has been suggested that many microbial products ("polyclonal activators," especially lipopolysaccharides) can stimulate B cells, including self-reactive B-lymphocytes. In contrast to a polyclonal activator, an antigen, when presented to lymphocytes in an appropriate manner, induces only one or a few clones of B or T cells. The immune system normally protects its lymphocytes against self-reactivity in several ways, e.g., suppressor T cells and anti-idiotype networks. The latter is a hypothesized network of receptors that regulate antibody responses. Any breakdown of T- suppressor cells and regulatory networks could allow autoimmune reactions to reach a point of causing disease. Thus, the conversion from a stable periodontal state to a progressive disease would involve polyclonal B-cell activation and regulation by suppressor T cells and T-cell macrophage interactions. The anti-idiotypic networks would tend to limit the reaction.

The immunopathologic potential of the lymphocyte-macrophage system is supported by studies of humans with immunodeficiencies (e.g., hypo- or agammaglobulinemia). Patients with deficient lymphocyte functions exhibited less gingival inflammation than controls. Conceptually, both protective and destructive immune responses would be involved in the lymphocyte-macrophage cell mediated immunity. Knowledge of the immunoregulatory role of lymphocytes and macrophages locally (at the level of gingival epithelium) may reflect cells which are the same or similar in function to Langerhans cells (immunologically competent keratinocytes) which react with helper T cells and perhaps Granstein cells (another type of dendritic antigen-presenting cell) which interact similarly with suppressor T cells to maintain normally a positive balance; this is generally the appropriate response to potentially harmful invaders. The presence of similar cells in the keratinized gingiva may help to resolve the question of the protective/destructive effects of immune responses in periodontal disease. The role of the lymphocyte-mac-

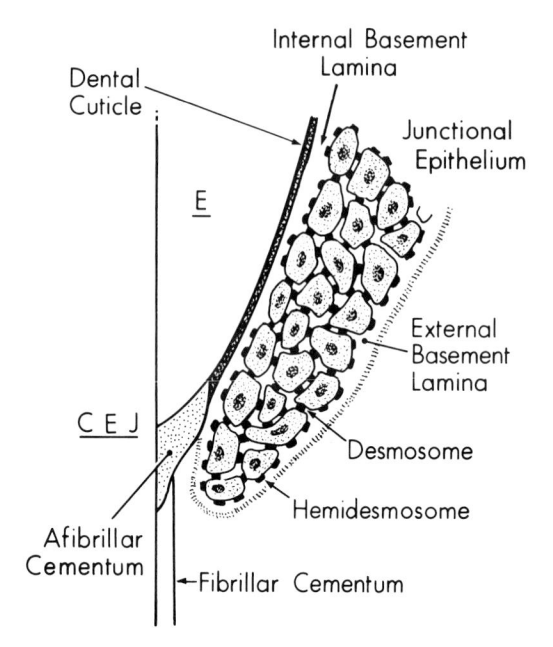

Fig. 13-16. Schematic drawing of junctional epithelium showing various structures. E, enamel; CEJ, cementoenamel junction.

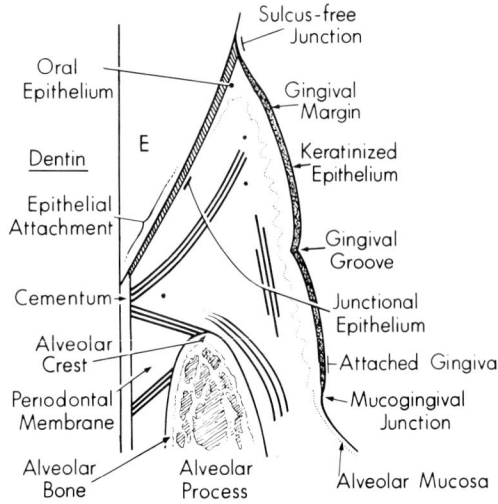

Fig. 13-17. Schematic representation of idealized sulcus-free dentogingival junction.

rophage system as a modifying factor in periodontal disease has yet to be clarified.

HISTOPATHOLOGY OF GINGIVITIS-PERIODONTITIS

The pathogenesis of inflammatory periodontal disease can be divided into initial, early, established, and advanced stages. Although such subdivisions are essentially arbitrary, and do not relate necessarily to the sequence of clinical events in the pathogenesis of the disease, a discussion of histopathologic changes which occur in the transition from a normal gingiva to gingivitis, and from gingivitis to periodontitis, may facilitate a better understanding of the pathogenesis of periodontal disease. Of particular significance is the dentogingival junction and the junctional epithelium.

DENTO-GINGIVAL JUNCTION

The dento-gingival complex is an anatomic and functional interface between hard and soft tissues and between systemic and local defense mechanisms. Of particular significance is the junctional epithelium (JE), which provides for the attachment of the gingiva to the enamel surface via numerous hemidesmosomes (Fig. 13-16). These attachment structures (p. 6) interface with the apatite crystals of the enamel surface through a fine layer of organic material.

Junctional Epithelium

The junctional epithelium represents a special type of interface between the gingiva and tooth surface. It extends from the cementoenamel junction to the free gingival margin or slightly beyond under controlled conditions, such as in germ-free animals where bacterial plaque is not present to cause reactive (inflammatory) changes. Under conditions of intense, regular and prolonged tooth cleaning in dogs, the junctional epithelium reaches the gingival margin and no gingival sulcus is present (Fig. 13-17). In a "normalized" sulcus-free healthy gingival state there is no gingivitis and no plaque present, the depth of the gingival crevice is zero, and there is a virtual absence of flow of crevicular fluid. A sulcus-free state in many may be seen when plaque is controlled chemically and there has been careful avoidance of any mechanical stimulation by brushing. However, even when the gingiva is clinically healthy, the gingival sulcus is found to be a shallow groove between the gingiva and tooth surface (Fig. 13–2). Thus, under favorable experimental conditions, the gingival sulcus may approach a depth of zero, but most frequently is found to be greater than 0 but less than 1 mm in depth. The accepted clinical standards for the depth of the gingival crevice have already been presented (p. 198).

When the gingival sulcus is present, the junctional epithelium forms the base of the sulcus and the oral sulcular epithelium forms the lateral wall. There may be only a few strata of cells forming the thickness of the junctional epithelium and its basal layer is parallel to the tooth surface. The superficial cells at the coronal edge of the junctional epithelium present a narrow surface along which all junctional epithelial cells desquamate. The turnover rate of the cells of the junctional epithelium is much higher than other types of oral epithelial cells, e.g., double the rate of the oral gingival epithelium. Thus, tears in the junctional epithelium may be repaired in a matter of 5 to 7 days.

The junctional epithelium is a highly permeable type of tissue as a consequence of wide intercellular spaces and short renewal time. It is the pathway for serum exudate containing antibodies and complement leaving inflamed gingiva, as well as the site for molecules diffusing into the connective tissues, including those which might provoke tissue responses that generate crevicular fluid and increased numbers of inflammatory cells. However, irrespective of the state of gingival health, polymorphonuclear leukocytes (PMNs) are always found in the junctional epithelium. Neutrophils are phagocytic at the surface of the plaque as well as within the junctional epithelium. In the presence of bacterial plaque, chemotactic substances are produced which stimulate neutrophils, and to a minor extent monocytes, to migrate through the junctional epithelium.

Gingival/Periodontal Pockets

The junctional epithelium is the site of cellular and humoral defenses. How well the gingival sulcus is maintained is dependent upon such variables as the virulence of the bacteria, mechanical removal of plaque (toothbrushing), proliferative rate of junctional epithelium and re-establishment of the epithelial attachment, and how effective the biologic defenses are against the injurious agents, e.g., clearing of bacteria from the junctional epithelium.

As long as the plaque does not extend apical to the gingival margin, apparently the gingival sulcus will remain as a narrow groove between the tooth surface and gingiva. However, when subgingival plaque is established, the gingival sulcus may change from a sulcus-free or shallow groove to a gingival pocket. Histologically, a gingival pocket is characterized by the presence of "pocket epithelium." The formation of a pocket occurs with the conversion of junctional epithelium to pocket epithelium (Fig. 13–18). Pocket epithelium is characterized by proliferation of rete pegs, microulceration, and loss of epithelial attachment. The pocket epithelium is infiltrated mainly by lymphocytes, T- and B-blasts, plasma cells, and transmigrating neutrophilic granulocytes (Fig. 13–19). When the loss of attachment extends apically beyond the cementoenamel junction and bone resorption takes place in the presence of periodontitis, the pocket is referred to as a periodontal pocket (Fig. 13–20).

Clinically a "pocket," gingival or periodontal, is present whenever the probing depth of the crevice around a tooth exceeds some standard, i.e., greater than 2 to 3 mm interproximally in a 35-year-old adult. However, it should be recognized that up to a probing depth of about 1 mm, histologic sections of a clinically healthy gingiva show oral, oral sulcular, and junctional epithelia

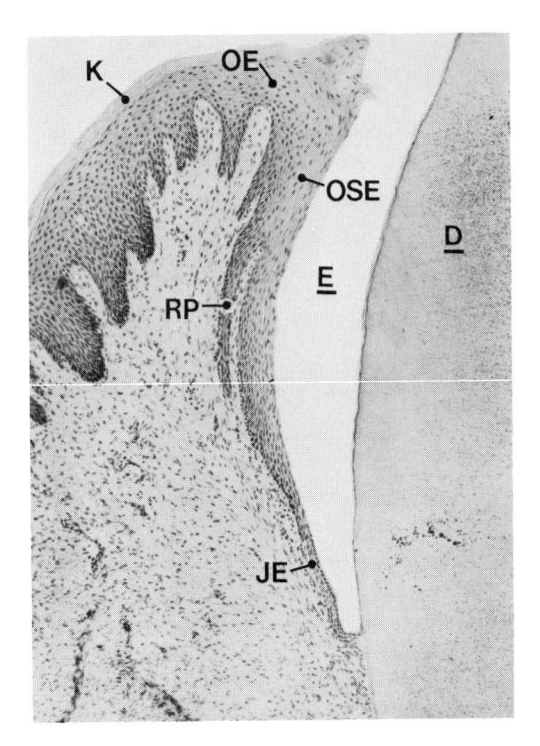

Fig. 13-18. *Photomicrograph of clinically healthy gingiva.* K, keratinized epithelium; OE, oral epithelium; D, dentin; RP, rete peg; JE, junctional epithelium.

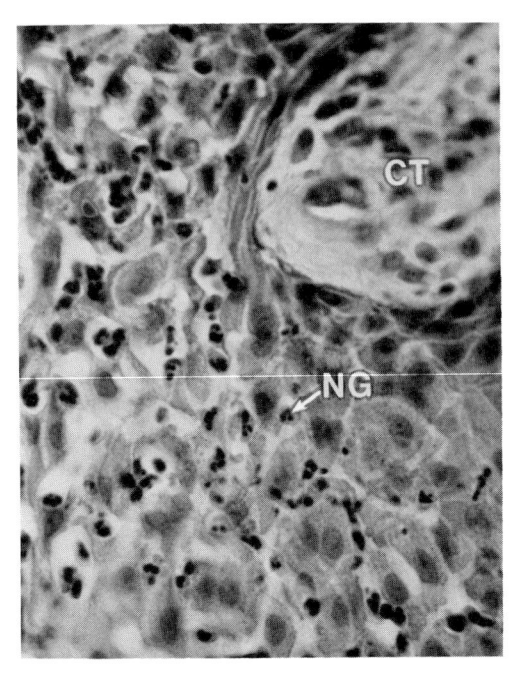

Fig. 13-19. Pocket epithelium with transmigrating neutrophils (NG). CT, Connective tissue.

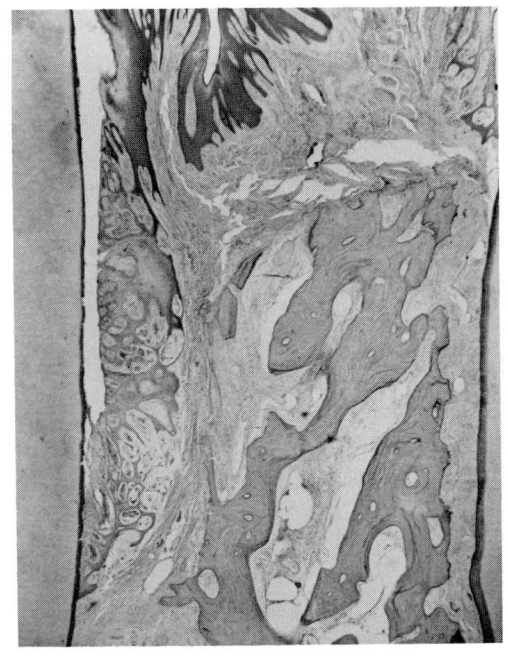

Fig. 13-20. Photomicrograph showing periodontal pocket with ulceration of pocket epithelium and loss of bone. Intrabony pocket is present.

but not pocket epithelium. With a gingival or relative pocket the attachment is at or coronal to the CEJ and the increase in depth of the crevice is due to gingival hyperplasia. An exception would be gingival recession.

The formation of a periodontal pocket, or more significantly the loss of attachment and supporting structures, is a reflection of injury produced by bacteria and/or their products, i.e., subgingival bacterial plaque. The mechanism by which pocket formation occurs has not been established. And although mediators and substances produced by bacterial plaque continuously penetrate the junctional epithelium in chronic gingivitis, periodontal breakdown does not occur. The transition from gingivitis to periodontitis is not simply a matter of bacterial plaque being present, although clinical studies indicate that most inflammatory

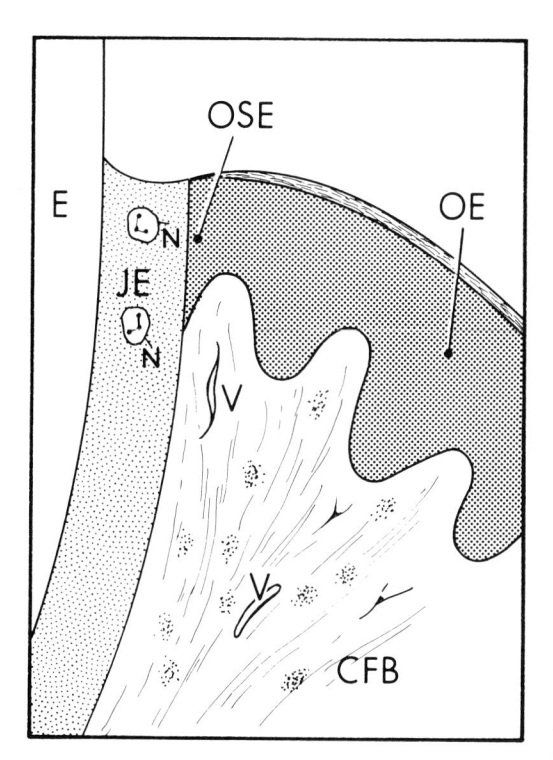

Fig. 13–21. Schematic of "normalized" gingiva with sulcus-free dentogingival junction. There are only a few neutrophils (N) present in the junctional epithelium after experimental reduction of plaque.

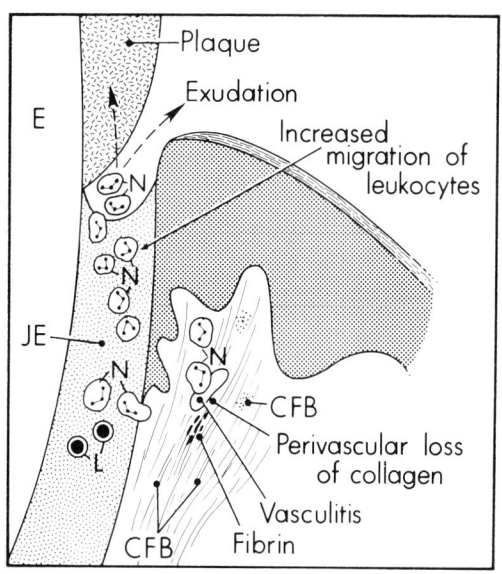

Fig. 13–22. Experimental gingivitis development following return of plaque (2 to 4 days) after reaching gingiva illustrated in Figure 13–2. Note formation of gingival sulcus and increased numbers of neutrophils (N). CFB, collagen fiber bundles.

periodontal diseases can be prevented or controlled by frequent plaque removal.

TRANSITION FROM GINGIVITIS TO PERIODONTITIS

Normal Gingiva

On the basis of microscopic or ultrastructural observations of the gingiva, and except in the experimental model where plaque is prevented from forming, it is hardly likely that the gingiva is free of some evidence of the inflammatory process. However, despite the presence of such minimal inflammatory changes in the gingiva, the clinical features still suggest a healthy gingiva. Thus, in the clinically healthy gingiva (Fig. 13–21), as defined by a gingivitis index score of zero (p. 202), only a few polymorphonuclear leukocytes will be found in the junctional epithelium. The junctional epithelium is everywhere in contact with the enamel. The subjacent connective tissue may show a small number of chronic inflammatory cells. However, in the dog model, in which there is intense and scrupulous control of plaque such that the gingival index score is zero and there is an absence of gingival sulcular fluid, inflammatory infiltration may be absent. However, it may not be possible to obtain complete health in all animals, nor in humans.

Gingivitis

The initial changes in the gingiva after 2 to 4 days of plaque accumulation after starting with a healthy gingiva include an acute exudative inflammation with vasculitis, gingival fluid exudation, extravascular fibrin deposition, some loss of perivascular collagen and the beginning of an inflammatory cell infiltrate into the junctional epithelium (Fig. 13–22). These changes are referred to as *initial gingivitis*. The gingiva may appear to be clinically healthy.

The histologic changes in *early gingivitis* involve the junctional epithelium and the most coronal part of the gingival connective tissues. There is an infiltration of lymphocytes, reduction in collagen fibers and proliferation of the basal layers of junctional epithelium. Rete peg formation from the oral sulcular and junctional epithelium may occur at this time.

The gingival crevicular fluid and number of leukocytes increase and reach a maximum between 6 to 12 days after the onset of clinical gingivitis. The junctional epithelium contains an increased number of polymorphonuclear leukocytes, especially from the basal layers to the surface layers (Fig. 13–19). Increasing numbers of monocytes, especially lymphocytes, are found at the inflammatory site, but the cells in the crevicular fluid are still mainly neutrophils (PMNs).

Within 2 to 4 weeks after the beginning of plaque accumulation, the gingivitis becomes established (Fig. 13–23). It is characterized by a preponderance of plasma cells within the connective tissues and is described as *chronic* or *established* gingivitis (Fig. 13–24). Even though the inflammation is chronic, the manifestations of acute inflammation persist as in the initial states of the inflammatory reaction. The plasma cells are present in the initial area of inflammation as well as in clusters adjacent to vessels and between fibers in the deeper connective tissues. Lymphocytes are present, macrophages are common, but only a few mast cells are present. The loss of collagen continues, but no bone loss is present in chronic or established gingivitis.

Periodontitis

At some point chronic gingivitis may progress to periodontitis, which is characterized by suppuration, bone loss, loss of attachment, pocket formation, tooth mobility, and loss of teeth. The characteristics of chronic gingivitis are also present in periodontitis. Active chronic inflammation with continued loss of collagen fibers, fibrosis, granulation tissue, and an inflammatory infiltrate of plasma cells is present throughout the tissues, but periods of quiescence and exacerbation of the inflammatory process occur.

At least two concepts of the development of periodontitis are evident: (1) destructive periodontal disease is a sequel to chronic gingivitis and thus the gingivitis-adult periodontitis is a continuum of the inflammatory

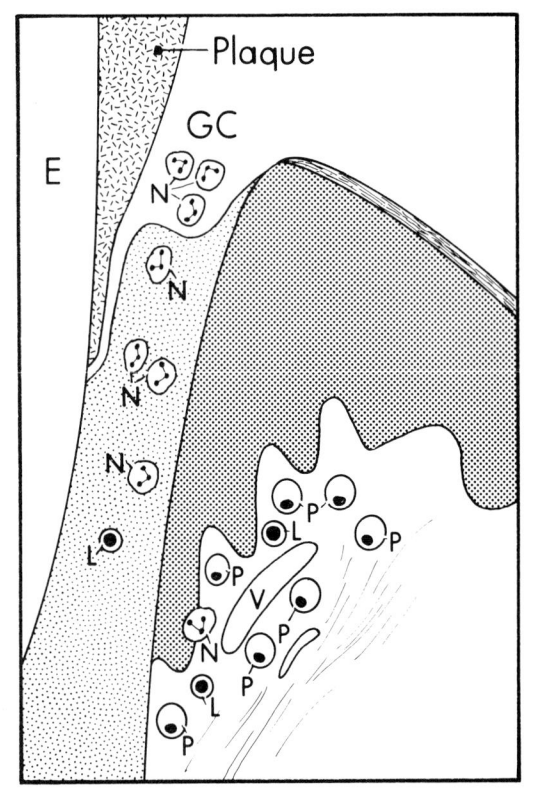

Fig. 13–23. Schematic illustration of chronic (established) gingivitis after 2 to 4 weeks of plaque accumulation of experimental gingivitis induction. GC, gingival crevicular fluid; N, neutrophil; L, lymphocyte; P, plasma cells; V, vessel dilated. Histologic characteristics include plasma cell preponderance, loss of collagen fibers, proliferation of junctional epithelium, extension of bacterial plaque and loss of attachment of junctional epithelium. CEJ, cementoenamel junction; E, enamel.

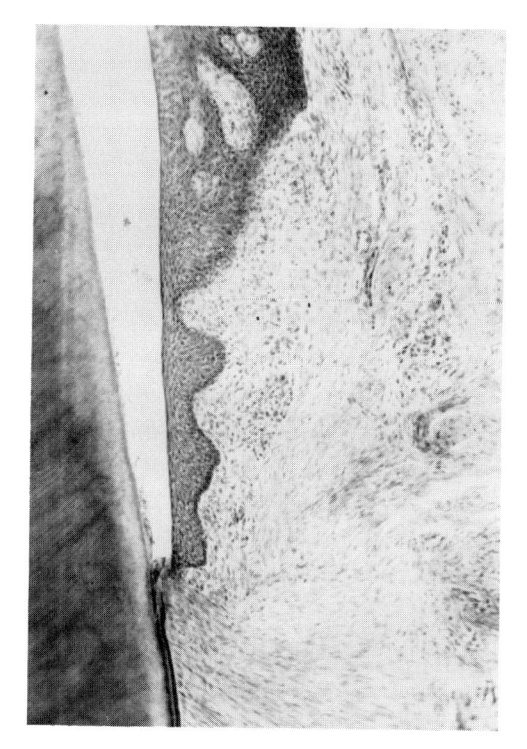

Fig. 13–24. Photomicrograph of chronic gingivitis showing lateral extension of junctional epithelium and development of inflammatory infiltration. Attachment does not extend apical to cementoenamel junction.

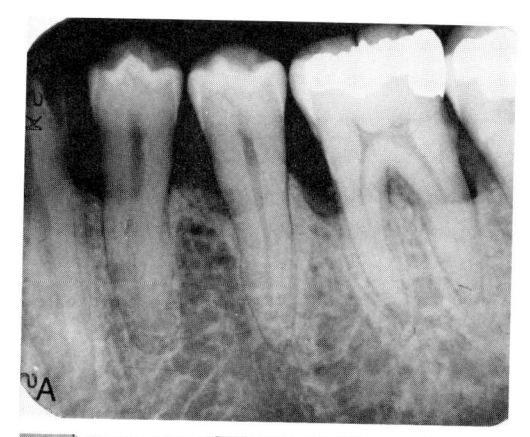

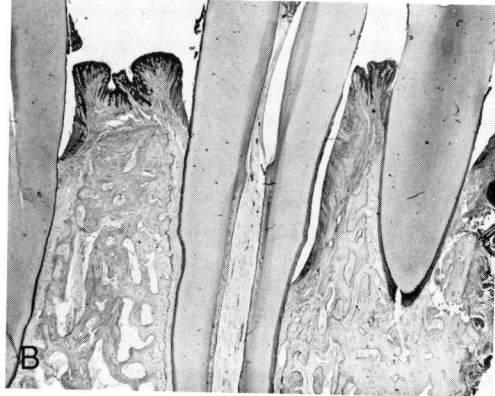

Fig. 13–25. *Advanced periodontitis.* A, photomicrograph showing loss of attachment and supporting bone; B, radiograph showing interdental loss of bone and generalized bone loss.

process involving first the gingiva and then the deeper supporting structures' and (2) the causative agent differs with time, individuals, teeth, and species, or the response of the host differs with time, individuals, teeth, and species. In the first concept the plaque can be composed of nonspecific bacteria or bacterial products that reach a level and duration of injury sufficient to cause destructive periodontal disease, or it could involve immune responses, wherein plaque would be the source of antigens that continuously challenge the gingiva. In the second concept, periodontitis would develop, for example, at some time in response to specific microorganisms or when a systemic modifying factor adversely affected the normal protective mechanisms of the host in the presence of specific bacteria. The possibility of either or both mechanisms being involved in the pathogenesis of periodontitis is not precluded.

Although there is a rather predictable response of the gingiva to plaque injury—the development of chronic gingivitis, which may persist for long periods of time without progression to periodontitis—the transition from an established lesion or chronic gingivitis to an advanced lesion or periodontitis with bone loss and pocket formation is not predictable. However, on the basis of clinical and histologic evidence, gingivitis precedes the transition to periodontitis. The hallmark of the advanced lesion is the destruction of supporting structures (i.e., periodontal ligament and alveolar bone), and eventually tooth loss.

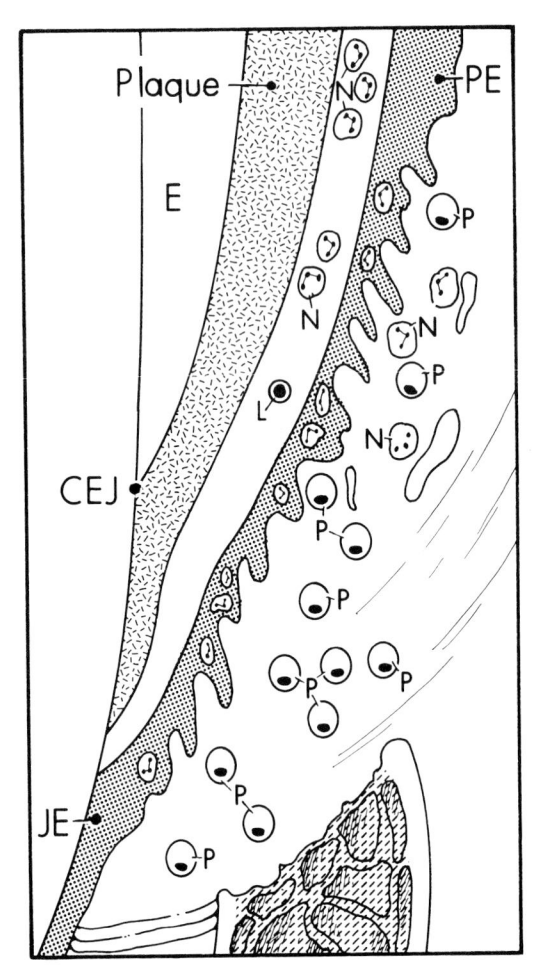

Fig. 13-26. *Schematic representation of periodontitis.* P, plasma cells; JE, junctional epithelium; L, lymphocytes; N, neutrophils; PE, pocket epithelium. Attachment is apical to CEJ (cementoenamel junction), the connective tissue fiber architecture has been replaced by granulation tissue or scar tissue, and the epithelial lining of the pocket shows ulceration and transmigration of neutrophils.

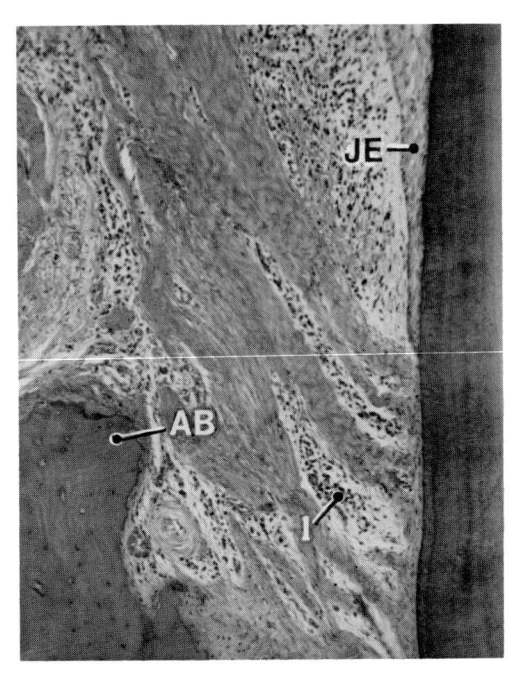

Fig. 13-27. Extension of inflammation into connective tissue with migration of junctional epithelium on the cementum. AB, alveolar bone; I, inflammatory infiltrate.

The characteristics that have been described for periodontitis (Fig. 13-25) include the presence of periodontal pockets; varying degrees of ulceration, suppuration, loss of gingival and periodontal fibers, gingival fibrosis, and fibrosis of the marrow spaces; and bone loss. Clinically there is a loss of attachment level; alterations in color, form, and density of the tissues, including varying degrees of hyperplasia and recession; bleeding with slight trauma; exudation, which may be frank pus; increased tooth mobility and drifting of teeth; and loss of teeth. The activity of the disease may not necessarily be reflected in the clinical characteristics, since they may only represent what is history, i.e., there is no assured method for determining whether the disease is active or not.

In periodontitis the inflammatory infiltrate is no longer related to the tissues subjacent to the base of the gingival crevice, as in gingivitis, but extends apically and laterally to form a band around the teeth. The junctional epithelium is located apical to the cementoenamel junction (Fig. 13-26), and strands of pocket epithelium extend apically into the connective tissues and apically along the root surface (Fig. 13-27). The junctional epithelium forms the base of the periodontal pocket and is attached to the root surface (Fig. 13-28). Plaque and

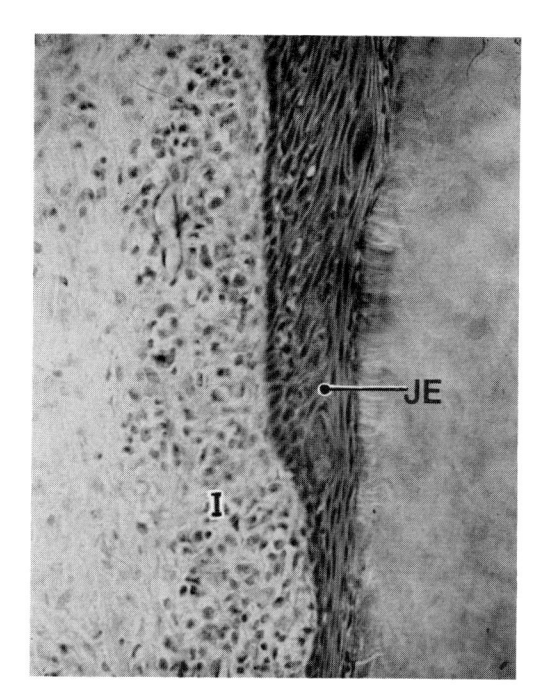

Fig. 13–28. Alteration of junctional epithelium (JE) and associated infiltration of inflammatory cells, mostly plasma cells.

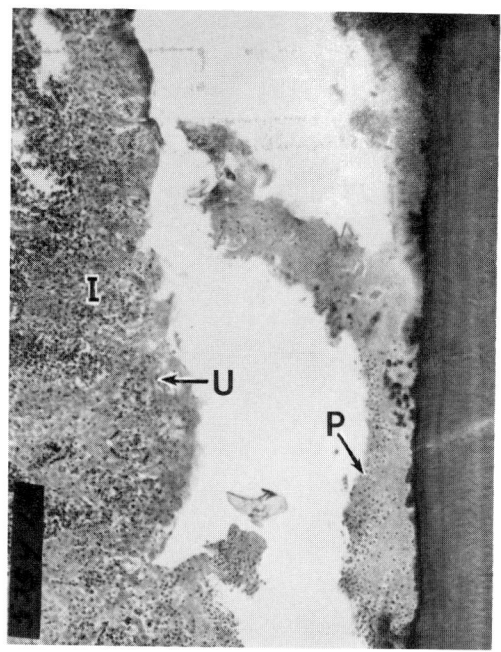

Fig. 13–29. *Plaque on root surface.* U, ulcerated pocket epithelium; I, polymorphonuclear leukocyte infiltration.

calculus are also present on the root surface (Fig. 13–29).

The normal architecture of the structural components of the gingival tissues is altered, and collagen destruction in the zone of dense inflammatory infiltration is almost complete, but fibrosis may be present in the adjacent areas. Although the fiber bundles of the gingiva are disorganized and lost, the transseptal fiber bundles are continuously regenerated in advance of the lesion or represent the residual collagen fibers that transverse the alveolar bone. The transseptal fibers remain in the presence of bone loss and appear to separate the inflammatory infiltrate from the remaining alveolar bone.

Bone resorption appears to be related to extensions of the inflammatory infiltrate around the blood vessels that enter the alveolar crest and to a lesser extent those that involve the periodontal membrane and periosteum. With the loss of alveolar bone proper, fibrosis of the marrow occurs, The resorption of bone is mediated by osteoclasts. Figure 13–30 summarizes the histologic changes in the transition from gingivitis to periodontitis.

It has become evident that periods of acute exacerbation of the disease may occur. With periods of quiescence and active destructive disease, the histologic appearance of the lesion may vary considerably. During an acute exacerbation, frank pus may be a prominent feature of the crevicular exudate; however, there is little evidence of tissue necrosis except in the presence of an abscess.

Often overlooked in histopathologic evaluations is the reparative phase of the inflammatory process. Granulation tissue, fibrosis, and scar tissue relate to repair and are important aspects of the host response to injury. The virtual absence of pain in the development is related to the nature of the tissue changes present.

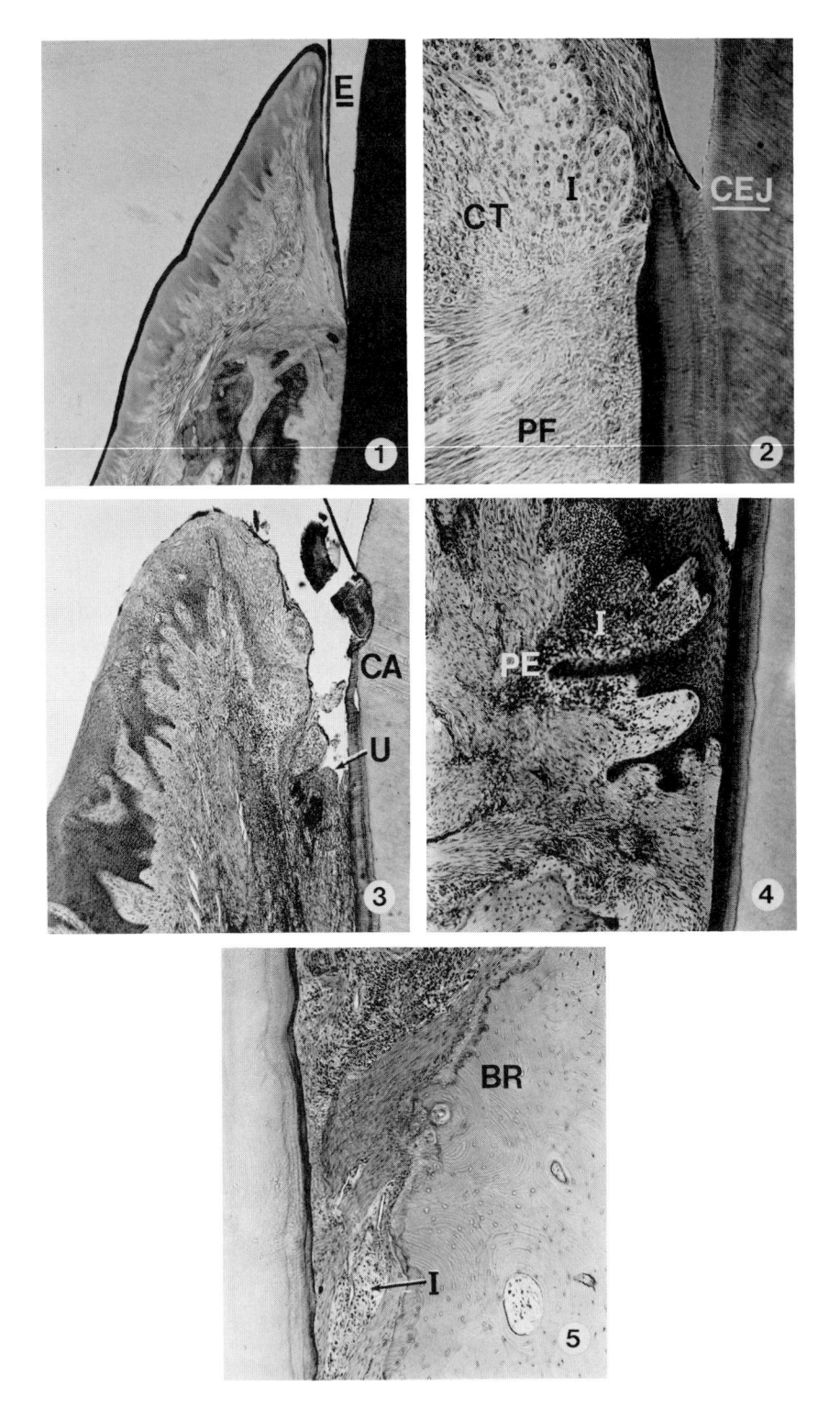

Fig. 13-30. *Progress of periodontitis.* (1) Normal gingival attachment (E) enamel space; (2) Inflammatory infiltration at cementoenamel junction (CEJ) with lateral proliferation of junctional epithelium; (3) Apical migration of attachment onto cementum, calculus (CA) present on nick in root surface below CEJ, ulceration of pocket epithelium (U), and heavy infiltration of inflammatory cells (active chronic inflammation); (4) Proliferating pocket epithelium (PE), heavy plasma cell infiltration, and loss of alveolar bone (AB); (5) Resorption of alveolar bone (RAB) and inflammatory cell response in the periodontal ligament apical to the alveolar bone crest.

Table 13-3. Classification
of Periodontal Diseases

Gingivitis
  Simple—No adverse systemic factors
  Complex—Modifying factors present
    Hyperplastic gingivitis
    Necrotizing ulcerative gingivitis
  Traumatic
Gingival Recession/Atrophy
Trauma from Occlusion
Periodontitis
  Simple—No adverse systemic factors
  Complex—Modifying factors present
    juvenile periodontitis, diabetes,
    vitamin C deficiency, etc.

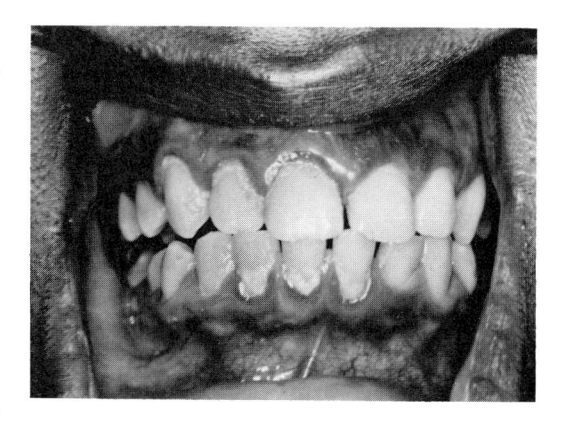

Fig. 13-31. *Simple hyperplastic gingivitis* associated with bacterial plaque.

CLASSIFICATION OF PERIODONTAL DISEASES

A classification of periodontal diseases given in Table 13–3 does suggest that most periodontal diseases are caused by bacterial plaque. However, to exclude other types of periodontal diseases from a classification would fail to recognize the significant incidence of direct injury to the gingiva by chemicals, heat, drugs, improper toothbrushing, and other trauma.

GINGIVITIS

Gingivitis is an inflammatory response of the gingiva primarily to bacterial plaque. Gingivitis may also occur in response to chemical, thermal, and mechanical injury and infrequently in response to allergenic agents (contact sensitivity). Gingival hyperplasia, gingival ulceration, and other alterations in color, form, bleeding, and crevice depth occur, but loss of attachment and bone are excluded in the gingivitis category. Gingivitis is present in periodontitis.

Simple Gingivitis

Simple gingivitis is a plaque-induced inflammation which begins at the dentogingival margins and interdental papillae (Fig. 13–31). It may begin at first in localized areas of plaque and calculus formation and spread to all areas of the mouth. Gingivitis increases in prevalence and severity with age and occurs at all ages. The transition from gingivitis to chronic destructive periodontitis does not occur invariably but is unpredictable, and therefore the significance of its treatment is obvious. Plaque-induced gingivitis can be prevented and treated effectively by control of bacterial plaque.

Complex Gingivitis

Complex gingivitis refers to forms of gingivitis in which local and/or systemic factors significantly influence the inflammatory response and/or response of the tissues to treatment.

Hyperplastic Gingivitis

Gingival hyperplasia includes gingival enlargement due to an increase in cellular elements, fibrous tissue, inflammatory cells, and blood vessels. Included in this category are mouthbreather's gingivitis, hereditary gingivofibromatosis, dilantin gingivitis, pregnancy gingivitis, and leukemic gingivitis.

Mouthbreather's gingivitis refers to an inflammatory hyperplasia of the labial gingiva of the anterior teeth (Fig. 13–14) associated with chronic mouthbreathing. The constant drying of the gingiva, especially in relation to anterior malocclusion and a "short lip line", may be the exciting factor although the exact mechanism of gingival injury is

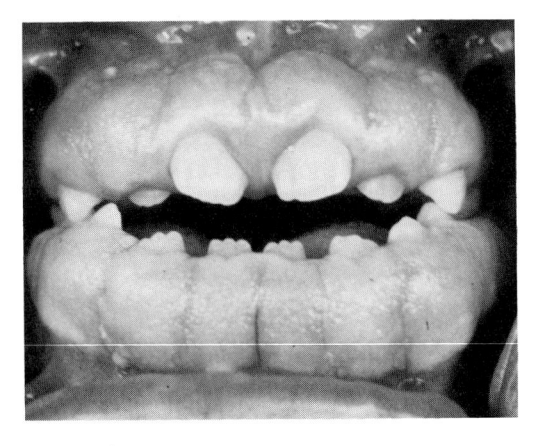

Fig. 13–32. *Hereditary gingival fibromatosis.*

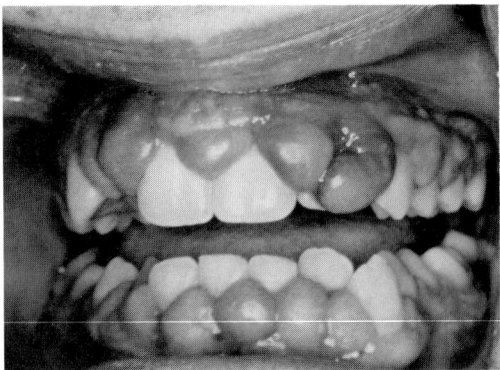

Fig. 13–33. *Dilantin gingivitis.*

not known. Control is related to elimination of hyperplastic gingiva (sometimes surgical), correction of malocclusion, and correction of the mouthbreathing habit.

Hereditary gingival fibromatosis is a rare gingival disease sometimes called elephantiasis gingivae and other descriptive names pointing out the severity of the gingival enlargement (Fig. 13–32). In instances there is a convincing history of family association and relationship to a hereditary anomaly transmitted by a dominant autosomal gene. The response of the tissues is dense fibrous enlargement rather than soft, edematous enlargement usually found in other forms of gingival enlargement. Inflammation is usually confined to the gingival crevice. The clinical and histologic features are not unique. Differentiation from dilantin hyperplasia is based solely on use of the drug for treatment of seizures. Surgical removal of the hyperplastic tissues may be necessary and bacterial plaque control appears to be essential for prevention, although the evidence for success is limited.

Dilantin gingivitis occurs in 40 to 50% of the patients taking phenytoin (Diphenylhydantoin sodium) for control of seizures (epilepsy). There is a significant correlation between the degree of hyperplasia and level of bacterial plaque. The diagnosis is based on a knowledge of the patient's use of the drug. Control of plaque is essential, but may be difficult for the patient. Surgical removal of redundant tissue is often necessary (Fig. 13–33). The mechanisms underlying connective tissue changes following the use of dilantin are not entirely clear. Clinically and histologically the appearance of the tissues is nonspecific and cannot be differentiated from that seen in simple hyperplastic gingivitis.

Pregnancy gingivitis is a term used to describe gingivitis aggravated by systemic factors during pregnancy (Fig. 13–34). It has been reported to be associated with *Bacteroides intermedius* and metabolic changes directly or indirectly related to the state of pregnancy. Under appropriate plaque control pregnancy gingivitis is not generally seen. Hormonal contraceptives

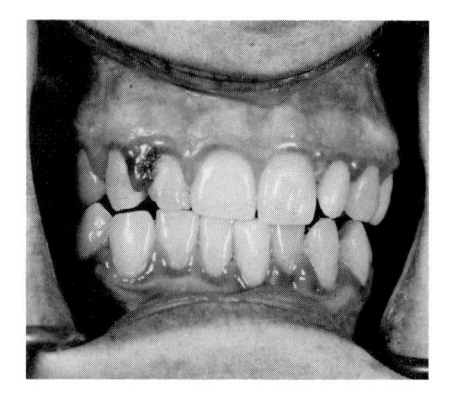

Fig. 13–34. Pregnancy gingivitis and granuloma pyogenicum (pregnancy tumor).

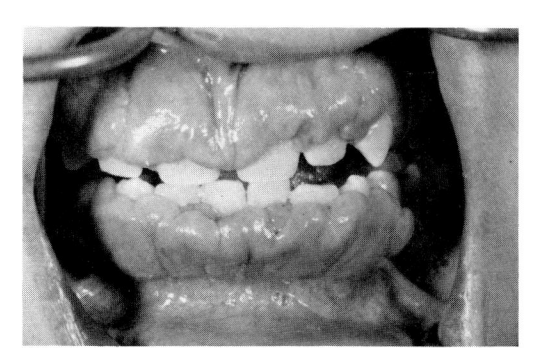

Fig. 13-35. Hyperplastic gingivitis associated with monocytic leukemia.

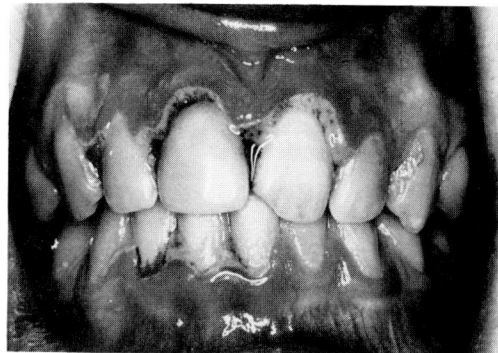

Fig. 13-36. *Ulcerative necrotizing gingivitis* (NUG). Note pseudomembrane covering area of necrotic tissue involving the free gingival margin of the maxillary central incisors.

may also induce gingival hyperplasia and easy bleeding on slight manipulation of the tissues. The clinical and histologic appearance of the gingiva demonstrates only nonspecific inflammatory hyperplasia, a positive history of pregnancy, or use of contraceptive drugs as prerequisites for the differential diagnosis of pregnancy gingivitis. Gingival changes respond to removal of bacterial plaque. The presence of localized gingival enlargement or so-called "pregnancy tumor" (p. 97) may require surgical removal.

Leukemic gingivitis is an inflammatory gingival hyperplasia associated with acute leukemias (Fig. 13-35), mainly monocytic and the acute myelogenous leukemias. The inflammatory response to bacteria is defective, possibly related to a lack of functional leukocytes. Histologically, there is a dense infiltration of immature leukocytes. Clinically, the tissues may be confused with secondary necrotizing ulcerative gingivitis. A history and blood studies are required to make the diagnosis. Treatment is palliative and control of plaque essential.

Necrotizing Ulcerative Gingivitis (NUG)

Necrotizing ulcerative gingivitis (Vincent's infection, Plaut-Vincent disease, trench mouth) is an acute localized or generalized gingivitis (Fig. 13-36) characterized by pseudomembranous ulceration of the free gingival margin and interdental papillae, formation of a pseudomembrane covering the ulcerated necrotic tissues, distinctive fetid odor of the tissues, bleeding of the gingiva that occurs so readily as to be called spontaneous, extremely painful gingival tissues, and interproximal cratering. Fever, malaise and lymphadenopathy are not consistent features of NUG.

Two species of bacteria, *Barrelia vincentii* (a spirochete) and *Bacillus vincentii* (a fusiform), have been implicated as the causative organisms in NUG as described by Vincent in 1882. More recently other bacteria, Bacteroides intermedius, as well as intermediate-sized spirochetes, have been implicated, but the general fusiform-spirochete character of the disease still remains valid.

Recurrent episodes of the disease (recurrent NUG) are sometimes referred to as chronic NUG; however, such episodes reflect an acute disease process with intercellular coagulation necrosis and pseudomembrane formation. NUG may involve one or two teeth or all the teeth (Fig. 13-37) and in a few instances may be found in other than the gingiva (Vincent's angina).

The histologic appearance of NUG is a fairly well demarcated necrotic ulcer covered by a fibrinous membrane incorporating dead cells, nuclear cell debris, numerous dead, dying, and living polymorphonuclear cells, plus a large number of

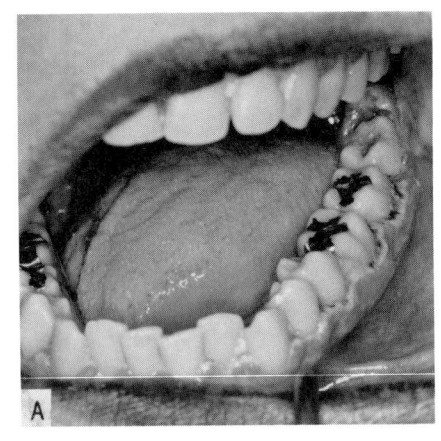

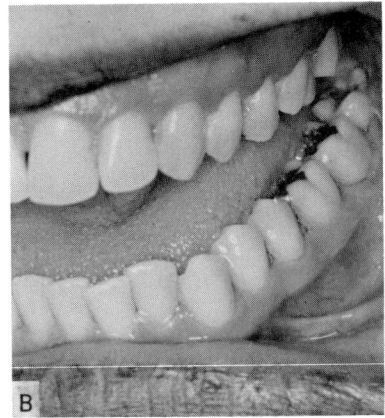

Fig. 13-37. A, Generalized acute ulcerative necrotizing gingivitis. B, After treatment.

bacteria, with a preponderance of fusiforms and spirochetes, but a variety of other organisms as well. The lesion is nonspecific and with light microscopy cannot be differentiated from a chemical or thermal burn. Bacteria have been observed within the tissues in the NUG lesions by both light and electron microscopy. The deepest penetration, extending for several cell layers into living connective tissue and epithelium, is by spirochetes. However, this penetration does not necessarily indicate that the spirochetes are the cause of the lesion. Gingival tissues with impaired microcirculation may undergo necrobiotic changes, and once the initial defense mechanisms of the tissues have been impaired, bacterial invasion may occur, with the deepest penetration by the most motile organisms rather than selective penetration by the organisms with the greatest potential for tissue destruction.

The epidemiology of NUG suggests that the incidence of NUG in Western countries has significantly decreased, perhaps related to the widespread use of antibiotics and improved oral hygiene. Predisposing factors which have been suggested are stress and heavy smoking. Stress has been implicated in the reduction of PMN phagocytosis and chemotoxis and attendant increases in cortisol and catecholamine levels which relate to relative ischemia of the tissues. Such factors are difficult to establish convincingly. The disease is not communicable, but occurs more frequently in individuals living under the same stressful conditions where oral hygiene and systemic defenses are less than optimal and "opportunistic" pathogens in the normal flora prevail.

The conditions under which NUG occurs appear to be increased bacterial virulence, decreased host resistance, and/or changes in oral hygiene. The role of specific microorganisms as initiating factors is difficult to establish, in part due to problems in culturing suspected pathogens individually. Although the several organisms cultured appear to be present in the ulcerative stage of NUG, sufficient evidence to demonstrate that these organisms *(Treponema, Bacteroides melaninogenicus ssp intermedius,* and *Fusobacterium)* initiate NUG has not been reported. Data showing appropriate and significant increases in antibody titers to putative causative organisms during the recovery phase are necessary to provide support for primary infection by one of these organisms.

Treatment of NUG is based on elimination of bacterial plaque and appropriate use of antibiotics when indicated. Recurrence of the disease occurs unless the dental plaque is removed, root surfaces scaled

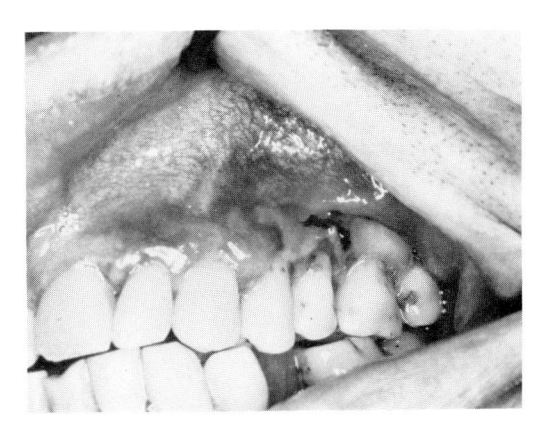

Fig. 13-38. *Chronic desquamative gingivitis.*

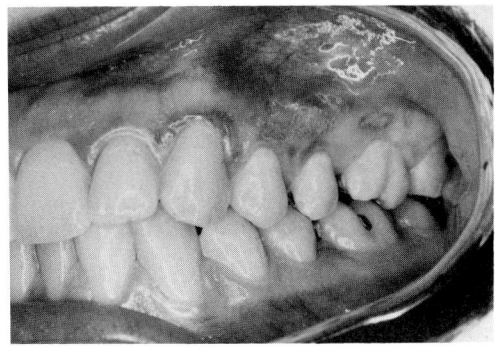

Fig. 13-39. *Toothbrush abrasion.*

and root planed, and good oral hygiene is maintained.

Chronic Desquamative Gingivitis

Chronic desquamative gingivitis (Fig. 13-38) is a term used to describe primarily gingival manifestations of a variety of diseases, most frequently dermatoses such as benign mucous membrane pemphagoid, pemphigus, and erosive lichen planus. Hormonal influences are less clear and therefore the emphasis on "hormonal gingivitis" has been reduced, although this type of gingivitis seen alone on the gingiva (with or without teeth) appears predominantly in women in the menopausal age.

The clinical features of chronic desquamative gingivitis depend somewhat upon the nature of the dermatosis, but as a descriptive term no attempt is made to differentiate between them here. Periods of remission and exacerbations give rise to various clinical appearances of the gingiva. Varying degrees of severity may also be encountered. The patient's history usually indicates a gingivitis of long duration with remissions of short duration. Clinically, there is superficial desquamation of the epithelium and a tendency for the epithelium to become ulcerated easily (Fig. 13-38). Areas of pronounced desquamation of the epithelium and loss of stippling give the gingiva a somewhat patchy appearance. The color of the gingiva is generally reddish and the surface is smooth and glossy, especially in areas of active desquamation. Areas of erosion may be present leaving a painful, denuded, bleeding surface. Minor trauma, slight thermal change, and foods are not well tolerated. Patients with chronic desquamative gingivitis complain of a burning sensation in the mouth and extremely painful areas of the gingiva which have been denuded. Palliative treatment of chronic desquamative gingivitis is directed toward the removal of irritation and trauma. However, a complete remission of the disease cannot be obtained usually, and specific treatment depends on a definitive diagnosis.

Traumatic Gingivitis

Traumatic gingivitis refers to gingival inflammatory changes caused by trauma by dental appliances, food impaction, and occlusal impingement (e.g., impinging overbite). These factors have already been considered earlier (p. 206). Trauma to the gingiva may also occur with faulty oral hygiene practice and other habits (Fig. 13-39). Prolonged faulty toothbrushing is more likely to give the appearance of gingival atrophy than a pronounced inflammatory reaction to injury.

Gingival Atrophy/Recession

A generalized atrophy of the mucous membranes and skin is usually attendant with aging. Although such atrophic changes may reduce stippling resulting in a smooth glistening appearance of the gingiva, there appears to be no decreased resistance to bacterial plaque or increased gingival inflammation. Other changes which are not uncommon are an associated reduction of salivation, dry mouth, and mild burning of the mouth, including the gingiva, when attempting to eat relatively spicy, hot or cold foods. Although referred to as atrophic gingivitis, there is little evidence of inflammatory changes.

Gingivitis characterized by gingival recession excessive for the age of the individual is also referred to as atrophic gingivitis, although gingivitis may not be present or related to the plaque present (Fig. 13–40). Young adults with little plaque and extensive recession sometimes appear to have large teeth and small alveolar base bone, i.e., a discrepancy between jaw size and tooth size, which are both genetically determined. These patients may reflect the earlier age of the *atrophic gingivitis* seen in older people. Recession associated with toothbrushing and root caries may complicate the diagnosis and treatment of gingival atrophy.

TRAUMA FROM OCCLUSION

Trauma from occlusion has been mentioned earlier in relation to the classification of periodontal diseases (p. 219). Progressive trauma from occlusion may in advanced periodontal disease accelerate tooth loss and complicate periodontal therapy. Continued discomfort, increased tooth mobility, and progressive loss of supporting structures may make treatment ineffective and unpredictable. Although the role of trauma from occlusion is still controversial in the pathogenesis of periodontal disease, control of increasing mobile, and sometimes painful teeth, requires appropriate occlusal therapy (Fig. 13–41). Appropriate therapy may effectively control progressive trauma so that progressive trauma, expressed as increased mobility, becomes self-limited.

PERIODONTITIS

The classification of periodontal diseases which has been considered (p. 219) suggests simple and complex categories to reflect significant differences between bacterial plaque-induced disease *without* apparent systemic and local modifying factors (simple) and disease *with* systemic and local factors present which adversely influence the defenses of the host. In this context, *adult periodontitis* or chronic destructive periodontitis fits into the category of *simple periodontitis* because it is consid-

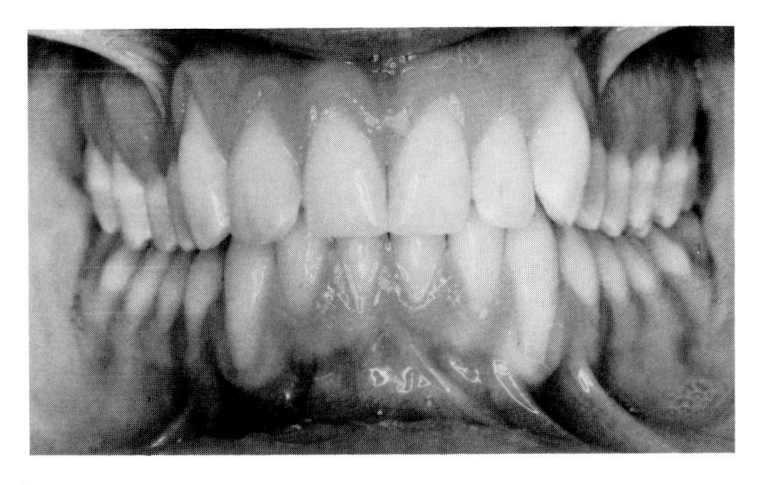

Fig. 13–40. *Gingival recession.*

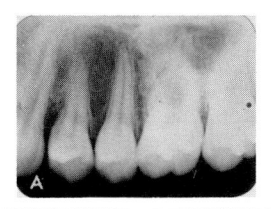

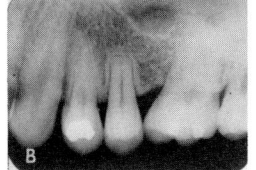

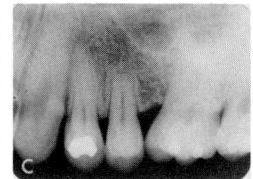

Fig. 13–41. *Trauma from occlusion.* A, Radiograph of premolars prior to placement of restoration; B, Radiograph taken 2 weeks later because patient complained of sore teeth. Note root resorption; C, Radiograph taken 6 months after occlusal adjustment.

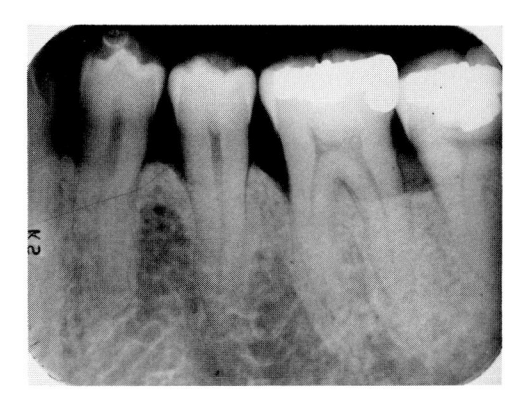

Fig. 13–42. Intra-intrabony pockets verified by clinical probing.

ered to be a continuation of simple gingivitis and therefore a part of the gingivitis-adult periodontitis axis. Of course any type of gingivitis may lead to, or be seen prior to, or be associated with, any kind of periodontitis. In the context of *complex periodontitis,* destructive periodontal disease in young individuals will be considered. Included in this category are *juvenile periodontitis* and *early onset periodontitis.*

Chronic Destructive Periodontal Disease in the Adult

The development of chronic destructive periodontal disease in the adult is generally slow, but progressive, often dependent upon the level of oral hygiene of the individual and systemic factors to account for "bursts" of disease activity.

The clinical characteristics of chronic destructive periodontitis show gingival changes and plaque, and loss of supporting structures. On periodontal probing, there is a deepening of the gingival crevice and the attachment is present on cemental surfaces, i.e., periodontal pockets are present.

Radiographically there is a loss of bone, either generally (horizontal bone loss) involving several or all the teeth, or locally with vertical bone loss. In the latter, the attachment may be apical to the height of the alveolar crest (determined by probing) and is called an infra- or intrabony pocket (Fig. 13–42).

Loss of structures between the roots of the teeth so that pockets extend into bi- and trifurcation areas are spoken of as "furcation involvement" (Fig. 13–43).

When bone loss and trauma from occlusion is sufficient, there is increased mobility of the teeth. Finally, the loss of supporting structures may be so extensive as to require extraction of involved teeth (Fig. 13–44). Root surfaces show extensive uneven surface topography (Fig. 13–45). The sequelae of periodontitis also include the development of subgingival plaque and calculus and sometimes the formation of periodontal

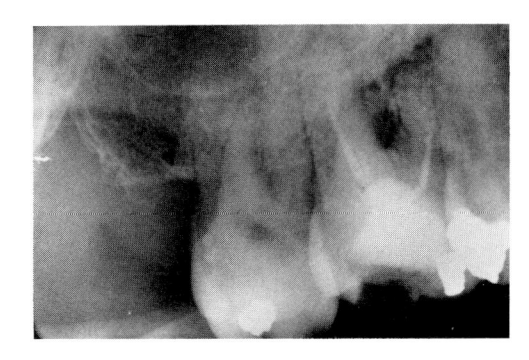

Fig. 13–43. *Trifurcation involvement with periodontitis.* Radiolucent areas and periodontal probing is needed to confirm the diagnosis.

abscesses as a consequence of foreign objects getting into the deepened crevices (Fig. 13–46).

Destructive Periodontal Disease in Young Individuals

Destructive periodontal disease may develop in individuals with systemic disease as well as those young people who are ostensibly healthy. On the basis of early onset, rapid progression, and to a certain extent the distribution of the lesions, several destructive forms of periodontal disease in apparently healthy young individuals (children, adolescents, young adults) have been provisionally identified. It should be recognized that young individuals having systemic diseases with compromised neutrophil or lymphocyte functions may also experience severe destruction of the periodontal tissues. The distinction between ostensibly well and diseased young individuals may reflect inadequate detection and a broad spectrum of disease manifestations.

Juvenile Periodontitis

Juvenile periodontitis is an uncommon disorder of the periodontium of otherwise healthy adolescents in which there is a severe loss of attachment and supporting bone around one or more of the permanent teeth. The clinical manifestations of the disease appear noticeably at early adolescence with involvement of the mesial or distal surfaces of one or more first permanent molars and additionally the incisors. The localized vertical bone loss and bifurcation involvement of maxillary and mandibular molars and additional involvement of inci-

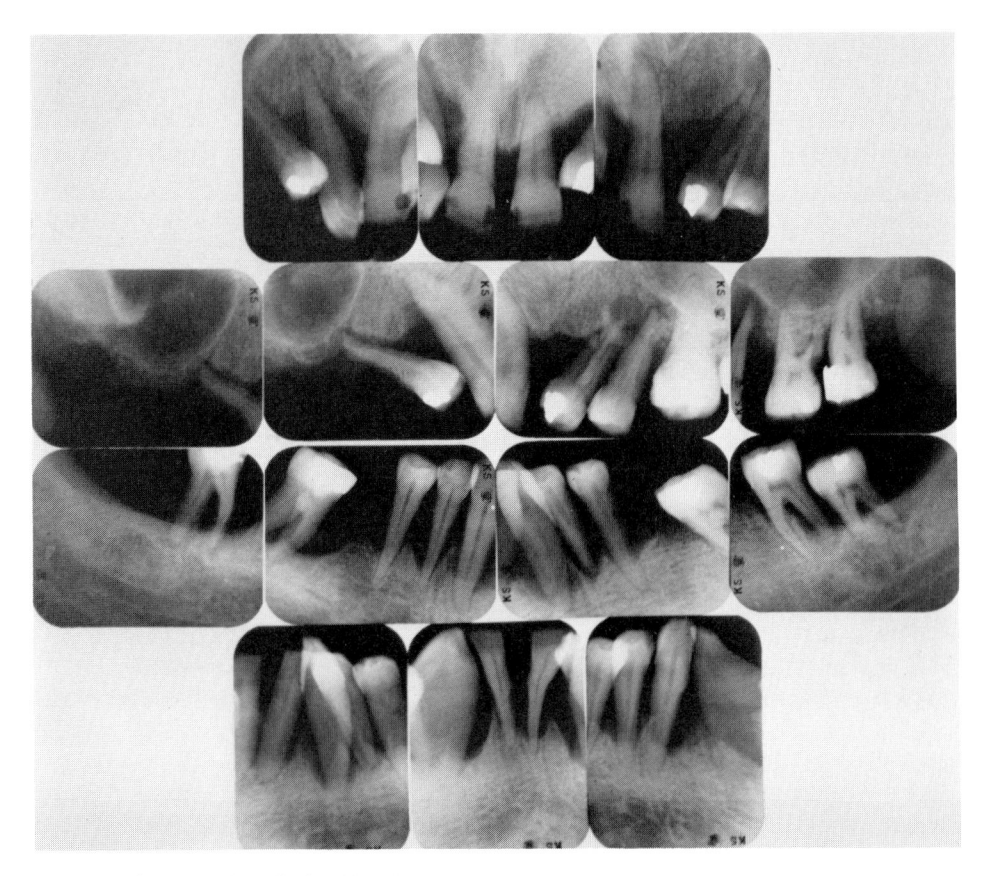

Fig. 13–44. Advanced periodontitis with potential loss of all the teeth.

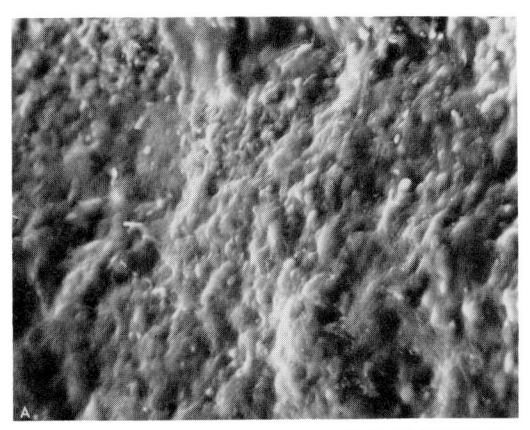

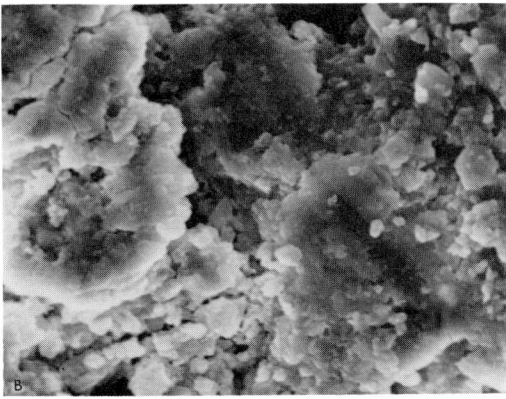

Fig. 13-45. Scanning electron microscopic appearance of a root surface. *A*, subgingival calculus with bacterial plaque present; *B*, subgingival calculus.

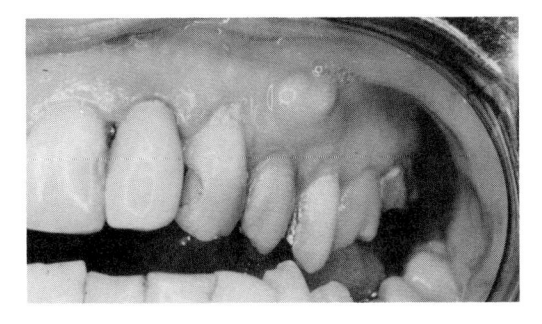

Fig. 13-46. Periodontal abscess above the roots of the cuspid and first premolar.

sors has suggested the term *localized juvenile periodontitis* (LJP). However, more generalized forms of juvenile periodontitis (JP) have been described and there is uncertainty whether LJP is a distinct entity or whether both the generalized and localized forms are manifestations of the same disease.

The prevalence of LJP varies considerably, perhaps because of the absence of adequate criteria. But even with the inclusion of debatable cases, the occurrence of the disorder is considered to be relatively rare, about 0.1% of adolescents. The prevalence of LJP appears to be somewhat greater in females than males, but epidemiologic studies do not substantiate this clinical impression.

Although a decreased chemotactic response of neutrophils (p. 65) and an altered immune response have been suggested as associated etiologic factors, there is increasing evidence that such mechanisms do not have the primary role in the etiology and pathogenesis of juvenile periodontitis. Rather, the evidence speaks for the hereditary nature of the disease involving an autosomal recessive (p. 16) mode of inheritance with full penetrance. Therefore, it is unlikely that there is an association between juvenile periodontitis and HLA (p. 78). Also it has not been shown that inheritance of juvenile periodontitis is linked with the major histocompatibility antigens, i.e., no immunogenetic basis for the disease exists.

Juvenile periodontitis is considered to be a reaction to injury (inflammation) and possibly associated with specific bacteria—Actinobacillus actinomycetemcomitans (A.a.) and Capnocytophaga species. Several factors possessed by A.a. could exert a direct effect, including epitheliotoxin, bone-resorbing toxin, a collagenase, and a fibroblast-inhibiting factor. Some strains are capable of producing leukotoxin which kills neutrophils.

It has been suggested that the susceptibility to juvenile periodontitis is genetically determined in neutrophil function and that because of a functional defect in the neutrophil, the host's defenses are compromised to the point that A.a. is allowed to establish itself in the gingival sulcus. These organisms as well as other anaerobic gram-negative microorganisms do not release chemotactic factors, but produce substances which are capable of inhibiting neutrophil chemotaxis (p. 65). Therefore, bacteria which are capable of inhibiting the function of neutrophils which already have an intrinsic defect could be expected to have a selective advantage in colonizing the host. Even so, the etiology and pathogenesis of juvenile periodontitis is not clear. Treatment of the disease utilizes a repeating regimen of tetracycline therapy and surgical/non-surgical procedures. Re-establishment of A. actinomycetemcomitans is associated with a recurrence of the disease. The continued use of antibiotics has severe limitations because of the possible development of resistant strains (p. 153).

Early Periodontitis

The loss of attachment and bone on one or more surfaces of the teeth (usually only one or two sites) in adolescents or young adults that are otherwise well, is referred to as early periodontitis. The diagnosis is dependent upon careful probing of the gingival crevice and radiographic evaluation. It is not unusual to find 1 to 2 mm of loss of attachment on the proximal surfaces of first molars and incisors even in adolescents where oral hygiene and professional care is limited.

Cyclic Neutropenia

Cyclic neutropenia is a form of agranulocytosis which occurs in a rhythmic pattern. The polymorphonuclear leukocyte count is low for a short period of time and the severe infection seen in prolonged forms of agranulocytosis is not usually present. However, severe forms of gingivitis and periodontitis are seen (Fig. 13–47), especially in adolescents and prepubertal children. Professional periodontal care and use of antibiotics is helpful, but there is no specific treatment for the cause of the disease.

Chédiak-Higashi Syndrome

The Chédiak-Higashi syndrome is a genetic disease transmitted as an autosomal recessive trait (p. 16). The clinical features include albinisms, photophobia, and recurrent infections. Destructive periodontitis related to neutrophil dysfunction occurs, as well as ulcerations of the mucosa and tongue. The disease is often fatal in early life. There is no specific treatment for the disease, but professional periodontal care and antibiotic therapy are helpful.

Papillon-Lefèvre Syndrome

Papillon-Lefèvre syndrome is characterized by severe destructive periodontal disease (Fig. 13–48) which may involve both primary and permanent dentitions. Skin lesions consist of keratosis of the palmar and plantar surfaces, but are not always obvious. It appears to be inherited as an autosomal recessive disease. There is a neutrophil disorder, possibly a defect in locomotion. Periodontal professional care and plaque control are helpful.

Down's Syndrome

Down's syndrome is found in individuals with an extra autosomal gene (p. 17). Severe destructive periodontitis is often present, possibly due to reduced neutrophil phagocytosis. Professional periodontal care and control of plaque is necessary.

PREVENTION OF PERIODONTAL DISEASES

The prevention of gingivitis can be accomplished through the control of bacterial plaque by simple mechanical and chemical methods. Accumulating evidence suggests that gingivitis is the precursor of chronic destructive periodontal disease and that control of plaque by these methods can control and prevent, to a significant degree

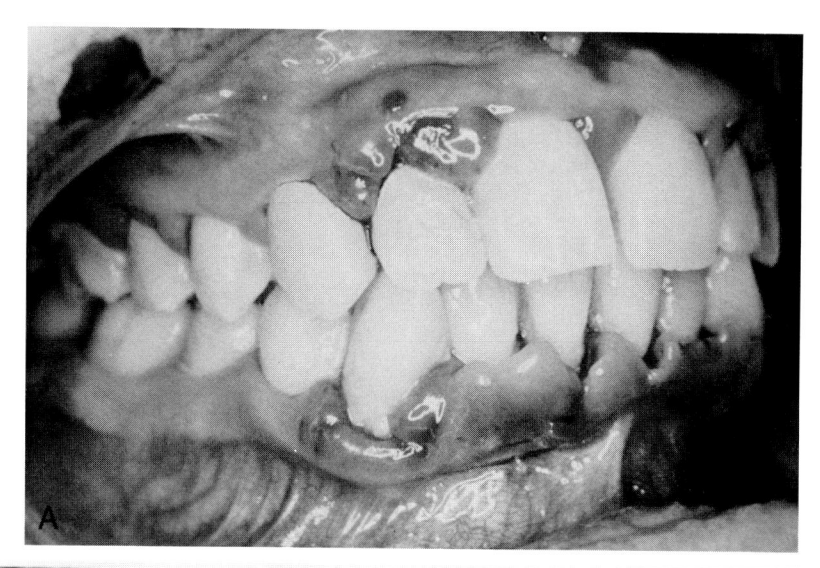

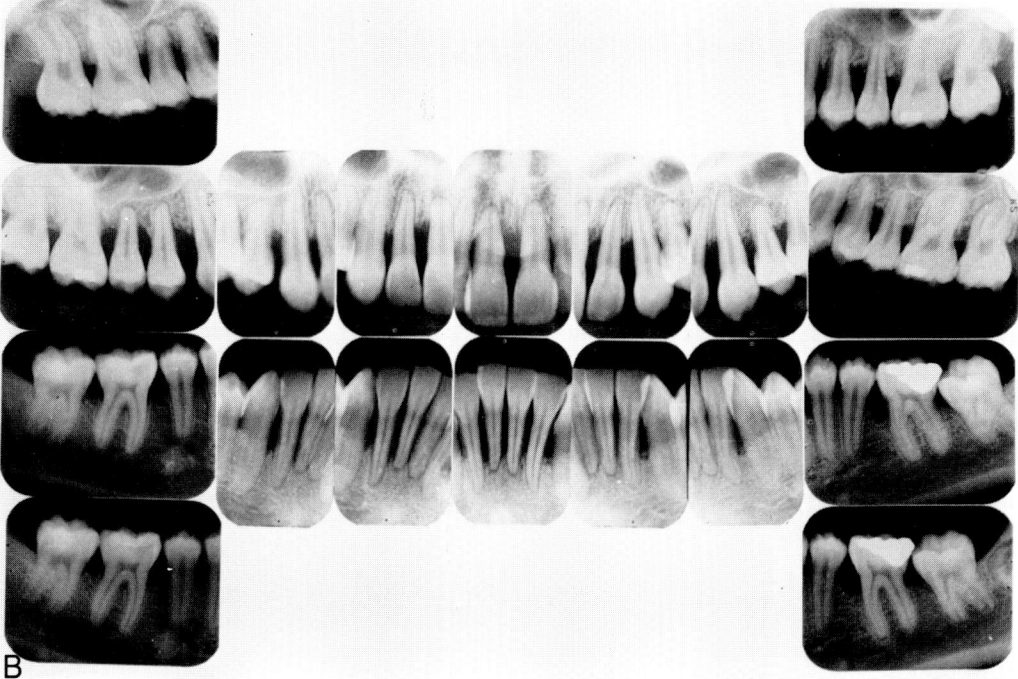

Fig. 13–47. Periodontitis associated with cyclic neutropenia. *A*, Radiographs showing extensive bone loss in 14-year-old girl; *B*, gingival tissues are soft, edematous, and do not respond well to subgingival scaling.

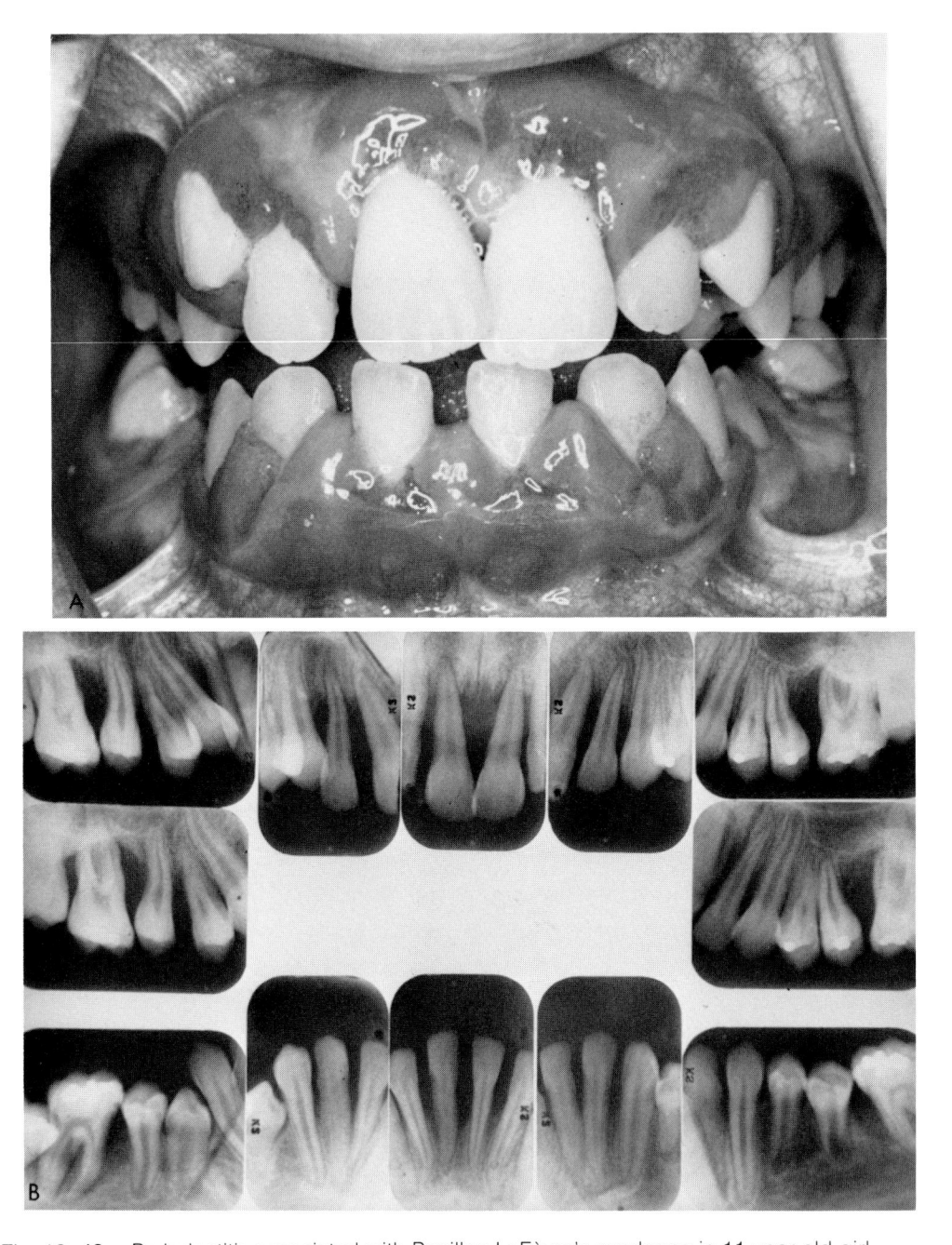

Fig. 13–48. Periodontitis associated with Papillon-LeFèvre's syndrome in 11-year-old girl.

in individual patients and populations, chronic gingivitis and slow progressive adult periodontitis, i.e., those periodontal diseases which constitute the major quantitative dental care problem. The concept of immunization for juvenile periodontitis appears warranted, but there are a number of reasons for doubting whether such a disease can be controlled by immune responses. However, with the development of precise criteria for assessing disease activity and identifying patients at risk, preventive methods may become more specific.

SUMMARY

The main response of the periodontium to injury by plaque microorganisms and their products is inflammation. The characteristics of the inflammatory response depend upon the nature of the injury and the modification of the response by intrinsic or systemic factors. The nature of the dentogingival complex (Fig. 13–49) and the supporting structures is unique and has special defensive needs against bacterial plaque.

Age or aging has not been demonstrated to modify the inflammatory response, nor do stress and psychologic factors appear to directly modify the responses of the host to dental plaque. A correlation between necrotizing ulcerative gingivitis and stress has yet to be clarified.

Several systemic diseases appear to influence the response of the host to local irritants, including leukemia, neutropenia, Chédiak-Higashi syndrome, diabetes mellitus, and Down's syndrome. Although the importance of the direct effects of dental plaque (enzymes, toxins, etc.) on the initiation of gingivitis is supported by a convincing body of evidence, the significance of systemic factors in modifying the inflammatory response has not been clearly demonstrated for chronic destructive periodontal disease.

Bacterial plaque is considered to be the primary etiologic exciting factor in gingivitis and periodontitis, and may be a focus of B-

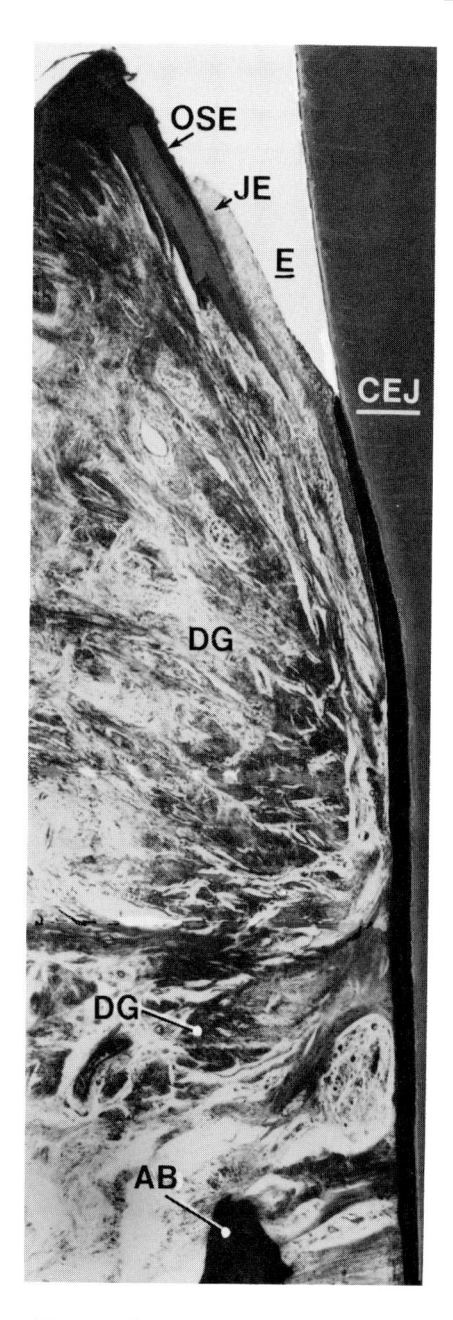

Fig. 13–49. Histologic features of periodontium. OSE, oral sulcular epithelium. JE, junctional epithelium. E, enamel space. CEJ, cementoenamel junction. DG, dentogingival connective tissue fibers. AB, alveolar bone crest.

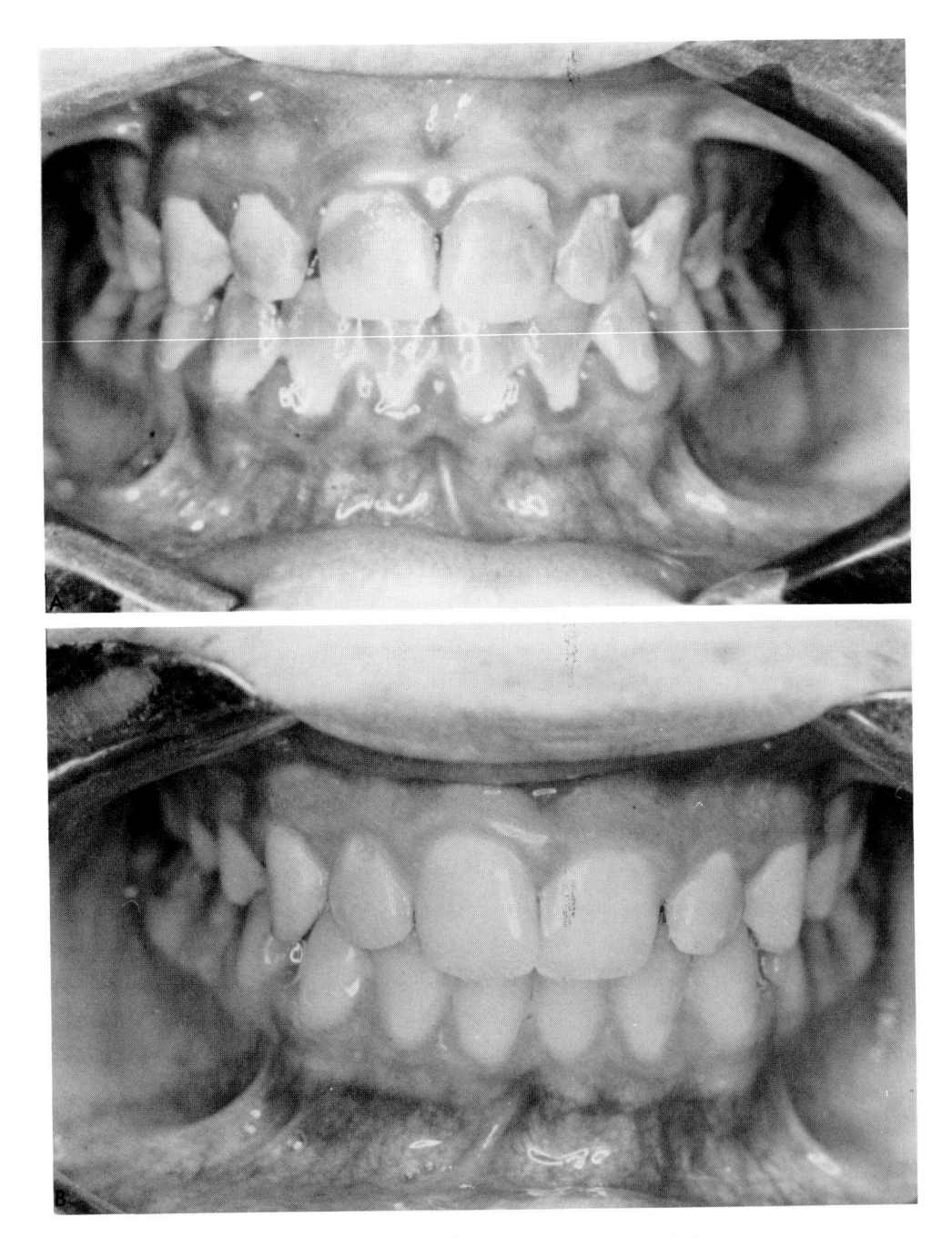

Fig. 13–50. *A*, Gingivitis related to plaque. *B*, Resolution of gingivitis following professional care and home care maintenance of oral hygiene.

cell mitogens and T-cell antigens, which modulate immune responses. Several mechanisms have been implicated in the loss of periodontal supporting structures, including phagocytosis by macrophages, enzymatic activity, lysosomal action, bacterial products, and the complement system.

Host responses to bacterial plaque include immuno-inflammatory reactions which are protective and potentially destructive. But it would be incorrect to assume that immune responses are not under control simply on the basis of their potential to cause destruction. Since inflammation and immunity are physiologic defense mechanisms rather than undesirable responses of pathologic destructive processes, their presence does not indicate a cause and effect relationship between inflammation and destructive periodontal disease.

The initial gingival lesion of gingivitis is an acute inflammation with lymphoid cell infiltration subsequently becoming superimposed upon the acute inflammatory reaction. Although the early gingival lesion which occurs during the first week of experimental gingivitis exhibits some of the morphologic features of a delayed hypersensitivity reaction, these features are only transient. Within 2 or 3 weeks, plasma cells and granulocytes continue to dominate the lesion throughout its course. The early lesion, seen 4 to 7 days after plaque accumulation, has features of the initial gingival lesion, i.e., altered fibroblasts, collagen loss, and an inflammatory infiltrate, 75% of which are lymphocytes. In the established lesion, there is continued loss of collagen, plasma cell infiltration at the bottom of the crevice, and perivascular infiltration. In the advanced lesion, there is further collagen loss, osteoclastic activity, and presence of plasma cells, lymphocytes, and macrophages. These features are considered to be consistent with, but not indicative of, immune complex disease and cell-mediated immunity.

Models constructed to demonstrate the potential relationship between immune responses and periodontal disease must of necessity—for want of sufficient information—remain largely conjectural at this time. It would not be surprising if some elements of an immune response complex involved in inflammation were inadequately controlled and led to destruction rather than protection. However, there is no convincing body of evidence that immune responses initiate periodontal disease (e.g., autoimmune disease). Immuno-inflammation is a manifestation of defense mechanisms that contribute to the homeostasis of the host. Alterations in neutrophil function and/or number appear to be significant factors in how well the host responds to bacterial plaque and play a significant role in the pathogenesis of plaque induced periodontal diseases.

The prevention and treatment of periodontal diseases is accomplished to a significant degree through the control of bacterial plaque by professional care and appropriate home care procedures (Fig. 13–50).

BIBLIOGRAPHY

Alexander, A.G.: Habitual mouthbreathing and its effects on gingival health. Parodontologie, 24:49, 1970.

Ash, M.M., Gitlin, B.N., and Smith, W.A.: Correlation between plaque and gingivitis. J. Periodontol., 35:5, 1964.

Axelsson, P., and Lindhe, J.: The effect of a preventive programme on dental plaque, gingivitis and caries in school children. Results after one and two years. J. Clin. Periodont., 1:126, 1974.

Baer, P.N.: The case for periodontosis as a clinical entity. J. Periodontol., 42:516, 1971.

Bissada, N.F., et al.: Neutrophil functional activities in juvenile and adult onset diabetic patients with mild and severe periodontitis. J. Periodont. Res., 17:500, 1982.

Caffesse, R.G., and Nasjleti, C.E.: Enzymatic penetration through intact sulcular epithelium. J. Periodontol., 47:391, 1976.

Cahn, L.R.: The penetration of the tissue of Vincent's organisms. J. Dent. Res., 9:695, 1929.

Carranza, F.A., and Kenney, E.B.: *Prevention of Periodontal Disease*. Chicago, Quintessence Publ. Co., 1981.

Cimasoni, G.: *Crevicular Fluid Updated,* Basel, Karger, 1983.

Courtley, R.L.: Vincent's infection. Br. Dent. J., 74:34, 1943.

Davies, R.M., et al.: Destructive forms of periodontal disease in adolescents and young adults. Br. Dent. J., 158:429, 1985.

Eichel, B., and Shahrich, H.A.: Tobacco smoke toxicity, loss of human oral leukocytic function and fluid cell metabolism. Science, 166:1424, 1969.

El-Ashiry, G.M., et al.: Comparative study of the influence of pregnancy and oral contraceptives on the gingivae. Oral Surg., 30:472, 1970.

Emerson, T.G.: Hereditary gingival hyperplasia. A family pedigree of four generations. Oral Surg., 19:1, 1965.

Genco, R.J., and Slots, J.: Host responses in periodontal diseases. J. Dent. Res., 63:441, 1984.

Glickman, I., and Lewitus, M.: Hyperplasia of the gingiva associated with Dilantin (sodium diphenylhydantoinate) therapy. J.A.D.A., 28:199, 1941.

Gorman, N.J.: Prevalence and etiology of gingival recession. J. Periodont., 38:316, 1967.

Hall, W.B.: Dilantin hyperplasia, a preventable disease. J. Periodont. Res., Suppl. 4:36, 1969.

Heijl, L., Rifkin, B.R., and Zander, H.A.: Conversion of chronic gingivitis to periodontitis in squirrel monkeys. J. Periodontol., 47:710, 1976.

Heylings, P.: Electron microscopy of acute ulcerative gingivitis (Vincent's type). Demonstration of the fusospirodental complex of bacteria within the pre-necrotic epithelium. Br. Dent. J., 122:51, 1967.

Horton, J.E., Oppenheim, J.J., and Mergenhagen, S.E.: A role for cell-mediated immunity in the pathogenesis of periodontal disease. J. Periodontol., 45:351, 1974.

Jacobson, L.: Mouthbreathing and gingivitis. J. Periodont. Res., 8:269, 1973.

Kenney, E.B., Saxe, S.R., and Bowles, R.D.: The effect of cigarette smoking on anaerobiosis in the oral cavity. J. Periodont., 46:82, 1976.

Lindhe, J., and Bjorn, A.-L.: Influence of hormonal contraceptives on the gingiva of women. J. Periodont. Res., 2:1, 1967.

Listgarten, M.A., and Lewis, D.W.: The distribution of spirochetes in the lesion of acute necrotizing ulcerative gingivitis: an electron microscopic and statistical survey. J. Periodontol., 38:379, 1967.

Lite, T., Dimaio, D.J., and Burman, L.R.: Gingival patterns in mouthbreathers. Oral Surg., 8:382, 1955.

Loe, H.: Closing Remarks: Microbial and immunological aspects of oral diseases. J. Dent. Res., 63:476, 1984.

Loe, H.: Periodontal changes in pregnancy. J. Periodontol., 36:37, 1965.

Manor, A., et al.: Bacterial invasion of periodontal tissues in advanced periodontitis in humans. J. Periodontol., 55:567, 1984.

Manson, J.D., and Lehner, T.: Clinical features of juvenile periodontitis (periodontosis). J. Periodontol., 45:636, 1974.

McCarthy, F.P., McCarthy, P.L., and Shklar, G.: Chronic desquamative gingivitis: A reconsideration. Oral Surg., 13:1300, 1960.

McIndoe, A., and Smith, B.O.: Congenital familial fibromatosis of the gums with the teeth as a probable aetiologic factor. Br. J. Plast. Surg., 11:62, 1958.

O'Leary, T.J., et al.: The incidence of recession in young males: A further study. J. Periodontol., 42:264, 1971.

Page, R.C., and Schroeder, H.A.: Pathogenesis of inflammatory periodontal disease. A summary of current work. Lab. Invest., 33:235, 1976.

Pearlman, B.A.: An oral contraceptive drug and gingival enlargement; the relationship between local and systemic factors. J. Clin. Periodont., 1:47, 1974.

Pindborg, J.J.: Gingivitis in military personnel with special reference to ulceromembranous gingivitis. Odont. Tidskr., 59:407, 1951.

Pittard, A.J.: Contribution of molecular biology to the understanding and control of microbial infections. J. Dent. Res., 63:374, 1984.

Ramfjord, S.P., and Ash, M.M.: *Periodontology and Periodontics*. Philadelphia, W.B. Saunders, 1979.

Ramfjord, S.P., Emslie, R.D., Greene, J.C., Held, A.J., and Waerhaug, J.: Epidemiological studies of periodontal diseases. Parodontologie, 2:109, 1968.

Ramfjord, S.P., Kerr, D.A., and Ash, M.M. (Eds.): *World Workshop in Periodontics*. Ann Arbor, The University of Michigan Press, 1966.

Roitt, I.M., and Lehner, T.: *Immunology of Oral Diseases*. Oxford, Blackwell Scientific Publications, 1980.

Rosan, B., and Wicken, A.J.: Workshop Report: Biologically active components of oral bacteria, particularly in relation to oral disease. J. Dent. Res., 63:472, 1984.

Saxen, L., et al.: Periodontal disease associated with Down's syndrome: an orthopantomy-

ographic evaluation. J. Periodontol., *48*:337, 1977.
Schluger, S.: Necrotizing ulcerative gingivitis in the army: Incidence, communicability, and treatment. J.A.D.A., *38*:174, 1949.
Schroeder, H.E.: Histopathology of the gingival sulcus. In T. Lehner (eds.), *The Borderland Between Caries and Periodontal Disease.* London, Academic Press, 1977.
Schroeder, H.E., and Attstrom, R.: Pocket formation: An hypothesis. In T. Lehner, and Cimasoni, G. (eds.), *The Borderland Between Caries and Periodontal Disease II.* London, Academic Press, 1980.
Seymour, G.J., and Mestecky, J.F.: Workshop Report: The Periodontium as a watershed between mucosal and systemic immunology. J. Dent. Res., *63*:474, 1984.
Shannon, I., Kilgore, W.G., and O'Leary, T.: Stress as a predisposing factor in ANUG. J. Periodontol., *48*:240, 1969.

Silness, J., and Loe, H.: Periodontal disease in pregnancy. II. Correlation between oral hygiene and periodontal condition. Acta Odont. Scand., *22*:121, 1964.
Sims, W.: Streptococcus mutans and vaccines for dental caries: A personal commentary and critique. Community Dental Health, *2*:129, 1985.
Vincent, H.: Sur l'etiologie et sur les lesions anatomopathologique de la pourriture d'hospital. Ann. Inst. Pasteur, *10*:448, 1896.
Walker, S.L., and Ash, M.M.: A study of root planning by scanning electron microscopy. Dent. Hyg., *50*:109, 1976.
Weski, H.: Elephantiasis gingivae hereditaria. Deutsch. Monatschr. Zahnheilkd., *38*:557, 1921.
Zachin, S.J., and Weisberger, D.: Hereditary gingival fibromatosis. Oral Surg., *14*:828, 1961.

14

STOMATITIS, INFECTIONS AND IMMUNOLOGIC DISTURBANCES

Lesions of the oral mucosa may be manifestations of systemic and local diseases caused by viruses, bacteria, fungi, and by physical and chemical agents. To be considered briefly are systemic and dermatologic diseases that have oral manifestations and which can complicate dental or periodontal therapy. In some instances oral lesions precede systemic manifestations. Several of the diseases considered may present some degree of hazard for contracting disease by direct contact and/or reflect life-threatening disease.

VIRAL INFECTIONS

The viral infections to be considered here are those due to herpes simplex virus (HSV), herpes varicella-zoster (VZ) virus, coxsackie virus, mumps virus, and HTLV-III (AIDS) virus.

Herpes simplex viruses are among the most common infectious agents, being transmitted usually by close personal contact. Considering all herpes, herpesviridae comprise more than 70 viruses. Besides other common characteristics, importantly they have the capacity to persist in their primary host for its lifetime. On the basis of host range, short duration of reproductive cycle, and usual establishment of latency in nerve ganglia, HSV have been classed as a subfamily (alphaherpesviridae) which on the basis of several tests, can be differentiated into two distinct human types: HSV-1 and HSV-2. HSV-2 is most often acquired by venereal contact or from passage of the neonate through the birth canal of a mother with herpetic vulvovaginitis. HSV-1 can also involve the genitals as a result of oral-genital contact, including autoinoculation or contact between two individuals. HSV-1 is most often acquired for the first time by nonvenereal means during childhood.

Both primary HSV-1 and HSV-2 infections may cause clinical manifestations; however, the primary infection may be asymptomatic or at least go unnoticed. Thus an initial clinical manifestation (e.g., fever blisters) of HSV-1 may not represent a primary HSV infection. Commonly diagnosed sites for HSV-1 are the oral cavity, lips, eyes, and trigeminal sensory nerve ganglia ("above the waist"); common sites for HSV-2 are the genitalia ("below the waist"); and sites in which both HSV-1 and HSV-2 occur with about equal frequency are the hands.

After a virus gains access to the tissues of the host, usually via the skin, the eye, or the mucous membranes, a latent infection is established (especially after symptomatic primary disease) in both sensory and autonomic nerve ganglia. An infection is considered latent if the virus can be isolated from ganglia cells grown in tissue culture. Evidence for latency in other tissues, such as at the site where the virus gained access to the tissues, is not clear.

A number of questions remain unanswered about the mechanisms that control latency and reactivation of latent infection (e.g., periodic herpetic fever blisters). Thus the mechanism by which there is the production of a recrudescent lesion by viruses located within neuronal cell bodies of ganglia (e.g., trigeminal) has to be clarified. The term "recrudescence" is used to indicate clinical lesions arising in peripheral tissues (e.g., lips) due to recurrent virus. Recurrence suggests that the virus appears in peripheral tissues (e.g., lips) without clinical lesions.

The control of HSV latency may be related to immune responses, but very probably the physiological state of the neuron may be a key factor. It is generally accepted that host responses are involved in suppressing virus replication and maintaining latency.

To summarize the general statements made about HSV-1 and HSV-2, these viruses are different from most other viruses inasmuch as they establish latency at the time of the primary infection, whether or not manifestations of the infection are clinically evident or not. After the virus is established it may remain dormant for variable periods of time, up to the lifetime of the host. After reactivation in the nerve ganglia, the virus may migrate to the site of the original infection where it causes recrudescent disease or a subclinical infection. Recurrent disease occurs most often as a result of endogenous reactivation of virus latent in nerve ganglia.

Herpes Simplex Virus—Type 1

The natural history of HSV-1 for the majority of the individuals who encounter this virus for the first time begins with development of immunity through a subclinical infection. Others begin with an *acute herpetic gingivostomatitis* (Fig. 14–1) which is seen most frequently in children who have no HSV-1 antibodies. Primary herpetic gingivostomatitis may occur in adults (Fig. 14–2) who do not develop adequate circulating antibodies during childhood.

Primary herpetic gingivostomatitis is characterized by the development of a high fever (102 to 104°F), regional lymphadenopathy (enlargement of lymph nodes) and "sore throat." Within a day or two, a gen-

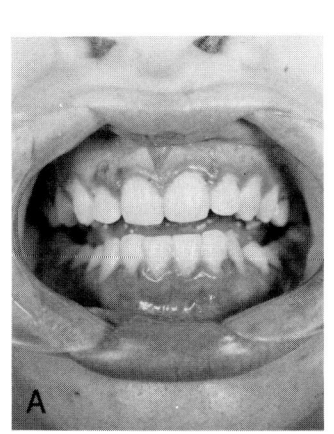

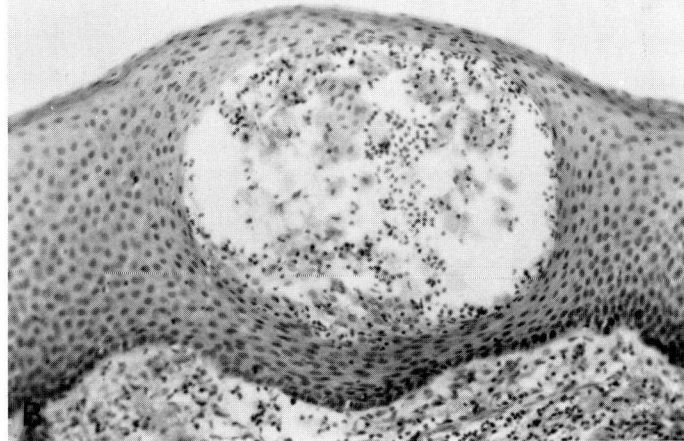

Fig. 14–1. *A,* Acute herpetic gingivostomatitis. *B,* Intraepithelial vesicle of the type seen in herpetic gingivostomatitis.

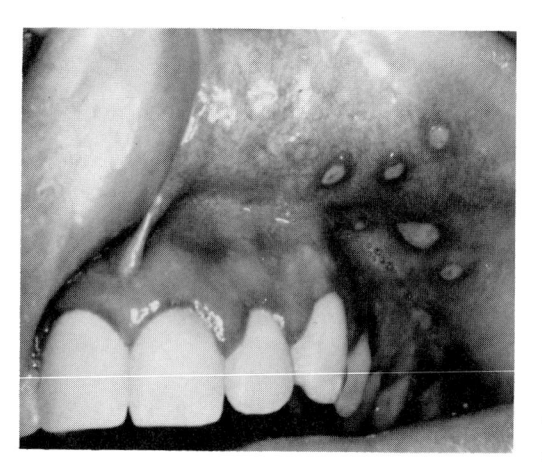

Fig. 14–2. *Acute herpetic gingivostomatitis.* Primary infection in an adult.

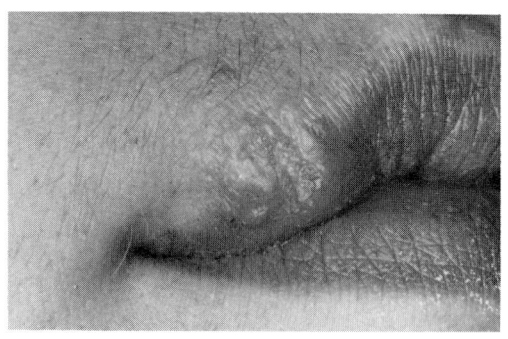

Fig. 14–3. Early herpetic lesions of lip with edema and vesicle formation at mucocutaneous junction.

eralized sore mouth develops, along with diffuse, erythematous (red) and swollen gingiva. All of the oral mucosa is tender and eating is painful. After 2 to 3 days the fever begins to subside (with or without antibiotics) and vesicles, which are difficult to see because they rupture early, form throughout the mouth. The ruptured vesicles form painful ulcers. Eating, drinking, and oral hygiene procedures are difficult. Because of the initial fever and "sore throat", which does not appear like "strep throat" but is frequently diagnosed as such, antibiotic therapy is instituted. However, the disease is self-limiting and resolves in 7 to 10 days without antibiotics. But ulcers may become secondarily infected and the after effects continue for another 1 to 2 weeks. In such cases antibiotics are helpful. The clinical manifestations are essentially the same for adults. Licensed anti-herpes compounds include vidarabine, acyclovir, and interferon.

A recurrence of infectious HSV-1 with recrudescent lesions involves most frequently the lips (Fig. 14–3), nose and adjacent skin (mucocutaneous junction) which is in contrast to the largely intraoral site for the clinical manifestations of primary herpetic gingivostomatitis. There are circulating HSV-1 antibodies present, but their influence on maintenance of latency is not clear. The lesions in recrudescent disease recur frequently at the same site, beginning with a burning, tingling sensation and then the formation of vesicles which frequently coalesce (Fig. 14–4). Subsequently, the vesicles rupture and crusting of the surface occurs. These lesions are often called "fever blisters" because recurrent herpetic infections are often reactivated by fever. The crusted lesions are also called "cold sores" because the common cold, or lowered "resistance" which leads to the coryza ("cold"), may trigger the recurrence of the lesions. A number of factors, such as sunlight, menstruation, dental treatment (local trauma), and apparently stress or anxiety, can trigger reactivation of the virus and recrudescent lesions. Recurrent lesions subside in 7 to 10 days. Prevention of these lesions by immunization and topical application of drugs during the prodromal period has met with limited success. Close contact during dental treatment of patients with pri-

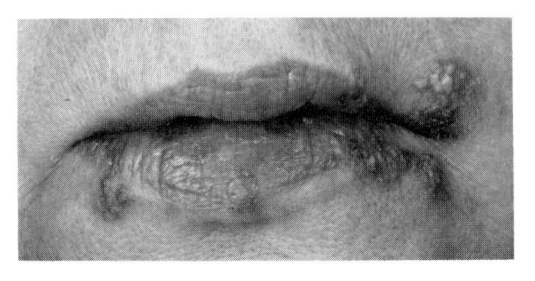

Fig. 14–4. *Herpes labialis* ("cold sores").

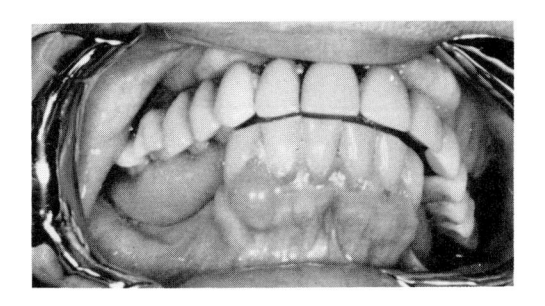

Fig. 14–5. *Vesiculobullous lesion of Varicella-Zoster virus.*

mary or recrudescent disease constitutes a risk to dental personnel because the disease is transmissible.

Varicella-Zoster (VZ) Virus

Another childhood-adult viral disease axis is chickenpox (varicella), which is seen as a primary VZ infection in children, and shingles (zoster), which is seen as a secondary VZ infection in adults. These varicella-zoster axis infections are similar to primary and secondary HSV-1 infections. Intraoral vesicular lesions may precede the skin lesions by a day or two, and involve most frequently the gingiva (Fig. 14–5) and palate. The vesicles soon rupture to form ulcers with an erythematous halo, also not unlike other ulcers of viral origin. There is general fever present in chickenpox, but may not reach that degree of fever seen in HSV-1. The cutaneous (skin) lesions tend to occur in crops, generally lasting 7 to 10 days. However, a few deep lesions, both intra- and extraoral, may persist for another week. Deep seated lesions on the palate or gingiva may be quite painful and persist for 2 to 3 weeks before healing takes place. Because these lesions are generally solitary and persist for so long after the initial disease, the diagnosis may be confused—both in the adult and child.

After the primary attack, the varicella-zoster (VZ) virus appears to have a latent existence in neural tissue and with subsequent activation may give rise to clinical manifestations of shingles (zoster). Secondary clinical manifestations are not common compared to HSV-1. Although shingles may occur clinically in the oral cavity apparently subsequent to dental procedures, cutaneous lesions which follow the distribution of peripheral nerves are more characteristic of the disease. However, because of intense pain which may precede the appearance of mucocutaneous vesicles and appear to involve the teeth, a misdiagnosis of acute pulpititis is possible. The unilateral distribution and vesicular nature of the lesions, intense pain associated with the disease, age of the patient, and presence of cutaneous lesion suggest the diagnosis of shingles.

Coxsackie Viruses

A number of types of coxsackie group A viruses are thought to be the cause of vesicular oral lesions such as *herpangina,* a disease which starts somewhat like HSV-1, i.e., high fever and sore throat with associated difficulty in swallowing (dysphagia) and anorexia (loss of appetite). However, the vesicular lesions are generally limited to the posterior part of the mouth, e.g., soft palate, pharyngeal walls, and posterior part of the tongue and buccal mucosa. The disease is self-limiting and subsides within 7 to 10 days without treatment. Severe ulceration following rupture of superficial vesicles is unusual.

Hand, foot and mouth disease is caused by several strains of Coxsackie virus A. It is a vesicular and ulcerative disease, sometimes appearing in epidemic form, and primarily affecting children. The skin lesions affect the hands, arms, legs, feet and sometimes the buttocks; and the oral lesions occur most frequently on the buccal mucosa, hard palate and tongue, but may occur anywhere. Mouth lesions occur in all cases, and in 10 to 15% of the cases only oral lesions occur. There is no cervical lymph node involvement, the fever is mild, and the mucous membranes are not erythematous as in herpetic gingivostomatitis. However, in mild cases differentiation may be difficult on a clinical basis. The disease is self-limiting but contagious, and regresses in 7 days to 2 weeks.

Mumps Virus

Mumps (epidemic parotitis) is an acute infection of the salivary glands (unilateral, bilateral), most often evident by involvement and enlargement of the parotid gland(s). Although seen primarily in children, infection of adults does occur with a tendency for complications involving other tissues (e.g., orchitis with occasional complete sterility). Because the virus is present in the saliva of patients with epidemic parotitis, infection by drop dissemination occurs. The incubation period for the virus is 14 to 28 days.

The onset of the disease begins with pain below the ear, especially with stimulation of salivary flow with citrus juices, followed by headache, chills, and moderate fever. Then the salivary glands begin to enlarge and may reach a point where the whole face and neck appear grossly altered. In other cases the swelling may be minor by comparison. The swelling subsides in 7 to 10 days. Other complications of the disease include encephalitis, mastitis, and deafness.

With the introduction of the mumps virus vaccine, incidence of the disease has decreased markedly. A number of noninfectious causes for parotid enlargement have been reported and should be considered when the reason for swelling of the parotid gland is not apparent.

AIDS Virus

Human T-cell lymphotropic viruses (HTLVs) include HTLV-I and HTLV-II, which cause human leukemias or lymphomas, and HTLV-III, which causes acquired immune deficiency syndrome (AIDS). The AIDS virus has been designated as HTLV-III, LAV (Lymphadenopathy-associated virus), or ARV (AIDS-associated retrovirus). The term ARC (AIDS-related complex) refers to an early or mild form of AIDS). HTLV-III preferentially infects and kills lymphocytes of the T4 subclass which includes "helper" cells needed for many immune responses.

AIDS is a disease which reflects a wide range of clinical disturbances including: (1) opportunistic infections by viruses (e.g., *Herpes simplex, hepatitis B, cytomegalovirus, Epstein-Barr virus,* etc.), by bacteria (e.g., atypical mycobacteria), by parasites *(Pneumocystis carinii)*, and by fungus (Candida albicans); (2) some unusual malignant processes (e.g., Kaposi's sarcoma); and (3) milder forms of AIDS-related syndromes in which there are consistent features of lymphadenopathy, fever, and weight loss.

In fully developed AIDS virtually all cellular and humoral immune responses are depressed. The major subset of lymphocytes, defined phenotypically as T4, and functionally as the helper population, is preferentially depleted. The decrease in T4 cells leaving a normal number of T8 cells (functionally suppressor cells) is one of the hallmarks of the disease, i.e., inversion of the normal T4/T8 ratio. Thus, the helper/suppressor balance in the T cell population of lymphocytes becomes severely disturbed. In addition to the inversion of the normal T4/T8 cell ratio, the T4 cells have an intrinsic defect in their ability to recognize and respond to soluble antigen. Normal individuals have about two T4 cells for every T8 cell.

In a normal individual the immune response is activated by a small number of precursor cells committed to respond to antigen. This central role in regulating the immune response is considered to be accomplished by the T4 helper/inducer cell population. This subset of cells responds to soluble antigen by proliferating, induces B cells to produce antibodies, and causes precytotoxic cells to become cytotoxic. Interactions between T4 and T8 lymphocytes are necessary to induce suppressor cells to down regulate the immune response.

T4 helper cells recognize antigen only in association with MHC. Thus, antigen is recognized in the context of the major histocompatibility complex (MHC), e.g., HLA- (Class I) and HLA-A,B (Class II) gene products. This aspect has been discussed earlier (p. 77). The activation of T4 cells involves the triggering of the T cell–MHC receptor complex which leads to the secretion of interleukin-2, a chemical mediator (lymphokine) which regulates the proliferation of T cells. Thus an early consequence of T-cell activation is the turning on of the gene coding for interleukin-2 which stimulates T-cell division. Along with proliferation of T cells and release of cytokines, T8 cytotoxic cells are generated. The T8 cytotoxic cells are involved in the destruction of virus-infected cells via recognition of viral antigens in association with Class I gene molecules. Also, after antigen triggering of the T-cell-MHC receptor complex, cytokines released by T4 cells activate macrophages and natural killer (NK) cells which respond to infection and tumors. NK cells are a group of lymphocytes which have the ability to recognize and destroy some virally infected cells and some tumor cells.

As indicated, HTLV-III/LAV selectively infects T4 cells, resulting in virus production and cell death. But HTLVs are retroviruses (RNA is their genetic material rather than DNA) and whether or not DNAs are integrated into the genomes (total genetic material contained in the cell) of infected cells they can remain without the genes being expressed when there is no cell division taking place. Because viral proteins (antigens) are not made, these latent viruses are not recognized and the infected cells eliminated by the immune system. However, the expression of the viral genes and reproduction of viruses is triggered by normal antigenic activation of infected lymphocytes. Thus the HTLV-III infected cells begin producing the virus and then die when the cells are stimulated to divide.

Only about 10% of T4 cells contain HTLV-III/LAV, but as these cells respond to foreign antigens, the virus will reproduce leading to death of these cells and the spread of virus to new cells until ultimately the immune system can no longer function because of the loss of T4 cell function. Apparently the individuals at greatest risk for developing AIDS are homo- or bisexual men who have many sex partners, drug addicts, and hemophiliacs because of their high exposure to foreign antigens. Thus virus infectivity appears to be enhanced when infected T4 cells proliferate and implies that other infections may enhance susceptibility to HTLV-III/LAV. The recognition of the T4 molecule by HTLV-III/LAV and the existence of tropism for the T4 cell suggests that the role of T4 cells in inducing antibody production by B cells, and in inducing cytotoxic T8 cells, as well as interleukin-2 and other cytokines, can explain many of the immunologic manifestations of AIDS or ARC.

Although the specific responses of the cellular and humoral immune system are the most drastically disturbed in AIDS, nonspecific immunity, such as the ability of phagocytosis carried out especially by macrophages or other antigen presenting cells, is relatively well preserved. However, the activity of nonspecific immune NK cells, which destroy targets by initiating chemical processes and are capable of recognizing virus infected cells, has been found to be depressed especially in the later stages of AIDS. Interferon, named for its ability to interfere with the replication and proliferation of viruses, appears to have impaired production in the disease.

Preliminary reports suggest that individuals who are infected with HTLV-III/LAV may initially become sick with symptoms resembling acute mononucleosis (the most common cause of mononucleosis is the Epstein-Barr virus in the United States), with fever, sore throat, painful joints and muscles, rash, and swollen lymph nodes. This syndrome appears to resolve in time leaving the patient with antibodies to HTLV-III as evidence of the continued presence of the virus, i.e., the infection seems to be permanent, and from the standpoint of prevention, may be considered potentially infectious to others. Some of these people will develop the

AIDS-related complex (ARC) with generalized swelling of the lymph nodes, diarrhea, and persistent fever. The ARC may persist for a long period of time, resolve, or progress to full-blown AIDS. Pneumonia, candidiasis (thrush), and bluish or purple-brown nodules appearing on the skin from Kaposi's sarcoma (usually a rare malignancy having an indolent, seldom fatal course) may herald the development of AIDS. The average incubation is measured in years and may take as long as 5 years for the disease to become manifest.

Oral "hairy" leukoplakia is a viral leukoplakia of the tongue in immunosuppressed male homosexuals who have or may develop the features of AIDS, including pneumonia associated with Pneumocystis carinii. Clinically the lesions appear as white, slightly raised "hairy" plaques on the tongue, ranging in size from a few millimeters to 2 centimeters. They usually produce no symptoms and do not rub off to leave a bleeding surface as may be seen in candidial lesions. It has been reported that both human papilloma virus, which causes warts on the skin and contiguous mucous membranes, and the Epstein-Barr virus are found in these tongue lesions.

The method of spread of AIDS is not clear, but there is general agreement that the disease appears to be acquired by direct exposure of the host's blood vascular system to blood, semen or saliva containing the virus. Therefore, a high risk of exposure and direct contact with the blood carrying the virus, places in high risk groups: hemophiliacs who receive blood products, intravenous drug users who share inadequately sterilized needles, and homosexually active men who are exposed to AIDS via receptive anal intercourse. The latter currently make up the largest fraction of AIDS patients. Inasmuch as saliva can contain HTLV-III virus the question of contagion by kissing has been raised. Any exposure of mucous membranes to blood, semen or saliva involves some risk of acquiring AIDS.

The risk of contracting AIDS from health-care staff or from patients does not appear to be appreciable if suitable precautions are taken. However at the current rate of new cases being reported to the Center for Disease Control (CDC) in Atlanta, there will be 100,000 people infected with HTLV-III by 1987 and the development of effective programs of precautions, care and support may be required. The development of a vaccine for AIDS is a scientific possibility, but many difficult scientific problems must be solved.

RECURRENT APHTHOUS STOMATITIS

Recurrent aphthous stomatitis (RAS) is a term used to describe recurrent oral ulcers of obscure etiology, yet having early intraepithelial degenerative changes consistent with both a viral and immunological basis. This basis of disease is compatible for roles of HSV-1, Streptococcus sanguis, and autoimmunity against epithelial cells in the etiology of RAS.

Recurrent aphthous stomatitis has been classified by severity of clinical symptoms, character of the lesions, and association with other disturbances having extra-oral manifestations. The most common type, which is found in about 20% of the population, has been called RAS minor (Fig. 14–6) or more commonly by patients as "canker sores." A more severe variant, but far less common is RAS major, formerly called periadenitis mucosa necrotica recurrens (Fig. 14–7). Another designation is given to uncomplicated aphthous ulcers when associated with Behçets disease, e.g., RAS associated with Behçets syndrome.

The aphthous ulcer usually begins as a superficial erosion covered by a grayish membrane having a well demarcated erythematous border. There may be one or more lesions present involving any of the nonkeratinized oral mucosa, i.e. all mucosa not bound to underlying periosteum. The lesions tend to heal in one to two weeks. Healing is dependent upon location, trauma

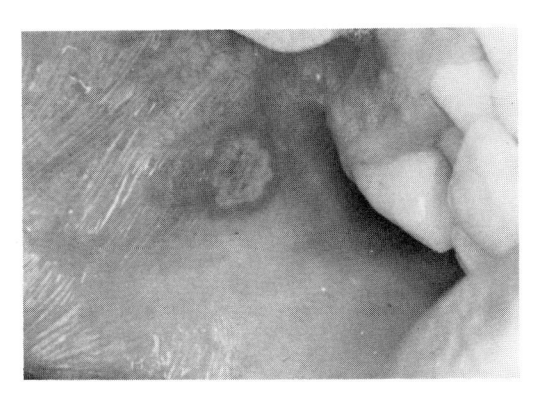

Fig. 14-6. Recurrent aphthous stomatitis ("canker sore").

involved, and size and number of lesions. Precipitating factors suggested include trauma, allergy to certain foods or drugs, and perhaps psychic stress. The lesions of RAS-major are deep seated, involving mucous glands, muscle and connective tissue. Unlike the lesions of RAS minor, which heal in 4 or 5 days, those of RAS major may persist for months and heal with scarring. These major aphthae may involve genital tissues with associated rheumatoid arthritis or conjunctivitis.

The onset of RAS may involve a variety of manifestations, including low-grade fever, lymphadenopathy and paresthesia. The frequency of attack is also quite variable within and between patients. Some

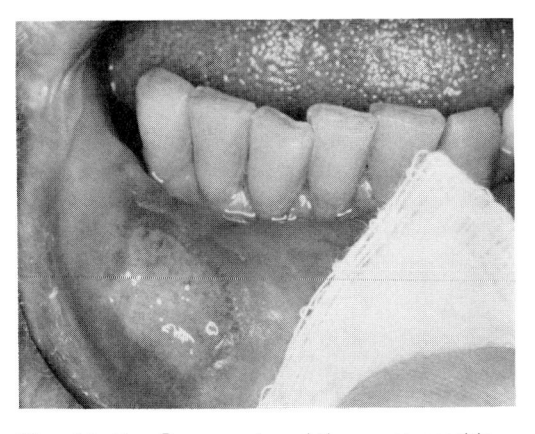

Fig. 14-7. Recurrent aphthous stomatitis—major (periadenitis mucosa necrotica recurrens).

have the attacks regularly 1 or 2 times a month or only once or twice a year. The patient with RAS major is seldom free of active lesions, which are much more painful than those in RAS minor. There is no specific treatment for RAS.

The histologic appearance of RAS during premonitory stages is characterized principally by subepithelial accumulations of lymphocytes. Changes in the epithelium consist of vacuolation, with degeneration of the epithelium and ulceration; the predominant feature is acute inflammation. Lymphocytes and plasma cells may be prominent in the deeper layers of the lesions. The microscopic picture is nonspecific and a careful history is required to make a diagnosis of recurrent aphthae.

Reiter's syndrome is a disease of unknown etiology with typical manifestations of urethritis, arthritis, conjunctivitis, and mucocutaneous lesions. All are not always present together. Lesions of the buccal mucosa, lips and gingivae may be mistaken for recurrent aphthae and lesions of the tongue may resemble "geographic tongue." Diagnosis is dependent upon the extra-oral manifestations, i.e., recurrent ocular lesions and/or genital ulcerations.

SYSTEMIC DISEASES WITH ORAL MANIFESTATIONS

A number of systemic and cutaneous diseases have oral manifestations, some involving immunologic mechanisms and often of unknown cause. Only a brief consideration will be given and no attempt is made to include all such diseases.

Lichen Planus

Lichen planus is a relatively common dermatologic (skin) disease with oral manifestations in about one-third of the cases. The clinical oral manifestations vary from flat or slightly elevated lesions with striae (Fig. 14-8) to extensive areas of ulceration or erosion (erosive lichen planus). Except for the erosive type, the oral lesions are seldom

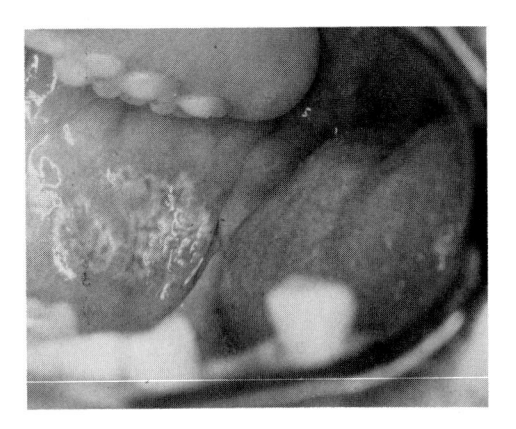

Fig. 14–8. *Lichen planus.*

a diagnostic problem or require treatment. The presence of skin lesions helps to make a diagnosis in erosive lichen planus.

Pemphigus

Pemphigus is a vesiculobullous disease (vesicles = small blister-like lesions and bulla = large blister-like lesions) involving both the skin and oral mucosa. Lesions commonly involve the oral mucosa first and are non-healing lesions. The autoimmune nature of pemphigus is well established. The mechanism of blister formation is antibody binding which results in the release of proteolytic enzymes from epithelial cells leading to an intraepithelial split and formation of a blister. Several forms of pemphigus exist. About 30 to 40% of the patients will die of the disease, although long periods of remission may occur in some forms of the disease.

Benign Mucous Membrane Pemphigoid (BMMP)

BMMP is a rare benign vesiculobullous cicatricial (scar forming) disease which is considered to be an autoimmune disease with clinical manifestation of blister formation followed by scarring of mucosal surfaces. Its relationship to desquamative gingivitis has already been considered (p. 223), i.e., chronic desquamative gingivitis may be a manifestation of pemphigus, erosive lichen planus, pemphigoid, and erythema multiforme. The diagnosis of BMMP rests on biopsy and immunofluorescence studies. Unlike pemphigus, the mortality rate is not high.

Erythema Multiforme

Erythema multiforme is a disease of uncertain cause with bullous erosive involvement of the oral mucous membranes. Infections, including HSV, drugs and environmental factors, have been implicated in its pathogenesis. Both early skin and mucosal lesions may subside in a few days to a week, leaving hemorrhagic papules. The bullous erosive involvement of the oral mucosa is seen as chronic desquamative gingivitis (Fig. 13–38).

Crohn's Disease

In ulcerative colitis and in Crohn's disease oral mucosa may be involved as well as the area of primary involvement in the intestinal mucosa. Crohn's disease may involve the oral mucosa and lips (e.g., aphthous type ulcers and/or raised nodules) with or without apparent associated intestinal disturbances.

BACTERIAL INFECTIONS

The bacterial infections to be considered here include gonorrhea and syphilis. The number of other diseases which may have oral lesions and could be included, such as leprosy, tuberculosis, actinomycosis, and diphtheria, are infrequently seen except in special circumstances and therefore will not be discussed.

Gonorrhea

Gonorrhea is one of the most common reportable infectious diseases, with numbers in the population exceeding one million annually. It is a venereal disease of the genitourinary tract, but extragenital lesions involving the lips and tongue are being seen with increasing frequency as a result of oral-genital contact and autoinoculation. Dissemination to the temporomandibular joint occurs also. Involvement of the parotid gland has also been reported. Lesions involving the oral and paraoral structures are not specific and gonococcal stomatitis may be similar to the oral lesions of vesicular and vesiculobullous diseases such as erythema multiforme. Fever and regional lymphadenopathy are common symptoms. An accurate diagnosis is based on a careful history and when indicated a bacteriologic evaluation. The identification of all lesions of the lips and mouth should be made before any periodontal treatment begins. The examination should be conducted as with any potentially infective disease.

Syphilis

Syphilis (Lues) is an infectious disease caused by the spirochete, Treponema pallidum, and compared to the incidence of this disease before the advent of antibiotics, it is uncommonly seen. However, there has been a serious increase in the overall incidence of the disease recently. The increase has been over-shadowed by the rise of AIDS, but syphilis is still a disease with serious consequences. Of interest to the dental profession are the primary lesions (chancre) which occur on the lips, tongue, palate and gingiva as a result of autoinoculation or oral-genital activity. A chancre is nodular, indurated and ulcerated, and there is generally an associated enlargement of local lymph nodes. The lip lesion often has a crusted appearance whereas the intraoral lesion is generally covered by a grayish-white membrane. A chancre is highly infectious and abounds in spirochetes demonstrable on dark field microscopy. Serologic tests may not be positive at this time. Chancres tend to heal spontaneously in weeks to months.

A secondary stage occurs about 6 weeks after the primary stage and the serologic test is positive. There are skin lesions (papules) present and oral lesions called "mucous patches" (Fig. 14–9). These are also highly infectious lesions. Such secondary lesions are generally irregular, multiple, grayish-white plaques on the oral mucosa. Spontaneous remissions occur, lasting weeks, to months or years.

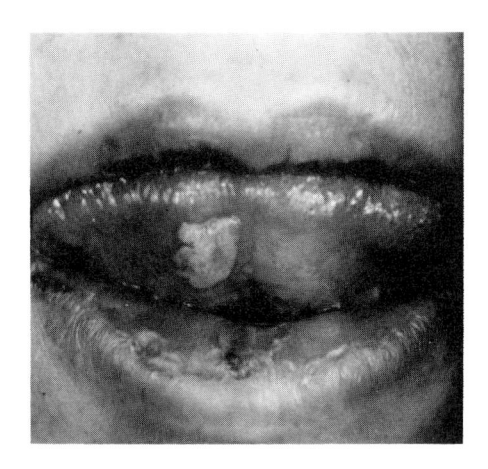

Fig. 14–9. "Mucous patch" lesion of secondary syphilis.

A tertiary or late stage of syphilis occurs usually several years after the secondary stage. It is not infectious. There is often involvement of the central nervous system (with paresis), cardiovascular system, and other organs. The skin and mucous membrane may have localized lesions called *gumma*. Involvement of the palate leads to perforation of the palate because of central necrosis of the nodular mass. Tongue lesions tend to undergo transformation into cancer.

Syphilis acquired at birth from infected mothers has been largely controlled, but a slight increase has occurred. If the infected mother is treated by the fourth month of pregnancy, approximately 95% of the newborn will be free of the disease. A triad of manifestations, which include hypoplasia of the molars ("mulberry molars") and incisors (screwdriver shaped), eighth nerve deafness, and eye damage (interstitial keratitis), are considered to be specific (pathognomonic) signs and symptoms of congenitally acquired syphilis.

FUNGUS INFECTIONS

Many forms of fungal infection seen in some developing countries are not seen commonly in Western industrialized countries although certain forms are more often present in subclinical states than formerly suspected, e.g., *histoplasmosis,* which is endemic in the Mississippi Valley and northeastern United States where a high percentage of the population have had a primary but subclinical infection; and *coccidioidomycosis,* which is endemic in the southwestern part of the United States where the majority of the population have had a subclinical infection. Probably the most common fungal infection seen in the dental office is *candidiasis* (moniliasis) and for that reason will be considered in more detail than other fungal infections. Most forms of candidiasis may be seen in AIDS.

Candidiasis

Candidiasis is caused by *Candida (Monilia) albicans,* as well as other species of Candida. Candida species are frequent oral commensals, but the mere presence of these yeast-like fungi is not sufficient to produce the disease candidiasis. There has been a marked increase in this opportunistic infection with the prevalent use of antibiotics and introduction of immunosuppressive drugs, e.g., corticosteroids. This disease may occur in chronic or acute form, at any age, and be local or systemic in nature. It is considered by some investigators to be a significant indication of an underlying immunodeficiency.

Candidiasis has been classified as *mucocutaneous candidiasis* and *systemic candidiasis.* Included in the first category is *oral candidiasis,* which has been classified into acute and chronic forms of the disease and into several subtypes (Lehner, 1966): oropharyngeal candidiasis (thrush), intestinal candidiasis, candidal balantitis, candidal vulvovaginitis, and paronchial (nail) candidiasis. The systemic category includes infection in the eyes, skin, kidneys, lungs and other viscera. The classification of oral candidiasis includes the following consideration and clinical features.

Acute pseudomembranous candidiasis

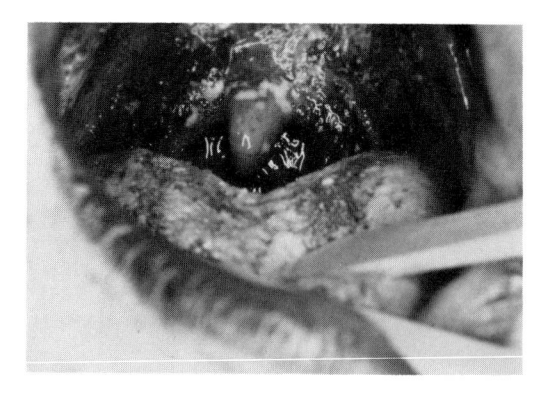

Fig. 14–10. *Acute pseudomembranous candidiasis.*

(thrush) is a common form of the disease, termed "thrush" when found in infants. It may also be present in debilitated patients, in patients treated with antibiotics, corticosteroids, immunosuppressive drugs, and radiation therapy to the head and neck region, and in patients with diabetes and malignant disease. The clinical features are white, loose, curd-like accumulations on the mucosa which can be detached, leaving an erythematous bleeding surface (Fig. 14–10).

Acute atrophic candidiasis is an uncommon type, a complication of broad-spectrum antibiotic therapy, in which the lesions do not have the pseudomembrane curd-like covering, but have a smooth, atrophic erythematous appearance, and the tongue is

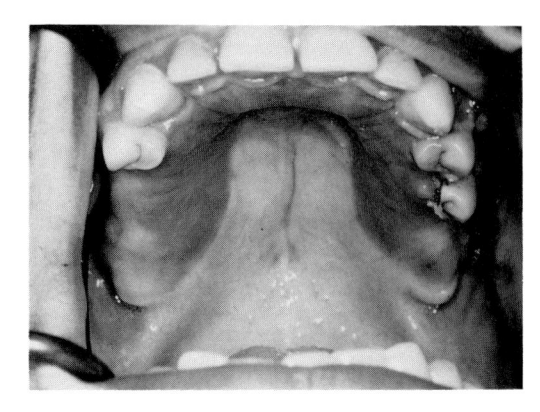

Fig. 14–11. *Chronic atrophic candidiasis* (denture stomatitis).

depapillated. Angular cheilitis (corner of the lips) may also be present. Pain is almost always present.

Chronic atrophic candidiasis (denture stomatitis) is a common form of candidiasis in which the mucous membranes under dentures are erythematous and spongy (Fig. 14-11). The inflammatory response varies from tiny red dots to diffuse erythematous tissues to papillary hyperplasia. There may be actual penetration of the tissues by Candida, although superficial. There may be no symptoms or the patient may complain of burning sensations. It is not clear what causes the tissue response: tissue invasion by the organisms, response to toxins released by the fungus, or a hypersensitivity reaction to antigens from Candida albicans. An ill-fitting denture is an exciting or contributing factor and must be replaced in addition to treatment with antifungal agents, e.g., nystatin troches. An existing denture should be sterilized and antifungal therapy conducted to determine the effect before starting a new denture. The diagnosis is made on the basis of clinical appearance of the lesion and response to antifungal therapy.

Chronic mucocutaneous candidiasis is characterized by chronic candidal involvement of the skin, mucous membranes, nails and scalp, resistance to common forms of treatment, and a wide range of immunologic defects, including impaired cell-mediated immunity and failure of anticandidal antibody response. But immunological defects alone do not explain the pathogenesis of the disease. Other factors include low levels of serum iron transferrin and blood folate, high glucose levels in diabetes mellitus, and granulocyte defects. The four clinical subtypes (Lehner, 1966) include: (1) *chronic oral hyperplastic candidiasis (candidal leukoplakia),* which is a firm, white, persistent plaque on the mucosa that is difficult to distinguish from other forms of leukoplakia (p. 242); (2) *chronic localized mucocutaneous candidiasis,* which begins in childhood by involving the oral mucosa and then the skin and nails; (3) *chronic localized mucocutaneous candidiasis with granuloma,* which is a long-lasting oral candidiasis starting in infancy and characterized by candidal granulomatous involvement of the face and scalp; and (4) *chronic localized mucocutaneous candidiasis with endocrinopathy,* which as the term implies, is associated with endocrine disorders, often multiple endocrinopathies. Endocrine deficiencies may not appear clinically for several years after the appearance of thrush in infants. Enamel hypoplasia has been associated with autoimmune polyendocrinopathy-candidiasis.

Histoplasmosis

Histoplasmosis is a fungus infection usually acquired by inhalation of dust containing spores of the fungus *(Histoplasma capsulatum).* Approximately one-third of the presenting complaints for this generalized infection involve oral lesions. Systemic involvement and symptoms relate to granulomatous infection (p. 71) and involvement of the phagocytic cells of the monocyte-macrophage (reticuloendothelial system), e.g., lymph node, spleen, liver enlargement. Chronic low-grade fever and cough also may occur. The oral lesions are nodular, ulcerated or vegetative lesions occurring at various sites on the lips and in the mouth. Subcutaneous lesions and involvement of the joints may occur. Although the generalized form often terminates fatally, most infections are mild. Pulmonary disease may be present for long periods of time, sometimes resolving spontaneously. Chemotherapeutic treatment is relatively effective.

Coccidioidomycosis

Coccidioidomycosis (San Joaquin Valley Fever) is a relatively common, but usually subclinical infection, transmitted by inhalation of dust containing the spores of the fungus *(coccidioides immitis).* A primary form of the disease is self-limiting with resolutions of systemic manifestations con-

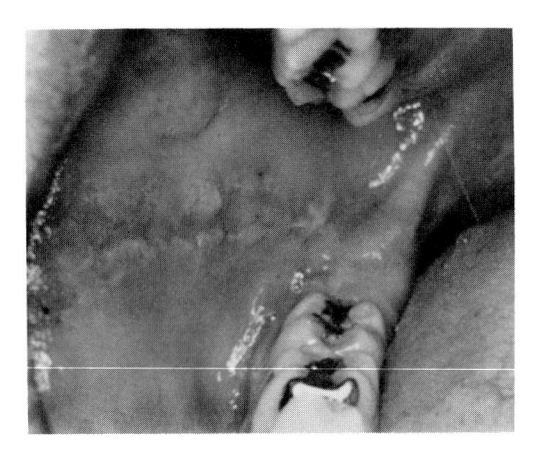

Fig. 14-12. *Injury from cheek chewing.*

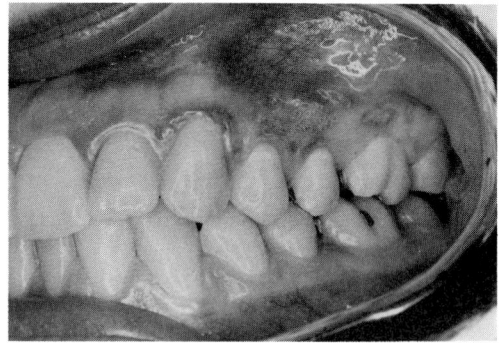

Fig. 14-13. *Toothbrush abrasion.*

sistent with a respiratory disease (cough, headache, etc.) in about 2 weeks. Intraoral lesions as well as skin lesions may occur but are generally nonspecific, sometimes resembling the lesions of erythema multiforme. Established lesions are ulcerated proliferative granulomatous nodules which histologically reflect specific granulomatous inflammation in response to endospores of the fungi present. A disseminated form of the disease occurs rarely, but has a high mortality rate. Chemotherapeutic control has been effective.

TRAUMATIC STOMATITIS

Mechanical Injury

One of the common forms of mechanical stomatitis is produced in the buccal and vestibular mucosa as the result of repeated or habitual cheek-biting. The changes produced by cheek-biting are seen in the buccal mucosa along the line of occlusion of the teeth extending from the most posterior teeth to the commissure and just inside the vermilion border of the upper and lower lips (Fig. 14-12). In more severe cheek-chewing, the mucosa shows a more severe hyperkeratosis; it is grayish-white and shaggy and has irregular small erosions where the superficial layers of the mucosa have been stripped away by being grasped between the teeth while the cheek is pulled away.

The lips may be irritated by contact with irregular, sharp anterior teeth or by habitual chewing. The changes are the same as those present in the buccal mucosa.

Mechanical injury is frequently produced in the gingiva owing to the vigorous use of a stiff toothbrush. The onset of tenderness is rather rapid and is due to the presence of multiple small ulcers of circular or linear configuration (Fig. 14-13). The stiff bristles of the brush either perforate or lacerate the gingiva, depending upon the method of application. The lesions are most severe at the height of contour of the gingiva over the roots of the teeth and at the gingival margins. They may occur on the labial, buccal, palatal, or lingual aspects of the gingiva. Toothbrush injury is accompanied by a burning type of tenderness of the entire area involved. The ulcers heal in 3 to 5 days if the injury is not repeated.

Mechanical injury also occurs under dentures, especially upper dentures which occlude against all natural teeth or against a few natural teeth and a partial denture. This type of injury occurs most frequently under areas of abnormal denture pressure on the anterior maxillary ridge and the vault of the palate. In the anterior ridge area the tissue becomes red, swollen, and flabby. The tissue has a tendency to be thrown into folds and may be crowded over the labial flange of the denture. In the palatal area the tissue

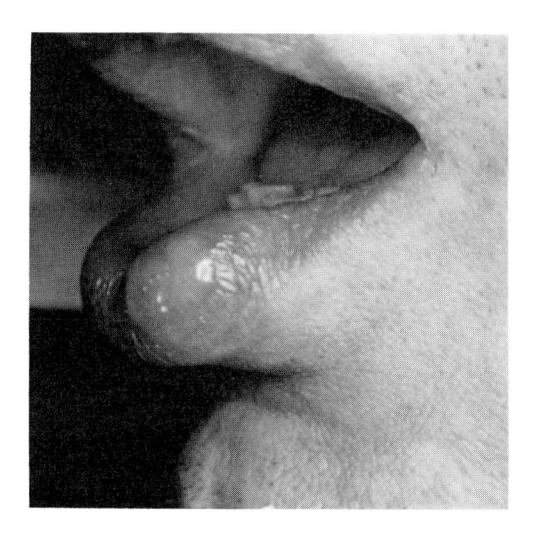

Fig. 14–14. *Thermal injury.* Second degree burn with blister formation.

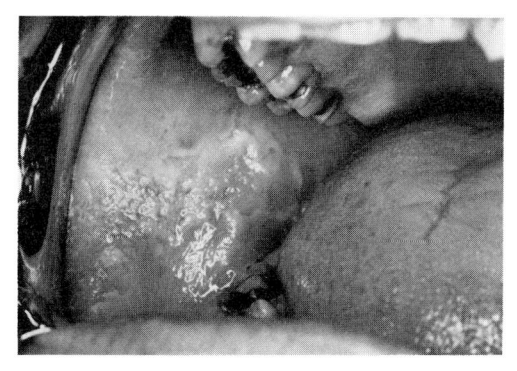

Fig. 14–15. *Chemical injury.* Sloughing of mucosal surface due to detergent in dentifrice.

becomes intensely red, smooth, and tender. There is hyperplasia of a polypoid character which produces a pebbly or cauliflower appearance to the surface.

Thermal Injury

Thermal irritation is usually produced by taking hot foods into the mouth. The degree and location of the burn depend on the type and temperature of the food. In the areas where hot, sticky material contacts the tissue, the burn is localized and superficial ulcers follow vesiculation (Fig. 14–14). The vesicles rupture almost as soon as they are formed and therefore are rarely observed.

Chemical Injury

Various chemical substances due to either repeated or prolonged contact may produce irritation of the oral mucosa. Mild change may be produced by dentifrices containing strong flavoring or detergent materials (Fig. 14–15). The changes are most marked in the buccal mucosa and to a lesser degree in the floor of the mouth, but are usually not produced in the area of the mucosa which is keratinized. The mucosal surface is covered by a thin slimy, grayish, slightly opaque film which can be rubbed or peeled away. When hydrogen peroxide is used persistently as a mouthwash, it produces keratinization of the tongue with an accentuation of the filiform papillae, giving the tongue the appearance of being covered with a brown fur.

Mild chemical burns may be produced by the repeated application of "toothache drops" (Fig. 14–16). They produce redness in the area of application and may, with overzealous use, produce ulceration. Chemical burns may be produced by the intentional or accidental application of caustic agents to the mucosa. Silver nitrate, phenol (Fig. 14–17), trichloroacetic acid and zinc chloride are all examples of agents which may be used that can cause chemical injury. Aspirin burns are frequently produced by patients holding aspirin tablets in con-

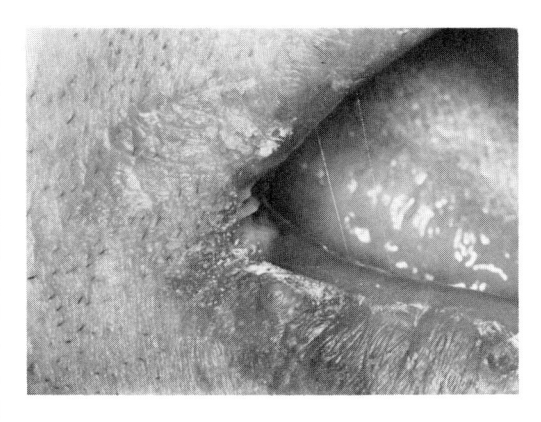

Fig. 14–16. *Chemical injury*—toothache drops.

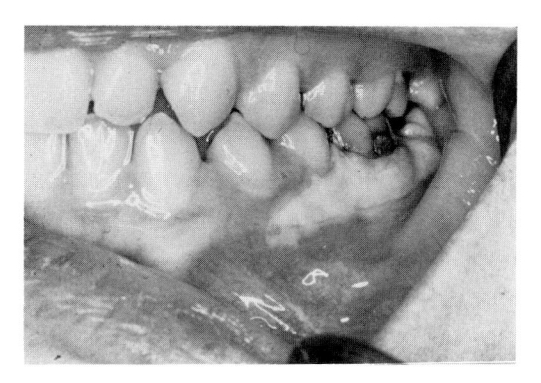

250 STOMATITIS, INFECTIONS AND IMMUNOLOGIC DISTURBANCES

Fig. 14–17. *Chemical injury*—phenol. Eschar-like lesion of gingiva.

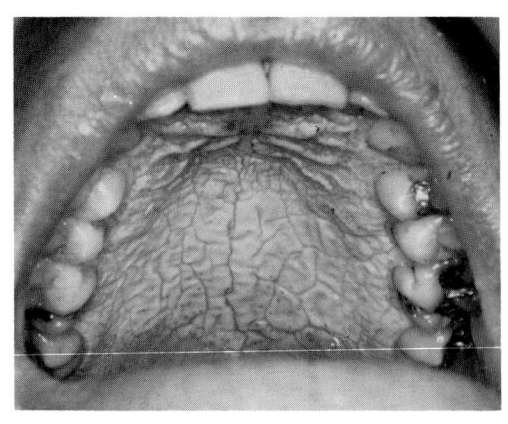

Fig. 14–19. *Smoker's stomatitis.* Hyperkeratosis and thickening of palatal mucosa.

tact with the mucosa for pain relief (Fig. 14–18).

Chemical irritation may be produced by smoking or chewing tobacco. In smoking the changes are produced in the palate, buccal mucosa, and the tongue. The orifices of the palatal glands appear as red pinpoint perforations. These changes are due to hyperkeratinization and hyperplasia of the palatal epithelium and slight dilatation of the duct orifice. When the process is more severe and of a more chronic nature, the palate is whiter and numerous papules (1 to 2 mm in diameter) appear on the surface (Fig. 14–19). In severe cases the papular lesions may be close together and produce a pattern of fissuring. When the smoking is intense and of long duration, the buccal mucosa and tongue become grayish-white and leathery owing to hyperkeratinization.

The changes produced by the use of chewing tobacco or snuff are those of hyperkeratinization and hyperplasia in the area contacted by the tobacco. The tissue is grayish-white in color and slightly folded or wrinkled. In persons who use chewing tobacco, the changes are in the buccal mucosa of the buccal pouch and involve the gingiva. In individuals using snuff, the alteration is usually in the anterior mucobuccal fold on either side of the midline and involves gingival and vestibular mucosa of a limited area because the individual habitually holds the snuff in the same location. Continuous use of chewing tobacco or snuff over protracted periods of time results in intense changes, and a warty appearance of the lesions suggests the development of a verrucal carcinoma. Verrucal carcinoma is a particular type of carcinoma resulting from the prolonged use of tobacco.

ALLERGIC STOMATITIS

Almost any drug may cause an allergic response in some individuals following injection or ingestion of even small amounts of the medicament. These responses may involve the skin or oral mucosa and are re-

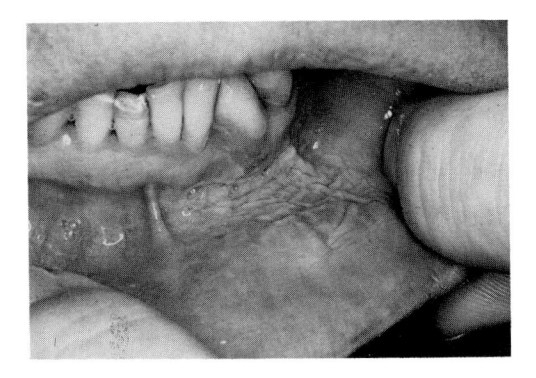

Fig. 14–18. *Chemical injury*—aspirin "burn." Necrosis of mucosa due to holding aspirin next to painful tooth.

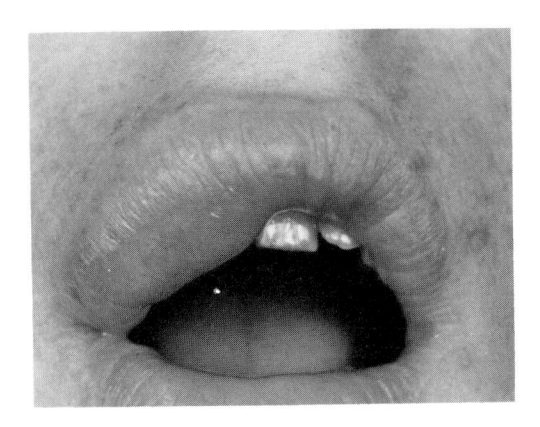

Fig. 14-20. *Allergic stomatitis*—angioneurotic edema of the lip.

ferred to as stomatitis and/or dermatitis medicamentosa. The oral lesions usually consist of multiple areas of erythema, erosion and angioneurotic edema (Figs. 14-20 and 14-21). Skin lesions, arthralgia (joint pain), fever, and lymphadenopathy may be manifestations of an allergic response as well. Localized reactions in response to contact with drugs (stomatitis venenata or contact stomatitis) also may occur. Certain dentifrices, oil of cloves, oil of wintergreen, and other dental therapeutic agents may elicit an allergic response of redness and swelling (urticaria). Surgical dressings containing essential oils also may produce an allergic stomatitis.

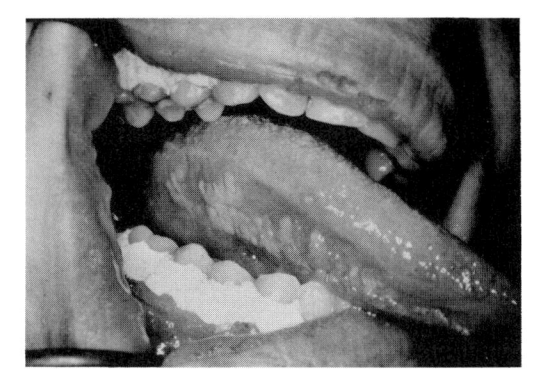

Fig. 14-21. *Allergic stomatitis*—response to periodontal dressing.

SUMMARY

Oral manifestations of diseases due to microorganisms and physical and chemical agents may complicate periodontal therapy and a few may pose some hazard to health-care personnel in the dental office, and/or indicate the presence of a serious, even life-threatening disease for the patient.

A common contagious viral disease is herpes simplex, most commonly recurring episodes of infection with HSV-1 involving the lip (mucocutaneous junction) in the form of "cold sores." Primary infections with HSV-1 may be severe with the development of full-blown herpetic gingivostomatitis with high fever, regional lymphadenopathy and vesicles which quickly rupture to form ulcers. The manifestations of HSV-1 generally subside in 7 to 10 days.

The recent epidemic of AIDS is more than a question of numbers. It is the first recognized communicable disease that directly attacks the host's defenses leading to a number of opportunistic infections, which are sometimes untreatable, and to malignancies. The "risk" groups include sexually active homosexuals, intravenous drug abusers, and hemophiliacs. AIDS is caused by HTLV-III, a virus which virtually eliminates all T-helper (T4) cells. The initial manifestations of the disease resemble acute mononucleosis with fever, pain in muscle and joints, lymphadenopathy, sore throat and rash. This mono-like syndrome subsides in time leaving the individual with antibodies to HTLV-III. The term ARC (AIDS-related complex) refers to an early or mild form of AIDS. Pneumonia, candidiasis (thrush) and Kaposi's sarcoma may develop in full-blown AIDS. Oral "hairy" leukoplakia of the tongue may be a manifestation of AIDS. The risk of health-care staff for contracting disease does not appear to be appreciable if suitable precautions are taken. The development of a vaccine for AIDS is scientifically possible.

Gonorrhea and syphilis are other diseases which are potential risks to health-care personnel; gonorrhea appears now to be much more common than syphilis. The lesions of these diseases are not specific enough to allow a clinical diagnosis on the basis of their appearance alone. Generally these diseases can be controlled by antibiotic treatment.

Fungus infections caused by Candida albicans have increased with the use of antibiotics and immunosuppressive drugs. Most forms of candidiasis are seen in AIDS. A common form of candidiasis is associated with denture stomatitis.

Traumatic stomatitis may be caused by a number of mechanical, thermal and chemical agents. These disturbances do not generally present difficult diagnostic problems and usually heal quickly after removal of the offending agent.

Allergic stomatitis may occur in response to ingestion of foods and/or drugs, or in response to contact of these agents with the oral mucosa. Elimination of the agents usually leads to resolution of the stomatitis, but some forms may be refractory.

BIBLIOGRAPHY

Adler, J.L., Mostow, S.R., Mellin, H., Janney, J.H., and Joseph, J.M.: Epidemiologic investigation of hand, foot, and mouth disease. Am. J. Dis. Child., *120*:309, 1970.

Antoon, J.W., and Miller, R.L.: Aphthous ulcers—a review of the literature on etiology, pathogenesis, diagnosis, and treatment. J. Am. Dent. Assoc., *101*:803, 1980.

August, M.J., Nordlund, J.J., and Hsiung, G.D.: Persistence of herpes simplex virus types 1 and 2 in infected individuals. Arch. Dermatol., *115*:309, 1979.

Banks, P.: Nonneoplastic parotid swelling: a review. Oral Surg., *25*:732, 1968.

Baum, G.L., Schwarz., J., Bruins Slot, W.J., and Straub, M.: Mucocutaneous histoplasmosis. Arch. Dermatol., *76*:4, 1957.

Bernstein, M.L., and McDonald, J.S.: Oral lesions in Crohn's disease: report of two cases and update of the literature. Oral Surg., *46*:234, 1978.

Borsanyi, S., and Blanchard, C.L.: Asymptomatic enlargement of the salivary glands. J.A.M.A., *174*:20, 1960.

Cawson, R.A., and Binnie, W.H.: Candida Leukoplakia and carcinoma: a possible relationship: in I.C. Mackenzie, E. Dabelsteen, and C.A. Squier: *Oral Premalignancy.* Iowa City, University of Iowa Press, 1980, p. 59.

Cohen, L.: Etiology, pathogenesis and classification of aphthous stomatitis and Behçet's syndrome. J. Oral Pathol., *7*:347, 1978.

Conte, J.E. (Jr.), et al.: Infection-control guidelines for patients with acquired immunodeficiency syndrome (AIDS). N. Engl. J. Med., *309*:740, 1983.

Curran, J.W., et al.: The epidemiology of AIDS: Current status and future prospects. Science, *229*:1352, 1985.

Fiese, M.J.: *Coccidioidomycosis.* Springfield, Charles C Thomas, 1958.

Fiumara, N.J., and Lessell, S.: Manifestations of late congenital syphilis. Arch. Dermatol., *102*:78, 1970.

Francis, D.P., and Petricciani, J.C.: The prospects for and pathways toward a vaccine for AIDS. N. Engl. J. Med., *313*:1586, 1985.

Francis, T.C.: Recurrent apththous stomatitis and Behçet's disease. Oral Surg., *30*:476, 1970.

Goodwin, R.A., Jr., Shapiro, J.L., Thurman, G.H., Thurman, S.S., and Des Prez, R.M.: Disseminated histoplasmosis: clinical and pathologic correlations. Medicine, *59*:1, 1980.

Graykowski, E.A., and Hooks, J.J.: Aphthous stomatitis—Behçet's syndrome workshop. J. Oral Path., *7*:341, 1978.

Greenspan, J.S., et al.: Replication of Epstein-Barr virus within the epithelial cells of oral "hairy" leukoplakia, an AIDS-associated lesion. N. Engl. J. Med., *313*:1564, 1985.

Guideline for infection control in hospital personnel. Infect. Control, *4*:326, 1983.

Hirsch, M.S., and Schooley, R.T.: Treatment of Herpesvirus infections. N. Engl. J. Med., *309*:963, *309*:1034, 1983.

Honma, T.: Electron microscopic study on the pathogenesis of recurrent aphthous ulceration as compared to Behçet's syndrome. Oral Surg., *41*:366, 1976.

Huebner, R.J., Cole, R.M., Beeman, E.A., Bell, J.A., and Peers, J.H.: Herpangina. J.A.M.A., *145*:628, 1951.

Huebsch, R.F.: Gumma of the hard palate, with perforation: report of a case. Oral Surg., *8*:690, 1955.

Igo, R.M., Taylor, C.G., Scott, A.S., and Jacoby, J.K.: Coccidioidomycosis involving the mandible: report of a case. J. Oral Surg., *36*:72, 1978.

Katz, S.I.: Blistering skin diseases, New Insights. (Editorial), N. Engl. J. Med., *26*:1657, 1985.

Lehner, T.: Pathology of recurrent oral ulceration

and oral ulceration in Behçet's syndrome: light, electron and fluorescence microscopy. J. Pathol., 97:481, 1969.

Indem: Immunologic aspects of recurrent oral ulcers. Oral Surg., 33:80, 1972.

Indem: Immunological aspects of recurrent oral ulceration and Behçet's syndrome. J. Oral Pathol., 7:424, 1978.

Levy, B.M.: Oral manifestations of histoplasmosis. J. Am. Dent. Assoc., 32:215, 1946.

Liebmann-Smith, R.: *The Question of AIDS in New York.* New York, The New York Academy of Sciences, 1985.

Loriaux, D.L.: The polyendocrine deficiency syndrome. N. Engl. J. Med., 312:1568, 1985.

Marx, J.L.: The slow, insidious natures of the HTLVs. Science, 231:450, 1986.

McGhee, J.R., Michalek, S.M., and Cassell, G.H.: *Dental Microbiology.* Philadelphia. Harper & Row, 1982.

McKinney, R.V.: Hand, foot, and mouth disease: a viral disease of importance to dentists. J. Am. Dent. Assoc., 91:122, 1975.

Meyer, I., and Shklar, G.: The oral manifestations of acquired syphilis. A study of eighty-one cases. Oral Surg., 23:45, 1967.

Myllarniemi, S., and Perheentupa, J.: Oral findings in the autoimmune polyendocrinopathy-candidosis syndrome (APECS) and other forms of hypoparathyroidism. Oral Surg., 45:721, 1978.

Nally, F.F., and Ross, I.H.: Herpes zoster of the oral and facial structures. Report of five cases and discussion. Oral Surg., 32:221, 1971.

Renner, R.P., Lee, M., Andors, L., and McNamara, T.F.: The role of C. albicans in denture stomatitis. Oral Surg., 47:323, 1979.

Roed-Petersen, B., Renstrup, G., and Pindborg, J.J.: Candida in oral leukoplakias. Scand. J. Dent. Res., 78:323, 1970.

Rogers, R.S., III, and Tindall, J.P.: Herpes zoster in children. Arch. Derm., 106:204, 1972.

Rowe, N.H., Heine, C.S., and Kowalski, C.J.: Herpetic whitlow: an occupational disease of practicing dentists. J. Am. Dent. Assoc., 105:471, 1982.

Sacks, J.J.: AIDS in a surgeon (Correspondence). N. Engl. J. Med., 313:1017, 1985.

Sande, M.A.: Transmission of AIDS: The case against casual contagion (Editorial). N. Engl. J. Med., 314:380, 1986.

Schmidt, H., Hjorting-Hansen, E., and Philipsen, H.P.: Gonococcal stomatitis. Acta Derm. Venereol., 41:324, 1961.

Scully, C.: Orofacial manifestations of chronic granulomatous disease of childhood. Oral Surg., 51:148, 1981.

Silverman, S.R., and Beumer, J.: Primary herpetic gingivostomatitis of adult onset. Oral Surg., 36:496, 1973.

Stevens, D.A. (ed.): *Coccidioidomycosis. A Text.* New York, Plenum Medical Book Co., 1980.

Stiff, R.H.: Histoplasmosis. Oral Surg., 16:140, 1963.

Turner, R., Shehab, Z., Osborne, K., and Hendley, J.O.: Shedding and survival of herpes simplex virus from "fever blisters." Pediatrics, 70:547, 1982.

Update: Prospective evaluation of health-care workers exposed via the parenteral or mucous membrane route to blood or body fluids from patients with AIDS. MMWR, 34:101, 1985.

Young, S.K., Rowe, N.H., and Buchanan, R.A.: A clinical study of the control of facial mucocutaneous herpes virus infections. I. Characterization of natural history in a professional school population. Oral Surg., 41:498, 1976.

15

ENDOCRINOPATHY AND METABOLIC DISEASES

The term endocrine system refers to a group of discrete glands which synthesize chemical messengers called hormones and then secrete them into the blood stream for transportation to distant sites where they exert action on "target cells."

In addition to enzymes produced by the classical endocrine system, chemical messengers produced elsewhere also modulate the activity of target cells. *Neuromediators* such as acetylcholine and the catecholamines (epinephrine, norepinephrine, and dopamine), which are synthesized by nerve cells and released at nerve endings, are also chemical transmitters of information. In addition, hormonal peptides found diffusely throughout tissues and organs induce a wide range of responses at the local level.

Of particular interest in the pathophysiology of pain are the *endorphins* and *enkephalins,* which are morphine-like peptides found in many areas of the body. The endorphins, which are found mostly in the CNS, are thought to be involved in pain perception and emotions. The enkephalins are found in the gastrointestinal tract as well as the CNS and are involved in gastrointestinal mobility as well as pain.

Prostaglandins are also chemical messengers. They modulate the action of neuromediators and hormones. These substances are released from different cell membranes in response to a wide range of agents and processes that involve vasodilatation, capillary permeability, inflammation, immunologic reactions, pain, and fever. Because certain prostaglandins appear in high concentration in the synovial fluid, anti-inflammatory agents such as indomethacin have been used in certain forms of TMJ arthritis to suppress the synthesis of prostaglandins.

Hormones act by binding to specific receptors on the surface of the "target cells." This provides for a specific hormone to bind (attach) to a specific tissue, e.g., receptors on the thyroid gland are specific for thyroid stimulating hormones. The response of the target cell depends upon the number of receptors on the cell membrane and the affinity of the hormone for the receptor. The number of receptors on a target cell may vary in relation to obesity, hypoglycemic ("blood sugar") drugs, and antibody responses.

One hormone-receptor interaction which modulates cell activity occurs via fixed cell membrane receptors. Binding of the hormone to the receptor on the target cell membrane causes the release of a second messenger (e.g., cAMP) within the cell that sets into play a series of enzyme reactions that modulate cell function. Some of these fixed messenger interactions relate to glucagon, insulin, and epinephrine, which are involved in the control of intermediary metabolism.

Another receptor mechanism involves hormones that pass through target cell membranes to attach to an intracellular "mobile" receptor. These hormone-receptor complexes are then activated in the cytoplasm and enter the nucleus of the cell to promote protein synthesis. This type of mobile receptor mechanism is involved in the action of such hormones as steroids and thyroid hormones.

Mechanisms for regulating the release of hormones involve feedback regulatory systems in which information is transmitted from cell to cell and from organ to organ. Levels of many of the hormones are regulated by feedback mechanisms like that of the *hypothalamic-pituitary-target cell system* (Fig. 15-1), a network which integrates the nervous system and endocrine system. A *primary* defect in hormone function originates in the target gland responsible for producing the hormone. In a secondary defect the structure of the target gland is normal, but the level of stimulating hormone is abnormal and the function of the gland is altered. For example, in the hypothalamic-pituitary axis, removal of the adrenal gland causes a primary deficiency of adrenocorticoid hormones. Removal of the pituitary gland decreases stimulation of the adrenal cortex and causes a secondary deficiency. Still other control mechanisms involve the level of substances in the blood. The production of each hormone is regulated directly or indirectly by the metabolic activity of the hormone. The regulation involves negative feedback loops. In the endocrine system, sensors monitor the level of hormone and adjust hormone secretion to maintain an appropriate level.

DISTURBANCES OF ENDOCRINE FUNCTION

Endocrine disorders have been perceived to result from an excess or deficiency of circulating hormones. However, there are instances when inactivation of the hormone, inadequate receptor function, and impaired cellular response can cause an endocrinopathy even though there is adequate circulating hormone. Even so, most clinically apparent endocrine disorders can be considered in terms of an excess or deficiency of particular hormones. Hyperfunction may result from hyperplasia of endocrine glands or hormone-producing tumor.

It should be kept in mind that endocrine manifestations of nonendocrine disease do occur. Thus an ectopic hormone syndrome may relate to the production of hormones by tissues other than tissues known to produce the hormone, usually a tumor. Hypofunction may occur as a result of infection, inflammation, autoimmune responses or tumors, as well as receptor defects and impaired cellular responses.

Pituitary Function

Pituitary growth hormone (GH) or somatotropin, induces growth in growing tissues, sustains protein synthesis, decreases glucose utilization, and increases utilization of fatty acids. A *deficiency* of growth hormone in the child leads to dwarfism, but the body is well-proportioned. The most common cause is a benign tumor. In pituitary dwarfs the eruption of the teeth is delayed. An *excess* of growth hormone occurring prior to puberty and before fusion of the epiphyses of the long bones leads to gigantism. In the adult, an excess of GH results in *acromegaly*. Patients with advanced acromegaly have prognathism (protruding lower jaw), large hands and feet, an enlarged tongue, spaces between the teeth, broad nose, prominent supraorbital ridge, and often a hunched back.

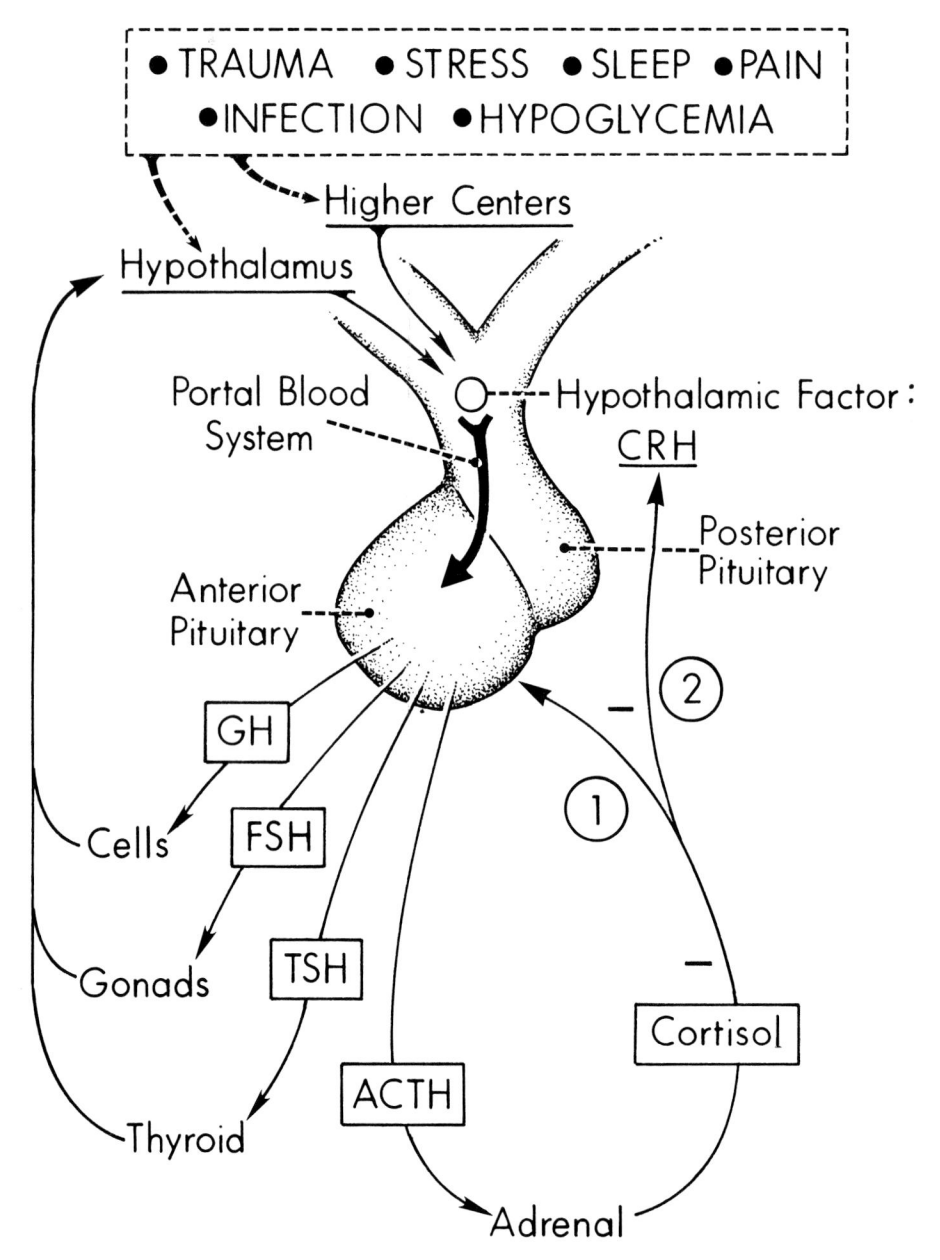

Fig. 15–1. Hypothalamic-pituitary-target cell control system. Hormones of target glands regulate release of hormones from anterior pituitary via a negative feedback system. A large number of factors may influence the system. CRH = corticotrophin releasing hormone (hypothalamic factor). GH = gonatropic hormone. FSH = follicle stimulating hormone. TSH = thyroid stimulating hormone. (1) dominant feedback (negative) control on the pituitary gland; (2) feedback control on hypothalamus.

Thyroid Function

The control of thyroid hormone secretion is regulated by the *hypothalamic-pituitary-thyroid feedback system* (Fig. 15–2). In this system the thyrotrophin-releasing hormone (TRH), which is produced by the hypothalamus, regulates the secretion of thyroid stimulating hormone (TSH) from the anterior pituitary gland.

Hypothyroidism may be due primarily to defects in the gland itself, or secondarily to pituitary or hypothalamic dysfunction. A deficiency of thyroid function at birth is called *cretinism*. If the disturbance occurs in the child, *juvenile myxedema* occurs, and in the adult, *adult myxedema* occurs. The primary manifestations of cretinism are related to the lack of growth and mental and sexual development. There is a lack of growth of

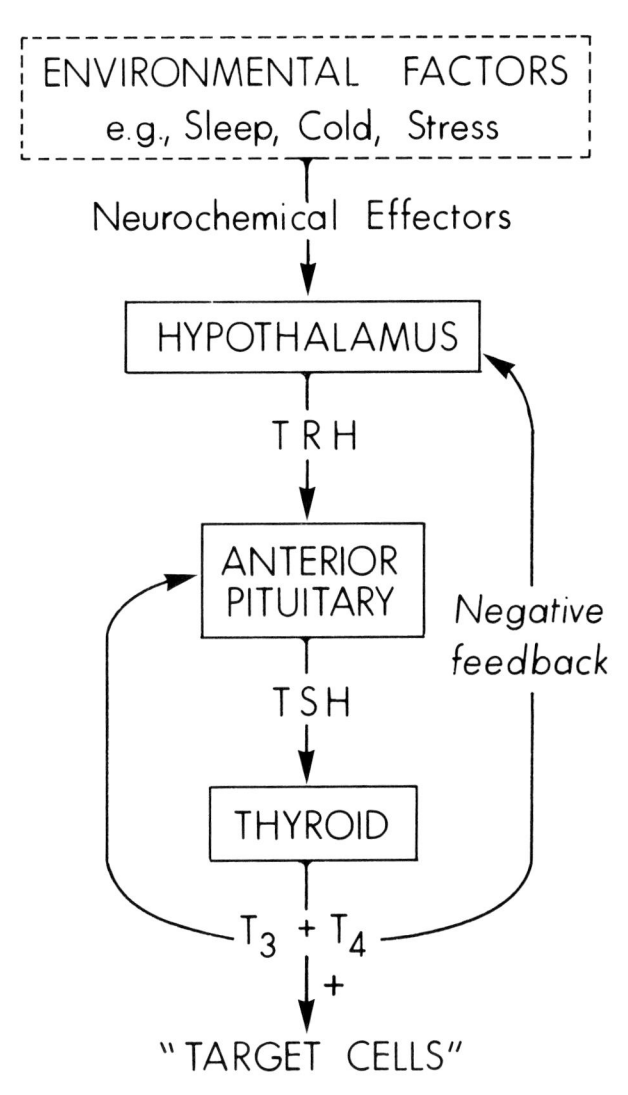

Fig. 15–2. Hypothalamic-pituitary-thyroid feedback control system which regulates thyroid hormone. TRH = thyrotrophin-releasing-hormone; TSH = thyroid-stimulating-hormone. T_3 = active form of thyroid hormone; T_4 = thyroxine. Environmental factors increase the production of thyroid hormone.

long bones, the mandible is underdeveloped, the base of the skull shortened, the hair is sparse and brittle, and the sweat glands atrophic. The clinical findings in myxedematous patients relate to swelling of the soft tissues of the face and mouth due to the accumulation of a mucopolysaccharide substance in the interstitial spaces. Causes of hypothyroidism include thyroidectomy, therapeutic irradiation, drugs, and secondary disturbances such as hypothalamic dysfunction and pituitary dysfunction. Treatment involves replacement with purified hormones.

Hyperthyroidism or thyrotoxicosis results from too much circulating thyroid hormone. Causes include hyperplasia, adenoma, and goiter. Clinical manifestations are due to increased metabolism and an increase in sympathetic nervous system activity. Clinical features are prominence of eyes ("stare"), increased irritability, heat intolerance, tremor, and in some forms of the hypofunction, Graves' disease (exophthalmos, goiter, and hyperthyroidism, i.e., bulging eyes, enlarged thyroid gland and excess thyroid hormone production). Treatment involves surgery or drugs to decrease thyroid function.

Parathyroid Function

The parathyroid glands produce parathyroid hormone (PTH), which acts to maintain serum calcium levels. The hormone calcitonin, which is secreted by C cells in the thyroid gland, inhibits calcium mobilization from bone and has an effect opposite to PTH. Of importance is the reciprocal relationship of calcium and phosphate concentration in the extracellular fluids, i.e., when calcium levels are high, phosphate levels are low, and calcium excretion from the kidneys is reciprocally related to phosphate excretion. Thus the regulation of serum calcium and phosphate is accomplished by vitamin D, parathyroid hormone, and calcitonin.

Hypoparathyroidism

A decrease in the secretion of parathormone may be due to various diseases, including neoplasms, or to accidental removal of the parathyroid glands at the time of thyroidectomy. The clinical manifestations of hypoparathyroidism include muscle cramps, aches and pains, convulsions, laryngeal spasms, dry scaly skin, frequent headaches, irritability, association with candidiasis, and paresthesias—numbness and tingling sensations). It has been reported that an insufficient secretion of parathyroid hormone in infancy results in defective enamel formation (aplasia, hypoplasia) and blunting of the roots of the molar teeth.

Hyperparathyroidism

Hypersecretion of the parathyroid hormone may result from neoplasms involving the parathyroid glands or from diffuse hyperplasia of the parathyroid glands. Hypersecretion may also result secondarily from hyperplasia of the parathyroid glands owing to calcium deprivation or renal disease. In the first instance, the dysfunction is called primary hyperparathyroidism; in the case of the compensatory response to a deficiency of calcium or to renal disease, the dysfunction is called secondary hyperparathyroidism.

The effects of hyperparathyroidism may be related to the musculoskeletal system and to the genitourinary system. Also involved less prominently is the gastrointestinal system. Musculoskeletal symptoms include localized or generalized pains in the bones, spontaneous fracture, tumors of the extremities and jaws, and bone deformities. Genitourinary symptoms include renal stones and infections secondary to obstruction by the stones, hematuria, renal insufficiency, and polyuria. Gastrointestinal symptoms include nausea, loss of weight, vomiting, constipation, and anorexia (loss of appetite).

The most prominent effect of hyperparathyroidism is decalcification of the bones, osteoporosis, and marked deformity of the bones. In areas of decalcification, there is replacement of the bone by newly formed fibrous tissue with the production of small, pseudocystic lesions in bone; the process is termed osteitis fibrosa cystica. Fibroblastic replacement of bone may be accompanied by hemorrhage and numerous multinucleated giant cells producing a "brown tumor" which histologically is typical of hyperparathyroidism. Radiographically, the bone lesions appear to have a "ground-glass" appearance.

Adrenal Function

The adrenal glands consist of an inner (medulla) portion, which secretes epinephrine and norepinephrine and is associated with the sympathetic nervous system, and an outer (cortical) part, which secretes three hormones: glucocorticoids, mineralocorticoids, and sex hormones. *Aldosterone* is the principal mineralocorticoid, *cortisol* (hydrocortisone) is the principal glucocorticoid, and several steroids with weak androgenic (male sex hormone) activity are sex hormones. Major disorders of the adrenal cortex occur with deficiencies or excesses of one or more of the steroids. An excess of glucocorticoid causes *Cushing's syndrome,* an excess of mineralocorticoid causes *Conn's syndrome* (aldosteronism), and an excess of androgens causes *virilization. Addison's disease* reflects a deficiency of all three. These diseases will be considered later.

Glucocorticoids are adrenal steroids having a predominant action on intermediary metabolism, i.e., anabolic and catabolic phases of metabolism determined by hormones. The anabolic phase is mediated primarily by insulin and the catabolic phase is initiated by glucagon. In the anabolic state substrates of ingested foods are transported to be stored as structural protein, fat and glycogen; however, some of the exogenous substrate is used at the time for energy. In the catabolic phase, or during the postabsorptive state, initially the glycogen stored in the liver is broken down to glucose and released as needed by the brain and central nervous system for energy. Later new glucose is derived from other peripheral sources via gluconeogenesis. Also free fatty acids are derived from adipose (fat) tissue and hepatic ketogenesis is activated in the liver. In terms of fasting, after a few days, free fatty acids and ketones are used for energy by most tissues, leaving glucose for the brain and other parts of the central nervous system. Thus in the first hours of fasting, glycogenolysis is predominant; but after the first day, catabolic processes involve gluconeogenesis and protein breakdown with accelerated use of fat stores. This postabsorptive metabolic adaptation provides for energy in the absence of exogenous substrates and is hormonally induced in response to a fall in insulin release and a rise in epinephrine, glucagon, cortisol, and growth hormone.

Aldosterone is an adrenal steroid having a primary role in regulating extracellular fluid volume and a major determinant of potassium metabolism. The mineralocorticoid effects of aldosterone include sodium conservation and potassium loss in the kidney. The secretion of aldosterone is controlled by the renin-angiotensin system, serum potassium, and ACTH (adrenocorticotrophic hormone). *Renin,* which is an enzyme produced by the kidney when there is a decrease in renal blood flow, combines with the plasma protein angiotensin to form *angiotensin I.* This complex then circulates to the lung to be activated and become *angiotensin II,* a vasoconstrictor, and in turn decrease the output of the renin. Angiotensin II stimulates the adrenal cortex to release more aldosterone, which increases sodium resorption by the kidney, resulting in increased water retention and vascular volume. Potassium ions regulate aldosterone independent of the renin-angiotensin system, i.e., an increase in oral potassium increases plasma levels of aldosterone. ACTH seems to have a minor role in aldosterone control in normal humans.

Adrenal androgens are peripherally interconvertible with the androgen testosterone produced in the testes. Androgens are the major determinants of hair distribution and virilizing syndromes may occur with adrenal overandrogenization due to adrenal hyperplasia, carcinoma, adenoma, or Cushing's syndrome (p. 261). Virilization refers to excessive androgen-dependent hair (terminal hair involving the upper lip, chin, anterior chest in women) plus other changes such as amenorrhea, frontal balding, deepening of the voice, and muscular hypertrophy). Ovarian virilization may also reflect a serious underlying disease.

Hypofunction of Adrenal Cortex

Adrenocortical hypofunction with a deficiency of adrenal steroid hormones may be due to a primary disturbance in elaborating the hormones or secondarily to a failure of ACTH elaboration by the pituitary gland. Primary adrenocortical deficiency (Addison's disease) involves combined glucocorticoid and mineralocorticoid deficiencies whereas secondary insufficiency involves only glucocorticoid deficiencies.

The manifestations of primary adrenocortical insufficiency (cortisol and aldosterone) include slowly progressive fatigue, weakness, loss of appetite, nausea, vomiting, weight loss, and hyperpigmentation of skin (diffuse brown or bronze) and in many patients, bluish-black hyperpigmented patches on the mucous membranes (Fig. 15-3). A primary insufficiency is relatively rare but secondary adrenocortical insufficiency is seen with increasing frequency because of increasing use of steroid therapy. The primary disease is most often due to idiopathic adrenal atrophy probably related to an autoimmune mechanism. Concomitant parathyroid and adrenal insufficiency with mucocutaneous moniliasis (p. 246) constitute a distinct familial autosomal recessive syndrome.

When a disease being treated with potentially harmful steroids no longer requires glucocorticoid therapy, steroid withdrawal may expose the patient to acute adrenocortical insufficiency especially in relation to stress, including periodontal surgical procedures. The withdrawal symptoms may be similar to those of chronic adrenocortical insufficiency.

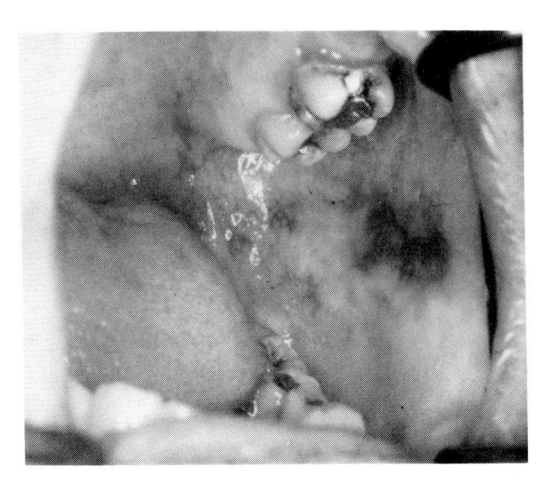

Fig. 15-3. Melanin pigmentation associated with Addison's disease.

Hyperfunction of Adrenal Cortex

The clinical syndromes associated with excess adrenocortical hormones include *Cushing's syndrome* related to an excess of cortisol, *aldosteronism* involved in an excess production of aldosterone, and *adrenal virilization* due to excessive production of adrenal androgens. There is generally overlapping of these syndromes.

Cushing's syndrome results from the overproduction of glucocorticoid when there is a malfunction of one of the components of cortisol production, i.e., hypothalamus, pituitary, adrenal cortex. The effects of excess cortisol (hypercortisolism) relate to the stimulation of gluconeogenesis by cortisol, i.e., production of increased glucose at the expense of protein anabolism. Manifestations include a "moon face," protruding abdomen, and a "buffalo hump" on the back just below the neck, associated with altered fat metabolism. There are also purple striae (stretch marks) of the thin skin over the protruding abdomen. Because of protein breakdown, there is muscle weakness and wasting. Also present is osteoporosis, an increased susceptibility to infection, and overt diabetes mellitus in some instances. Personality changes, hypertension, and gastric ulceration may be manifestations. An overproduction of adrenal androgen may lead to hirsutism (increase in androgen-dependent hair in women), acne and occasionally virilization.

Cushing's syndrome is caused in one-third of the cases by an overproduction of ACTH by the pituitary gland in response to a pituitary adenoma. Adrenal adenomas produce clinical manifestations of an excess of glucocorticoids, not mineralocorticoid or adrenal androgens.

An excess of mineralocorticoid occurs most commonly from an overproduction of aldosterone. *Primary hyperaldosteronism* may be caused by hyperplasia of the adrenal cortex or by an aldosterone-producing adenoma (Conn's syndrome). Secondary pathologic aldosteronism may occur in congestive heart failure, hypertension, and unilateral renal disease. The increase in the production of aldosterone by the adrenal gland occurs in response to the activation of the renin-angiotensin system. Most patients who exhibit secondary aldosteronism have an associated hypertension or underlying edema disorder. The manifestations of *primary aldosteronism* include frequent mild frontal headache, chronic fatigue, muscle weakness, frequent urination, hypertension, impaired insulin secretion caused by hypokalemia (abnormally low serum potassium), and sodium retention. The clinical features of *secondary aldosteronism* are primarily those of the cause of the disease, including hypertension (progressive), use of oral contraceptives, and toxemia of pregnancy to add a few not already mentioned. Edema is relatively common in secondary aldosteronism.

Hypertension is an abnormal maintained elevation of arterial blood pressure. In terms of measuring arterial pressure with an arm cuff (sphygmomanometer) the criteria for screening of hypertension is based on pressures that exceed 140 to 160 mm Hg systolic and 90 to 95 mm Hg diastolic. Hypertension may be primary (essential), where the cause is largely unknown, or secondary, where the chronic elevation of blood pressure is due to kidney disease associated with increased renin levels and present in aldosteronism, arteriosclerosis, and perhaps alcohol consumption. *Malignant* hypertension is a progressive, accelerated form of hypertension which is potentially fatal and is usually a disease of younger individuals. Manifestations of this form of hypertension are diastolic values of 120 mm Hg and above with headache, visual disturbances, motor and sensory deficits, and symptoms related to kidney damage. Drugs used in the control of hypertension include beta-blocking drugs and enzyme inhibitors which prevent conversion of angiotensin I to angiotensin II. A number of drugs are used in the treatment of hypertension that have frequent side-effects of interest, such as dry mouth (xerostomia) that may occur with the use of methyldopa (Aldomet) and clonidine (Catapres).

GONADAL DYSFUNCTION

The testes and ovaries produce hormones which control secondary sex characteristics, the reproductive cycle, and the growth and development of accessory reproductive organs. Testosterone is the principal naturally occurring male hormone and the chief androgen of the testis. The two principal hormones of the ovary are the follicular hormone (estradiol) and luteal hormone (progesterone). Gonadal dysfunction in both men and women may be due to failure of the pituitary gland to stimulate the gonads or adrenal glands, or to dysfunction of the gonads.

Hypogonadism

The effects of hypogonadism in men depend upon the age at onset of the disturbance. When there is a complete loss of testicular function as the result of inflammation, surgery, injury, or other causes before sex maturation takes place, secondary sex characteristics fail to appear. In the presence of a pituitary deficiency of gonadotropin and other pituitary hormones, dwarfism and hypogonadal changes may result if the pituitary deficiency occurs prior to puberty.

Hypogonadism may be related directly to ovarian insufficiency or may be secondary to a deficiency of gonadotropic hormone secretion by the anterior pituitary gland. The principal effects of ovarian insufficiency are amenorrhea, menopausal symptoms, hot flushes, gain in weight, sweating, nervous tension, and, less frequently, osteoporosis and hirsutism. Naturally occurring ovarian insufficiency between the ages of 45 and 50 years is the menopause. The symptoms of the menopause are numerous and include irregularity and cessation of the menses, emotional disturbances, arthralgia, fatigue, hot flushes, sweating, and headaches. Hirsutism and osteoporosis are not uncommon. Secondary ovarian insufficiency is related to a disturbance of gonadotropin secretion by the pituitary gland and to the action of the hypothalamus on the pituitary.

Hypergonadism

An overproduction of ovarian hormones may result in abnormal menstrual changes. It must be recognized that relative hypergonadism is common during the active reproductive period and is usually of no importance. However, uterine bleeding prior to puberty and after menopause may be due to neoplasms. Prepubertal hypergonadism results in precocious puberty with premature onset of menses, secondary sex characteristics, and rapid skeletal growth. In some instances, such hypergonadism is due to tumors of the ovaries. Postpubertal hypergonadism may be primary or secondary in origin and is characterized primarily by changes in the menstrual cycle. A few ovarian neoplasms are functional and give rise to masculinization, feminization, or precocious puberty and menstrual bleeding.

POLYGLANDULAR DISORDERS

Disorders reflecting hyper- or hypofunction of multiple endocrine glands may refer to multiple hormonal deficiencies resulting from interference with central control of pituitary hormone secretion, or to autonomous dysfunction of more than one endocrine gland in relation to neoplasia or immunologic abnormalities.

Multisystem Hyperfunction

The major multiple endocrine neoplasia syndromes are: Type I (MEN-I), which is characterized by multiple tumors of the pituitary, parathyroid, and pancreatic islet cells and a high incidence of peptic ulcer; Type II (MEN-II), which is characterized by carcinoma of the thyroid gland, pheochromocytoma (tumor of the sympathetic nervous system), and parathyroid hyperplasia; and Type III (MEN-III), which resembles Type II in that thyroid carcinoma and pheochromocytoma are present, but may also include manifestations of disfiguring neuromas of the lips, tongue, and buccal mucosa, and café-au-lait spots, and neurofibromas of the skin.

Multisystem Hypofunction

The major polyglandular deficiency syndromes include Schmidt's syndrome and the candidiasis-endocrinopathy syndrome.

The principal features of Schmidt's syndrome include Addison's disease, lymphocytic thyroiditis, "primary" failure of other endocrine glands such as the parathyroids, gonads, and nonendocrine abnormalities presumed to be of autoimmune origin.

The characteristics of the candidiasis-endocrinopathy syndrome that differentiate this disturbance from the Schmidt syndrome include the early onset of chronic monilial infection followed by the development of idiopathic (cause not determined) adrenal insufficiency or hypoparathyroidism or both. The fungal infection is refractory to conventional chemotherapy. Candida albicans has not been isolated from the affected endocrine gland.

METABOLIC DISEASE

Some metabolic diseases are closely related to endocrinologic problems and will be discussed briefly. Considered will be diabetes mellitus, which is a prototype for multifactorial disorders, disorders of bone metabolism (osteitis deformans; osteoporosis), and disturbances of purine metabolism (gout).

Diabetes Mellitus

Diabetes mellitus is a term used to describe a constellation of metabolism abnormalities which appear to be caused by an absolute or relative insulin deficiency in association with a relative or absolute excess of glucagon. Glucagon is produced by the pancreatic alpha cells of the islets of Langerhans and has actions which are diametrically opposite to those of insulin. Whereas insulin, which is produced by the beta cells, provides for glucose storage, increases protein synthesis and prevents fat breakdown, glucagon increases gluconeogenesis, increases lipolysis and enhances the breakdown of proteins. Ingested glucose or glucose mobilized from body stores cannot be assimilated into fat or muscle cells and builds up in the blood (hyperglycemia) or is excreted in the urine (glycosuria). When sufficient insulin is present, glucose is stored as glycogen in the liver or muscle cells, and stored in fat cells as triglycerides. When glucose stores are depleted, the liver is able to synthesize glucose from amino acids (glyconeogenesis). Stored fatty acids cannot be converted to glucose, but are used as a source of energy directly, or converted to ketones by the liver. The brain and other parts of the central nervous system can only utilize glucose or ketone bodies for energy. Excess ketone production results in ketoacidosis (a disturbance of diabetes mellitus which tends to add acid to body fluids, e.g., ketones). The clinical manifestations of diabetes mellitus include polyphagia (frequent eating), polydipsia (frequent fluid intake), and polyuria (frequent urination). These are closely related to an elevated blood sugar (hyperglycemia) and sugar in the urine (glycosuria).

Diabetes mellitus has been classified by the National Diabetes Data Group of the National Institute of Health into two categories: *Type-I, Insulin-dependent* diabetes mellitus (IDDM), which previously has been classed as juvenile-onset diabetes; and *Type-2, Non-insulin-dependent* diabetes mellitus, which has been described previously as adult-onset diabetes mellitus. Type-2 is not insulin dependent or ketosis-prone, although insulin may be required occasionally. Another category is *other types of diabetes,* which includes diabetic disturbances secondary to pancreatitis, hormones, insulin receptor anomalies, and drug or chemical induced diabetes mellitus.

The criteria for diabetes mellitus are established in terms of "blood sugar" (plasma glucose) still present at selected intervals of time after ingestion of a glucose load. The oral glucose tolerance test (OGTT) is able to demonstrate that diabetic individuals respond inadequately to an increase in the blood sugar by releasing too little insulin to facilitate storage. Therefore, the blood glucose is greater initially and remains elevated longer in diabetic persons than in normal individuals. Other home methods are available to monitor blood glucose levels so that the diabetic patient may adjust insulin, food, and activity to meet each day's program, including stressful situations.

The normal fasting blood sugar (plasma glucose in mg/dl) is less than 115. An OGTT is never above 200 and is below 140 at 2 hours after a beverage containing a precise amount of glucose has been given to a person who had fasted overnight. With impaired glucose tolerance, fasting values are below 140, and the OGTT values may be over 200 once and between 140 to 199 at 2 hours. For a diabetic the fasting value is 140 more than once (repeat testing), and the OGTT is over 200 at 2 hours and at one earlier time.

A complication of type I diabetes (IDDM) is ketoacidosis. A patient with advanced ketoacidosis and dehydration may be nauseated, vomit, breathe rapidly and deeply, and his/her breath may have the sweetish odor of acetone. Such patients may go into a coma. Ketoacidosis does not occur in Type-2 diabetes (NIDDM) although a coma may result from high blood sugar in elderly individuals.

The complications of chronic hyperglycemia and attending biochemical changes that accompany diabetes mellitus include structural defects in the basement membrane of small blood vessels and capillaries, thickening of the walls of nutrient vessels that supply nerves, demyelinization of nerve cells and problems with tissue oxygenation. The kidneys, the retina, and the extremities appear to be most sensitive to the small blood vessels in these structures.

The treatment of diabetes mellitus involves insulin control or keeping blood sugar as normal as possible. Such control can be accomplished in many instances by having the patient monitor the blood sugar level throughout the day and using an insulin pump to provide insulin as appropriate in small droplets at a rate consistent with monitored needs. Tight control of blood sugar with insulin has its hazards. An insulin reaction may occur, either mild or leading to a coma. Insulin reactions can be warded off by drinking fruit juice or something sweet, but if this is not possible, an injection of glucagon can offset the effects of insulin and raise the blood sugar.

Metabolic Bone Disease

Bone is a dynamic tissue which has a mechanical function as well as being a store of calcium, phosphorus, sodium, magnesium and other ions used in mineral metabolism and homeostatic functions. Bone consists of an organic matrix, principally collagen, and a solid mineral phase comprised of calcium and phosphate. Bone is formed by osteoblasts that secrete the matrix which is then mineralized and surrounds the secreting cell which becomes an osteocyte connected by canaliculi to its blood supply. Bone resorption is carried out by mononuclear cells and multinucleated giant cells. Factors that alter calcium metabolism and the activities of bone cells provide the basis for understanding metabolic bone disease.

Factors that decrease bone formation include hypophosphatasia, glucocorticoid excess (Cushing's syndrome), aging, and a deficiency of growth hormone. Factors that increase bone resorption include aging, gonadal hormone deficiency, hyperparathyroidism, osteolytic neoplasms, glucocorticoid excess, prostaglandin E, and a deficiency of calcium or phosphate (dietary or renal loss). Pharmacologic and therapeutic agents may be related to a decrease in bone resorption.

Paget's disease of bone (osteitis deformans) is a chronic skeletal disease in which at some stage resorbed bone is replaced by coarse-fibered, dense trabecular bone organized in a haphazard way. The etiology of osteitis deformans is still unknown. The disease occurs predominantly in patients over 40 years of age, and may only be discovered by accident or as the result of such complaints as bone pain, headache, deafness, visual disturbances, weakness, mental disturbances, and facial paralysis. Any skeletal bone may be involved.

Involvement of the jaw bone is common with a predilection for the maxilla which exhibits progressive enlargement. The radiographic appearance of the bone has been described as being like "cotton-wool" in appearance in the osteoblastic phase.

The serum alkaline phosphatase level may be extremely elevated in the osteoblastic phase and during formation of new bone when there is polyostotic involvement.

The formation of bone and hypercementosis associated with this disease sometimes results in obliteration of the periodontal membrane.

The complications of osteitis deformans include pathologic fractures, the development of osteosarcoma, and symptoms already mentioned.

Osteoporosis is a generalized disorder of the skeleton in which there is an excess of bone resorption over bone formation, eventually leading to loss of bone mass, bone fragility and fractures. The cause of osteoporosis is certain in only a few disorders, such as Cushing's syndrome. Osteoporosis is seen most frequently in postmenopausal women although the relationship to menopause is not certain. Risk factors for osteoporosis include postmenopausal state, hypogonadism in males, poor calcium intake, inactivity, heavy smoking, heavy coffee consumption, anticonvulsant therapy, and adrenal corticosteroid therapy. Osteoporosis accounts for a significant mortality rate (16%) in elderly patients with hip fracture associated with osteoporosis.

Gout is a group of diseases in which there is hyperuricemia (increased serum urate, i.e., greater than 7.0 mg/dl), inflammatory arthritis, and in some patients, kidney disease, and deposits of urate crystals (tophi). Primary gout (in contrast to secondary gout where the reason for urate overproduction is known) is genetically determined. The excessive amounts of circulating urates have a predilection for the joints, often the big toe (p. 112).

SUMMARY

Disturbances of the endocrine system may be easily recognized in some instances because the clinical picture is so distinctive, but in other instances the endocrinopathy may be subtle and easily overlooked. Hormones are produced under feedback control, with the most simple systems regulated by the plasma concentrations of the substance that the hormone regulates. The most complex control mechanisms involve cascades of hormones activated by neurologic or neuroendocrine systems. The hypothalamus and the pituitary gland along with the nervous system and endocrine system controls many of the other glands. An excess of a particular hormone, whether related to a *primary* or *secondary* disorder, may produce a deficiency or an excess of the hormone.

A deficiency of growth hormone in a child leads to dwarfism, and an excess in a child leads to gigantism. An excess of the hormone in an adult causes acromegaly. A deficiency of thyroid results in myxedema and when present at birth is called cretinism. An excess of adrenal cortical function leads to Cushing's syndrome, whereas an insufficiency causes Addison's disease. Other disturbances of endocrine function include hypogonadism and hypergonadism. Polyglandular endocrinopathies occur.

Diabetes mellitus, insulin-dependent and noninsulin-dependent forms of the disease, is a disorder of insulin availability. Disturbances associated with the disease involve most of the body and chronic complications include changes in the retina, blood vessels, and peripheral nervous system. Periodontal considerations have already been considered in Chapter 13.

Metabolic bone disease and bone disturbances is best described in terms of factors altering calcium metabolism and activities of bone cells. A common disturbance is osteoporosis, a disease primarily of postmenopausal women. The potential risk for fracture of the hip in the elderly should be considered, and preventive treatment considered. Another disturbance is Paget's disease (osteitis deformans). Bony deformities of the legs, headache, deafness, pain, and pathological fractures occur commonly in this disease.

Oral manifestations of endocrinopathies are not commonly seen except for diabetes mellitus. Candidiasis may be seen with the candidiasis-endocrinopathy syndrome, and multiple neuromas of the lips and tongue seen in adrenal pheochromocytoma—a tumor of the sympathetic nervous system, thyroid or other endocrine glands.

The patient with diabetes mellitus may be susceptible to infection and develop multiple periodontal abscesses in response to deep scaling. The organism, *Capnocytophaga*, has been implicated in advanced periodontitis in "juvenile diabetics." Prevention of infection may require antibiotic coverage.

BIBLIOGRAPHY

Biglieri, E.G.: A perspective on aldosterone abnormalities. Clin. Endocrinol., 5:399, 1976.

Carlson, H.E. and Hershman, J.M.: The hypothalamic-pituitary-thyroid axis. Med. Clin. North Am., 59:1045, 1975.

Foster, D. and McGarry, J.: The metabolic derangements and treatment of diabetic ketoacidosis. N. Engl. J. Med., 309:159, 1983.

Irvine, W.J.: Autoimmunity in endocrine disease. Recent Prog. Horm. Res., 36:59, 1980.

Kuehl, F.A., Jr. and Egan, R.W.: Prostaglandins, arachidonic acid and inflammation. Science, 210:978, 1980.

National Diabetes Data Group. Classification and diagnosis of diabetes mellitus and other categories of glucose intolerance. Diabetes, 28:1039, 1979.

Nordin, B.E., et al.: Osteoporosis and osteomalacia. Clin. Endocrinol. Metab., 9:177, 1980.

West, K., et al.: A detailed study of risk factors for retinopathy and neuropathy in diabetes. Diabetes, 29:501, 1980.

16

HEMATOLOGIC AND HEMATOPOIETIC DISEASES

The pathophysiology of blood and the vascular system reflects a study of the formed elements of the blood, the vessels, the fluid phase of the blood, the active bone marrow, the spleen, lymph nodes, and the macrophage system. Therefore, hematologic and hematopoietic diseases include a wide range of manifestations due to: (1) too few red cells in the circulation *(anemias)*, or too many *(polycythemia* or erythrocytosis); (2) too few white blood cells *(neutropenia,* granulocytopenia), or too many white blood cells *(leukocytosis; leukemia)*; (3) a deficiency of platelets *(thrombocytopenia)*, or abnormal platelet function *(thrombocytopathia);* (4) vascular factors such as increased blood vessel permeability or fragility (e.g., hereditary hemorrhagic telangiectasia, Kaposi's sarcoma) with bleeding into the skin and mucous membranes; and (5) disorders involving eosinophils, plasma cells, lymphocytes, monocyte-macrophage system, and primitive precursor cells of the immune system (e.g., Hodgkin's disease (p. 130), Langerhan's cell (eosinophilic) granulomatosis). These categories will be considered only briefly.

FORMATION OF BLOOD CELLS

All types of blood cells are produced in the bone marrow and, with the exception of lymphocytes, no blood cells are produced outside the bone marrow. The production of new cells (hematopoiesis) in the red bone marrow occurs in response to the need to replace the cells that die each day. The source of the replacement is the hematopoietic stem cell system which encompasses *erythrocytes* (red blood cells) and *thrombocytes* (platelets), as well as leukocytes (all white blood cells) and certain cells not ordinarily included, i.e., macrophages, mast cells, and perhaps osteoclasts. The term *myeloid* pertains to the bone marrow and myeloid hematopoiesis occurs only in the bone marrow in the normal adult. Extramedullary hematopoiesis may occur in a number of diseases, but routinely only with such diseases as leukemia.

RED BLOOD CELLS

Red blood cells are produced by the pluripotent stem cell in the bone marrow. Pluripotent indicates that granulocytes, monocytes and platelets evolve as well as red blood cells from this progenitor cell. A stem cell is capable of self-renewal and differentiation. Under the influence of *erythropoietin* (hormone produced by the kidney), erythroid stem cells differentiate into red cell precursors, and after several cell divisions, the red cell nucleus is removed and the *reticulocyte* is formed. The reticulocyte stays in the blood for 24 hours before losing its mitochondria and ribosomes and becomes a mature red blood cell. At any one time reticulocytes constitute only a small fraction of the total count of red blood cells (Table 16–1).

The primary role of the red blood cell is to transport oxygen from the lungs to tissues and carbon dioxide from the tissues, which is accomplished by hemoglobin in the red blood cells (RBC). The steps in the biosynthesis of *heme* (iron complexed with a pigment called protoporphyrin IX), which is assembled with globin to form hemoglobin, is a delicately coordinated series of biochemical events. The normal erythrocyte survives for 120 days and is then ingested by phagocytes of the monocyte-phagocyte (reticuloendothelial) system. The form of the mature erythrocyte is that of a biconcave disk with an average diameter of 8 μ. Disorders of erythrocytes are classified in many ways and can be involved. The rather simple classification used here is based on the morphologic aspects of the erythrocytes.

ERYTHROCYTE DISORDERS

NORMOCYTIC, NORMOCHROMIC ANEMIAS. In these types of anemias the patient has red blood cells of normal size and normal hemoglobinization, but is suffering from blood loss, hemolytic, aplastic, or myelophthisic anemias. Increased red cell destruction is the cause of *hemolytic anemias,* bone marrow failure is the cause of *aplastic anemias,* and replacement of bone marrow by malignancy, fibrosis, or granulomas is the cause of myelophthisic anemia. The mean cell volume (MCV) and mean cell hemoglobin concentration (MCHC) values are normal (Table 16–1).

MICROCYTIC, HYPOCHROMIC ANEMIAS. The characteristic morphologic features of the erythrocytes in these anemias are small, incompletely hemoglobinized red blood cells. These defects are related to defective production of hemoglobin. Most of these anemias are seen in patients with a deficiency of iron, with a defect in heme synthesis, or with defective globin synthesis. MCV and MCHC values are low.

MACROCYTIC NORMOCHROMIC ANEMIAS. These anemias are characterized by large red blood cells. This defect in erythrocytosis leads to premature cell death. Such anemias are most often associated with deficiencies in vitamin B_{12} or folic acid. In some instances these anemias are due to liver disease or related to leukemia. MCV values are high, but MCHC values are normal.

In terms of pathogenesis, erythrocyte disorders can be classified as being due to: (1) stem cell disorders such as polycythemia and aplastic anemia; (2) DNA disorders, including vitamin B_{12} deficiency or megaloblastic anemia; (3) heme and globin disorders such as porphyria, sickle cell anemia, and thalassemias; and (4) eryth-

Table 16–1. Normal Blood Values

Plasma volume:	39–40 ml/kg/body weight
Hemoglobin:	Male, 16.0 ± 2.0 g/dl
	Female, 14.0 ± 2.0 g/dl
Red blood cells (RBC):	Male, 5.4 ± 0.9 millions/mm³
	Female, 4.8 ± 0.6 millions/mm³
White blood cells:	4,300 to 10,000/mm³
Platelets:	150,000 to 440,000/mm³
Reticulocytes:	0.1% to 1.5% of total RBC
Mean cell volume (MCV):	82–101 femtoliters/cell (fl.)
Mean cell hemoglobin conc (MCHC):	32–36 g/100 ml (gm/dl)

rocyte survival disorders such as erythroblastosis fetalis.

Polycythemia vera is a chronic disease in which erythrocytosis results in an increase in red cell mass with an increase in blood viscosity and blood volume. Clinical manifestations include headache, tinnitus (ringing in the ears), epistaxis (nose bleeding), vertigo (dizziness), and ruddy cyanosis (reddish-blue tinge in the color of the skin or mucosa). Oral manifestations involving the oral mucous membranes include the cyanotic (deep purple-red) appearance of the tongue and gingiva.

Aplastic anemia is a bone marrow disturbance in which there is a reduction in stem cells and active bone marrow. The bone marrow is replaced by fatty tissue and *pancytopenia* results, i.e., not only red cells but white cell production is affected. The manifestations resulting from the pancytopenia include: general weakness and fatigue; fever and infections; and hemorrhages into the skin, mucosa, and gingiva. Aplastic anemia is caused by drugs, irradiation, and immunologic and neoplastic disorders. In many cases the cause is unknown (idiopathic), but in the past one-fourth of the cases were due to the use of the antibiotic chloramphenicol.

Megaloblastic anemias occur as a result of defective DNA synthesis and ineffective erythropoiesis. In all but a few cases of this type of anemia, defective DNA synthesis is secondary to a deficiency of vitamin B_{12} or folic acid. The intestinal absorption of vitamin B_{12} (extrinsic factor) is dependent upon its being complexed with an intrinsic factor (IF) produced by the parietal cells of the stomach. B_{12} and folic acid are interrelated as coenzymes in cell DNA synthesis. Common causes of vitamin B_{12} deficiency include partial gastrectomy, pernicious anemia and sprue (malabsorption syndrome). Other possible causes of macrocytic erythrocytes include antimetabolites such as 6-mercaptopurine used in cancer chemotherapy, and phenytoin therapy (p. 220).

Pernicious anemia is associated with vi-

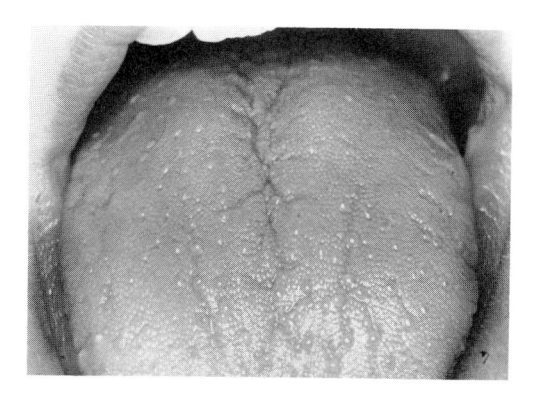

Fig. 16-1. *Pernicious anemia.* There is loss of filiform papillae and the fungiform papillae are reduced in number and size. The apparent prominence of the fungiform papillae is secondary to atrophy of the filiform papillae.

tamin B deficiency and is an anemia resulting from defective secretion of intrinsic factor. The characteristics of pernicious anemia are pancytopenia, atrophy of the papillae of the tongue (Fig. 16-1) and ineffective erythropoiesis. Also present are neurologic symptoms such as paresthesia and loss of position and vibratory sense. Treatment of vitamin B_{12} deficiency is parenteral injection of the vitamin. Megaloblastic anemias due to other causes require treatment of the primary disease after initial B_{12} therapy.

Iron deficiency anemia is a common form of anemia which occurs with chronic gastrointestinal blood loss, inadequate intake of iron and with achlorhydria (decreased stomach juices). The symptoms of this microcytic hypochromic anemia are weakness, fatigue, lassitude and light-headedness. With severe, prolonged iron deficiency anemia, patients may develop the Plummer-Vinson syndrome, i.e., dysphagia due to membranous webs at the postcricoid area. In addition to these esophageal strictures there is angular cheilitis (cracking of the angles of the mouth), painful atrophic glossitis (Fig. 16-2), and spoon-shaped fingernails (koilonychia). There appears to be a relationship between Plummer-Vinson syndrome and the development of oral car-

270 HEMATOLOGIC AND HEMATOPOIETIC DISEASES

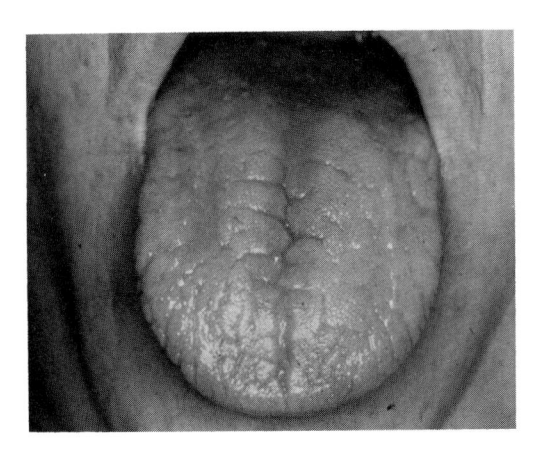

Fig. 16–2. Atrophic changes in tongue associated with Plummer-Vinson syndrome.

cinoma. Therapy for iron deficiency anemia is the administration of iron salts (e.g., ferrous sulfate).

Congenital erythropoietic porphyria is a rare recessively inherited defect with severe accumulation of porphyrins in the bones and teeth (Fig. 16–3) during fetal development. The teeth are discolored red and the urine is pink or red in color. Severe scarring of the fingers, ears and nose may occur. In addition to these lesions, there is hemolytic anemia and severe photosensitivity.

Sickle cell anemia is caused by a structurally abnormal hemoglobin (HbS) which causes erythrocytes to undergo distortion (sickling) under reduced partial pressure of oxygen. The erythrocyte sickling causes chronic hemolytic anemia and periodic bouts of vaso-occlusive (closing of vascular structures) phenomena in the microvascular system of tissues and organs. These bouts cause excruciating crises of pain. Organ damage from the occlusion of micro- and sometimes macrovasculature (arteries and veins) is cumulative. There is a susceptibility to infection. This anemia is inherited as a mendelian dominant, non-sex-linked characteristic. Carriers of sickle cell trait are asymptomatic except for hematuria due to renal infarction. Therapy is essentially symptomatic. Roentgenograms of the skull may show perpendicular radiating trabeculations which give the skull the appearance of having bone standing on end and resembling hair standing on end ("hair-on-end"). This pattern is also seen in thalassemia.

Thalassemias are usually inherited disorders of erythrocytes in which there is a deficiency in the rate of synthesis of specific globulin chains during the formation of hemoglobin. The disease is inherited as an autosomal dominant trait. There are two types: thalassemia minor or thalassemia trait, which is a mild form of the disease; and thalassemia major, which is a severe form of the disease. Other forms do exist. Thalassemia major (Cooley's anemia) is usually seen early in life with the patient being small in size, having progressive anemia, jaundice, chronic leg ulcers and mongoloid facies, i.e., eyes wide apart, nose flattened, bossing of the skull, hypertrophy of the maxilla, and prominent malar eminences. Radiographs of the skull show the hair-on-end striations. Thalassemia trait does not have clinical manifestations and no treatment is required. Transfusions remain the treatment for thalassemia major, but survival beyond the second decade does not occur.

Erythroblastosis fetalis (congenital hemolytic anemia) is an erythrocyte disorder due essentially to the inheritance from the

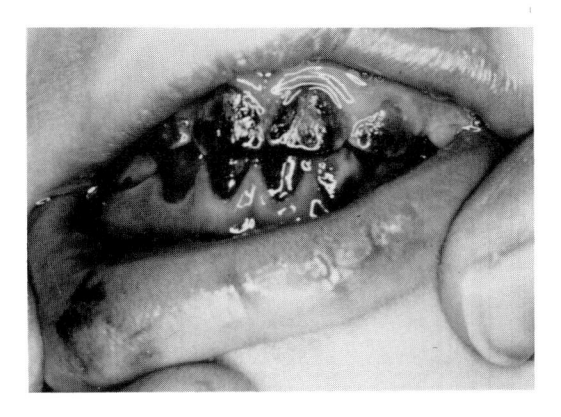

Fig. 16–3. Pigmentation of the teeth consistent with porphyria.

Table 16-2. Differential White Cell Count

Cell Type	%	International Unit (× 10⁹/L)
Neutrophils (Segs)	54–62	—
Neutrophils (Bands)	5–10	—
Neutrophils (total)	40–75	1.50– 7.5
Eosinophils	0– 3	0.00– 0.60
Basophils	0– 1	0.00– 0.05
Monocytes	1– 7	0.00– 0.80
Lymphocytes	18–35	0.60– 5.00
Total WBC	—	4.00–11.00

father of a blood factor which acts as a foreign antigen to the mother. This disturbance has been discussed in an earlier chapter (p. 78). Oral manifestations include staining of the enamel and dentin of developing primary teeth, giving them a green, brown, or blue hue. Also enamel hypoplasia involving the incisal edges of the anterior teeth may occur.

WHITE BLOOD CELLS

The role of white blood cells in preventing and fighting infections has been discussed in earlier chapters and will not be repeated here. To be considered here are qualitative and quantitative disorders of granulocytes and lymphocytes, and proliferative and malignant diseases of leukocytes. The diseases that cause anemia may also affect the white blood cells, and the anemia may be clinically more important than a quantitative abnormality of the leukocyte.

The total white blood cells (WBC) count in the circulating peripheral blood and the differential white cell count (neutrophils, lymphocytes, monocytes, eosinophils and basophils) for normal humans is shown in Table 16–2.

Neutrophils (granulocytes) in the peripheral blood are usually segmented leukocytes (polymorphonuclear leukocytes) but less mature cells may also be found in normal blood, e.g., "stab" or "band" neutrophils.

Leukopenia refers to a WBC less than 4.0 × 10⁹/L; *granulocytopenia* or *neutropenia* means an absolute count less than 3.0 ×

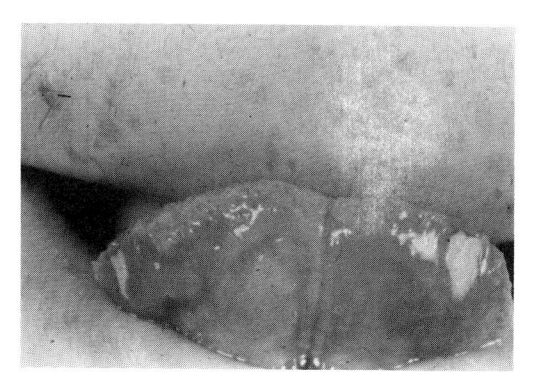

Fig. 16–4. Ulcerations of tongue associated with agranulocytosis.

10⁹/L; and *agranulocytosis* refers to granulocytopenias in which the bone marrow reserve has been depleted. When the absolute number of neutrophils reaches only 1000/mm³ the patient becomes vulnerable to infection, but serious risk occurs at counts of less than 500/mm³. *Cyclic neutropenia* is a periodic granulocytopenia with aggravated periodontitis (p. 228). The syndrome of agranulocytosis consists of fever, sore throat, depressed granulocyte count, and ulcerations of the oral mucosa (Fig. 16–4).

Granulocytopenia may reflect an increased destruction of neutrophils caused by hypersplenism, viral and bacterial infections, drugs and other agents, or a decreased production of granulocytes caused by drugs and ionizing radiation. Common drugs causing granulocytopenia include alcohol, aminopyrine, antibiotics (e.g., chloramphenicol, sulfa drugs, etc.), diphenylhydantoin (p. 220), 6-mercaptopurine, nitrogen mustard (Fig. 16–5), and other cancer chemotherapy agents, tricyclic antidepressants, indomethacin (anti-inflammatory agent), phenothiazines, and tolbutamide.

Granulocytosis is present when the granulocyte count exceeds 10,000/mm³ or greater than 11.0 × 10⁹/L. When the granulocyte count is over 30,000/mm³ the term *leukemoid reaction* is often used. The causes of granulocytosis are numerous, in-

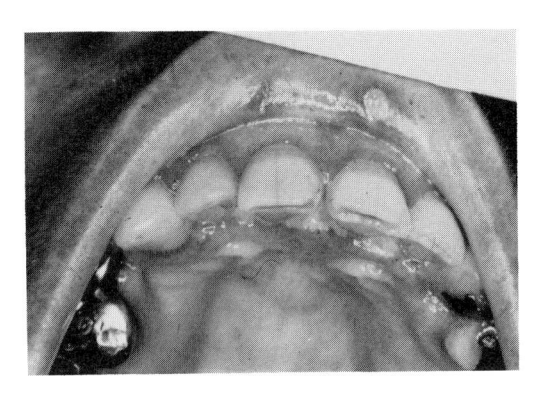

Fig. 16–5. Lesions of the lip and palate related to chemotherapy with nitrogen mustard. The neutropenia was 1,675 white cells. RBC was normochromic, normocytic.

cluding infections, stress, pregnancy, and cigarette smoking.

Eosinophilic granulocytosis or *eosinophilia* refers to greater than 0.6×10^9/L eosinophils in the peripheral blood. Eosinophilia occurs most often in association with allergic or dermatologic disturbances involving antigen-antibody complexes. Other causes of eosinophlia include Hodgkin's disease, X-irradiation therapy, and malignancy.

Basophilia is present when the basophil count is greater than 0.05×10^9 cells per liter. Basophilia may occur in asthma, chronic myelocytic leukemia and hypersensitivity reactions. Low basophil counts may occur as a result of thyroid hormones, radiation, and chemotherapy.

Monocytosis is defined as an "absolute" monocyte count greater than 0.50×10^9/L (>500/mm^3) in patients with tuberculosis, subacute bacterial endocarditis, myelocytic leukemias, lymphomas, and myeloproliferative disorders (e.g., overgrowth of bone marrow cells).

Lymphocytosis is defined as an increase in the absolute lymphocyte count above 5.0×10^9/L (>4000/mm^3) in adults. Infectious mononucleosis is associated with modest lymphocytosis. Lymphocytosis occurs in carcinoma, several infections, malignant lymphomas, and hypopituitarism to name a few disorders.

Lymphopenia is a decrease in the number of circulating lymphocytes (<1500/mm^3) and is seen in a number of infections, neoplastic and connective tissue diseases. Lymphopenia is also seen as a result of therapy with cytotoxic drugs, irradiation, corticosteroids, and immune deficiency diseases.

LEUKEMIAS

Leukemias are malignant diseases of leukocytes in which there are large numbers of leukocytes present in the circulating blood and infiltration of organs and tissues by mature and immature leukocytes. In *acute* leukemia the bone marrow and peripheral blood are filled with immature granulocytes or lymphocytes. In *chronic* leukemia the lymphocytes or granulocytes are mature. Myelocytic and lymphocytic types of leukemia occur. As the names indicate, lymphocytic leukemia involves mature and immature lymphocytes and myelocytic anemia involves large numbers of mature or immature granulocytes or related cells. The time course of acute leukemia is measured in months, whereas it is measured in years in chronic leukemia.

The etiology of leukemias is unknown. Present evidence suggests that they are clonal in origin. Thus leukemia arises from the malignant transformation of one cell. For most patients with leukemia no cause or predisposition can be found.

Acute myelocytic leukemia (AML) is a malignant neoplasm and patients may die within a few days of diagnosis. The median survival time is 2 months. Patients usually have anemia, infection and bleeding (Fig. 16–6A). The diagnosis of AML is made on the basis of changes in the peripheral blood and bone marrow. Gingival hyperplasia may occur in AML (Fig. 16–6B). Unusual manifestations are mucosal ulcerations, dental abscesses, enlargement of salivary glands and hearing loss. Cytotoxic therapy

HEMATOLOGIC AND HEMATOPOIETIC DISEASES 273

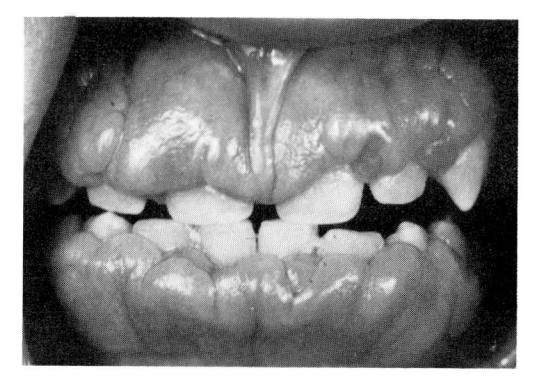

Fig. 16–7. Hyperplastic gingivitis related to monocytic leukemia.

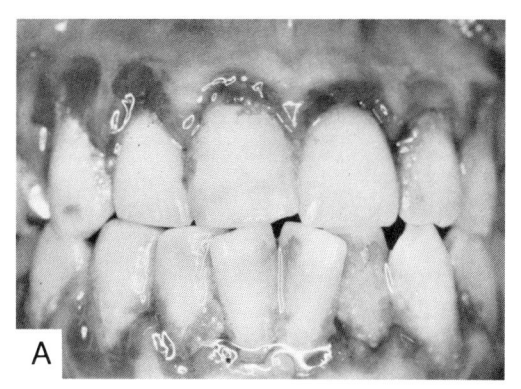

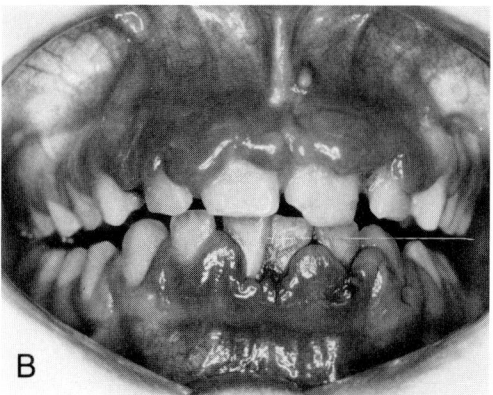

Fig. 16–6. A, Marked gingivitis in patient with acute myelogenous leukemia. B, Hyperplastic gingivitis in patient with chronic myelogenous leukemia.

renders the patient "aplastic" for several weeks before the hematopoietic stem cell (HSC) system begins to produce cells again. Remission may last for months.

Chronic myelocytic leukemia (CML), or chronic myelogenous leukemia, shows increased mature neutrophils in the blood as well as neutrophil precursors found normally only in the bone marrow. Red cell production is decreased. The typical patient is relatively asymptomatic, although a crisis similar to AML may develop.

Acute lymphocytic leukemia (ALL) is usually seen in children with symptoms of anemia, bleeding, or fever. Patients often have severe thrombocytopenia with petechiae and purpura of the skin and mucous membrane. The disease is characterized by large numbers of lymphoblasts and immature lymphocytes in the blood, bone marrow, lymph nodes and spleen. There are a number of subclasses of acute lymphocytic leukemia including T-ALL and B-ALL which have a poor prognosis compared to ALL.

Chronic lymphocytic leukemia (CLL) occurs generally in the elderly patient and is characterized by the accumulation of functionally incompetent lymphocytes. In later stages of CLL, susceptibility to infection develops. Most elderly patients only survive for less than 5 years, but some survive for 10 to 15 years.

Acute monocytic leukemia is characterized by large numbers of monocytes in the blood and bone marrow. Gingival hyperplasia is a common clinical manifestation in this rather rare form of leukemia (Fig. 16–7). In *chronic monocytic leukemia* the manifestations are fatigue and weight loss. Pure monocytic leukemia is rare. Patients may live for months to years, but monocytic leukemia does not respond well to treatment.

Generally the oral manifestations of leukemia include gingivitis, hemorrhage, ulceration and hyperplasia.

THROMBOCYTIC DISORDERS

Excessive bleeding may occur as a result of disorders of platelets, blood vessels or coagulation factors. The coagulation factors have been discussed in chapter 4 in relation to inflammation.

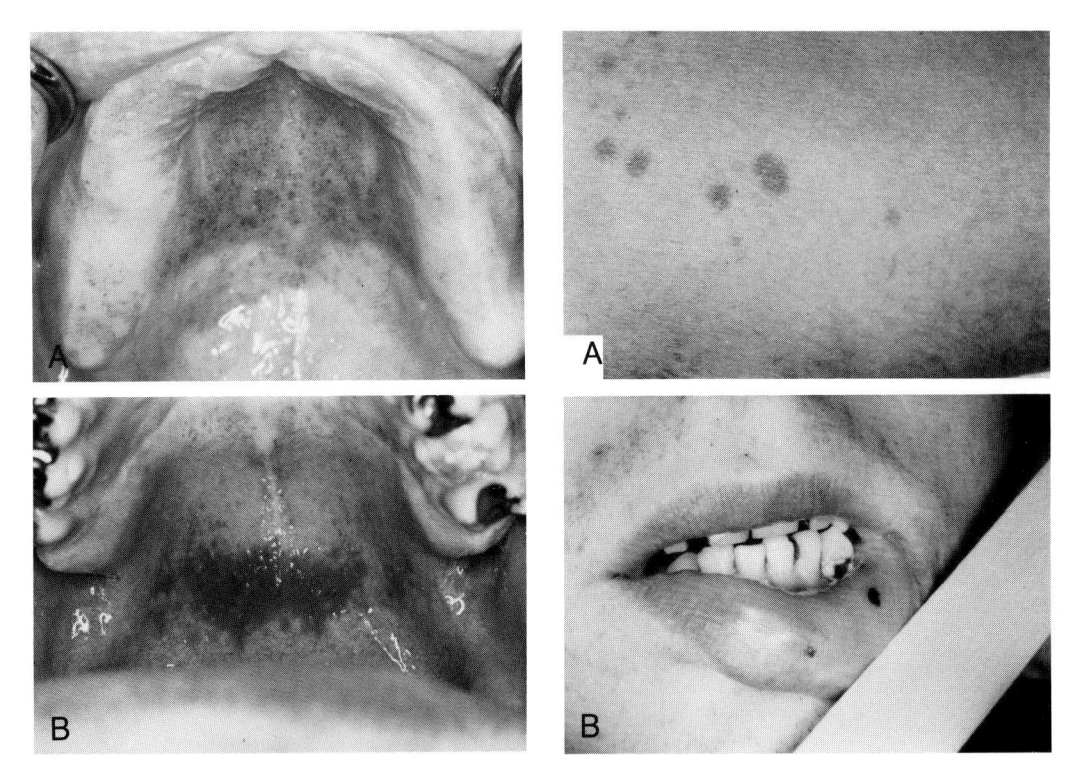

Fig. 16–8. *A,* Petechial hemorrhage associated with anticoagulant therapy and trauma from denture. *B,* Ecchymosis related to coughing.

Fig. 16–9. *A,* Petechiae in skin of the arm of a patient with thrombocytopenic purpura secondary to leukemia. *B,* Petechiae of idiopathic thrombocytopenic purpura.

Functional or numerical inadequacies of platelets result in petechiae, hemorrhages, prolonged bleeding time, and impaired clot retraction. Petechiae (Fig. 16–8A) and ecchymosis or purpura are the hallmark of platelet deficiency disorders. Petechiae and ecchymosis (Fig. 16–8B) are small to large discolorations of the skin and mucous membrane due to hemorrhage. Petechiae and ecchymosis are the general types of purpura. Petechiae usually refers to smaller lesions compared to ecchymosis.

Normal hemostasis requires about 50,000 platelets/mm³, but spontaneous hemorrhage (no trauma) probably does not occur until the platelet count reaches 20,000 platelets/mm³.

Thrombocytopenia may be due to decreased or increased production of platelets. The manifestations of acquired thrombocytopenia include toxic, nutritional and neoplastic disturbances of bone marrow hematopoiesis. Thrombocytopenia is a complication of chronic alcoholism, the use of drugs such as some antibiotics and morphine, and immune reactions which result in increased destruction. Idiopathic thrombocytopenic purpura (ITP) is characterized by an increased platelet destruction in an ostensibly well person. Acute ITP occurs usually following viral infections in children. Chronic ITP occurs commonly in adults, usually in association with other diseases reflecting defective immune responses (e.g., Hodgkin's disease, systemic lupus erythematosus). Compared to the drug-induced immune thrombocytopenia which has a sudden onset, that of chronic ITP is less abrupt. The clinical manifestations of thrombocytopenia relate to purpuric manifestations of the skin (Fig. 16–9A) and oral mucosa (Fig. 16–9B) after minor trauma, including coughing or periodontal scaling, and leukemia.

VASCULAR FACTORS

Vascular factors in hematologic disease include increased permeability and fragility of blood vessels. A number of purpuric and bleeding disorders occur in the absence of platelet coagulation disorders, including diseases of impaired collagen synthesis such as in the hereditary disorder, Ehlers-Danlos syndrome, or in scurvy (p. 140).

Ehlers-Danlos syndrome is a number of disorders characterized by hyperextensibility of the joints, hyperelasticity of the skin, fragility of blood vessels and oral manifestations which may be some of those in osteogenesis imperfecta and dentinogenesis imperfecta (p. 57).

Hereditary hemorrhagic telangiectasia is an autosomal dominant disorder which causes localized dilatations of small vessels. Small vascular spots appear on the mucous membranes of the mouth and nose and on the skin of the fingers and nose. Bleeding may occur from these sites, especially in older patients.

Another hereditary autosomal dominant disorder is *von Willebrand's disease (vWD)* in which there is excessive bleeding with a prolonged bleeding time but normal platelet count. The disturbance involves defective endothelial factors resulting in excessive post-traumatic bleeding, "spontaneous" bleeding from the gingiva, and menorrhagia. Fractions of normal blood plasma may be required to arrest bleeding or prepare for surgery.

Immunologic damage to endothelial cells lining blood vessels leads to purpuric lesions, often with urticarial (welts or hives) raised lesions. These lesions may occur following the use of medication.

As already indicated, there has been a marked increase in Kaposi's sarcoma with the acquired immunodeficiency syndrome (AIDS). These lesions involve dilated blood vessels with endothelial hyperplasia, local hemorrhage, and macrophage ingested iron from the hemorrhage that occurs. These hemosiderin deposits give substance and color to the nodular lesions of Kaposi's sarcoma.

COAGULATION DISORDERS

Disturbances in hemostatic mechanisms that lead to bleeding may be related to defects in platelets, the vascular system or plasma coagulation factors. Coagulation factors have been discussed in relation to inflammation and although hereditary deficiencies of each of the ten clotting factors have been described in the literature, all are rare except classical hemophilia A, hemophilia B, and von Willebrand's disease. The latter involves impaired platelet adhesion and has been considered under *Vascular Factors*.

Hemophilia A is a hereditary deficiency of Factor VIII (antihemophilic factor), and *hemophilia B* (Christmas disease) is a hereditary deficiency of Factor IX (Christmas factor). Both are sex-linked and transmitted via asymptomatic carrier females to one-half their sons. One-half their daughters are carriers. Sons of hemophilic fathers are normal, but daughters are obligate carriers. The clinical disorder is seen only in affected males.

Hemophilia A and B are clinically the same, i.e., both are characterized by bleeding into the joints (hemarthroses), especially ankles, knees, and elbows. Patients with mild hemophilia may only have minor joint hemorrhage. Spontaneous and post-traumatic bleeding may occur. Oropharyngeal bleeding is a dangerous complication of hemophilic hemorrhage because of potential respiratory obstruction.

Control of bleeding is by Factor VIII replacement using concentrates such as cryoprecipitate or highly purified freeze dried concentrates. These concentrates can elevate the Factor VIII level to 60% of normal. However, the occurrence of antibodies to

Factor VIII coagulant activity poses serious problems for some patients. Treatment of hemophiliacs with an antibody to Factor VIII is difficult.

von Willebrand's disease is a hereditary hemorrhagic disorder due to a deficiency of Factor VIII and an associated platelet functional defect. It is transmitted as an autosomal dominant trait from parent to child irrespective of their sex. The severity of this disorder is variable, but there is usually mild bleeding into the skin and mucous membranes. Platelet adhesion in injured blood vessels is impaired and the bleeding time prolonged. Joint hemorrhage is unusual. Cryoprecipitate is the treatment of choice.

Hypercoagulable states are disturbances in which there is a thrombotic tendency, i.e., diseases affecting the blood flow, or vascular integrity. Included in such hypercoagulable states are prosthetic heart valves, atherosclerosis, sickle cell disease, pregnancy, oral contraceptive use, and congestive heart failure.

MONOCYTE-MACROPHAGE DISORDERS

Disorders of the monocyte-macrophage system or reticuloendothelial system (RES) include quantitative and qualitative disturbances, as well as malignant diseases. Malignant disorders include chronic monocytic leukemia. Chronic independent proliferation of completely differentiated macrophages is found locally as *eosinophilic granuloma,* or as now called, *Langerhans cell (eosinophilic) granulomatosis*. Also the term Hand-Schüller-Christian disease is probably synonymous with the term multifocal Langerhans cell granulomatosis. The term histiocytosis X has been challenged also.

The oral manifestations of multifocal Langerhans cell granuloma include single or multiple radiolucent areas that may resemble cysts, periapical granulomas, or periodontal disease. Histologically the lesions consist of masses of histiocytes or eosinophils. Langerhans cell granulomatosis is a benign disease and may have an immune basis.

Malignant lymphoma (Hodgkin's type) has been considered in Chapter 8 (Neoplasia). It is a malignancy of the lymphatic system. *Non-Hodgkin's lymphomas* are mostly neoplasms of B cell lines. Several variations exist, including histiocytic, lymphocytic, and mixed histiocytic-lymphocytic types. The most common clinical manifestation of non-Hodgkin's lymphoma is painless enlargement of one or more of the peripheral lymph nodes. These lymphomas are sensitive to irradiation and chemotherapy.

SUMMARY

The hemopoietic tissues are the sites of production of differentiated blood cells. Some of these cells appear in the circulating blood only, whereas others appear in the tissues in a different form, e.g., basophils as mast cells and monocytes as macrophages. The number of cells, erythrocytes or white cells, are normally present in a certain range that reflects homeostasis. Disturbances may be seen as too many or too few cells in the circulating blood and clinical manifestations relate to a quantitative as well as a qualitative disorder of the cells, including malignancy. The pathophysiology of these disorders may be related to hereditary and/or acquired factors. The causes of many of the disturbances involving the pathophysiology of blood are not entirely clear and treatment may be symptomatic.

Anemia can be viewed as a reduction in the oxygen transporting capacity of the blood. In general the consequences of severe anemia are pallor of skin and mucosa and jaundice when there is excessive destruction of red blood cells as in hemolytic anemias. The manifestations of disorders causing the anemia are those of the underlying diseases, i.e., nutritional deficiencies affecting the tongue, mucosa, purpura, or bruising consistent with accompanying thrombocytopenia.

The numbers of white blood cells in the circulating blood indicate the needs of the body for defense against foreign agents. An increase may suggest that infection or a malignancy is present. If there is a bacterial infection or oral ulceration, there will be leukocytosis in most cases. Granulocytopenia is observed in patients with disorders causing marrow replacement or marrow aplasia. An acute granulocytosis may occur after exposure to acute infections, trauma, or emotional or physical stress.

Uncontrolled proliferation of bone marrow cells may reflect polycythemia vera with large numbers of erythrocytes being produced, or large numbers of white cells as in several of the acute and chronic leukemias involving one of the white cell types, e.g., chronic myelogenous leukemia or acute leukemias such as myelogenous or lymphocytic leukemia.

Disturbances in platelets include thrombocytopenia with clinical manifestations of petechiae, hemorrhages, prolonged bleeding time, and impaired blood clot retraction. Thrombocytosis occurs in response to a number of illnesses, e.g., anemia, leukemia, and chronic inflammatory disorders.

The breakdown of hemostatic mechanisms resulting in bleeding may involve disturbances in platelets, plasma coagulation factors, and vascular factors. A number of hereditary and acquired diseases occur that lead to bleeding, ranging from minor blemishes (petechiae) to such life-threatening states as hemophilia.

Neoplastic and nonneoplastic diseases related to disturbances in the monocyte-macrophage system are not common disorders, although they present diagnostic difficulties for the pathologist. Concepts concerning their origin and classification continue to be revised and their relationship to immune responses clarified. It is important to recognize that radiographic demonstration of radiolucent lesions involving the jaw may have more than local significance and alter dental treatment.

Hematologic and hemopoietic disturbances comprise a broad spectrum of diseases that need to be recognized and considered in dental treatment, not only because of potential adverse effects for the patient such as bleeding, infection, and delay in treatment of unrecognized disease, but potential hazards for those engaged in treatment of patients at risk for acquired immune deficiency diseases.

BIBLIOGRAPHY

Ahlbom, H.E.: Simple achlorhydric anemia, Plummer-Vinson syndrome, and carcinoma of the mouth, pharynx and oesophagus in women. Br. Med. J., 2:231, 1936.

Birch, C.L., and Snider, F.F.: Tooth extraction in hemophilia. J. Am. Dent. Assoc., 26:1933, 1939.

Boggs, D.R., and Winkelstein, A.: *White Cell Manual,* 4th ed., Philadelphia, F.A. Davis Co., 1983.

Cook, T.J.: Blood dyscrasias as related to periodontal disease: with special reference to leukemia. J. Periodontol., 18:159, 1947.

Curtis, A.B.: Childhood leukemias: initial oral manifestations. J. Am. Dent. Assoc., 83:159, 1971.

Erslev, A.J., and Gabuzda, T.G.: *Pathophysiology of Blood,* 3rd ed., Philadelphia, W.B. Saunders Co., 1985.

Friedman-Kien, A.E., et al.: Disseminated Kaposi's sarcoma in homosexual men. Ann. Intern. Med., 96:693, 1982.

Goldenfarb, P.B., and Finch, S.C.: Thrombotic thrombocytopenic purpura. A ten-year survey. J.A.M.A., 226:644, 1973.

Gorlin, R.J., and Chaudhry, A.P.: The oral manifestations of cyclic (periodic) neutropenia. Arch. Dermatol., 82:344, 1960.

Hayward, J.R., and Capodanno, J.A.: Trigeminal neurologic signs in leukemia. J. Oral Surg., Anesth. Hosp. Dent. Serv., 21:499, 1963.

Lewis, J.H.: Coagulation defects. J.A.M.A., 178:1014, 1961.

Livingston, R.J., White, N.S., Catone, G.A., and Hartsock, R.J.: Diagnosis and treatment of von Willebrand's disease. J. Oral Surg., 32:65, 1974.

Millard, H.D., and Gobetti, J.P.: Nonspecific stomatitis—a presenting sign in pernicious anemia. Oral Surg., 39:562, 1975.

Novak, A.J.: The oral manifestations of erythroblastic (Cooley's) anemia. Am. J. Orthod. Oral Surg., *30*:539, 1944.

Pogrel, M.A.: Thrombocythemia as a cause of oral hemorrhage. Oral Surg., *44*:535, 1977.

Poyton, H.G., and Davey, K.W.: Thalassemia. Changes visible in radiographs used in dentistry. Oral Surg., *25*:564, 1968.

Reich, P.R.: *Hematology, Physiopathologic Basis for Clinical Practice*, 2nd ed., Boston, Little, Brown & Co., 1984.

Rosenberg, R.D., and Rosenberg, J.S.: Natural anti-coagulant mechanisms. J. Clin. Invest., *74*:1, 1984.

Weiss, H.J.: Platelet physiology and abnormalities of platelet function. N. Engl. J. Med., *239*:531, 1975.

17

PATHOPHYSIOLOGY OF TEMPOROMANDIBULAR JOINTS AND MUSCLES OF MASTICATION

Disturbances of the temporomandibular joints (TMJ) and muscles of jaw movement, as well as those associated with the posture of the head and neck, have been described as functional disturbances and given a number of names such as *TMJ/muscle dysfunction, myofascial pain dysfunction syndrome (MPD), craniomandibular dysfunction,* and *mandibular* dysfunction, to name but a few. A term may reflect a concept of etiology or merely provide the user with a shorthand description of a set of symptoms (syndrome) that occur together with the functional disturbance.

The most common set of *symptoms* which involve the temporomandibular joints and muscles of mastication will be referred to here as *TMJ/muscle dysfunction syndrome*. The term does not dictate the primary disorder nor the state of the disturbance, e.g., masticatory muscle spasm being the primary factor responsible for the manifested signs and symptoms. Common manifestations are: (1) *pain* (described as a dull ache or as sharp) that is present in front of the ear (preauricular), or at the angle of the mandible, and which often radiates to the temple region of the head, and occasionally to the neck and shoulder area; (2) *tenderness of muscles* of mastication to palpation; (3) *TMJ clicking, popping or crepitus* sounds on jaw movement; and (4) *limitation of jaw movement*. Because of the morphologic and neuromuscular basis for these manifestations, a brief review of the temporomandibular joints and muscles is included here.

MASTICATORY SYSTEM AND CONTROL

The temporomandibular joint (Fig. 17–1) has a complex (hinge and glide) articulation capable of limited free movements, i.e., open and close, protrusive, retrusive, and lateral movements. An articular disk is interposed between the condyle of the mandible and the glenoid (mandibular) fossa of the temporal bone (Fig. 17–2). The temporal bone has a concave part (glenoid fossa) and an anterior convex part (articular tubercle or eminence). The joint is surrounded by a capsule attached to the neck of the condyle and around the border of the articular surface of the temporal bone.

The articular disk consists of dense col-

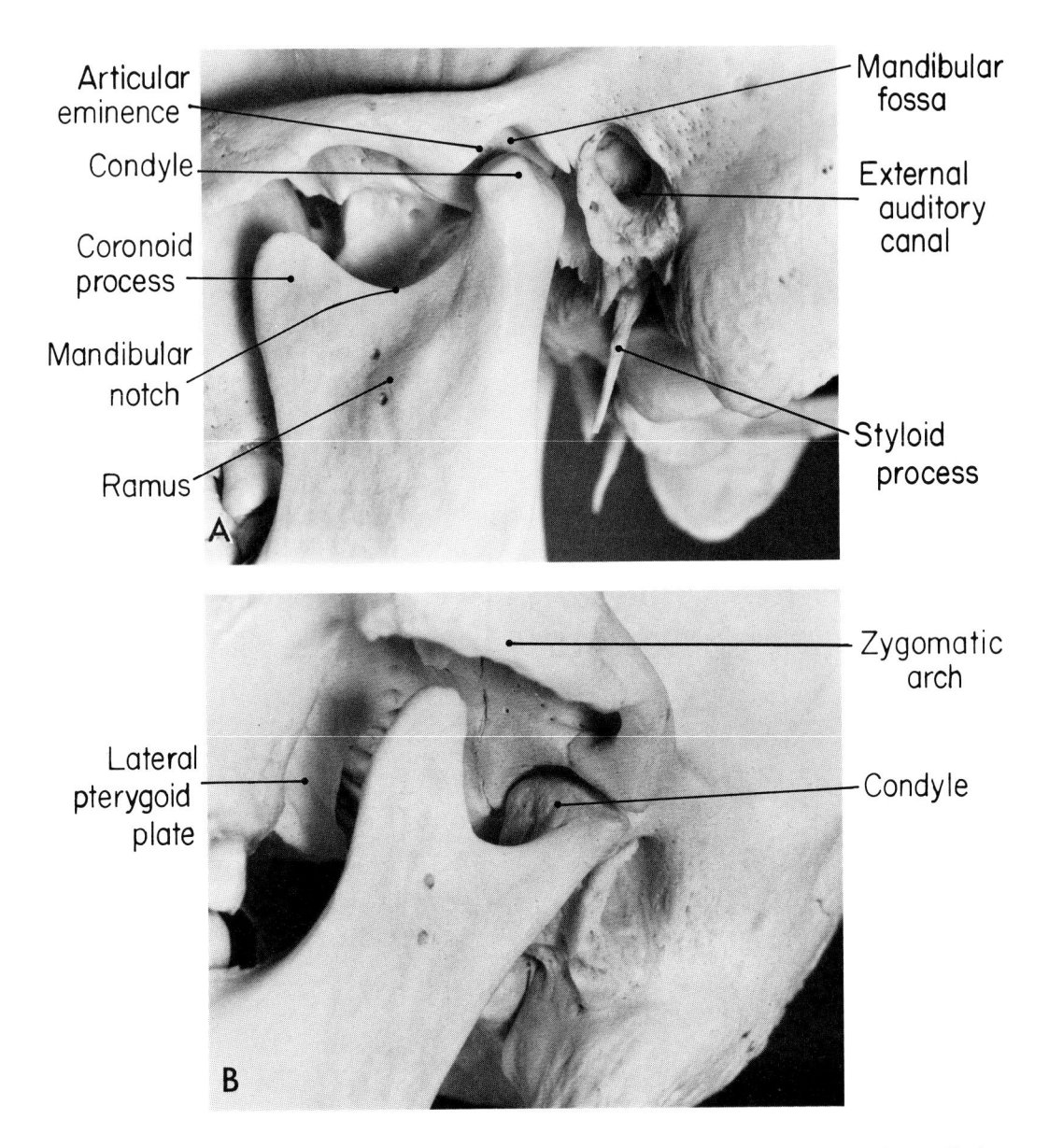

Fig. 17–1. *A,* Osseous structures of the TMJ. *B,* Shape of condyle and medial wall of mandibular fossa (glenoid fossa).

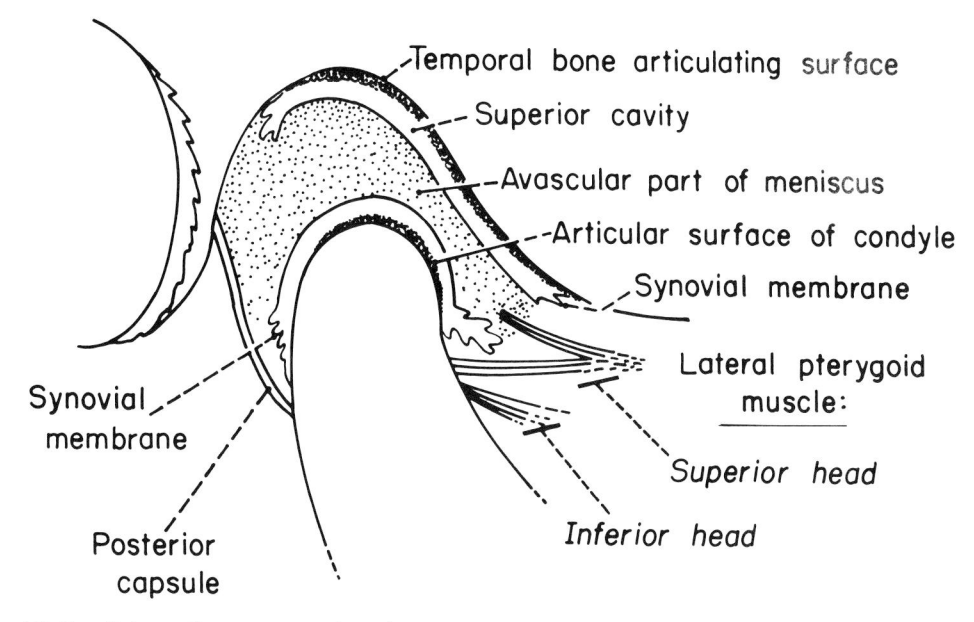

Fig. 17–2. Schematic representation of temporomandibular joint. Lateral pterygoid muscle (upper) attaches to disk and neck of condyle.

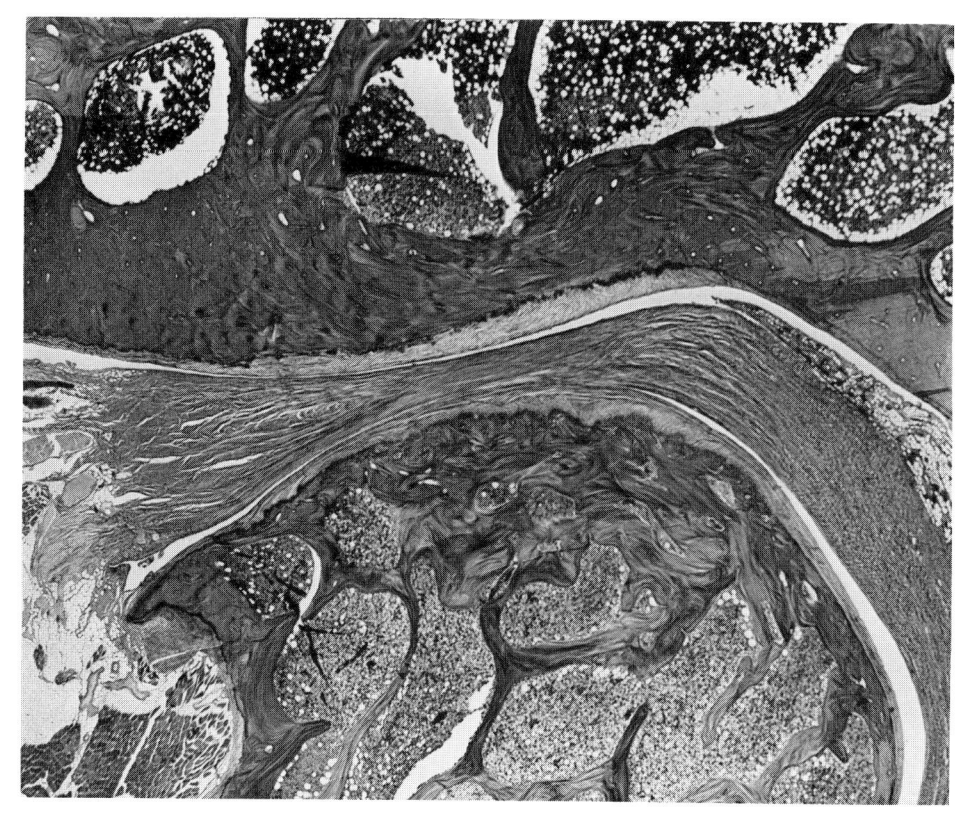

Fig. 17–3. *Histologic aspects of the disk and articulating surface of the condyle.* Articular surface is a fibrous layer. Note anterior "lipping" without pathologic changes in the TMJ.

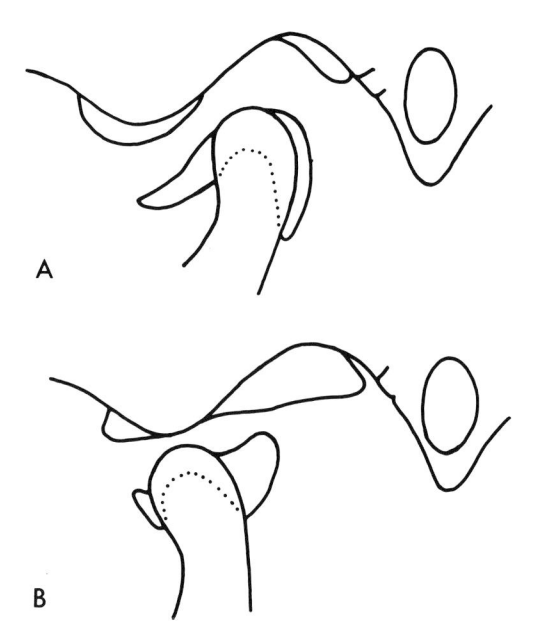

Fig. 17-4. A, Schematic representation of relationship between condyle disk and eminence with the teeth in centric occlusion. B, Advancement of disk with condyle in protrusive movement.

lagenous connective tissue (Fig. 17-3). The anterior part is collagen fiber bundles interspersed with the tendon of the lateral pterygoid muscle and is innervated and vascularized. The central part is dense, fibrous, avascular connective tissue devoid of innervation. The posterior part of the disk is loose connective tissue containing nerves and is richly vascularized. The disk may be pulled forward by the upper head of the lateral pterygoid muscle, but posterior movement may depend on thickened elastic fibers in the posterior part of the disk. Both the upper and lower joint cavities are lined by synovial cells which secrete a complex fluid that acts as a lubricant.

During mandibular opening, the disk advances with the condyle (Fig. 17-4). With pure rotation up to 20 to 25 mm there is little if any movement. When the jaws are in maximum occlusal contact (centric occlusion) the condyles contact the disks and the disks contact the posterior slopes of the articular eminence and the glenoid fossae. In extremely wide opening the contact of the joint is on the distal part of the condyle. Radiographically the condyle moves from a position seated in the mandibular fossae to the articular eminence and sometimes beyond (Fig. 17-5).

The masticatory muscles include the masseter, pterygoid, temporalis, and digastric muscles (Fig. 17-6). The digastric and lateral pterygoid muscles are usually classed as jaw openers or depressors, and the masseter, temporal, and medial pterygoid muscles as jaw closers or elevators. However, this is an oversimplification inasmuch as the same muscle may consist of muscle fiber types with different response characteristics.

Mandibular movements occur on a postural stage of jaw, head and body positions which are being continually and largely "automatically" set in relation to function or dysfunction. Because of such postural and functional relationships it may be possible to account for clinical manifestations of dysfunction which occur outside the muscles of mastication. Thus posture during typewriting, fingernail biting, and bruxism (purposeless grinding or gnashing of teeth) to name a few relationships, may relate to craniomandibular dysfunction with headache and neck/shoulder pain because of hyperactivity of the muscles of these areas distant from the muscles of mastication.

The control of jaw positions and movements depends on programs in the central nervous system and from peripheral input via receptors of information in the muscle (position sensors), periodontium (pressure, touch, etc.), and joints (position, pressure). Such movements as chewing and probably bruxism are highly programmed and dependent on inherent and learned information, but peripheral modulation of jaw movements is possible and probable.

Modulation of jaw position can relate to reflexes which work to position the condyle disk assembly into an ideal position. At the same time reflexes to optimize the intercuspal occlusal relations are at work as

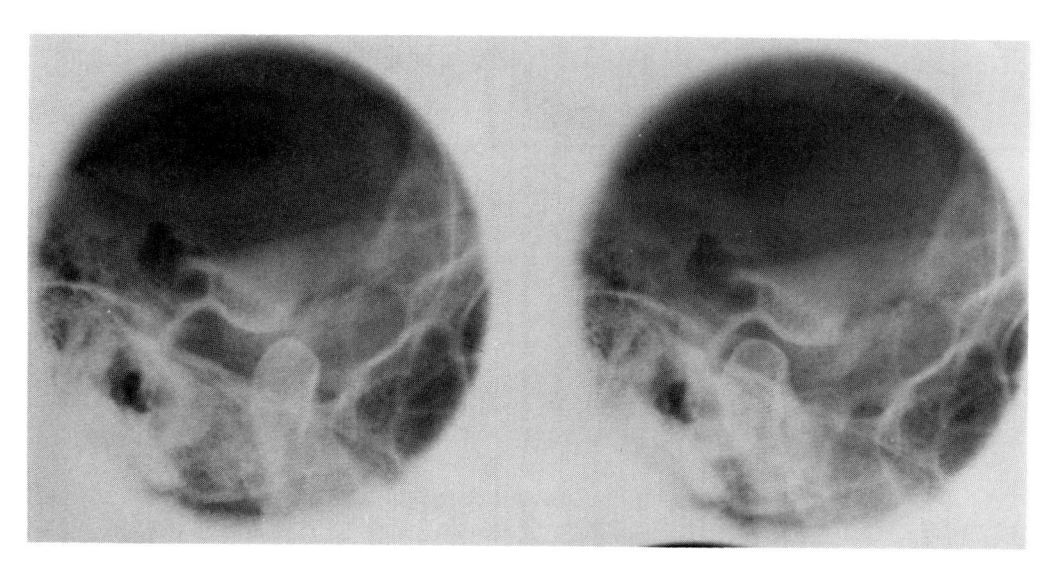

Fig. 17–5. Transcranial radiographs of right TMJ in open jaw position (left side) and closed position with teeth in the intercuspal position (right side).

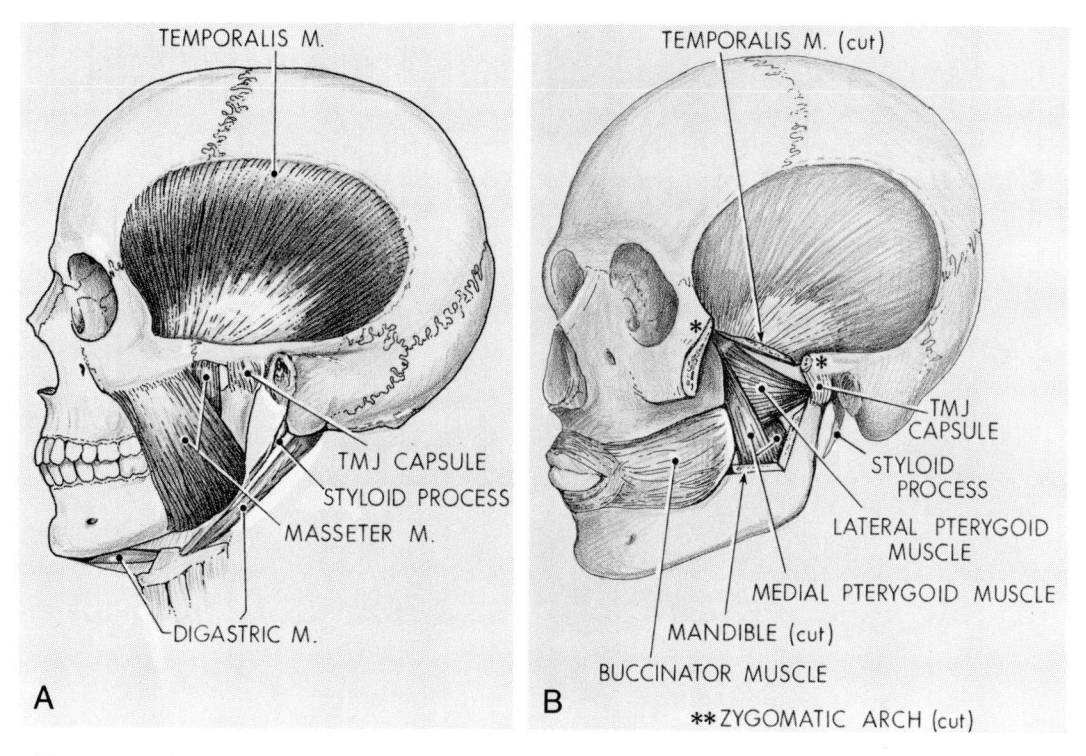

Fig. 17–6. A, Temporalis, masseter, and digastric muscles. B, Lateral pterygoid and medial pterygoid muscles.

well. These two reflexes in the presence of occlusal interferences (Fig. 17-7) may result in reflexes working to different ends. Although such occlusal disharmony does not usually cause dysfunction, occasionally TMJ/muscle pain dysfunction does result, especially in the presence of a compromised joint. Adaptation of the teeth by movement or modulation of movement by reflexes to avoid occlusal disharmony appears likely, but adaptation of the adult joint seems less likely. Functional (movement) adaptation of the condyle-disk assembly for slight "last minute" adjustments for occlusal interferences does appear likely, but requires study.

The active and passive positioners of the jaws and disks are muscles, whereas the teeth are passive physical guidances. Final positioning of the disk and mandible close to the intercuspal position may be modulated by reflexes.

EPIDEMIOLOGY OF TMJ/MUSCLE DYSFUNCTION

The most common symptom of the TMJ/muscle dysfunction syndrome appears to be painless clicking, which has been estimated to occur in about 70% of the population at one time or another. However, joint sounds in children up to the age of high school seniors may be far less (10%). The incidence of major symptoms of TMJ/muscle dysfunction in adolescents (10 to 18 years) was found to be less than 10% in a recent study. Other studies have reported up to 20%. Such a range of values probably reflects cultural and socio-economic, as well as measurement, differences.

Epidemiologic studies of subjects in the age group of 15 to 74 shows that more than half reported some symptom of dysfunction; about one-third had two or more symptoms, and only about 12% had pain during jaw movement. Difficulty in opening the mouth wide was reported by 7% and joint sounds were reported by 39% of the population reviewed. The occurrence of TMJ/muscle dysfunction appears to be cumulative and such cross-sectional data does not provide information on the natural history of the disease.

Such epidemiologic data suggest that the prevalence of disease increases with age, but that the incidence may reach a peak in the 20- to 40-year-old group. Considering active disease as being present only with pain, the incidence of TMJ/muscle dysfunction may not be greater than 10 to 12%, and probably less if transient pain and headache from other causes could be excluded. Even so, the prevalence of TMJ/muscle dysfunction reflects a major dental public health problem.

ETIOLOGY

There are a number of hypotheses about the primary causes of TMJ/muscle dysfunction syndrome, but there is little disagreement that the causes reflect a heterogeneous, multifaceted etiological phenomenon (Fig. 17-8).

The most common underlying cause of TMJ/muscle dysfunction is acute or chronic trauma from extrinsic and intrinsic sources. External sources include injury from contact sports, accidents, general anesthesia with intubation, prolonged jaw opening, and difficult dental procedure. Intrinsic sources are abnormal muscle action associated with psychic stress, occlusal disharmony, and bruxism (purposeless gnashing of teeth), especially in the presence of an already compromised joint.

The vicious cycle of muscle hyperactivity and injury involved in bruxism, fingernail biting, and other habits plays an important role in the development of traumatic TMJ arthritis and associated disk disturbances. Occlusal interferences, psychic tension, a compromised (injured) joint, and a lack of adaptive capacity is undoubtedly associated with excessive forces and traumatic TMJ arthritis, with or without pain in the muscles.

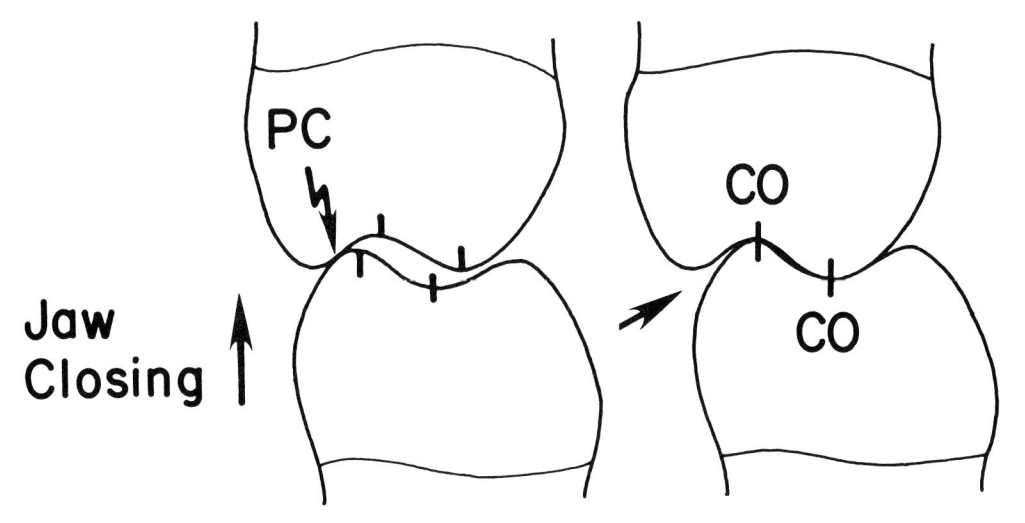

Fig. 17-7. Occlusal interference to harmonious jaw closure into centric occlusion (CO) requiring functional and/or structural adaptation. PC, premature contact to maximum intercuspation, causing anterior and lateral shifting (functional adaptation, i.e., avoidance movement).

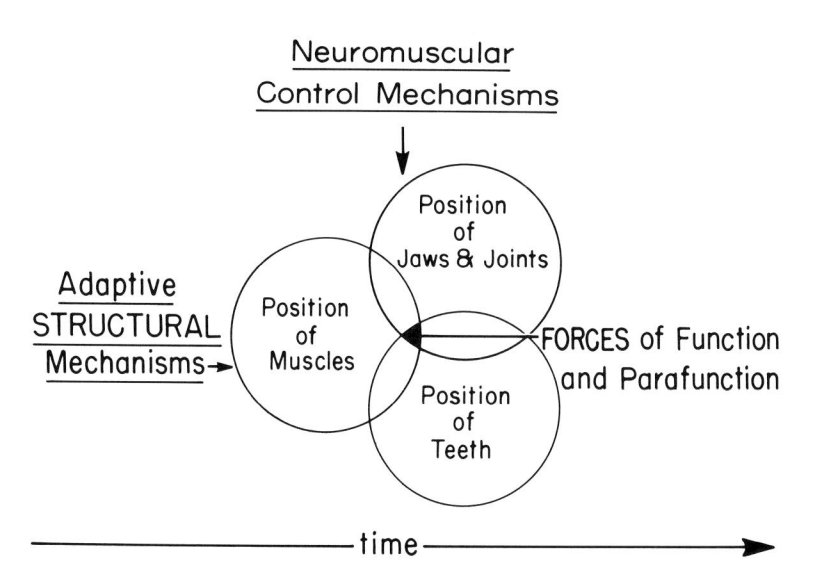

Fig. 17-8. Forces of function and/or parafunction may reach a destructive level when neuromuscular control and adaptive structural mechanisms do not provide for harmonious relationships between the joints, disks, muscles, and teeth.

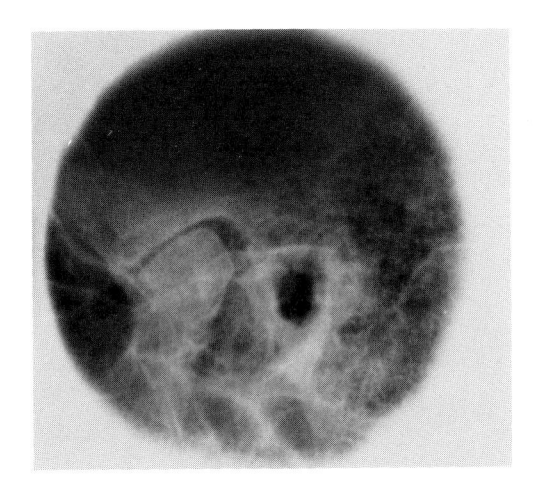

Fig. 17-9. Osteoarthritis with reduction of joint space.

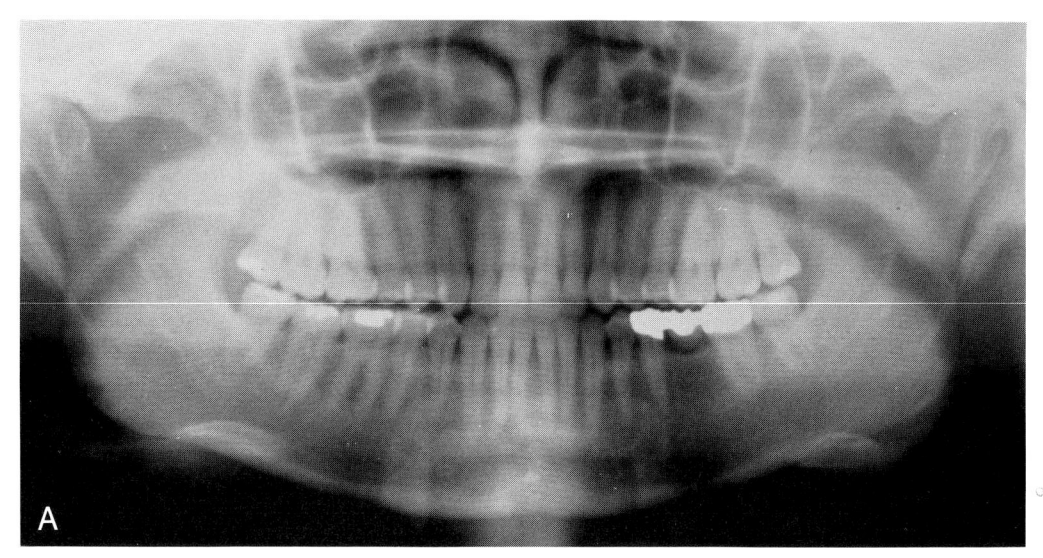

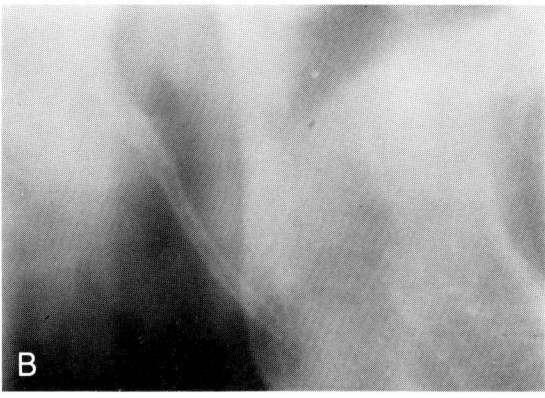

Fig. 17-10. *A*, Panoral radiograph showing calcified stylomandibular ligament. *B*, Close-up view of symptomatic calcified ligament (Eagle syndrome).

SIGNS AND SYMPTOMS

The manifestations attributed to TMJ/muscle dysfunction syndrome are extensive and include TMJ pain, joint sounds, muscle tenderness, locking and/or limitation of jaw motion, headache, ear symptoms, and neck and shoulder discomfort. Symptoms of degenerative and inflammatory TMJ disease complicate the symptom complex of TMJ/muscle dysfunction. The clinical symptoms of degenerative osteoarthritis may be the same as those of TMJ/muscle dysfunction which is initially often without radiographic evidence of osseous changes compared to osteoarthritis (Fig. 17–9). Also the symptoms of TMJ/muscle dysfunction may be secondarily induced by a primary disturbance such as neoplasia, migraine, cracked tooth syndrome, or Eagle syndrome (Fig. 17–10), all of which may produce symptoms similar to TMJ/muscle dysfunction.

Internal derangement generally suggests an anterior displacement of the disk associated with posterior-superior displacement of the condyle with the teeth in the intercuspal position. Anterior displacement is often divided into displacement with reduction and displacement without reduction. Repositioning of the disk to a normal position (displacement with reduction) has been related to clicking and failure of the disk to reposition (displacement without reduction) has been associated with locking (Fig. 17–11). For example, a patient may not be able to open the mouth more than 15 to 20 mm because of disk derangement (as well as pain or muscle dysfunction). Conceptually the disk in an anterior position is considered to prevent condylar translation ("locking"). Radiographic evidence of disk displacement is seen in arthrograms (Fig. 17–12). Normally, mandibular opening is greater than 40 mm measured between the maxillary and mandibular incisors. Lateral movements may be 10 mm or more to the left and right. Restricted movement opening and lateral movements may be due to pain, unilateral or bilateral disk derangement, muscle spasms, or ankylosis related to degenerative joint disease.

Contributory factors which relate to TMJ/muscle dysfunction are the signs of bruxism (Fig. 17–13) and trauma from occlusion related to occlusal interferences (Fig. 17–14).

Roentgenographic changes associated with osteoarthritis of the temporomandibular joints include (1) lack of definition of the anterior aspect of the condyle, (2) peripheral lipping of the condyle (Fig. 17–15), (3) bone resorption, and (4) other changes requiring special technique such as fragmentation and dystrophic calcification of disk.

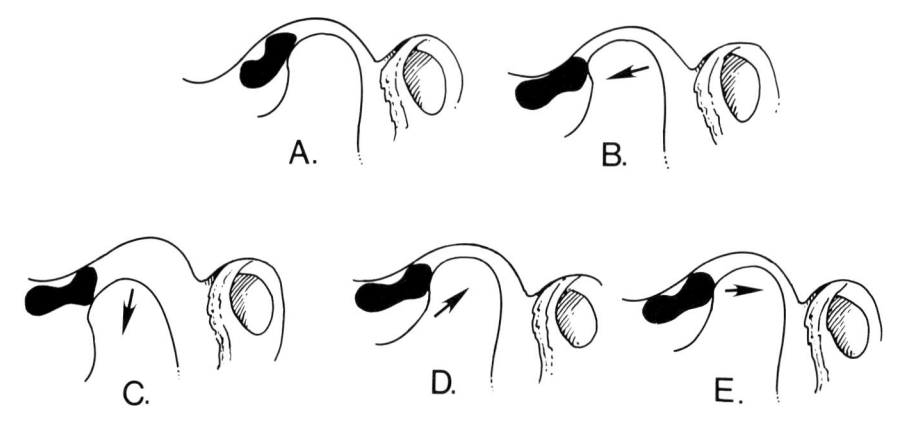

Fig. 17–11. *Schematic representation of "closed lock."* A, Anteriorly displaced disk with teeth in centric occlusion. B, Beginning translation of condyle. C, Opening movement stopped. D, Closing and retrusion to intercuspal position at E.

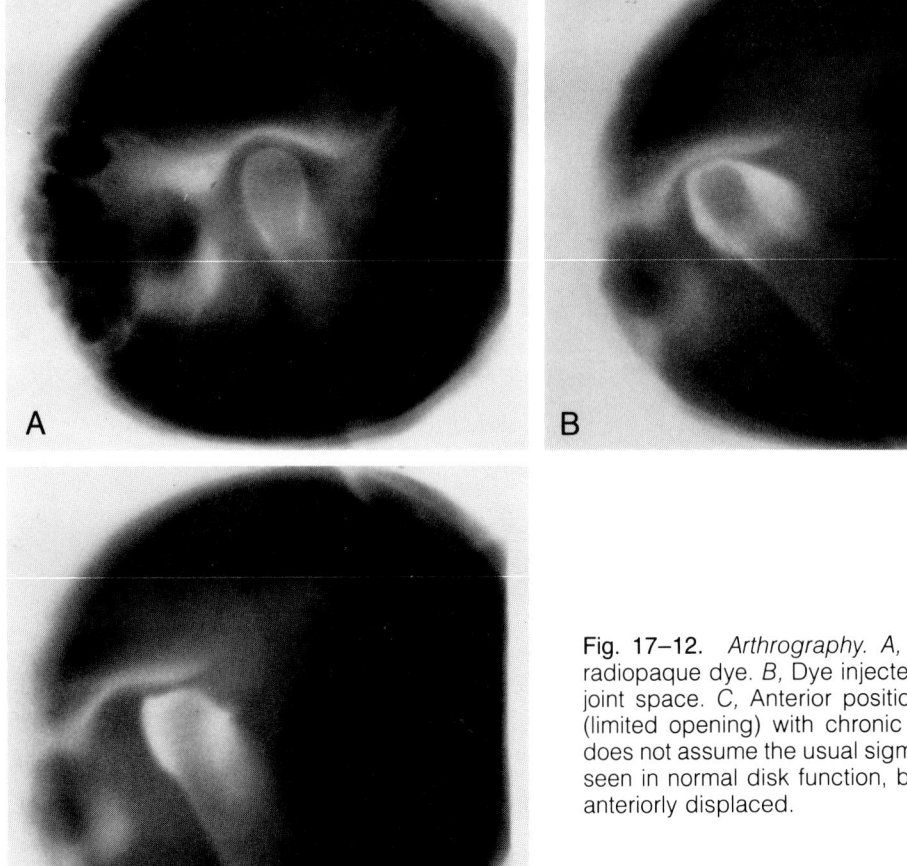

Fig. 17-12. *Arthrography.* *A,* Joint without radiopaque dye. *B,* Dye injected into inferior joint space. *C,* Anterior position of condyle (limited opening) with chronic locking. Dye does not assume the usual sigmoid shape as seen in normal disk function, but disk is not anteriorly displaced.

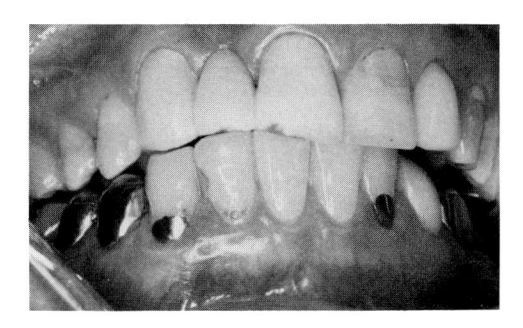

Fig. 17–13. *TMJ/muscle dysfunction caused by bruxism.* Newly placed bridge interfered with bruxing habit involving the cuspid. Attempts to brux in the usual position resulted in fracture of bridge and TMJ trauma.

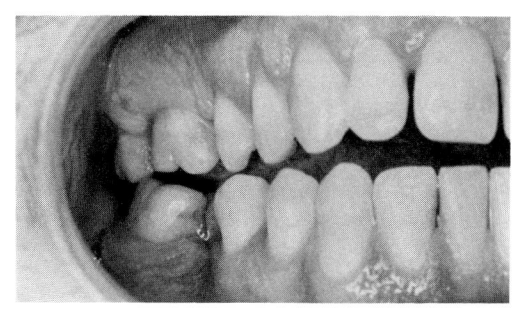

Fig. 17–14. *Protrusive interference related to TMJ/muscle dysfunction.* Occlusal adjustment resulted in elimination of pain and muscle hyperactivity.

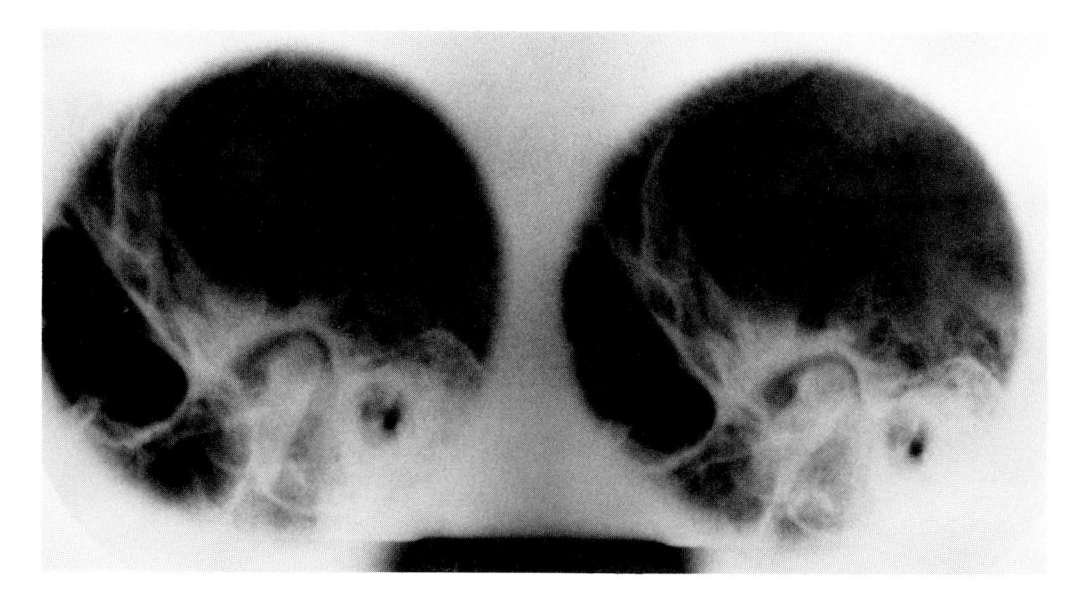

Fig. 17–15. Osteoarthritis of the temporomandibular joint with marked deformity of condyle.

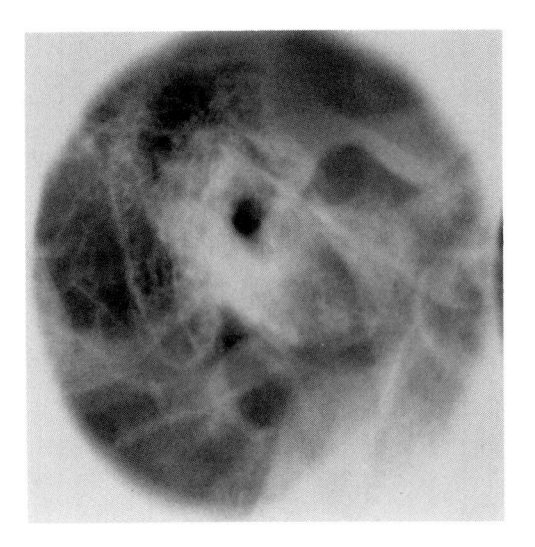

290 PATHOPHYSIOLOGY OF TEMPOROMANDIBULAR JOINTS AND MUSCLES OF MASTICATION

Fig. 17-16. Surgical removal of part of condyle as treatment of disk derangement. (Symptoms did not abate.)

Radiographic changes of the TMJ may also be related to surgical procedures (Fig. 17-16). Teflon pads, condylectomy, meniscectomy and augmentation of the articular eminence alter the normal radiographic appearance of the joint.

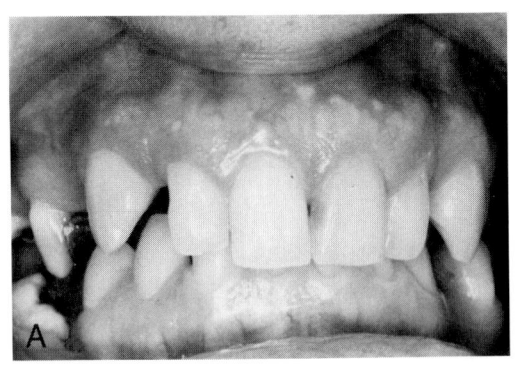

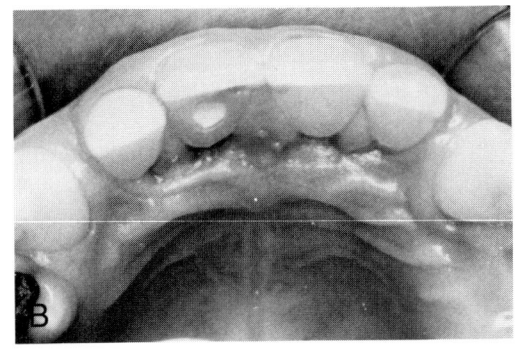

Fig. 17-17. *A*, Malocclusion with impinging overbite. *B*, Trauma to gingiva.

TRAUMA FROM OCCLUSION

Trauma from occlusion refers to injury to any part of the masticatory system as a result of abnormal occlusal contact relations and/or abnormal function. Predisposing factors include malocclusion, loss of teeth, faulty dental restorations, loss of periodontal support, and habits.

Malocclusion such as impinging overbite leads to soft tissue injury (Fig. 17-17). The concept that a class II malocclusion (retrognathic mandible) predisposes to TMJ dysfunction has not been substantiated.

Faulty dental restorations with occlusal interferences (Fig. 17-13) may lead to trauma of the supporting structures of the teeth involved or the temporomandibular joints. Restorative treatment may predispose to bruxing with "jiggling" of a tooth

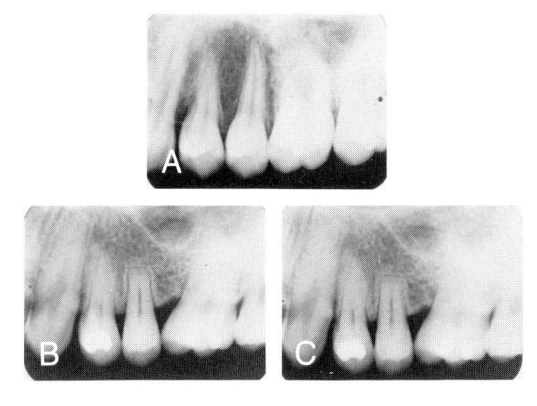

Fig. 17-18. *Trauma from occlusion following placement of restoration.* Upper radiograph prior to placement of restoration. *Left,* loss of root following placement of restoration in the first premolar. *Right,* followup after occlusal adjustment to eliminate trauma from occlusion and pulpitis in the premolar.

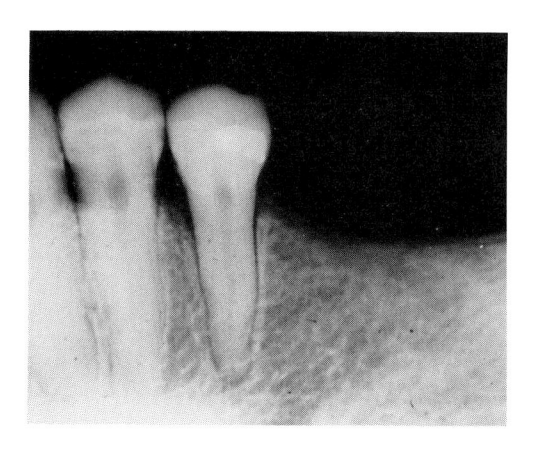

Fig. 17–19. Increased width of periodontal membrane space associated with hypermobility of the premolar. Pain and discomfort continued as a result of continued trauma.

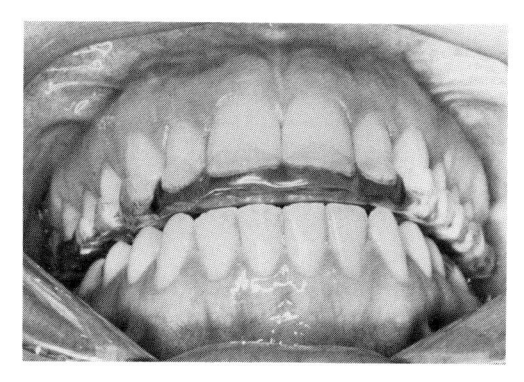

Fig. 17–21. Occlusal bite plane (stabilization) splint.

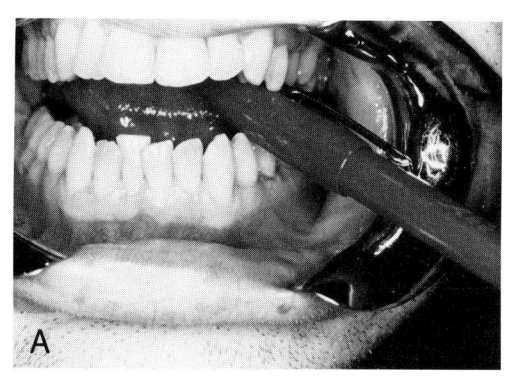

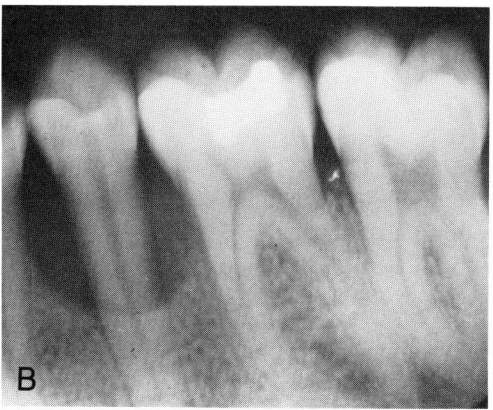

Fig. 17–20. Trauma from occlusal habit. A, chronic biting of pen. B, Loss of support seen on radiograph.

because of pulpitis as well as occlusal interference by the restoration (Fig. 17–18).

The diagnosis of trauma from occlusion can only be made if the proposed cause of the injury is eliminated and the signs and symptoms of the trauma are eliminated (Fig. 17–19). In order to make a diagnosis of trauma from occlusion, the signs and symptoms of trauma must be related in time to the dysfunction. For example, increased mobility of a tooth that is seen clinically and radiographically as an increase in width of the periodontal membrane space (Fig. 17–20) may reflect adaptation, not progressive injury. Thus, trauma from occlusion means that there is evidence of continued trauma, e.g., continued pain or discomfort.

Habits such as fingernail biting, pencil or pen chewing (Fig. 17–20), and pipe stem chewing may cause trauma, loss of periodontal support, and TMJ/muscle dysfunction.

TREATMENT

A wide spectrum of treatment modalities has been advanced for the control of TMJ/muscle dysfunction and trauma from occlusion. Treatment includes the use of drugs such as muscle relaxants, tranquilizers, anti-inflammatory agents and analgesics.

Physiotherapy measures include hot moist packs, exercises, cold sprays, ultrasonography, electrical stimulation, dia-

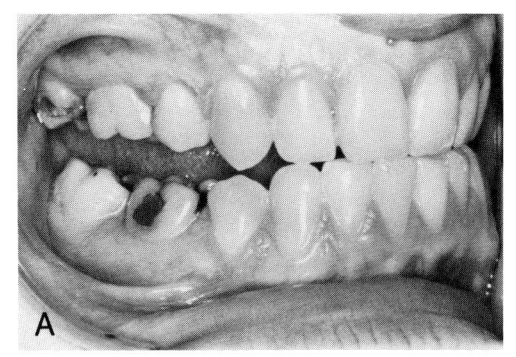

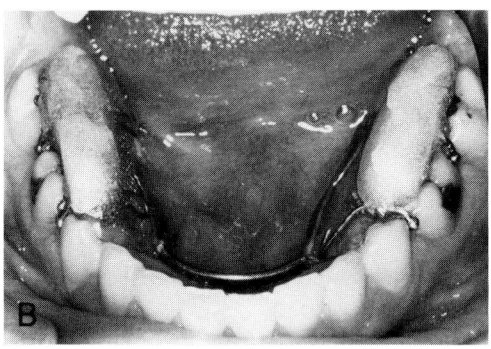

Fig. 17-22. A, Posterior open bite created by repositioning device. Such repositioning often requires orthodontic finalization of the occlusion. B, Mandibular anterior repositioning appliance.

thermy, and massage. Behavioral modification with the use of feedback techniques is generally directed toward muscle relaxation.

Occlusal therapy includes the use of occlusal bite plane splints (Fig. 17-21), which are considered to be reversible appliances, and occlusal adjustment which is considered to be irreversible treatment.

Repositioning devices to advance the mandible (Fig. 17-22) are considered to be conditionally irreversible appliances in as much as they may permanently reposition the mandible forward and require follow-up orthodontics or reconstruction to finalize the occlusion.

Orthodontics and orthognothic surgery are irreversible procedures. In general, these procedures are not initial forms of treatment for TMJ/muscle dysfunction.

TMJ surgery is considered to be irreversible treatment and is not often an initial form of treatment. Some forms of injections (cortisone, etc.) may lead to irreversible changes in the joints.

The initial form of therapy generally recommended is reversible treatment. The average length of treatment is 4 to 6 months.

SUMMARY

TMJ/muscle dysfunction and trauma from occlusion are functional disturbances of the masticatory system. The signs and symptoms of TMJ/muscle dysfunction syndrome are: pain (preauricular), noise in the joints, tenderness of masticatory muscles, and limitation of jaw motion. Other symptoms such as headache, salivary gland enlargement, hearing changes, and pain extending to the neck and shoulders, may occur.

The etiology of TMJ-muscle dysfunction is related to extrinsic and intrinsic trauma, as well as systemic factors such as rheumatoid arthritis. Muscle hyperactivity can be due to central induction by psychologic stress, or from occlusal factors (malocclusion, occlusal interferences, developmental disturbances), or from postural problems involving occupations. Thus the cause of TMJ/muscle dysfunction syndrome and trauma from occlusion is a multifactorial phenomenon, and a specific diagnosis may not be possible.

The provisional diagnosis of TMJ/muscle dysfunction may emphasize the joint, as with the pain of disk derangement, or the muscles, as with myofascial pain. Many patients may have residual effects of past episodes of dysfunction, e.g., clicking, crepitus, and limited jaw motion, but no evidence of pain or progressive disease. These patients may only require physiotherapy to increase jaw opening. Others may require palliative treatment for pain and definitive treatment of malocclusion and occlusal instability. In some instances, surgery of the TMJ because of pain and destruction of the joint may be necessary.

BIBLIOGRAPHY

Agerberg, G. and Carlsson, G.E.: Functional disorders of the masticatory system I. Distribution of symptoms according to age and sex as judged by investigation by questionnaire. Acta Odont. Scand., 30:397, 1972.

Ash, M.M.: An appraisal of current concepts of treatment for TMJ/muscle dysfunction. J.M.D.A., 66:307, 1984.

Ash, M.M.: Current concepts in the etiology, diagnosis, and treatment of TMJ and muscle dysfunction. J. Oral Rehabil., 13:1, 1986.

Ash, M.M.: Occlusal adjustment: An appraisal. J.M.D.A., 67:9, 1985.

Griffiths, R.H.: Report of the President's conference on the examination, diagnosis, and management of temporomandibular disorders. J. Am. Dent. A., 106:75, 1983.

Grosfeld, O. and Czarnecka, B.: Musculo-articular disorders of the stomatognathic system in school children examined according to clinical criteria. J. Oral Rehabil., 4:192, 1977.

Helkimo, M.: Epidemiological surveys of dysfunction of the masticatory system. Oral Sci. Rev., 7:54, 1976.

Nilner, M. and Sven-Akelassing: Prevalence of functional disturbances and disease of the stomatognathic system in 15–18 year olds. Swed. Dent. J., 5:189, 1981.

Ogura, T., et al.: An epidemiological study of TMJ dysfunction syndrome in adolescents. J. Pedodontics, 10:22, 1985.

Ramfjord, S.P., and Ash, M.M.: *Occlusion,* 3rd ed. Philadelphia, W.B. Saunders Co., 1983.

Ramfjord, S.P., and Ash, M.M.: *Periodontics and Periodontology.* Philadelphia, W.B. Saunders Co., 1979.

Richards, L.C.: An assessment of radiographic methods for the investigation of temporomandibular joint morphology and pathology. J. Austr. Dent. J., 30:323, 1985.

Storey, A.T.: Neurobiology of Occlusion. In Johnston, L.E. (ed.), *New Vistas in Orthodontics.* Philadelphia, Lea & Febiger, 1985.

INDEX

Page numbers in *italics* indicate a figure; those followed by *t* indicate a table.

Abrasion, of teeth, 108-109, *109*
Abscess, as inflammatory response, 67, *67*
   definition of, 28
Acid etching, in dental caries control, 192
Acidogenic theory, of caries production, 182-183
Acquired immunodeficiency syndrome. *See* AIDS
Acromegaly, 255
Actinobacillus actinomycetemcomitans, in juvenile periodontitis, 227
   in periodontal disease(s), 202
Actinomyces, in carious lesions, 189
Actinomyces naeslundii, in caries, by site, 179
Actinomyces viscosus, in caries, by site, 179
Acute lymphocytic leukemia (ALL), 273
Acute myelocytic leukemia (AML), 272-273, *273*
Acute necrotizing ulcerative gingivitis. *See* Necrotizing ulcerative gingivitis (NUG)
Acute pulpitis, 171-172
Addison's disease, definition of, 260
   dysfunction of adrenal glands and, 259, 265
   manifestations of, 260, *260*
   pigment metabolism and, 116, *260*
Adenine, in biochemical basis of heredity, 7
Adenocarcinoma, 124-125, *125*
Adenoma, 124-125, *125*
   adrenal, Cushing's syndrome and, 261
   pleomorphic, definition of, 124
Adenosine triphosphate, function of, 3
   mechanisms of transport and, 4
   requirement for, in cellular injury, 11
Adherence, bacterial. *See* Bacterial adherence
Adhesion, definition of, 73
   See also Bacterial adherence
Adrenal cortex, hyperfunction of, 260-261
   hypofunction of, 260
Adrenal function, 259-260
Adrenal gland(s), structure of, 259
Aerobic bacteria, definition of, 146
A-fiber(s), in dentin-pulp complex, 166-167
Agenesis, in developmental disturbances of teeth, 51
Agent(s), antimicrobial, in dental caries control, 190
   of disease, 15-34. *See also* specific agents
      chemical, 31-32
      drugs and hormones as, 33
      environmental, 32-33
      infectious, 27-31
      physical, 22-27
   teratogenic, 19, 19*t*
Aging, alterations in cells and tissues related to, 103
   and disease, 103-108
      specific, 106-116
   etiology of, 103
      theories of, 104
   normal, 104, *105*
   organ changes in, 104-106
   retrogressive changes and dysfunction and, 103-116
Agranulocytosis, cause of, 33

   drug-induced, periodontal disease and, 205
   syndrome of, 271, *271*
AIDS, 86-87
   clinical disturbances and, 240
   course of development of, 241-242
   epidemiologic pattern and aspects of, 86
   groups at risk for, 86, 241, 242
   guidelines for treatment of patients with, Council of American Dental Association on Dental Therapeutics recommended, 86-87
   incubation period for, 86
   marker diseases for, 86
   method of spread of, 242
   possiblity of vaccine for, 87
   virus causing, 240-242, 251
AIDS-related complex, 240, 242
Air pollution, as physical agent of disease, 32
Akinesia, definition of, 106
Alcoholism, vitamin deficiency and, 137
Aldosterone, functions and regulation of, 259
Aldosteronism, cause of, 259
   hyperfunction of adrenal cortex and, 260
   manifestations of, 261
Allele(s), definition of, 16
Allergy. *See* Hypersensitivity
Alpha-adrenergic receptor(s), in pulp, 168
Alveolar bone, anatomy of, 200, *200-201*
Alveolar process, anatomy of, 200, *200*
Alveolar ridge, carcinoma of, 124
Alzheimer's disease, 106-107
   diagnosis of, 106
   possible causes of, 106
Ameloblast(s), definition of, 48
   function of, in embryology of teeth, 49, *49*
Ameloblastoma, 125-126, *126*
   as developmental neoplasm, 120
Amelogenesis imperfecta, 54, *54*
American Heart Association, dietary fat recommendations of, 135
Amniocentesis, in prenatal diagnosis, 20-21
Amplification, in activation of oncogene, 17-19
Amputation neuroma, description of, 101
Amyloidosis, 111
Anaerobic bacteria, definition of, 146
   facultatively, growth of, 146-147
   obligate, growth of, 147
Androgen(s), adrenal, 260
Anemia, 267-271, 276
   hemolytic, vitamin K and, 138
   iron deficiency and, 136
   manifestations of disorders causing, 276-277
   See also specific types
Angiodysplasia, definition of, 136
Angioma(s), of tongue, 127
   See also specific types
Ankyloglossia, 42, *42*
Anodontia, in developmental disturbances of teeth, 51-52

INDEX

Anorexia nervosa, definition of, 31
Anoxia, cellular, 23
Antibiotic(s), as physical agent of disease, 33
　interference of, with protein synthesis, 9-10
　microbial resistance to, 153-154
Antibody(ies), in immune response, 76, 78-79
　in phagocytosis, 66-67, *81*
　in serum of patients with periodontal disease, 156
　potential adverse effects on bacteria of, 155
　prototypic structure for IgGl (κ) molecule, *79*
Antigen(s), 77
　composite view of immune response to, *85*
　in phagocytosis, 67, *81*
　See also specific types
Antigenic determinant(s), CTL response to, 82-83
　in immune system, 76, 84, *85*
Anti-idiotype network(s), immune mechanisms and, 209
Antimicrobial agent(s), in dental caries control, 190
Antitoxin, definition of, 77
Anxiety neurosis, description of, 21-22
Aphasia, definition of, 106
Aphthous ulcer(s), possible causes of, 1
Aplastic anemia(s), 269
　cause of, 268
Apraxia, definition of, 106
Argyria, definition of, 115
Argyrosis, 115-116, *116*
Arteriosclerosis, 114-115
Arthritis
　rheumatoid. *See* Rheumatoid arthritis
Articular disk(s), displacement of, 287, *287, 288, 290*
　structure and function of, 279-282, *280, 281, 282,* 284
Ascorbic acid. *See* Vitamin C
Aspirin "burn," 249, 250, *250*
Atherosclerosis, 114-115
　definition of, 104
　risk factors for, 115
ATP. *See* Adenosine triphosphate
Atrophy, 109-111
　definition of, 109
　fatty. *See* Fatty atrophy
　of lip, 111, *111*
Attrition, of teeth, 108, *108*
Autoanalyzer, biochemical profile of serum findings made by, *13*
Autoimmune disease(s), 88-90
　definition of, 76
　major histocompatibility complex and, 78
　oral manifestations of, 88-89
　probable mechanisms for, 88
　See also specific diseases
Auto-immunity theory, of caries production, 183
Autosomal dominant disorder(s), definition of, 16
Autosomal recessive disorder(s), definition of, 16-17

Bacilli, description of, 28
Bacillus vincentii, necrotizing ulcerative gingivitis and, 221
Bacteremia, transient, definition of, 61
Bacteria, accumulation of, shift in population of, 163
　adherence of. *See* Bacterial adherence
　antibiotics and, 153-154
　as physical agent of disease, 27-29
　coexistence of in plaque, substrate requirements and, 147
　distribution in sulci of, from health to increasing severity of periodontal disease, 149-150
　division into groups of, 27-28
　in carious lesions, 188-189
　invasion of, periodontal disease and, 207-208
　killing of, in immune response to plaque, 156
　potential mechanisms of, for destruction of periodontal tissues, 153
　　for evading host defenses, 152
　predominance of, in periodontal disease, 145, 145*t*

　See also Microbiota; Microorganisms; specific types
Bacterial adherence, adverse influences on, 151-152
　specificity of, 151
　therapeutic importance of, 145
Bacterial nutrient(s), on tooth surface, source of, 147
　See also Substrate(s)
Bacterial plaque. *See* Dental plaque
Bacteriocidins, as ecologic factor in dental plaque, 151-152
Bacteroides, necessary growth factors for, 152
　nutritional requirements of, 147
Bacteroides gingivalis, antibodies to, adult periodontitis and, 156
　role of, in periodontal disease(s), 202
Bacteroides intermedius, necrotizing ulcerative gingivitis and, 221
　role of, in periodontal disease(s), 202
Barodontalgia, definition of, 23
Basal cell, in basal layer of gingiva, 7
Basal cell carcinoma, 122-123
　cause of, 119
Basal metabolic rate, definition of, 133
Basophil(s), definition of, 63
Basophilia, 272
B-cell(s). *See* B-lymphocyte(s)
Behçet's syndrome, 242
Bell stage, of tooth development, 46, *48*
Benign mucous membrane pemphigoid (BMMP), 244
Beta-adrenergic receptor(s), in pulp, 168
B-fiber(s), in dentin-pulp complex, 167
Bifid tongue, 42
Bilirubin, pigment metabolism and, 116
Binding site, bacterial adherence and, definition of, 151
Birth defect(s), causes of, 15
Birthmark(s), 127
Bleeding, intestinal, causes of in aging, 136
Bleeding disorder(s), 70, 74
Blood, normal values of, 268*t*
Blood cell(s), formation of, 267
　red. *See* Erythrocyte(s)
　white. *See* White blood cell(s); specific types
Blood group antigen(s), 78
B-lymphocyte(s), differentiation of, 82
　distinguishing features of, 79
　humoral immunity and, 80
　in periodontal disease, pathogenesis of, 209
Boil(s), definition of, 28
Bone(s), decalcification of, hyperparathyroidism and, 258-259
　formation of, factors that decrease, 264
　fractures of. *See* Fracture(s)
　metabolic diseases of, 265
　repair of, 73, 74
　resorption of, factors that increase, 264
　structure of, 264
　temporal, 279, *280, 281, 283*
Bone marrow, acute leukemia and, 129
Borrelia vincentii, necrotizing ulcerative gingivitis and, 221
Botulism, effect of bacterial toxicity in, 28
Branchial bar, formation of, 35, *36*
Branchial cyst(s), 39
"Brown tumor," hyperparathyroidism and, 100, 259
Bruxism, definition of, 108, 282
　periodontal disease and, 205
　TMJ/muscle dysfunction and, 287, *289, 290*
Buffer systems, acid production in plaque and, 184
Bulimia, definition of, 31
Burkitt's tumor, as non-Hodgkin's lymphoma, 130
Burnishing, of dentin. *See* Smear layer

Caisson disease, 23
Calcification, radicular, 113-114, *114*
Calcium, absorption of, 135-136
　and phosphate concentration, regulation of, 258
　in demineralization process, 184

INDEX

Calculus, 159-161, *159*
  attachment of, 161
  composition of, 159
  formation of, mechanisms of, 160-161
  ground sections, in studies of, 159, *160*
  saliva and, 160, 161
Callus, definition of, 92
  in bone healing, 73, *74*
Cancer, 17-19
  chemotherapy for, *130*, 131
  definition of, 122
  immunotherapy for, 131-132
  incidence of, 117-118, 118*t*
  oral, oral pathology and, 2
  radiation therapy for, 131
  therapy for, and complications of, 131-132
    principles of, 131
  See also Neoplasia; Neoplasm(s); specific types
Candida albicans, 246
Candidiasis, 246-247, 252
  acute atrophic, 246-247
  acute pseudomembranous, 246, *246*
  chronic atrophic, *246*, 247
  chronic mucocutaneous, 247
  classification of, 246
  oral pathology and, 2
Candidiasis-endocrinopathy syndrome, characteristics of, 262-263
Canker sore(s), 242, *243*
Capillary(ies), in pulp, 168
Capnocytophaga, in juvenile periodontitis, 227
  in periodontitis, 266
  role of, in periodontal disease(s), 202
"Capnophilic" bacteria, nutritional requirements of, 147
Carbohydrate(s), metabolism of, 134
Carbon monoxide, in gas homeostasis, 22-23
Carbuncle(s), definition of, 28
Carcinogen(s), definition of, 119
Carcinoma(s), origin of, 122
  See also Squamous cell carcinoma
Cardiovascular system, age-related changes in, 105-106
Caries. *See* Dental caries
Caseation necrosis, 113
Catarrhal exudate, 67
Catatonia, description of, 21
Cell, absorption in, 5
  adaptation of, 10-11
  as basis of life and disease, 3-10
  basal, in basal layer of gingiva, 7
  differentiating, ultrastructure of, *10*
  differentiation of, 5
  immunocompetent, definition of, 76
  in inflammation, 61-63
  injury of, 11
    clinical correlates of, 13
    response to, 10-13
  mast, 65
  odontogenic, ultrastructure of, *7*
  structure and function of, 3-5
Cell cycle, 6-7
  mitotic phase of, cancer therapy and, *131*
Cell membrane, structure and function of, 3-4, *4*, *5*
Cellulitis, definition of, 67
  pulp disease and, 174
"Cementopathia," periodontal disease and, 208
Cementum, developmental disturbances of, 59-60, *59*
  periodontal disease and, 200
Center for Disease Control, projection for incidence of HTLV-III infection, 242
Central nervous system, age-related changes in, 106
  viral diseases of, 29
Chancre, in syphilis, 245
Change(s), retrogressive. *See* Retrogressive change(s)
Chédiak-Higashi syndrome, periodontitis and, 228

Cheek-chewing, injury from, 248, *248*
Cheilitis, solar or aging, definition of, 111
Cheilosis, angular, riboflavin deficiency and, 139, *139*
Chemical(s), as teratogenic agent(s), 20
  neoplastic causal factors in, 119
Chemico-parasitic theory, of caries production, 182
Chemotaxis, definition of, 65
Chicken pox, lesions in, 239
Chlamydiae, description of, 31
Chlorhexidine, chemical control of plaque and, 153
  in dental caries control, 190
Cholecalciferol. *See* Vitamin D
Cholesterol, average value for Americans of, 115
  coronary heart disease and, risk factors in, 135
  lipoproteins and, 134-135
  nicotinic acid and, 139
Christmas disease, 275
Chromium, requirement for, 137
Chromosomal disorder(s), 17
Chromosome(s), injury to, 11
Chromosome translocation, definition of, 19
Chronic desquamative gingivitis, classification of, 223, *223*
Chronic lymphocytic leukemia (CLL), 273
Chronic myelocytic leukemia (CML), 273, *273*
Cleft(s), 37-39, *38*
Cleft palate, fetal developmental disturbances and, 1
Cleidocranial dysostosis, definition and description of, 52-53
"Closed lock," 287, *287*
Clotting. *See* Coagulation
Cloudy swelling, as degenerative change, 111
  impairment of homeostatic control and, 11
Coaggregation, definition of, 151
Coagulation, 69-70, 74
  disorder(s) of, 70, 74
    in hematologic and hematopoietic diseases, 275-276
  process of, 69, *69*
Coagulation factor(s), 69-70, *69*, 69*t*
  hereditary defects in, 70
  hemophilia and, 275-276
Coagulation necrosis, *71*, 113
Coat, of tongue, 42-43
Cobalamin, 140
Cobalt, requirement for, 137
Cocci, description of, 28
Coccidioidomycosis, 247-248
  areas endemic in, 246
Codon(s), definition of, 9
"Col," description of, 197, *197*
Cold sores, 238, *238*, 251
  oral pathology and, 1-2
Collagen, formation of, 10, *10*
"Collagen disease," 112
Colonization, adverse influences on, 151-152
  bacterial, 148-152
  by Streptococcus mutans, 150
  initial, of subgingival area, 149
  mechanisms of, 150-151
Complement, activation of. *See* Complement fixation
  plasma-protein fractions of, as mediator of vascular permeability, 65
Complement cascade, 80, *80*. *See also* Complement fixation
Complement fixation, complement receptor region of antibody and, 79
  immunoglobulin(s) and, 79
  pathways of, 80, *80*
Complement system, 79-80, *80*
  activation of, by plaque components, 156
  in inflammatory response to injury, 65
  major components of, 80, *80*
Concrescence, definition of, 59-60, *59*
Condyle(s), displacement of, 287, *287*, *288*, 290
  structure and function of, 279-282, *280*, *281*, *282*, 284
Congenital, definition of, 15

Conjugation, antibiotic-resistant bacteria and, 153-154
Conn's syndrome. *See* Aldosteronism
Contusion(s), definition of, 25
Cooley's anemia, 270
Copper, dietary, 136
Coronary heart disease, decreased incidence of, high-density lipoproteins and, 115
Cortisol, Cushing's syndrome and, 260
    effects of excess, 260
    in adrenal function, 259
Coxsackie virus, infections by, oral lesions in, 239-240
Creatine phosphokinase (CPK), diagnostic value of, 13
Cretinism, 257-258, 265
Crevicular fluid, 155-156
Crohn's disease, 244
Cushing's syndrome, adrenal adenoma and, 261
    cause of, 259, 265
    manifestations of, 260-261
    mechanism of, 260
Cyanosis, description of, 23
Cyclic adenosine triphosphate (cAMP), in vascular response to injury, 65
Cyclic neutropenia, periodontitis and, 228
Cyclosporine, immunosuppression and, 88
Cyst(s), types of, 39-41, *40, 41*
Cystic fibrosis, tetracycline pigmentation of teeth and, 57
Cytogenic disorder(s), 15
Cytokine(s), types of, 84
Cytomegalic inclusion (CMV), as physical agent of disease, 29
Cytoplasm, of differentiating cell, *10*
    structure of, 3, *4*
Cytoplasmic membrane, of differentiating cell, *10*
Cytosine, in biochemical basis of heredity, 7
Cytotoxic reaction(s), in hypersensitivity, 87
Cytotoxic T-cell(s) (CTL), in immune response, 82-83

"Dead tracts," of dentin, 170, *170*
Defect(s), fissural. *See* Fissural defect(s)
Deficiency(ies), nutritional, 133. *See also* specific elements; types of
    combined, 141
Degeneration(s), definition of, 111
    infiltrations and dysfunction and, 111-113
    See also types of
Dehydration, causes of, 24
Dementia, definition of, 106
Demineralization, acid production in plaque and, 184
"Dens in dente," 53, *53*
Dental caries, 178-195
    acid production in plaque and, 183-184
    characteristics of lesions, 184-189
        advancing lesions, 187-188, *188-189*
        initial enamel lesion, 184-187, *185-186*
        microorganisms in, 188-189
        remineralization phenomena and, 187, *187-188*
        root surface lesions, 189
    control of, 146, 189-192
        dietary sugar control, 190-191
        fissure sealants and, 192
        fluoride mechanisms, 191-192
        immunization and, 191
        mechanical and chemical plaque control, 190
        microorganism replacement therapy, 191
        natural defense mechanisms, 191
    definition of, 178
    diet and, 181-182
    epidemiology of, 179
    etiology of, 182-183
    fluoride and, 136-137
    host response in, 154
    mechanisms of, 178
    microbiology of, 182
    prediction of, 192
    prevalence of, 179
    prevention of, 3
    sites of, 179-180, *179-180*
    summary about, 192-193
    target populations of, 180-181, *180*
    xerostomia and, 2
Dental crypt, definition of, 50
Dental cuticle. *See* Enamel cuticle
Dental floss, in dental caries control, 190
Dental health, operational definition of, changes in, 2
Dental lamina, definition of, 46
    development of primary and secondary teeth and, 50, *51*
    in embryology of teeth, 46, *47, 48,* 50, *51*
Dental papilla, definition of, 47
    histodifferentiation of teeth and, 48, *48*
    in bell stage of developing tooth, *48*
Dental plaque, and microbiota, calculus, stains and disease and, 144-165, *145*
    host responses to, 154
    pathogenicity and virulence of, 144, 152-158
    bacterial accumulation in, 148
    bacterial studies of, 145
    clinical aspects of, 146
    coexistence of bacteria in, substrate and, 147
    components of, associated with immune responses, 154
    control of, mechanical, 146
    definition of, 144, 163
    development of, bacterial adherence in, 145
    disease and, 158-159
    ecologic determinants of, 146-148, *147*
    flora of, identification of, 158
    formation of, 148-152
    immune responses to, 154
    immunosuppressive agents in, 157
    limitations on thickness of, 147
    mineralization of, 160-161
        prerequisite for, 160
    role of, in periodontal disease(s), 202-203, *203,* 204t
    subgingival, 149-150, *150*
        characterized by, 145t, 149
        zones of, 149
    supragingival, "corncob" appearance of, 151
Dental restorations, as modifying factor, in periodontal disease, 205-206, *206*
    trauma from, *289,* 290-291, *290*
Dental sac, in embryology of teeth, 50
Dental tubule(s), in dentin-pulp complex, 167-168, 169-170
    permeability of, 170
Denticle(s). *See* Pulp stone(s)
Dentifrice(s), chemical injury from, 249, *249*
Dentin, calcified, odontogenic tumors and, 127-129, *129*
    characteristics of, *167-168,* 169-170, *170-171*
    "dead tracts" of, 170, *170*
    dysplasia of, 59, *59*
    formation of, 49, *49,* 50, *51*
        disturbances in, 57-59, *58*
    irregular secondary, 170, *171*
    peritubular, in carious lesions, 186
    reactive, 170, *171*
    sclerosis of, 113, 170, *170*
    translucent, in carious lesions, 185
    See also Dentin-pulp complex
Dentinogenesis imperfecta, 57-59, *58*
    characteristics of, *58,* 59
    classification of, 57
Dentin-pulp complex, circulation in, 168-169
    composition of dentin in, 169-170, *168*
    description of, 166-170
    innervation of, 166-168, *168*
    pulp disease and, 170-172, *173*
    sequelae of, 172-176, *173-176*
    summary about, 176
Dento-enamel membrane, formation of, 49

INDEX

Dentofacial malrelation(s), 44-46, *44-46*
   causes of, 46
   orthodontic evaluation of, *45*, 46
Dento-gingival junction, histopathology of, in periodontal disease, 210-213, *210-213*
Denture(s), mechanical injury under, 248-249
Denture stomatitis, *246*, 247
Deoxyribonucleic acid. *See* DNA
Desmosome(s), 6, *6, 7*
Developmental disturbance(s), 35-60
Diabetes mellitus, 263-264, *265*
   classification of, by National Diabetes Data Group, 263
Diagnosis, prenatal, of developmental disturbances, 20-21
Diazepam, effect of, 20
Diet, dental caries and, 181-182
   control of, 190-191
   See also Food
Differentiating cell, ultrastructure of, *10*
Differentiation, in facial embryology, definition of, 35
Digestive tract, age-related changes in, 106
Dilaceration, description of, *52*, 53
Dilantin gingivitis, classification of, 220, *220*
Diphenylhydantoin, periodontal disease and, 205
Diphtheria, 67
Disease, agents of, 15-34
   development at site of plaque formation of, bacteria and, 144
   extrinsic factors in, 22-33
   genetic factors in, 15-16
   hematologic and hematopoietic. *See* Hematologic and hematopoietic disease(s)
   intrinsic factors in, 15-19
   metabolic. *See* Metabolic disease(s)
   psychological factors in, 21-22
   systemic, with oral manifestations, 243-244
Disjunction, definition of, 17
Disk, articular. *See* Articular disk(s)
Disorder(s). *See* specific types
Disseminated intravascular clotting (DIC), 70
Disturbance(s), developmental, 35-60. *See also* specific developmental disturbances, structures
   nutritional, 133-143
      clinical considerations in, 141-142
DNA, definition of, 7
   function of, in response to cellular injury, 11
   hybridization of, use of new methods of, 79
   injury to, 11
   replication of, in life cycle of cell, 6
   synthesis of, megaloblastic anemia and, 269
Dominant trait, expression of, 16
Down's syndrome, 17
   periodontitis and, 228
Drug(s), as agents of disease, 33
   as modifying factor, in periodontal disease, 205
   as teratogenic agent(s), 20
   selection of in cancer therapy, relationship of to cell cycle, *130*, 131
Dry mouth. *See* Xerostomia
Dwarfism, of teeth, as developmental disturbance, 53-54, *54*
   pituitary, 255, 265
Dysostosis, cleidocranial, 52-53
Dysplasia, ectodermal, 51
   of dentin, 59, *59*

Eagle syndrome, TMJ/muscle dysfunction and, *286*, 287
Ecchymosis, platelet disorders and, 274, *274*
Ectodermal dysplasia, in developmental disturbance of teeth, 51
Edema, causes of, 25
   definition of, 64
Ehlers-Danlos syndrome, 275
Electrical energy, as physical agent of disease, 26-27
Electroencephalography, in cell injury, 13
Electromyography, in cell injury, 13

Elephantiasis gingivae, 220, *220*
Embolism, definition of, 23
Embolus, definition of, 23
Embryology, of face, 35-37, *36*
   of teeth, 46-51, *47, 48, 49, 51*
Emigration, definition of, 65
Enamel, calcified, odontogenic tumors and, 127-129, *129*
   formation disorders of, 54-57, 60. *See also* specific disorders
   formation of, 49-50, *49*
   mottling of, fluoride and, 137
   surface structure(s) of, 51
Enamel cavitation, in carious lesions, 187, *188*
Enamel cuticle, 50-51
Enamel epithelium, in bell stage of developing tooth, 46, *48*
Enamel hypoplasia, 54-57, *54, 55, 56*
   candidiasis and, 247
   causes of, 55-57
   erythroblastosis fetalis and, 271
   variation in involvement of teeth, 55
Enamel organ, definition of, 46
   in embryology of teeth, 48-49, *51*
   results of variations in development of, 50
Enamel pearl(s), *59*, 60
Endocrine system, definition of, 254
   diseases of. *See* Endocrinopathy(ies)
   disturbances in function of, 255-261, 265
   multiple neoplasia syndromes of, 262
   neuromediators of, 254
   polyglandular disorders of, 262-263
Endocrinopathy(ies), and metabolic diseases, 254-266
   chronic localized mucocutaneous candidiasis with, 247
   oral manifestations of, 265-266
Endoplasmic reticulum, of differentiating cell, *10*
   structure and function of, 3, *4*
Endorphin(s), in pathophysiology of pain, 254
Endothelium, definition of, 65
Energy, dietary, expression of total daily requirement for, 133-134
   maintenance of cellular activity and, 133
Enkephalin(s), in pathophysiology of pain, 254
Environment, as physical agent of disease, 32
Enzyme(s), diagnostic value of, *12*, 13
   lysosomal, basic types of, 66
      in phagocytosis, 66-67, 74, *81*
Eosinophil(s), definition of, 63
Eosinophilia, 272
Eosinophilic granuloma, 276
Epidemic parotitis, 240
Epithelial attachment, definition of, 50
Epithelium. *See* specific types
Epstein-Barr virus, diseases associated with, 29
   rheumatoid arthritis and, 88
Erosion, of teeth, 109, *109*
Erythema multiforme, *223*, 244
Erythroblastosis fetalis, 270-271
   oral manifestations of, 271
Erythrocyte(s), classification of, 268-269
   disorders of, 268-271
   formation of, 267-268
   primary role of, 268
Erythropoietin, in formation of red blood cells, 267
Estrogen, exogenous, as physical agent of disease, 33
   osteoporosis and, 136
Exostosis(es), 101, *101*
Exudate(s), as inflammatory response, 67
   definition of, 64
   See also specific types
Exudation, definition of, 64
Eye(s), age-related changes in, 104
   changes in, vitamin A deficiency and, 137

Face, embryology of, 35-37, *36*
   upper, developmental disturbances of, 37-41

Fat(s), and lipids, nutritional effects of, 134-135
Fatty acid(s), essential, 134
Fatty atrophy, 112
    definition of, 111
Fatty degeneration, 112
Fermentation, lactic acid production and, 183
Fertilization, description of, 16
Fetus, developmental disturbances of, cranio-facial malformations in, 1
Fever blisters. *See* Cold sores
Fiber, dietary, 133
Fibrinolysin, 69-70
Fibrinolysis, 68, 69-70
Fibrinous exudate, as inflammatory response, 67
Fibroblast(s), capabilities of, following injury, 72
Fibroma(s), *126*, 127
    odontogenic, 127
    See also specific types
Fibromatosis, hereditary gingival, classification of, 220, *220*
Fibronectin, in dental pulp, description of, 166
    in immune response to plaque, 157
Fissural defect(s), 39-41, *40*
Fissure sealants, in dental caries control, 192
Fistula, definition of, 39
    pulp disease and, 174, *175-176*
Fluid, crevicular, 155-156
    in dental tubules, pain and, 168-170, *168*
Fluoride, dietary, 136-137
    in dental caries control, 191-192
Fluorosis, *56*, 57
    systemic, 137
Folacin, nutritional disturbances and, 140, *140*
Food, changes in consumption of, emergence of opportunistic pathogens and, 164
    specific dynamic action of, definition of, 133-134
    See also Diet
Fordyce's spots, 39-41, *41*
Fracture(s), compound, definition of, 25
    of bones, healing of, 73, *74*
Functional epithelium, permeability of, 155
Fungus(i), as physical agent of disease, 31
"Furcation involvement," in periodontal disease, 225, *225*
Furrowed tongue, 43, *43*
Furuncle(s), definition of, 28
Fusion, lines of, disturbances in, 39-41, *40*
    of teeth, definition of, 60
Fusobacterium, role of, in periodontal disease(s), 202

Gangrene, cellular injury and, 11
Gangrenous necrosis, 113
Gas homeostasis, as physical agent of disease, 22-23
Gating, 6
Geminism, definition of, 60, *60*
Gene(s), mutant, effect of location of, 16
Gene expression, 7-10
Gene locus, definition of, 16
Genetic, definition of, 15
Genetic code. *See* Heredity, biochemical basis of
Geographic tongue, 43-44, *43*, *44*
Giant cell(s). *See* Macrophage(s)
Giant cell granuloma, central, description of, 99-100, *100*
    radiographic features of, 100, *100*
    peripheral, description of, 97-99, *99*
    histologic features of, 98
    recurrence of, hyperparathyroidism and, 100
Giantism, of teeth, as developmental disturbance, 53, *53*
Gigantism, excess of growth hormone and, 255, 265
Gingiva, anatomy of, 196-199, *197-199*
    attached, description of, 197, *197*
    clinical evaluation of, 198-199, *198-199*
    in polycythemia vera, 269
    marginal, description of, 196-197, *197*
    normal, histology of, 213, *213*
    pigmentation of, 198, *198*
    response of, to plaque irritants, antigens, or mitogens, 156
        to very little plaque, 155
    toothbrush abrasion of, 248, *248*
    unattached (free), definition of, 197
    varicella-zoster lesions in, 239, *239*
Gingival atrophy/recession, classification of, 223-224, *224*
Gingival crevice, description of, 196
Gingival fibromatosis, hereditary, classification of, 220, *220*
Gingival hyperplasia, in myelocytic leukemia, 272, *273*
Gingival Index (GI), definition of, 202
Gingival sulcus, description of, 196, *197*
    histopathology of, in periodontal disease, 210-211, *210*
Gingivitis, acute necrotizing ulcerative. *See* Gingivitis, necrotizing ulcerative (NUG)
    chronic desquamative, as manifestation of disease, *223*, 244
    classification of, 219-224, *219-224*
        atrophic or recessive, 223-224, *224*
        chronic desquamative, 223, *223*
        complex, 219
        hyperplastic, 219-221, *220-221*
        necrotizing ulcerative (NUG), 221-223, *222*
        simple, 219, *219*
        traumatic, 223, *223*
    clinical, initiation of, 149
    cyanosis in, 23
    experimental, bacterial colonization and, 148-149
    histology of, 213-214, *213-215*
    histopathology of, 210-217
    hyperplastic, mouthbreathing and, 205, *206*
    initiation of, calculus and, 161
    plaque-induced, changes in plasma cells and, 155
    results of, 157
    scorbutic, *140*
    transition to periodontitis, 213-217
Gingivostomatitis, herpetic, 237-238, *237*, *238*
Glenoid fossa. *See* Mandibular fossa
Globular process, formation of, *36*, 37
Globulomaxillary cyst(s), 39
Glossitis migrans. *See* Geographic tongue
Glucagon, functions of, 263
Glucan, synthesis of, colonization by Streptococcus mutans and, 150
Glucocorticoid(s), metabolic function of, 259
Glucose, metabolism of, in diabetes, 263
    nutritional disturbances and, 134
    oral tolerance test for, 263-264
Glycocalyx, description of, 4, *4*
Glycogen, nutritional disturbances and, 134
Glyconeogenesis, definition of, 263
Glycosuria, definition of, 263
Goiter, 136
Golgi apparatus, of differentiating cell, *10*
Golgi complex, structure and function of, 3, *4*
Gonad(s), dysfunction of. *See* Gonadal dysfunction; specific disorders and organs
Gonadal dysfunction, 261-262
Gonorrhea, 244-245
Gout, 112, *112*
    as metabolic bone disease, 265
Granulation tissue, in healing, 72, 73, *73*
Granulocyte(s), description of, 62, *62*
Granulocytopenia, 271, *272*
Granulocytosis, 271-272, 277
Granuloma(s), chronic localized mucocutaneous candidiasis with, 247
    definition of, 71
    periapical, pulp disease and, 173
    See also specific types
Granuloma pyogenicum, 205, *205*, 220-221, *220*
Granulomatous disease(s), hypercalcemia and, 136
Ground substance, in dental pulp, description of, 166
Guanine, in biochemical basis of heredity, 7

Gum boil, pulp disease and, 174, *175*
Gumma, 245
Gut-associated lymphoid tissue (GALT), local immune responses and, 155

Hair-on-end, roentgenographic pattern of, 270
Hairy tongue, *42*, 43
Hand, foot and mouth disease, 239-240
Hand-Schüller-Christian disease, 276
Hapten(s), definition of, 77
Healing, by primary intention, 72
　by secondary intention, 72, 73, *73*
　repair and regeneration and, *64*, 71-73
Health, requirements for, 133
Hearing, age-related changes in, 106
Hebephrenia, description of, 21
Hemangioma(s), description of, 127, *128*
Hematologic and hematopoietic disease(s), 267-278
　causes of manifestations of, 267
　vascular factors in, 275-276
　See also specific diseases
Hematopoiesis, definition of, 267
　extramedullary, 267
Heme, biosynthesis of, 268
Hemidesmosome(s), 6, 7
Hemidesmosome-basement lamina complex, 6, 7
Hemoglobin, endogenous pigments from, 116
Hemolytic anemia(s), cause of, 268
　chronic, sickle cell anemia and, 270
　congenital, 270-271
　phenacetin and, 87
Hemolytic disease of newborn, cytotoxic hypersensitivity reaction and, 87
　Rh antigen and, 78
Hemophilia, 275-276
Hemorrhagic exudate, as inflammatory response, 67
Hemostasis, 68-69, 74
　breakdown of mechanisms of, 273-274, 277
　coagulation and fibrinolysis and, 68-70, 74
　stages of, 68
Hepatitis, viral, description of, 30-31
Heredity, biochemical basis of, 7-10
　dental caries susceptibility and, 181
Herpangina, 239
Herpes labialis, 238, *238*
Herpes simplex 1 (HSV-1), as physical agent of disease, 29
　natural history of, 237
　oral lesions in infection by, 237-239, 251
　recrudescent lesions in, 238, *238*
Herpes simplex 2 (HSV-2), as physical agent of disease, 29
Herpes simplex virus, classification of, 236
　common sites for, 236
　infections by, 236-239, 251
　latency of, 236-237
Herpes virus(es), avoidance of immune system by, 84
　infections from, 29
　See also specific viruses
Herpes zoster, as physical agent of disease, 29
Hertwig's sheath, formation of enamel pearl and, 60
Heterozygote(s), definition of, 16
High-density lipoprotein(s) (HDL), in decreased incidence of coronary heart disease, 115
Histamine, as mediator of vascular permeability, 65
Histodifferentiation, of enamel epithelium, definition of, 46-48
Histogenesis, classification of cancer and, 122
Histoplasma capsulatum, 247
Histoplasmosis, 247
　areas endemic to, 246
Hodgkin's disease, 130
　chemotherapy and, 131
Homeostasis, control of cellular adaptation to injury by, impairment of, 11
　mechanism(s) of, in repair of tissues, 68
　See also specific types of

Homozygote(s), definition of, 16
"Hormonal gingivitis," classification of, 223
Hormone(s), as agents of disease, 33
　binding to receptors of, modulation of cell activity and, 254-255
　control mechanisms for, 265
　defects in function of, 255
　mechanisms for regulating release of, 255
　testicular and ovarian, 261
Host defense(s), periodontal disease and, pathogenesis of, 208
HTLV-III. *See* Human T-cell lymphocytotrophic virus III
Human leukocyte antigen (HLA), 78, *78*, 90
Human T-cell lymphocytotrophic virus III, 86
　AIDS and, 240-242, 251
　　course of development of, 241-242
　enzyme-linked immunocompetent assay for, 87
　infection by, projections of Center for Disease Control for, 242
Human T-cell lymphotropic virus III. *See* Human T-cell lymphocytotrophic virus III
Hutchinson incisors, *55*, 56
Hyaline degeneration, 111
Hydrocortisone. *See* Cortisol
Hydrodynamic theory, of pain transmission, across dentin, 167-168, *168*
Hydrogen peroxide, chemical injury to tongue by, 249
Hydrophobia, 30
Hydropic degeneration, 111
　impairment of homeostatic control and, 11
Hydroxyapatite, in demineralization process, 184
Hypercalcemia, diseases associated with, 136
Hypercementosis, 92-93, *94*
Hypercoagulable states, 276
Hypercortisolism, 260
Hyperemia, active, definition of, 65
　types of, definition of, 23
Hyperglycemia, definition of, 263
　See also Diabetes mellitus
Hypergonadism, 262
Hyperkeratinization, tobacco use and, 250
Hyperkeratosis, 93-95, *94, 95*
Hyperlipidemia, treatment of, 115
Hypermagnesemia, 137
Hyperodontia, 51, 52
Hyperparathyroidism, 100, 258-259
Hyperplasia, 92-93
　hypertrophy versus, 93
　of gingival tissue, 92, *93*, *94*
　tobacco use and, 250
Hyperplastic gingivitis, classification of, 219-221, *220-221*
Hyperplastic pulpitis, 172, *173*
Hypersensitivity, 87-88, 90
Hypertension, 261
Hyperthyroidism, 258
　iodine excess and, 136
Hypertrophy, 93
Hypogonadism, 261-262
Hypomagnesemia, 137
Hypoparathyroidism, 258
Hypophosphatasia, 138
Hypoplasia, causes of, 55
　of enamel. *See* Enamel hypoplasia
Hypothalamic-pituitary target cell control system, 255, *256*
Hypothalamic-pituitary-thyroid feedback control system, 257, *257*
Hypothyroidism, 257-258
Hypoxia, clinical manifestations of, 23
Hysteria, description of, 22

Icterus, pigment metabolism and, 116
Idiopathic thrombocytopenic purpura (ITP), 274, *274*
Immune mechanisms, in periodontal disease, pathogenesis of, 209-210

INDEX

Immune response(s), and immune injury, 76-91
　cellular, T-lymphocytes in, 82-84, *82*
　characteristics of, 77
　genetic control of, 77-78
　in AIDS, 240-241
　normal activation of, 240-241
　regulation of, 157
　summary of, 84-86, *85*
Immune system, 76-84, 90
　age-related changes in, 107-108
　cells of, 80-83
　cellular components of, 77
　common mucosal, 155
　common to bacterial infections, 154
　humoral components of, 77
　impairment of. See also Immunologic disturbance(s)
　　cancer and, 120
　　origin of lymphomas and, 130
　See also Immunity; Immune response(s)
Immunity, antibody-mediated. See Immunity, humoral
　cell-mediated, *82*, 83-84
　humoral, *82*, 83
　types of, 77
Immunization, in dental caries control, 191
Immunodeficiency, definition of, 76
Immunodeficiency disease, 86. See also specific diseases
Immunogen(s). See Antigen(s)
Immunoglobulin(s), classes of, functions of, 79
　cleavage fragments of, 78-79, *79*
　definition of, 77
　See also Antibody(ies); specific types
Immunologic disturbance(s), infections and, 236-253
Immunopathology, 86-90
Incidence, of periodontal disease, definition of, 200
Incision, definition of, 25
Infant(s), dental caries in, as target population, 180
Infarction, definition of, 23
　zone of, 23, *24*
Infection(s), and immunologic disturbances, 236-253
　bacterial, 244-245, 251-252
　definition of, 27
　fungal, 245-248
　immunologic demonstration of, 13
　viral, 236-242
Infiltration(s), definition of, 112
Inflammation, acute, 63, 68, *71*
　　definition of, 68
　　initial phase of, 74
　　recurrent attacks of, 71
　　resolution of, *71*, 74
　as multicellular response, 73-75
　cells in, 61-63
　chronic, 70-71, *71*, 74
　　foreign bodies and, 71, *71*
　definition of, 61
　granulomatous, 71
　manifestations of, 61
　plaque-induced gingivitis and, immune response in, 156-157
　purulent, as response to injury, 67, *68*
　resolution of, 71-72, *71*
　subacute, definition of, 68
　vascular response to, 63-65, *64*
Inflammatory response(s), net effect of, 164
　types of, 67
　See also Inflammation
Influenza, pandemics of, 30
Inheritance, of genetic disease, modes of, 17t
Injury, chemical, 249-250, *249, 250*
　　as physical agent of disease, 31-32
　mechanical, 248-249
　　as physical agent of disease, 25
　response to, 61-75
　　cellular, *64*, 65

　reparative, *64*
　vascular, 63-65, *64*
　thermal, 249, *249*
Insulin, functions of, 263
　secretion of, protein-calorie deficiency and, 134
Intercellular communication, 6, *6*
Interdental ligament, description of, 198, *198*
Interdental papilla, description of, 197
Interferon(s), as antiviral defense mechanism, 84
Interferon, production of, in AIDS, 241
Interstitial pressure, in pulp, pain and, 169
Intestinal IgA, precursors of, 155
Iodine, dietary, 136
Iron, nutritional disturbances and, 136
Iron deficiency anemia, 269-270
Irradiation, development of cancer and, 119
Ischemia, definition of, 23

Jaundice, 116
Jaw, control of positions and movement of, 282-284
　in Paget's disease, 264
　metastatic tumors of, 129
　movement of, occlusion and, 282-284, *282, 283, 285*
　See also Mandible
Junction, intercellular, 6, *6*
Junctional epithelium, definition of, 50
　histopathology of, in periodontal disease, 210-211, *210*
　impermeability to bacteria of, 156
Juvenile periodontitis, classification of, 226-228

Kanamycin, in dental caries control, 190
Kaposi's sarcoma, in AIDS, 242
　lesions of, 275
Karyorrhexis, definition of, 95
Karyotype, definition of, 17, *18*
Keloid, definition of, 73
Ketoacidosis, definition of, 263
Ketone(s), metabolism of, diabetes and, 263
Kidney, age-related changes in, 106
Killer (K) cell(s), description of, 83
Kinin(s), as mediators of vascular permeability, 65
Kwashiorkor, protein-calorie deficiency and, 134

Laceration(s), definition of, 25
Lactic acid, production of, in plaque, 183-184
Lactobacillus, in carious lesions, 189
Lactobacillus count, in caries prediction, 192
Lactoferrin, as ecologic factor in dental plaque, 151
Lamina dura, definition of, 200, *200*
Lamina limitans,, description of, *167*, 169
Langerhans cell granulomatosis, oral manifestations of, 276
Latency, of viral infections, 236-237
Lectin(s), dietary, interference with bacterial adherence of, 151
Legionnaire's disease, effect of bacterial toxicity in, 28
Lesion(s), oral. See Oral lesion(s)
Leukemia(s), 272-273, 277
　acute, 129-130
　etiology of, 272
　oral manifestations of, 273
　origin of, 122
　See also types of
Leukemic gingivitis, classification of, 221, *221*
Leukemoid reaction, definition of, 271
Leukocyte(s), migration of, in cellular response to injury, 65
　types of, 62-63
　See also specific types
Leukocytosis, definition of, 61
　in response to inflammation, 61-62
Leukopenia, definition of, 271
Leukoplakia, candidal, 247
　"hairy," in AIDS, 242
　keratinization and, 95
Leukotriene(s), definition of, 65

Lichen planus, 243-244, *244*
Ligand(s), bacterial adherence and, 151
Linkage disequilibrium, definition of, 78
Lip, angioneurotic edema of, allergic stomatitis and, 251, *251*
  atrophy of, 111, *111*
  cancer of, sunlight and, 119-120, *120*
  carcinoma of, 123-124, *123, 124*
  cleft of, 37, *38*
  hemangioma of, *128*
  lesions of, granulocytopenia and, *272*
  multiple neuromas of, 265-266
Lipoma(s), description of, 126-127, *126*
  of oral region, 127
Lipoprotein(s), cholesterol and, 134-135
Liquefaction necrosis, 113
Lithiasis, definition of, 113
Liver, function of, vitamin K and, 138
Localized juvenile periodontitis (LJP), 227
  neutrophil dysfunction and, 157-158
Lymphangioma(s), description of, 127
Lymphocyte(s), 82-83
  antibody producing, language of, 79
  in immune response to plaque, 157
  types and function of, 63
Lymphocyte-macrophage system, in periodontal disease, as modifying factor of, 204
  pathogenesis of, 209
Lymphocytosis, 272
Lymphokine(s), factors of, 84
  in cell-mediated immunity, 83-84
  in cellular immunity, 82, *82*
  released in immune response to plaque, 156-157
Lymphoma(s), description of, 130
  immunodeficiency and, 120
  non-Hodgkin's, 130
    monocyte-macrophage disorders and, 276
  origin of, 122
  types of, 130
Lymphopenia, 272
Lymphoproliferative response, periodontal destruction and, 157
Lysozome(s), as ecologic factor in dental plaque, 151-152
  structure and function of, 3

Macrocytic normochromic anemia(s), 268-271
Macrophage(s), formation of, 66
  functions of, 80, *81*, 90
  in chronic inflammation, 71
  in immune response, 80-82
    to plaque, 156-157
  in phagocytosis, 66-67
  interaction of T-lymphocytes with, in cell-mediated immunity, 83
  response of, to injury, *71*
  See also Lymphocyte-macrophage system; Monocyte-macrophage system
Magnesium, deficiency of, 137
Major histocompatibility complex (MHC), 77-78, 90
Major histocompatibility region, regulation of immune system and, 157
Malformation(s), congenital, 19-21
  teratogenic agents as causes of, 19, 19*t*
  vitamin A and, 137
Malocclusion, classification of, *44*, 46, *46*
  definition of, 44
  trauma from, 290, *290*
  types of, description of, 44-46
Malrelation(s)
  dentofacial. *See* Dentofacial malrelation(s)
Mandible, formation of, 35, *36*
  movement of, postural and functional relationships and, 282

repositioning devices for, in TMJ/muscle dysfunction, 292, *292*
Mandibular condyle. *See* Condyle(s)
Mandibular fossa, of temporal bone, 279, *280, 281, 283*
Manganese, requirement for, 137
Manic-depressive psychosis, description of, 21
Marasmus, protein-calorie deficiency and, 134
Margination, definition of, 65
Mast cell(s), function of, 65
Mastication, muscles of, *281, 282, 283*
  system and control of, 279-284
  system of, trauma to, 290-291
Materia alba, definition of, 145
Maxilla, formation of, *36*, 37
Maxillary process, formation of, *36*, 37
Median process, formation of, *36*, 37
Median rhomboid glossitis, 42, *42*
Megakaryocyte(s), definition of, 68
Megaloblastic anemia(s), 269
Meiosis, definition of, 16
Melanin, oral pigmentation and, 116, *260*
Membrane receptors, function of, 5
Mendelian inheritance, 16-17
Menopause, 262
Mercury, as teratogenic agent, 20
"Mesenteric line," black stain of teeth, 162, *162*
Metabolic disease(s), 263-265
  endocrinopathy and, 254-266
  of bone, 264-265
Metabolism, diseases of. *See* Metabolic disease(s)
  inborn errors of, 15
  mineral, 113-114
  pigment, 115-116
Metaplasia, 95-96, *96*
Metastasis(es), definition of, 121
Metazoa, description of, 31
Methemoglobin, in gas homeostasis, 23
Microbiology of dental caries, 182
Microbiota, dental plaque, calculus, stains and disease and, 144-165
  indigenous, definition of, 144
    development of, 144-145
  See also Bacteria; Microorganisms; specific types
Microcytic hypochromic anemia(s), 268
Microflora
Microflora, indigenous. *See* Microbiota, indigenous
Micrognathia, definition of, 44
Microorganisms, as teratogenic agents, 20
  periodontal disease and, pathogenesis of, 206-207
  role of, in periodontal disease(s), 202-203, *203*
  See also Bacteria; Microbiota; specific types
Microphage(s). *See* Polymorphonuclear leukocyte(s)
Midpalatine cyst(s), 39, *40*
Mineral(s), nutritional needs for, 135-137
  trace *See also* specific trace minerals
    nutritional disturbances in, 136-137
Mineral metabolism, 113-114
Mitochondria, of differentiating cell, *10*
  of odontogenic cell, *7*
  structure and function of, 3, *4*
Mitogen(s), functions of, 154
Mitosis, definition of, 15
Molecules, types of, in biochemical basis for heredity, 7
Molybdenum, requirement for, 137
Mongolism. *See* Down's syndrome
Monocyte(s), formation of macrophages and, 66
  function of, 63
  migration of, in cellular response to injury, 65
Monocyte-macrophage system, disorders of, 276, *277*
Monocytic leukemia, 273, *273*
Monocytosis, 272
Monokine(s), in immune response to plaque, 157
Mononuclear phagocyte(s), in immune response, 80
Mononucleosis, infectious, 272

Morphodifferentiation, in embryology of teeth, 46
  in facial embryology, 35
Mottled enamel, 56, 57
Mouthbreather's gingivitis, classification of, 219-220
Mouthbreathing, as modifying factor, in periodontal disease, 205, 206
Mucinous degeneration, 111
Mucinous exudate, as inflammatory response, 67
Mucocele(s), 41, 41, 112, 112
"Mucous patch(es)," in syphilis, 245, 245
Mucous retention, 112, 112, 113
Mucous retention cyst(s), 41, 113, 113
Mulberry molars, 55, 56
Multiple endocrine neoplasia syndrome(s), 262
Multiple sclerosis, possible cause of, 84
Mumps virus, 240
Muscle(s), age-related changes in, 104, 106
Mutation(s), ionizing radiation and, 20
  occurence of, 16
Myeloid, definition of, 267
Myelophthisic anemia(s), cause of, 268
Myocardial infarct, enzymatic diagnosis of, 13
Myxedema, clinical findings in, 258
  types of, 257
Myxoma(s), odontogenic, 127

Nasal process(es), formation of, 36, 37
Nasmyth's membrane, 50
Nasopalatine cyst(s), 39, 40
National Diabetes Data Group, classification of diabetes mellitus by, 263
Natural defense(s), in dental caries control, 191
Natural killer (N_k) cell(s), in immunologic cytolysis, 83
Necrosis, cellular injury and, 11
  definition of, 23
  types of, 113
Necrotizing ulcerative gingivitis (NUG), classification of, 221-223, 222
  epidemiology of, 222
  etiology of, 221-222
  inflammatory response to injury and, 67, 68, 71
  treatment of, 222-223
"Negative bone factor," periodontal disease and, 208
Neoplasia, 117-132
  definition of, 117
  developmental factors in, 120
  epidemiology of, 117-118, 118t
  etiology of, 118-120
  extrinsic factor(s) in development of, 118-120
    chemicals as, 119
    irradiation as, 119
    mechanical irritation as, 118-119
    sunlight as, 119-120
  general characteristics of, 120-121
  hereditary factor(s) in development of, 118
  immunologic defects and development of, 120
  multiple endocrine syndromes of, 262
Neoplasm(s), benign, 120-121, 121
  differences between malignant and, 122t
  classification of, 121-130, 123t
  malignant, 121, 122
    differences between benign and, 122t
  odontogenic, 127-129
  of epithelial origin, 122-126, 123t
    metastatic, 129
  of mesenchymal origin, 123t, 126-129
Nerve(s), in dentin-pulp complex, 166-168, 168
Nervous system, central. See Central nervous system
Neurilemmoma(s), definition of, 127
Neurofibroma(s), 127
Neurogenic inflammation, P substance and, 169
Neuroma(s), multiple, of lip, 265-266
Neuromediator(s), of endocrine system, 254
Neutropenia, cyclic, 271
  classification of periodontitis and, 228, 229
  definition of, 271
  in lesions of lip and palate, 272
Neutrophil(s), as modifying factor, in periodontal disease, 204
  definition of, 62
  dysfunction of, in periodontal disease, 157
    mechanism of, 157-158
    susceptibility to periodontal disease and, 164
  function of, in periodontal disease, 156
  in disorders of white blood cells, 271
  periodontal disease and, pathogenesis of, 208
Niacin, 139-140
  deficiency of, 139-140, 139
  equivalents, dietary allowances for, 140
Nicotinic acid, pellagra and, 140
  vascular effects of, 139
Night blindness, vitamin A deficiency and, 137
Nitrogen toxicity, description of, 23
Normocytic, normochromic anemia(s), 268
Nucleolus, of differentiating cell, 10
Nucleotide(s), definition of, 7
Nucleus, of differentiating cell, 10
  of odontogenic cell, 7
  structure and function of, 3, 4
"Null cell(s)," 83
"Nursing bottle caries," 180
Nutrient(s), bacterial, 147
  necessary, 133-141. See also specific nutrients
Nutrition, as factor in disease, 31

Obesity, as factor in disease, 31
Obsessive-compulsive neurosis, 22
Occlusal trauma, as modifying factor, in periodontal disease, 205
  diagnosis of, 291, 291
  periodontal diseases and, 224, 225
Occlusion, therapy for, 291, 292
  trauma from, 289, 290-291, 290. See also Occlusal trauma
Odontoblast(s), dentin formation and, 49, 49, 50, 166, 167
Odontogenic cell, ultrastructure of, 7
Odontoma(s), 128-129, 129
-oma, definition of, 122
Oncogene(s), definition of, 17
Oncornavirus(es), definition and classification of, 29-30
Opsonin(s), phagocyte receptor for, 81, 81
Opsonization, 81-82, 81
  definition of, 77
Oral contraceptives, periodontal disease and, 205
Oral glucose tolerance test (OGTT), 263-264
Oral lesion(s), reactive, 96-102, 96t. See also specific lesions
Oral mucosa, chemical injury to, 249-250, 249, 250
  lesions of. See also specific diseases and infections
    as manifestations of disease, 236, 251
Oral pathology, scope of, 1-3
  cleft palate and, 1
Oral tissues, pathophysiology of, 2, 2
Organ transplantation, HLA typing in, 78
  immunologic rejection of, 88
Organelles, cellular, definition of, 3, 4
Orofacial pain, oral pathology and, 2
Orthodontic evaluation, 45, 46
Osseous callus, in bone healing, 73, 74
Osteitis deformans. See Paget's disease
Osteitis fibrosa cystica, definition of, 259
Osteoarthritis, 107, 107
  clinical symptoms of, TMJ/muscle dysfunction vs., 286, 287
  definition of, 105
  of TMJ, roentgenographic changes related to, 287, 289
Osteoblast(s), function of, 73
Osteoclast(s), function of, 73

Osteocyte(s), function of, 73
Osteomalacia, vitamin D deficiency and, 138
Osteomyelitis, pulp disease and, 176
Osteoporosis, as metabolic disease of bone, 265
  calcium deficiency and, 135-136
  definition of, 105
  risk factors for, 265
Ovarian insufficiency, hypogonadism and, 262
Ovary, principal hormones of, 261
Overbite, as modifying factor, in periodontal disease, 205, 206
Oxygen, microbial growth and, 146-147
Oxygen homeostasis, as physical agent of disease, 22-23
Oxygen toxicity, description of, 23

P substance, pulp circulation and, 169
Paget's disease, 264-265
  complications of, 265
Pain, orofacial, oral pathology and, 2
  severity of, pulpitis classification and, 171-172, 172
  transmission of, in dentin-pulp complex, 167-168, 168
Palate, cleft of, 37, 38, 39
  formation of, 36, 37
  lesions of, granulocytopenia and, 272
  tumor of, 125
Pancytopenia, in aplastic anemia, 269
Panic disorder, description of, 21-22
Papilloma, 122, 123
  fibroepithelial, 121
Papillon-Lefevre syndrome, periodontitis and, 228, 230
Paranoia, description of, 21
Parasite(s), as physical agent of disease, 31
Parathyroid function, 258
Parathyroid hormone (PTH), 258
Parulis, pulp disease and, 174, 175-176
Pathogenicity, definition of, 152
Pathogens, periodontal disease and, pathogenesis of, 206-207
"Peg lateral," 54, 54
Pellagra, 139-140, 139, 140
Pellicle(s), intraoral, description of, 148
Pemphigoid, 244
Pemphigus, 244
Penetrance, definition of, 19
Periapical abscess, pulp disease and, 174, 175
Periapical cyst, pulp disease and, 173-174, 174
Periapical granuloma, pulp disease and, 173
Periodontal disease(s), 196-235
  classification of, 219-228, 219t
    gingivitis, 219-224, 219-224
    occlusal trauma, 224, 225
    periodontitis, 224-228, 225-227, 229-230
  control of, 146
  dental plaque and, 164
  diagnostic profiling of pathogens in, 158-159
  epidemiology of, 200-202
  etiology of, 202-206, 203-206, 204t
  histopathology of gingivitis- periodontitis and, 210-217. See also Gingivitis; Periodontitis
  host response in, 154
  initiating factors in, 202-203, 203, 204t
  measurement of, 201-202
  modifying factors in, 203-206, 203, 204t, 205-206
  neutrophil dysfunction and, 157
  nutritional deficiencies and, 141-142
  pathogenesis of, 206-210
  periodontal anatomy and, 196-200, 197-201
  predominant bacteria in, 145, 145t
  prevention of, 228, 231
  significant bacteria in, 152
  specific vs. nonspecific plaque pathogens in, hypotheses for, 158-159
  summary of, 231-233, 231-232
Periodontal disease index (PDI), definition of, 201

Periodontal fiber(s), description of, 197-198, 197
Periodontal Index (PI), definition of, 201
Periodontal ligament, anatomy of, 199-200, 200
  formation of, 10
Periodontal membrane, formation of, 10
Periodontitis, antibodies to Bacteroides gingivalis in, 156
  classification of, 224-228
    Chédiak-Higashi syndrome and, 228
    chronic destructive disease in adult, 225-226, 225-227
    cyclic neutropenia and, 228, 229
    destructive disease in young individuals, 226
    Down's syndrome and, 228
    early, 228
    juvenile, 226-228
    Papillon-Lefevre syndrome and, 228, 230
  histology of, 214-217, 215-218
  in juvenile diabetes, 266
  localized juvenile. See Localized juvenile periodontitis (LJP)
  predominant genera in, 145t, 150
  spirochetes and, 149
Periodontium, anatomy of, 196-200
  alveolar bone, 200, 200-201
  cementum, 200
  gingiva, 196-199, 197-199
  periodontal ligament, 199-200, 200
  changes in, combined nutritional deficiencies and, 141
Periodontoblastic space, definition of, 169
Peripheral fibroma, description of, 97, 98
  ossifying, 97, 99
Pernicious anemia(s), 269
Petechiae, platelet disorders and, 274, 274
Pfluger molars, 55, 56
Phagocyte(s), surface receptors of, 81-82, 81
Phagocytosis, 66-68, 66
  definition of, 66
  phases of, 80-82, 81, 85
Phenacetin, in hypersensitivity cytotoxic reactions, 87
Phobia(s), description of, 22
Phosphate, in demineralization process, 184
Pigment metabolism, 115-116
Pituitary function, disturbances of, 255
Pituitary growth hormone (GH), disturbances of, 255
Plaque, acid production in, 183-184
  dental. See Dental plaque
Plaque Index (Pl.I), definition of, 202
Plasma protein(s), transport of, through dentin, 170
Plasmid(s), antibiotic-resistant bacteria and, 153-154
  definition of, 9
Plasmin, in fibrinolysis, 69-70
Plasminogen, 69-70
Platelet(s), function of, 68
Plaut-Vincent disease. See Necrotizing ulcerative gingivitis (NUG)
Plummer-Vinson syndrome, iron deficiency anemia and, 269-270, 270
PMA index, definition of, 201
PMNs. See Polymorphonuclear leukocyte(s)
Pocket(s), formation of, periodontal disease and, 208
  periodontal, histopathology of, 211-213, 212
"Pocket epithelium," histology of, 211, 212
Podagra, 112
Point mutation, in activation of oncogene, 17
Poliomyelitis, description of, 29
"Polyclonal activators," immune mechanisms and, 209
Polycythemia vera, 269
Polydipsia, definition of, 263
Polygenic disorder(s), 17
Polymorphonuclear leukocyte(s) (PMN), definition of, 62
  function of, 62-63
  in phagocytosis, 66-67, 66
  migration of, in cellular response to injury, 64, 65
  ultrastructural characteristics of, 62
Polyphagia, definition of, 263

Polyuria, definition of, 263
Porphyria, congenital, discoloration of teeth and, 163
    erythropoietic, 270, *270*
Porphyrin, excess of, 116, *270*
"Port wine stain(s)," 127
Potassium, deficiency of, 135
    excess of, persons at risk for, 135
    metabolism of, aldosterone and, 259
Preauricular cyst(s), 39
Pregnancy, as modifying factor, in periodontal disease, 204-205, *206*
Pregnancy gingivitis, classification of, 220-221, *220*
"Pregnancy tumor," 205, *205*, 220, *220*
    description of, 96-97, *97*
Prevalence, of periodontal disease, definition of, 200
Probing, periodontal, 198-199, *199*
Procallus, in bone healing, 73, *74*
Procollagen, formation of, 10
Progestin(s), effect of, 20
Prognathism, definition of, 255
Proliferation, in facial embryology, definition of, 35
Prostaglandin(s), as chemical messengers, 254
    as mediator of vascular permeability, 65
Protein, dietary requirements for, 134
    synthesis of, 8-9, *8*, *9*
Protein-calorie deficiency(ies), 134
Proteoglycan(s), in dental pulp, description of, 166
Proteolysis-chelation theory, of caries production, 183
Proteolytic theory, of caries production, 183
Prothrombin, abnormal, vitamin K deficiency and, 138
Protozoa, diseases caused by, 31
"Proud flesh," 72, *73*
Pseudomembrane, formation of, in response to injury, 67, *68*
Pulp, circulation in, 168-169
    dental, description of, 166, *167*
    necrosis of, 169
    See also Dentin-pulp complex
Pulp disease, 170-172
    classification of, 171
    sequelae of, 172-176
        cellulitis, 174
        osteomyelitis, 176
        parulis, fistula and gum boil, 174, *175-176*
        periapical abscess, 174, *175*
        periapical cyst, 173-174, *174*
        periapical granuloma, 173
Pulp stone(s), 113-114, *114*
Pulpitis, chronic, 171-172, *173*
    classifications of, 171-172, *172*
    hyperplastic, 172, *173*
Pus, definition of, 67
Pyogenic granuloma, description of, 96, *97*
Pyridoxine, 140

Rabies, description of, 30
Race, dental caries susceptibility and, 181
Rad(s), definition of, 19
Radiant energy, as physical agent of disease, 25-27
Radiation, as teratogenic agent, 19-20
    cervical caries and, 27
    chronic effects of, *26*
Radicular cyst. *See* Periapical cyst
Ranula. *See* Mucous retention cyst(s)
Receptor(s), bacterial adherence and, definition of, 151
Recessive trait, expression of, 16
Recognition marker. *See* Antigenic determinant(s)
Recommended daily allowance (RDA), adequate nutrition and, 133
Recommended Dietary Allowances, of National Academy of Sciences, factors not accounted for in, 133
Recrudescence, definition of, 237
Recurrence, of viral disease, definition of, 237
Recurrent aphthous stomatitis (RAS), 242-243, *243*
Reduced enamel epithelium, definitions of, 50

Reed-Sternberg cell(s), in diagnosis of Hodgkin's disease, 130
Regeneration, of tissue(s), 72
Reiter's syndrome, 243
Rem(s), definition of, 20
Remineralization phenomena, in dental caries, 187, *187-188*
Renin-angiotensin system, aldosterone regulation and, 259
    aldosteronism and, 261
Replacement therapy, in dental caries control, 191
Replication, in protein synthesis, 8, *8*
Resorption, of teeth, 109, *110*
Response(s), immune. *See* Immune response(s)
    inflammatory. *See* Inflammatory response(s)
    to increased function, irritation, and injury, 92-102
Reticulocyte(s), in formation of red blood cells, 268
Reticuloendothelial system (RES), disorders of, 276
    See also Monocyte(s); Macrophage(s); Monocyte-macrophage system
Retinoid(s), definition of, 137
Retinol, vitamin A and, 137
Retrogressive change(s), 108-116
    and dysfunction, aging and, 103-116
    types of, 108
Retrovirus, definition of, 19
Rheumatoid arthritis, 88-90, *89*
    amyloidosis and, 111
Riboflavin, deficiency of, 139, *139*, *140*
    requirements for, 139
Ribonucleic acid. *See* RNA
Rickets, vitamin D deficiency and, 138
    vitamin D-resistant, 138
Rickettsiae, description of, 31
RNA, forms of, 8
    functions of, in protein synthesis, 8-9, *8*, *9*
Roentgen, definition of, 19-20
Root surface caries, 189

Salicylate(s), toxic effects of, 33
Saliva, and calculus, 160, 161
    components of, interference with bacterial adherence of, 151
    immune mechanisms of, 154-155
    in spread of AIDS, 242
    in spread of mumps, 240
    major inorganic compounds of, 160
Salivary gland(s), neoplasm(s) of, 124-125, *125*
    obstruction of, 113
San Joaquin Valley Fever, 247
Sanguineous exudate, 67
Sarcoma(s), origin of, 122
Scar tissue, formation of, 72, *73*
Schizophrenia, description of, 21
Schmidt's syndrome, principal features of, 262
Schwannoma(s), definition of, 127
Sclerosis, definition of, 113
Scurvy, periodontal disease and, 205
    vitamin C deficiency and, 140-141, *140*
Secretory IgA (sIgA), in salivary immune response, 154-155
Selenium, requirement for, 137
Senescence, immune, 107-108
Septicemia, definition of, 61
Sequestration, of bone, definition of, 26
Serotonin, as mediator of vascular permeability, 65
Serous exudate, as inflammatory response, 67
Serum, tests for antibody of, 13
Serum hepatitis, cell-mediated immunity and, 84
Sex-linked inheritance, definition of, 17
Sharpey's fibers, 199
Shingles, oral lesions in, 239
Sialolith(s), definition of, 113
Sialolithiasis, definition of, 113
Sicca syndrome, 90
Sickle cell anemia, 270

Single-gene disorder(s), 16-17
Sinus, definition of, 39
Sjögren's syndrome, definition of, 2
　rheumatoid arthritis and, 90
Skeleton, lesions of, in aging, 104-105
Skin, age-related changes in, 104, *106*
　as element of immune system, 82
Slow progressive diseases (SPD), 84
"Slow virus(es)," 84
Smallpox, description of, 30
Smear layer, of dentin, pain transmission and, 168-170, *168*
Snyder colorimetric test, 192
Sodium, 135
Solar cheilitis, lip cancer and, 119-120, *120*
Somatic cell(s), formation of, 15
Somatotropin, 255
Sorbitol, acid production in plaque and, 183
　in dental caries control, 191
Specific cell-mediated immunity, 87-88
Spirochete(s), description of, 29
　in subgingival plaque, advanced destructive periodontitis and, 149
Squamous cell carcinoma, atypical proliferation of epithelium in, *122*
　of alveolar ridge, 124
　of lip, 123-124, *123, 124*
　of oral region, 123-124
　of tongue, 124, *125*
　x-ray burns and, 119, *119*
Squamous epithelium, in embryology of teeth, 48
　physiology of, 93-95, *94*
　replacement of respiratory epithelium by, 96
"Stab(s)," definition of, 63
Stain(s), 161-163
　black, 162, *162*
　endogenous, 162-163
　exogenous, 161-162
　green, 162, *162*
　metallic, 161-162
　nonmetallic, 162
　orange, 162
Staphylococci, description of, 28
Starch, acid production in plaque and, 183
Stellate reticulum, enamel formation and, 49, *49*
　in embryology of teeth, 48, *48, 49*
Steroid therapy, secondary adrenocortical insufficiency and, 260
Stomatitis, allergic, 250-251, *251, 252*
　denture, *246*, 247
　recurrent aphthous *See* Recurrent aphthous stomatitis (RAS)
　smoker's, 250, *250*
　traumatic, 248-249, *252*
Stratum germinativum, definition of, 93, *94*
Stratum intermedium, definition of, 48
Stratum spinosum, definition of, 93, *94*
Streptococci, reaction of tissues to, 28
Streptococcus mutans, antibiotic resistance of, transformation and, 153
　antibody potential and, 155
　in caries, by site, 179, *179*
　in carious lesions, advanced, 189
　in dental caries production, 182
　increased colonization by, excess sucrose consumption and, 164
　nutritional requirements of, 147
　oral colonization by, 150
　　presence of teeth required for, 145
　replacement of, in dental caries control, 191
　smooth coronal surface caries and, 158
　virulence mechanisms of, 153
Structure, loss of, 108-109
Substrate(s), bacterial growth in plaque and, 147-148
Sucrose, in diet, dental caries and, 181-182

Sucrose-chelating theory, of caries production, 183
Sugar, in diet, dental caries and, 181-182
　dental caries control and, 190-191
　pain stimulation and, 171
Supernumerary teeth, in developmental disturbances of teeth, 51, 52
Suppuration, definition of, 67
Swelling, cloudy. *See* Cloudy swelling
Syphilis, 29, 245, *245*
　congenital, enamel hypoplasia and, 55, 56
System(s). *See* specific system(s)
Systemic disease, oral pathology and, 2

T4/T8 ratio, inversion of, in AIDS, 240
Tartar. *See* Calculus
T-cell(s). *See* T-lymphocyte(s)
Telangiectasia, hereditary hemorrhagic, 275
Temperature, changes in, as physical agent of disease, 24
Temporomandibular joint(s). *See* TMJ
Teratogenic agent(s), 19, 19*t*
Testosterone, adrenal androgens and, 260
Tetracycline, effect of, 20
　pigmentation of teeth by, 57, *57*
Thalassemia(s), 270
Thalidomide, 20
Thiamin, 139
Thrombocytic disorder(s), 273-275
Thrombocytopenia, 274-275
　causes of, 70
Thrombosis, 23, *24*
Thromboxane(s), definition of, 65
Thrush. *See* Candidiasis
Thymine, in biochemical basis of heredity, 7
Thyroid function, 257-258
Thyroid-stimulating hormone (TSH), 257
Thyrotoxicosis. *See* Hyperthyroidism
Thyrotrophin-releasing hormone (TRH), 257
Tissue(s), classification of, 5*t*, 6
　definition of, 5-6
Tissue pressure, in pulp, pain and, 169
T-lymphocyte(s), cell-mediated immunity and, 80
　function of, 82, 90
　in immune senescence, 107-108
　in periodontal disease, pathogenesis of, 209
　interaction of macrophages with, in cell-mediated immunity, 83
　populations of, in cellular immune response, 82-84, *82*
　regulation of immune system by, 157
　source of, 82, *82*
TMJ, and muscles of mastication. *See also* TMJ/muscle dysfunction syndrome
　functional disturbances of, 279
　pathophysiology of, 279-293
　arthography of, *288*
　articulation of, 279. *See also* structures involved in
　osseous structures of, *280*
　osteoarthritic changes in, *107*
　positions of jaw and, *283*
　roentgenographic changes in, 290, *290*
　　osteoarthritis and, *286, 287, 289*
　traumatic arthritis of, 284
TMJ/muscle dysfunction syndrome, and occlusal trauma, treatment of, 291-292
　contributory factors related to, 284, *289*
　epidemiology of, 284
　etiology of, 284, *285*, 292
　manifestations of, 279, 292
　most common symptom of, 284
　occlusal disharmony and, 284
　protrusive interference related to, *289*
　provisional diagnosis of, 292
　signs and symptoms of, 287-290
　trauma from occlusal habits and, 291, *291*
Tobacco, chemical irritation from, 250, *250*

INDEX

Tobacco stain(s), of teeth, 162
Tocopherol, 138
Tongue, angiomas of, 127
  carcinoma of, 124, *125*
  developmental disturbances of, 42-44
  "hairy" leukoplakia of, in AIDS, 242
  hemangioma of, *128*
  in Plummer-Vinson syndrome, 269, *270*
  in polycythemia vera, 269
  injury from hydrogen peroxide to, 249
  multiple neuromas of, 265-266
  pernicious anemia and, 269, *269*
Tongue tie, 42, *42*
Tooth(Teeth), abrasion of, 108-109, *109*
  attrition of, 108, *108*
  colonization of, by Streptococcus mutans, 153
    concurrent processes of, 163
  developmental disturbances of, 50, 51-60. *See also* specific disturbances, structures
  embryology of, 46-51, *47, 48, 49, 51*
  erosion of, 109, *109*
  eruption of, disturbances in, 52
  formation of, disturbances in, 54-60
  impacted, definition of, 52
  in pituitary dwarfs, 255
  metallic staining of, causes of, 161
  number of, disturbances in, 51-53
  occlusal disharmony and, 284
  permanent, chronology of development of, 50, 51*t*
  pigmentation of, porphyria and, 270, *270*
  position of, disturbances in, 53
  resorption of, 109, *110*
  staining of, 161-163
    in erythroblastosis fetalis, 271
  succedaneous, 50, *51*
  supporting mechanism of, formation of, 50
  surface structure(s) of, 50-51
  vitamin-D resistant rickets and, 138
Tooth bud, development of, 46, *47, 48, 51*
Tooth germ, definition of, 46
  formation of, 46-48, *48*
"Toothache drops," chemical burns from, 249, *249*
Toothbrush, gingival abrasion from, 248, *248*
  gingivitis and, 223, *223*
Tooth-brushing, in dental caries control, 190
Tophus(i), definition of, 112-113
Torus mandibularis, *100*, 101
Torus palatinus, 100-101, *100*
Toxic immune complex, in hypersensitivity, 87
Trachoma, 31
Transcobalamin II, vitamin B_{12} deficiency and, 140
Transcription, in protein synthesis, 8-9, *8*
Translation, in protein synthesis, *8*, 9
Transport, mechanisms of, 4-5, *5*
  cellular injury and, 11
Transposon(s), antibiotic resistance of bacteria and, 154
Transseptal fiber(s), description of, 198, *198*
Transudate(s), definition of, 64
Transudation, definition of, 64
Trauma, definition of, 25
  from occlusion, 289, 290-291, *290, 291*
    periodontal diseases and, 224, *225*
Traumatic fibroma, description of, 97, *98*
Traumatic gingivitis, classification of, 223, *223*
Traumatic hemangioma(s), 101-102, *101*
Trench mouth. *See* Necrotizing ulcerative gingivitis (NUG)
Triglyceride(s), lipoproteins and, 134-135
Trisomy 21. *See* Down's syndrome

Tropism, definition of, 29
Tuberculosis, description of, 28-29
Turner's tooth(teeth), *56*, 57

Ulcer, aphthous. *See* Recurrent aphthous stomatitis
  granulation tissue in healing of, *72, 73*
Ultraviolet light, effects of exposure to, 25
Uric acid, deposition of, 112-113

Vancomycin, in dental caries control, 190
Varicella-zoster virus, infections by, oral lesions in, 239, *239*
Varix(ices). *See* Traumatic hemangioma
Vascular permeability, changes in, causes of, 64-65
  mediators of, 65
Veillonella, lactic acid use by, 184
Verrucal carcinoma, tobacco use and, 250
Vincent's angina, necrotizing ulcerative gingivitis and, 221
Vincent's infection. *See* Necrotizing ulcerative gingivitis (NUG)
Virilization, causes of, 259
  and effects of, 260
Virulence, definition of, 152
Virus(es), as physical agent of disease, 29-31
  oncogenic, 120
Vitamin(s), classification of, 137
  in bleeding disorders, 70
  nutritional disturbances and, 137-141
  supplementation of, 141
  See also specific vitamins
Vitamin A, 137
Vitamin B group, nutritional disturbances and, 138-140
  See also specific vitamins
Vitamin B_1, deficiency of, 139
Vitamin B_2. *See* Riboflavin
Vitamin B_6, nutritional disturbances and, 140
Vitamin B_{12}, deficiency of, anemia and, 269
  nutritional disturbances and, 140, *140*
Vitamin C, in collagen synthesis, 10
  nutritional disturbances and, 140-141
Vitamin C deficiency, 141, *142*
  as modifying factor, in periodontal disease, 205
Vitamin D, 138
  deficiency of, calcium absorption and, 135-136
    disorders associated with, 138
Vitamin E, dietary, 138
Vitamin K, nutritional disturbances and, 138
von Willebrand's disease (vWD), 275, *276*

Wandering rash. *See* Geographic tongue
Water balance, as physical agent of disease, 24-25
Water pollution, as physical agent of disease, 32
White blood cell(s), differential count of, 63, 63*t*, 271, *271*
  disorders of, 271-273
  See also specific types
"White spot" lesion, in dental caries, *185*, 186
Wilson's disease, copper excess and, 136
Wound, penetrating, definition of, 25

Xerostomia, aging and, 111
  dental caries and, 2
X-linked inheritance, definition of, 17
X-ray dermatitis, development of cancer and, 119, *119*
X-ray radiation, as physical agent of disease, 25-26, *26,27*
Xylitol, acid production in plaque and, 183
  in dental caries control, 191

Zinc, nutritional disturbances and, 136
Zone(s), in dental caries, 186, *186*
Zygote, 16